Auditory Processing Disorders

ASSESSMENT, MANAGEMENT, AND TREATMENT

EDITED BY

Donna Geffner, PhD, CCC-SLP/A
Debra Ross-Swain, EdD, CCC-SLP

Cover illustration by Richard H. Nodar, PhD, and Wendy Malan, MAPA

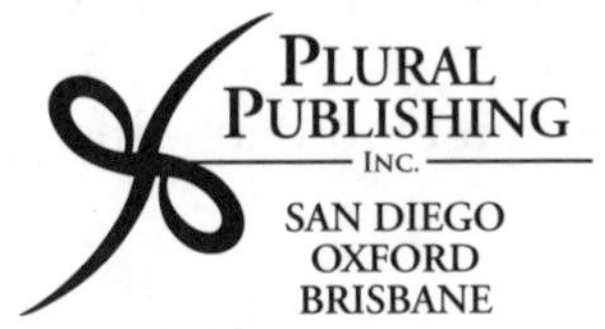

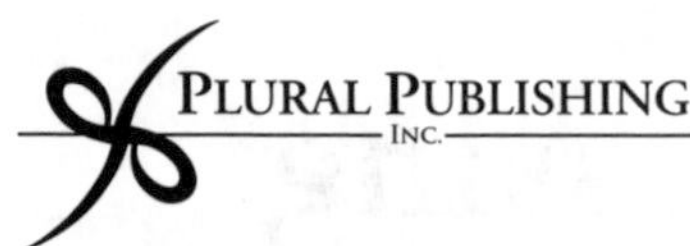

5521 Ruffin Road
San Diego, CA 92123

e-mail: info@pluralpublishing.com
Web site: http://www.pluralpublishing.com

49 Bath Street
Abingdon, Oxfordshire OX14 1EA
United Kingdom

Typeset in 10½/13 Palatino by Flanagan's Publishing Services, Inc.
Printed in the United States of America by McNaughton and Gunn

Library of Congress Cataloging-in-Publication Data:

Auditory processing disorders : assessment, management, and treatment
[edited by] Donna Geffner and Deborah Ross-Swain.
p. ; cm.
Includes bibliographical references and index.
ISBN-13: 978-1-59756-107-5 (pbk.)
ISBN-10: 1-59756-107-X (pbk.)
1. Word deafness. 2. Speech disorders. I. Geffner, Donna S. II.
Ross-Swain, Deborah.
[DNLM: 1. Auditory Perceptual Disorders—therapy. WV 270 A91648 2007]
RC394.W63A83 2007
617.8—dc22

2006103406

Auditory Processing Disorders

ASSESSMENT, MANAGEMENT, AND TREATMENT

Editor-in-Chief for Audiology
Brad A. Stach, PhD

Contents

Foreword

When Donna asked me to write a Foreword for this book, one request I made was that I wanted a prepublication copy to read and that I would not feel comfortable unless there was sufficient physiology, anatomy, and science backing the models to warrant my full reading. Needless to say, I will leave it to readers to decide if this volume meets their own particular standards. My rationale for the request was simple. Producing a germinal text on a topic as arcane, complex, and controversial as central auditory processing disorders is indeed a serious undertaking.

My interest was piqued by the topic because I decry the recent separation of Speech-Language Pathology from Audiology at the expense of our patients and want to see more common ground redevelop. To this end, I have personally suggested and hoped for a common convention every 3 to 5 years so that we can look at the new areas that have developed that require our mutual interaction on behalf of the patients. Auditory neuropathy/dys-synchrony and (C)APD are two of the areas that need this special attention and will become fertile meeting grounds for future connections.

There are those among us, and I count myself among them, who want to see the physiology, the anatomy, the solid data in the same class as temporal bone pathology and or Horseradish Peroxidase or Golgi tracings, and so on. These are available to us in the neurology and neuroscience literature, rarer in the speech-language and hearing domains, but they are thankfully not absent here.

There are others among us who put greater stock in the behavioral tests and special listening conditions (dichotic, diotic, speech in noise, competing and degraded messages, temporal psychophysics, etc.) to make the diagnosis and or assessment for us. Having contributed to the literature on dichotic listening and similar tests of central function, I view them with some jaundice because they are sometimes not test-retest reliable until there is a specific focal lesion, such as a temporal lobectomy or corpus callosum section. And even then, they change with plasticity of the CNS.

Yet some of the patients my associates and I reported on in 1972 of Roger Sperry's who had total hemispherectomies and corpus callosum sections, or who were Viet Nam brain-injured vets and had total temporal lobectomies, showed no APD other than dichotic asymmetries that we could measure back in the early 1970s. We also showed back then that changing the intensity of one ear released the other from suppression, but there was no everyday perceptual correlate that even vaguely resembled an auditory processing disorder. The patients had no problem hearing in noise, had normal MLDs, and seemingly carried on normal lives. But fortunately new procedures are now available that would probably have revealed those problems of which the patients were barely aware.

Both evoked potentials and fMRI sometimes converge to give us insight into brain function in these difficult cases, but Musiek's chapter on DIID opens new territories of both testing and management. His previous germinal work correlating auditory tests with focal and diffuse brain lesions achieved deserved widespread acknowledgment before he contributed to this text. And his clever application with Weihing of dichotic listening as a training tool is indeed innovative and important.

I was particularly pleased to see and read the chapter by Rance differentiating auditory neuropathy/dys-synchrony (AN/AD) from CAPDs. In my clinical and research experience, auditory neuropathy/dys-synchrony often masquerades as CAPD because the patients show poor hearing in noise, poor ability to localize sound, poor working memory based on poor signal salience, speech and language delays disproportionate to the "normal audiogram," and histories of hyperbilirubinemia, prematurity, and hypoxia. All of these signs of (C) APD are traceable to malfunction of inner hair cells and/or primary auditory nerve fibers. We now know that, if the diagnosis of "normal peripheral hearing" is done only with otoacoustic emissions and pure tone audiograms, AN/AD can be missed. I have many patients in my portfolio who spent years in fruitless therapies for "specific language impairment" or central auditory disorder because of poor hearing in noise, but who were correctly triaged with the simple addition of middle ear muscle reflexes. None of the "look-alikes" discussed in Chapter 3 show absent middle ear muscle reflexes and those that do should be re-examined for the ever-present specter of AN/AD—not just for academic purposes but because the neural dys-synchrony that is the hallmark of AN/AD can often be managed successfully with cochlear implants.

When the reflexes are absent or elevated above 95 dB, desynchronization of the afferent auditory signal should be suspected, and an ABR done with one positive and one negative polarity click to separate cochlear microphonic from true neural responses. Until the physiologic screening to include reflexes is added to our common assessment of CAPD, many such patients will be mismanaged as having CAPDs.

The careful reader will appreciate Dr. Geffner's again coming to grips in Chapter 2 with the definition, trying to rule out ADHD and be more specific about a diagnosis that resists specificity. In fact, more than half of what she uses to describe CAPD also describes mild or unrecognized cases of ANAD as well, hence the importance of the Rance chapter to me as bringing more physiologically based triage to the field.

As further evidence for the difficulty of the task, an entire additional chapter by Hamaguchi and Tazeau addresses "look alikes" with understandably few concrete suggestions on how to distinguish between them. It is indeed a difficult task with today's tools to be any more precise. The parable of the blind man and the elephant cited in the opening chapter and chapter 8 seems almost like an appropriately recurring theme.

Johnson, Bellis, and Billiet open their chapter with what by now is an obligatory reprise of trying to tease out a firm definition of (C)APD before they launch into their recommendations of what audiological tests uncover the condition. They wisely distinguish between assessment and diagnosis, and acknowledge that physiological tests may play some role here, but restrict themselves to tests that are available in common practice, here meaning schools and similar environments. Thus, evoked potentials are not recommended early in the chapter but the value of physiological results are described later in the chapter as they present the very lucid and meaningful Bellis/Ferre model. However, the addition of middle ear muscle reflexes to the basic pure tone and speech assessment would help alert the diagnostician to true neural or synchrony disorder.

The often repeated, but highly debatable, maxim that "many people lack middle ear muscle reflexes" assumes that they lack stapedius tendons. From my experience reviewing hundreds of human temporal bones at Stacy Guild's Temporal Bone Collection at the Johns Hopkins, I can assure the reader that only once did I ever see a temporal bone where the stapedius might have been absent, but just as likely skipped by the microtome in its sections. Thus, I would respectfully add the inclusion of middle ear muscle reflexes to the audiological test battery for APD, and, if they are absent, further physiological analysis would be recommended.

In Chapter 6, Rawool addresses the heart of the theoretically important issues in CAPD but I must reiterate that, without differentiating AN/AD from CAPD, one will find very poor temporal processing in both categories of patients as attested to by the works of Zeng et al. and Rance as cited in this book. Thus finding poor temporal processing without ruling out AN/AD physiologically is a dangerous maneuver, and as of yet there is much more peer-reviewed literature confirming the temporal disruption of patients with easily diagnosable AN/AD than there is confirming such disruptions in what may be difficult-to-diagnose CAPD.

In all the chapters that stress the importance of audiologic collaboration with SLPs, starting with Dr. Swain's, I can only express a hearty Amen. The separation between SLPs and Audiologists, whatever your opinion regarding its merits, certainly has caused problems for our patients, This is especially true with both AN/AD patients and the more controversial diagnosis of CAPD.

And then comes Marty Burns (Chapter 9) to clarify that many of these APD issues, including dyslexia, may in fact be connected to basic auditory processes underlying the auditory comprehension of spoken language and dealing with timing at the 40- to 70-msec level. The solid fMRI evidence of Temple et al. that she cites, and the post Fast ForWord© brain changes are indeed powerful counter-arguments to the criticism that this area of research lacks physiologic and anatomic support.

Phonemic synthesis training (Chapter 13) is advocated by Katz; broad metacognitive approaches by Hamaguchi; Dichotic Interaural Intensity Difference Training suggested by Weihing and Musiek; metalinguistic approaches by Jane Baran, and the Lindamood-Bell systems by Nancy Bell all offer management suggestions. The theory behind the systems range from APD as a special case of a language problem, or a brain engram problem, all the way to a result of auditory deprivation in childhood or genetic predisposition of some unspecified "brain malfunction." Surprisingly absent (or did I miss it in my haste to meet this deadline?) was a consideration of the interactive metronome as a technical management for the temporal as well as impulse management and motor control aspects of APD.

In Chapter 18, Medwetsky offers the coolest assessment of evidence-based practice, suggesting in part that no one has a complete management tool for

APD perhaps because both the subject selection and definitions as well as the theories are still lacking in coherence and universality. The selection of subjects and their proper nosology remain the most difficult part of the area. With respect to nosology, Wikipedia (as of January 2007) says:

> One of the main problems with nosologies is that diseases often cannot be defined and classified clearly especially when pathogenesis or causality is not known. So, diagnostic terms often are in fact only symptoms or sets of symptoms (syndromes).

Thus, it seems in parts of this text we will read that APD is not a language disorder, is a timing disorder, is not a timing disorder, but it very well may be under certain conditions. So we are back at the beginning, trying to define the problem while at the same time studying it.

Compiling this book was a serious undertaking, fraught with sturm und drang, hidden pitfalls, internal contradictions, turf wars, and even some physiologic and anatomic data. The reflective reader will appreciate with me the inherent problems involved and the sincerity of the authors in their attempts to bring more order and more solid framework to this and related fields where the professions of Audiology and Speech-Language Pathology may once again work in concert for the benefit or our CAPD as well as AN/AD patients.

Charles I. Berlin, PhD, CCC-A; CCC-SLP
License 005 State of Louisiana
Retired 9/1/02 from LSUHSC as
First Director of the Kresge Hearing Research Laboratory and
First Frances Barnes Bullington Professor of Hearing Science.
Professor of Otolaryngology, Head and Neck Surgery, Neuroscience,
After Hurricane Katrina . . .
Research Professor CSD
University of South Florida
Tampa Florida

Preface

It has been decades since Helmer Mylelbust introduced the concept of auditory processing disorder to our professions in 1954. Since that time, significant advances in the definition, description, assessment, diagnosis, and treatment of auditory processing and its disorders have been made. These tremendous advances have been the result of the work of respected researchers, professors, scientists, and clinicians including but not limited to to Jane Baran, Teri James Bellis, Charles Berlin, Gail Chermak, Jeanne Ferre, Jay Hall III, Jack Katz, Robert Keith, Frank Musiek, and more. Their contributions have resulted in the assimilation of unprecedented amounts of information reflecting both the breadth and depth of clinical and educational studies and publications.

The 25 chapters of this book comprise an anthology of the disorders of and rehabilitation for auditory processing disorders. It is a collection of professional papers from noted authorities regarding this ever expanding topic of interest. Beginning with a historical overview of auditory processing and its disorders in Chapter 1, the ensuing content offers the reader a sequential learning continuum of chapters that, on some level, tell the auditory processing story.

Written by both audiologists and speech-language pathologists, the content of this book is intended to provide our professions specific and practical information that will improve our understanding of auditory processing in terms of assessment, interpretation, management, and treatment in order to better serve the children, their parents, and adults with these disorders. In addition to audiologists and speech-language pathologists, this comprehensive book of information can serve a range of professionals in education, medicine, and clinical fields who are involved with children and adults who are experiencing auditory processing disorders and are responsible for the educational, medical, and clinical interventions. These professionals can include teachers, psychologists, neuropsychologists, physicians, educational therapists, occupational therapists, school nurses, resource specialists, school psychologists, and school administrators. We believe that the information provided here can be useful in university programs offering undergraduate and graduate courses in auditory processing and its disorders.

This book is divided into three sections. Section I introduces the historical perspective, definitions, comorbidities, assessment, including behavioral and physiological measurements, the differentiation between auditory and language processing, and the role of auditory processing in literacy. Section II explores management and practical strategies and guidelines for clients and parents. Section III presents a variety or treatment protocols, including computer applications, educational provisions, and resources. In some cases, nontraditional approaches are presented to heighten the reader's awareness.

From Chapter 1 in which the historical perspective of auditory processing and its disorders is presented to Chapter 2 where a detailed description of behaviors, symptoms, and observed classroom behaviors are described with a differential assessment of AD/HD, the reader is assisted in identifying impairments of auditory processing skills so that teachers and parents can recognize children at risk. Chapter 3 is devoted to comorbidity of APD and other disorders that *masquerade* or coexist with auditory processing disorders. This chapter enables the reader to become familiar with behaviors that may be a result of a neurobiological disorder and not necessarily attributable to auditory processing disorders.

Assessment of auditory processing skills can be performed by audiologists and speech-language pathologists. Chapter 4 is devoted to comprehensive assessment batteries from the perspectives of audiologists. Chapter 5 provides an insightful analysis of the prevalence and identification of neural dys-synchrony that may be co-occurring with, or mistaken for, an auditory processing disorder. Measures and assessment for auditory neuropathy are described with an emphasis on the electrophysiologic measures to show a neural transmission disorder. This chapter discusses auditory neuropathy and hearing loss and its relationship to auditory processing disorders. The clinical profile for affected individuals is presented to outline the pattern of auditory processing deficits typically associated with the condition. This chapter discusses similarities and differences between auditory neuropathy, hearing loss and auditory processing disorders and provides clinicians with guidelines for identifying a neural dys-synchrony to determine the need for medical referral.

Chapter 6 describes the various aspects of temporal processing, its measurements and its contribution to receiving the auditory signal. Various aspects of temporal processing, including temporal integration, resolution, modulation, separation, ordering, masking, summation, are described, along with measures to assess each. Chapter 7 presents an assessment from the perspective of a speech-language pathologist and the contribution that such a person makes to the overall assessment of this multimodality disorder. This chapter discusses scope of practice for diagnosis and assessment, screening procedures, assessment batteries and interpretation of results. Although there is no one battery for assessing auditory processing disorders, these chapters will guide clinical decision making for selecting the most effective assessment tools that will provide the clinician with the most useful data for interpretation and implementation.

Chapter 8 is devoted to assisting professionals in differentiating between language processing and auditory processing. All too often a child is described as having a "processing disorder" leaving professionals with more questions than answers. Disorders or deficits that result in a diagnosis of a processing disorder can range from a neuropathy to a linguistic deficit. The information in this chapter will assist clinicians as well as other professionals in determining specific differences between language processing and auditory processing so that intervention efforts can be more specific and effective.

The relationship between auditory processing disorder and literacy is discussed in Chapter 9. This chapter presents the often neglected and misunderstood role of sound, processing and hearing in the development and mastery of literacy skills. Literacy is inextricably entwined with sound and auditory processing. When children experience difficulty acquiring and mastering age-level appropriate literacy skills very often they are referred for tutoring assistance that may not assist in improving deficit skills because the underlying auditory processing problems have not been identified and addressed. This chapter will provide the reader with specific information that will guide assessment and intervention decisions for children with auditory-based literacy acquisition problems.

Significant clinical, educational, and technological advances have resulted in a better understanding of specific management strategies or treatment interventions for children with auditory processing disorders.

In Section II, Management, Chapter 10 discusses simple and practical day-to-day activities and behaviors that can positively influence the listening skills of children with auditory processing disorders. These practical suggestions can be used in a variety of settings that may include home, classroom, tutorial, or social and can assist in maximizing therapy interventions, minimize learning and communication obstacles and enhance listening skills for all listeners.

Chapter 11 describes management strategies from teaching compensatory strategies to environmental modification, to sound enhancement devices such as FM personal units and classroom amplification systems. Information provided in this chapter will assist clinicians in determining the appropriateness of an amplification system and provide specific criteria for its use. Parenting the child with auditory processing disorders can be daunting and challenging when considering educational, communication, behavioral and social implications and needs. Chapter 12 provides advice to parents, defines their role as team members, facilitators, strategists, and managers. Divided into six major sections this chapter provides the reader with practical information that includes: team membership for parents and roles; understanding legal terrain; communication facilitators and organization strategists; parents as facilitators of social-emotional growth; parents and children having fun; and future forecasting as children with auditory processing disorders become adults.

Chapters 13 through 22 are dedicated to specific treatment interventions that can be used with children and adults with auditory processing disorders. Treatment for auditory processing disorders is intended to remediate skills that are weak. The reader is cautioned to remember that, despite the success using one particular treatment with one child, the same treatment may not be successful with other children. Children respond differently to various treatments depending upon their auditory processing skill weaknesses. The treatment interventions that are presented to the reader include background information, the theoretical frameworks that were considered when developing the intervention, the use and application of the intervention, the population that would benefit from its use, and where applicable, a case study.

A variety of treatment approaches is presented from Phonemic Synthesis/Phonemic Training Programs (Chapter 13), Metacognitive Approaches, Chapter 14), Dichotic Interaural Intensity Difference (DIID) Training (Chapter 15), Metalinguistic Approaches (Chapter 16), Lindamood-Bell Learning Processes

(Chapter 17), Computer Software programs (Chapter 18), Fast ForWord (Chapter 19), to Technology (Chapter 20).

The use of assistive technology in the management and treatment of auditory processing disorders has achieved increased attention in clinical and educational setting. Assistive technology tools can range from highly specialized equipment to very simple applications that may be found in homes, classrooms and clinics. Chapter 20 defines assistive technology, discusses the process of procuring assistive technology for children with auditory processing disorders, describes evaluation for assistive technology, and offers a comprehensive listing of various assistive technology tools that help the child and adult with auditory processing disorders.

Chapter 21 is devoted to the controversial topic of medication use with children with auditory processing disorders and coexisting Attention Deficit Hyperactivity Disorder (ADHD). This chapter highlights, describes, and reviews four studies concerning medication and auditory processing disorders as well as offers the reader information that explains the mechanics and effects of medications on CNS. Recommendations regarding auditory processing disorders and medication are given.

Chapters 22 and 23 explore the use of alternative treatments such as sound therapies to remediate auditory processing deficits. Although such programs have not been typically embraced by the audiology and speech-language pathology community, they exist and warrant understanding by the professions.

Chapter 24 explores educational implications as defined by public laws and regulation in order to provide specific accommodations and modifications so children can meet with success in the classroom. Chapter 24 presents the history of federal laws for disability protection that has impacted the delivery of public education for children with auditory processing disorders. The information presented in this chapter details recent and current federal legislation that ensures these children receive a free and appropriate education. This chapter is intended to provide the reader with an understanding of federal laws (i.e., IDEA), resources ,and practical suggestions for modifications and accommodations. Chapter 25 is devoted to providing samples of reports with different types and styles summarizing evaluation results. The reader is cautioned to remember that there is no one reporting type and style that is written or expected. When clinicians generate reports many factors will influence the type and style of the report. Some factors may include: the type of evaluation (e.g., screening versus comprehensive); the specific tests that were administered; how the results are interpreted; quantitative versus qualitative analysis of the data; who is reading the report; how the findings will affect educational and treatment decisions; how the deficits are affecting the child's communication and learning abilities and the overall intent of the report (e.g., developing IEP goals and objectives; implementing a 504 plan; determining eligibility for interventions, etc.).

The Appendix provides a compilation of Web resources, Web sites, organizations, and supports for the reader to obtain more information or additional perspectives on auditory processing disorders.

Significant advances in assessment, diagnosis, differential diagnosis, treatment, and management of auditory processing disorders have taken place over the course of 50 years. The content of this book is intended to offer the reader current clinical trends that provide speech-language pathologists and audiologists with the ability to provide children and adults with auditory processing disorders the most valid and reliable assessments possible; interpretation of results that translate to functional abilities and outcomes; meaningful and effective treatment interventions, and advocacy for appropriate education. The comprehensive information contained in this book is a result of a collaboration of esteemed colleagues sharing years of clinical and research experience for purposes of expanding knowledge and understanding of auditory processing disorders in children and adults. Even after this book is read, we continue to strive for answers and solutions to improve the quality of our assessment and intervention tools that will eventually result in improving the lives of these children, adults, and their families.

Contributors

Jane A. Baran, PhD
Professor and Chair
Department of Communication Disorders
University of Massachusetts Amherst
Amherst, Massachusetts
Chapter 16

Nanci Bell, MA
Director
Lindamood-Bell Learning Processes
San Luis Obispo, California
Chapter 17

Teri James Bellis, PhD, CCC-A, FAAA, F-ASHA
Associate Professor and Chair
Department of Communication Disorders
Adjunct Associate Professor
Sanford School of Medicine
Division of Basic Biomedical Sciences
The University of South Dakota
Vermillion, South Dakota
Chapter 4

Cassie Billiet, MS
Doctoral Candidate
Department of Communication Disorders
The University of South Dakota
Vermillion, South Dakota
Chapter 4

Martha S. Burns, PhD
Adjunct Associate Professor
Northwestern University
Evanston, Illinois
Director
Clinical Specialist Market
Scientific Learning Corporation
Oakland, California
Chapters 9 and 19

Dorinne S. Davis, MA, CCC-A, FAAA, RCTC, BARA
President/Founder
The Davis Center
Mt. Arlington, New Jersey
Chapter 23

Jeanane M. Ferre, PhD, CCC-A
Audiologist
Private Practice
Oak Park, Illinois
Chapter 10

Donna Geffner, PhD, CCC-SLP/A
Director of Graduate Programs in Speech-Language Pathology & Audiology
St. John's University
Jamaica, NY
Chapters 2 and 11

Patricia McAleer Hamaguchi, MA, CCC-SLP
Founder and Director
Hamaguchi & Associates Pediatric Speech-Language Pathologists, Inc.
Cupertino, California
Chapters 3 and 14

Marni L. Johnson, AuD, CCC-A, FAAA
Assistant Professor
Department of Communication Disorders

The University of South Dakota
Vermillion, South Dakota
Chapter 4

Jack Katz, PhD
Director, Auditory Processing Service
Research Professor, University of Kansas Medical Center
Professor Emeritus, University of Buffalo
Parie Village, Kansas
Chapter 13

Dorothy A, Kelly, DA, CCC-SLP
Doctor of Arts in Communication Disorders
Professor, Speech-Language Pathology
St. Joseph's College
Patchogue, New York
Chapter 12

Rhandee Lipp, MS, CCC-SLP
Director
Speech and Language Services of Rohnert Park-Cotati
Cotati, California
Chapter 24

Jay R. Lucker, EdD, CCC-A/SLP, FAAA
Associate Professor
Department of Communication Sciences and Disorders
Howard University
Washington, DC
Private Practice Specializing in APD
Alexandria & Ashburn, VA, and Bethesda, Maryland
Chapter 1

Larry Medwetsky, PhD
Vice President, Audiology and Research
Rochester Hearing and Speech Center
Rochester, New York
Chapter 18

Frank E. Musiek, PhD
Professor and Director of Auditory Research
Department of Communication Sciences
Professor of Otolaryngology
School of Medicine
University of Connecticut
Storrs, Connecticut
Chapter 15

Gary Rance, PhD, MSc, DipAud, BEd, MAudSA(CC)
Associate Professor
Head of Academic Programs
The University of Melbourne
Department of Otolaryngology
East Melbourne, Australia
Chapter 5

Vishakha Waman Rawool, PhD, CCC-A
Faculty, AuD Program
Department of Speech Pathology and Audiology
West Virginia University
Morgantown, West Virginia
Chapter 6

Gail J. Richard, PhD, CCC-SLP
Professor and Chair
Communication Disorders & Sciences
Eastern Illinois University
Charleston, Illinois
Chapter 8

Thomas Rosati, EdD, A.T.P.
Teacher of Speech and Hearing
Eastern Suffolk BOCES
Professor St. John's University
Special Education Technology
Certification in Speech, Special Education
School Administration and Educational Assistive Technology

Nesconset, New York
Chapter 20

Deborah Ross-Swain, EdD, CCC-SLP
CEO, Clinical Director
The Swain Center
Santa Rosa, California
Chapters 7 and 25

Theresha A. Boomgarden-Szypulski, MA, CCC-SLP
Private Practice
Moline, Illinois
Chapter 22

Yvette N. Tazeau, PhD
Clinical Neuropsychologist
Clinical Private Practice
Los Gatos, California
Chapter 3

Kim L. Tillery, PhD, CCC-A
Associate Professor and Chair
Department of Speech Pathology and Audiology
State University of New York at Fredonia
Fredonia, New York
Chapter 21

Jeffrey A. Weihing, MA
Doctoral student
Neuroaudiology Lab
University of Connecticut
Storrs, Connecticut
Chapter 15

This book was written with the intention of contributing knowledge to the discipline of auditory processing from the perspective of both audiologists and speech-language pathologists. After all, the area of auditory processing has had a long history and journey from being an obscure entity, embroiled in questions as to its existence and substance, to becoming its own body of study. From the early days of Myklebust who recognized this phenomenon in children to the doubting eyes of others, auditory processing has succeeded in standing on its own merit. That is not due to any small feat but to the works of great audiologists and speech-language pathologists who have paved the way through their writings, investigations and rigorous study that enabled this area to become an entity in its own right. Auditory processing has a body of knowledge, consisting of assessment, management and treatment protocols- surely enough to make for a 25 chapter text, among other many fine texts, and even a graduate course of study at some universities. Nonetheless, this success or emancipation could not have happened without the greats of Charles Berlin, James Jerger, Jack Katz, Frank Musiek, Gail Chermak, Teri Bellis, Jane Baran, and Robert Keith. Most of these scholars have agreed, once again, to write yet another chapter. How fortunate for us that they have agreed and how wonderful that we were able to place their chapters among those of other renowned experts in audiology and speech-language pathology, such as Nanci Bell, Marty Burns, Jeanane Ferre, Patti Hamaguchi, Dorothy Kelly, Jay Lucker, Larry Medwetsky, Gary Rance, Vishakha Rawool, Gail Richard, Kim Tillery and their associates. This text introduces other fine writers as Cassie Billiet, Dorinne Davis, Marni Johnson, Rhandee Lipp, Tom Rosati, Trish Syzpulski, Yvette Tzaeau, and Jeff Weihing. After all, isn't the area of auditory processing one that truly bridges the two professions?

We want to express our sincere gratitude to all the outstanding authors whose professionalism was only surpassed by their expertise. Their skillful writing and knowledge have contributed significantly to the value of this text. We are ever grateful to the many authors and co-authors who so willingly accepted our challenge to write a chapter with such depth and fortitude.

Our acknowledgement also goes to our families who endured the many months of our diligence and commitment, often at the expense of other responsibilities, to see this project come to fruition. We extend our appreciation to our support staff for their help. A special thank you goes to Ewa Dynda, a bright, upcoming star in speech-language pathology, and Graduate Assistant to Donna Geffner, who was always there for me.

It has been an extraordinary learning experience for us and a truly exceptional opportunity to work with such greats. How fortunate for us to call them colleagues and friends.

We dedicate this book to those who have traveled before us and paved the way. Thank you. To those of you whose discoveries are yet to come and whose sites have been set high, know that you have been fortunate to stand on tall shoulders.

I

Identification and Assessment

1

History of Auditory Processing Disorders in Children

Jay R. Lucker

Overview

The beginning of Auditory Processing Disorders (APD) as a distinct category or disorder was first identified during the 1950s. However, APD described as an auditory processing dysfunction was not identified until an NIH monograph was published in the late 1960s.

Interest in APD in children became most evident during the first formal symposium held in Cincinnati, Ohio during the 1970s. At that time, the first APD test batteries specifically used with children were described. From that time forward, work on developing and refining the assessment of APD in children continued. Additionally, information regarding treatment options began to emerge.

Committees were formed to identify the present state of knowledge on APD in children including the development of two consensus statements. This work started in the 1990s and has proceeded into the 21st century.

Because attempts have been unsuccessful in coming to a consensus on what APD is, how it is to be assessed, and what treatments are available to help children identified with APD, there are varying views or approaches taken. Some focus on the auditory factors only. Others combine auditory and language factors without differentiating between the two. A few look at auditory, language, and cognitive factors as being integrated into the process we call auditory processing.

This chapter includes speculations regarding the future of APD. Some speculations include research in genetics, advances in neurobiology, and new methods for assessing neurophysiology. Perhaps we will find a day when a consensus among professionals will be attained. Until that day, we look back to the past to obtain an objective perspective for the future.

The Beginnings of APD as a Recognized Disorder in Children

For many parents, educators, and other professionals the area of auditory processing disorders (APD) seems relatively new. If we were to ask when do *you* believe APD was first identified as a specific disorder in children separate from more general learning problems, what would be your response? Would you say that APD was first described as a specific disorder in children only since the 1990s? Some might believe so, but APD was identified well before that time. How about since the 1980s? When I ask this same question at presentations some in the audience indicate they believe APD was first identified in children in the 1980s. But this is not true. It occurred much earlier than that.

How about the 1970s? As we will see, the first national conference on auditory processing disorders in children held in the United States was constituted in the late 1970s (see Keith, 1977). Thus, many people think that APD was first recognized as a disorder in children only since the mid-to-late 1970s, but they would be decades off.

It may come as a surprise to many that the identification of a disorder specific to auditory processing, separate from language disorders, hearing disorders, and intellectual or cognitive problems, was recognized approximately 50 years ago. In a book published in 1954, Helmer Mykelbust (1954) identified a problem he related to a disorder of auditory perception that looked like hearing loss but was found in children with normal hearing. He described auditory perceptual disorders as the inability to " . . . structure the auditory world and select those sounds which are immediately pertinent to adjustment" (p. 158). Later, in 1956, Mildred Berry and Jon Eisenson stated that children with auditory perceptual disorders *can* hear sound, but are unable to recognize the sounds they hear. Thus, auditory processing disorders in children (not called auditory processing disorders, nor the older term, central auditory processing disorders) were identified in the literature in the fields of audiology, speech-language pathology, psychology, and deafness over half a century ago.

What made auditory processing disorders unique was the distinction professionals made between these originally called "auditory perceptual" problems and other disorders of communication including hearing loss, language disorders, and cognitive problems. In the 1960s some professionals even referred to auditory processing problems as "aphasic deaf" meaning that the children could not process linguistic material and functioned as if they had hearing loss although audiological tests of their hearing yielded normal results.

Among the description of these auditory perceptual disorders were difficulties: understanding speech unexplained by the lack of a hearing loss, understanding speech in noise, and understanding distorted speech. It was not unusual for audiologists or speech-language pathologists to identify children as having auditory processing disorders when these children could not use or understand language and functioned as if they had hearing losses, but tested as having normal hearing. Because of the primary problem being an inability to understand spoken language, many of these children were given a diagnosis of "childhood aphasia," meaning an inability to use language in childhood. However, aphasia means a loss of language, whereas these children did not have a language to lose and some had good expressive language skills although their receptive language was the primary deficit area.

When I first graduated from college, one of the first job offers I received was as a teacher at the New York School for the Aphasic Deaf. Little did I know, at that time, that the world of auditory processing disorders in children would become my life-long work. My first introduction to these children presented school-age boys and girls who appeared to function as children with significant hearing losses, that is, misunderstanding what they heard or not responding when people called their names. These children were treated in many ways as children who were identified as "oral deaf," that is., children with significant hearing loss who were in oral focused educational programs where the emphasis of communication was listening and speaking. Thus, in the mid-to-late 1960s, we not only recognized that some children had significant educational and communication problems due to APDs, but we even set up special schools for those with such severe problems because they could not be educated in regular education classrooms; and this was well before the advent of Public Law (PL) 94-142, the federal law regarding children with educational handicaps, that has now become IDEA (the Individuals with Disabilities Education Act).

At that time, the 1960s, the focus was on aphasia (a language disorder) and brain injury. The few researchers who, at that time, investigated auditory perceptual disorders studied persons with known neurological problems. It was easier to establish a relationship between brain damage and auditory processing problems when the neurological disorder was known. This noted relationship led to the first description of tests to identify APD in both children and adults.

History of APD Testing

I have been surprised at times to meet people, including professionals in the fields of audiology, speech-language pathology, education, psychology, and even medicine, who ask me whether

I work with adults who might have APDs. I am even further surprised when professionals ask whether there are APD tests for adults, or whether one can assess auditory processing in adults as the tests and the area of APD is primarily for children.

Many professionals and adult individuals (and their families) who come to see me for APD assessment are surprised when I tell them that APD was originally a disorder recognized in adults, and the first tests for APD were developed for use with adults. (Actually, there is a test that can be considered an evaluative tool for assessing some aspect of APD with children that dates back to the late 1950s that is discussed below.)

In the mid-1950s and early 1960s, Bocca and Calearo and their colleagues published what are often considered the earliest articles documenting the evaluation of and identification of APD in adults (Bocca, 1958; Bocca & Calearo, 1963; Bocca, Calearo, & Cassinari, 1954; Bocca, Calearo, Cassinari, & Migliavacca, 1955; Calero & Lazzaroni, 1957). They described the use of distorted speech (filtered words) and speech with competing speech (such as speech-in-noise, auditory figure-ground, and competing sentences) that were used to assess patients who were later identified as having cortical and subcortical lesions (often tumors) involving the central auditory pathways and the auditory centers in the temporal lobe of the brain. One specific outcome of this early research was that certain tests (such as filtered-words tasks) were more sensitive to identification of cortical lesions whereas other tests (such as speech-in-noise) were more sensitive to subcortical lesions. However, these researchers only discussed the evaluation and identification of such lesions and uses of these original APD tests in adults. Their studies described the subjects as having cortical deafness or subcortical deafness, not using the term auditory processing or auditory perceptual disorders. These original publications sparked interest in the United States regarding auditory processing problems in adults with identified neurological disorders such as brain injuries, tumors, and strokes. The focus was to develop tests sensitive to identify the "site-of-lesion" or the specific part of the central nervous system that was impaired or malfunctioning. Therefore, the earliest tests for auditory processing were developed to identify neurological disorders in adults. What is interesting is that APD testing today is still used to help identify the neurophysiological problems some children and adults have when a probable neurological disorder is suspect.

Although typically not considered a test of auditory processing, the Wepman Auditory Discrimination Test (ADT) is probably the first widely used as a clinical measure of one aspect of auditory processing in children (i.e., auditory discrimination abilities or the ability for the child to determine whether two words are the same or different regarding their phonemic makeup). Joseph Wepman developed his first ADT in 1958 and revised it in 1973. The latter version continues to be used by some clinicians today in the assessment of auditory discrimination in children.

In their original edition of the *Handbook of Clinical Audiology* published in 1972, Katz and Illmer discussed the sensitivity of the Wepman ADT in identifying learning disabilities and reading problems in children. Essentially, Katz was describing the high sensitivity of the ADT in identifying APD problems in children back in the early 1970s.

Another test developed to look at the specific site of lesion of central auditory disorders in adults was the Staggered Spondaic Word (SSW) Test developed by Jack Katz originally in 1963. Dr. Katz described a complex "grid" to translate SSW test findings with different parts of the brain including both auditory regions (called auditory reception area or AR) and frontal, temporal, and parietal lobe regions of cortex (called nonauditory reception areas or NAR). It was not until nearly two decades later that Katz and colleagues developed his Buffalo Model designed specifically to identify auditory processing disorders in children (and adults) without focusing on the site-of-lesion approach. However, the original uses for the SSW test were with adults.

As interest in APD continued, tests were developed or modified to assess auditory processing disorders in adults. Some professionals were also investigating auditory processing problems in children. However, it was not until the mid-to-late 1960s that the National Institutes of Health (NIH) authorized the first formal study of APD in children. The committee that investigated APD in children was formed in 1963. The committee's research culminated in the first publication that focused on APD in children (Chalfant & Scheffelin, 1969). They labeled the disorder as a "Central Processing Dysfunction in Children," and specifically used the term "Auditory Processing." The committee described auditory processing as involving attention to auditory stimuli, sound versus no sound, sound localization, discriminating sounds, discriminating sound sequences, and auditory figure-ground (pp. 11–17). Furthermore, the committee describe what they called "Dysfunctions in the Synthesis of Sensory Information," including auditory synthesis, and described such synthesis as auditory integration, a term we still use today in describing auditory processing and APD. Although they describe various processes involved in auditory processing of information, they do *not* describe any specific assessment tools (i.e., tests) to evaluate such functions in children.

Because interest in central auditory dysfunction (later called central auditory processing) developed in children, various professionals began to administer tests originally developed for adults in the assessment of auditory processing and APD in children. Thus, the same filtered-speech tasks used by Bocca and colleagues was applied to children. Katz and his followers began to administer the SSW test to children. Speech-in-noise tasks were also used with children. Thus, the era of investigation of auditory processing abilities in children was launched and the 1970s started seeing publications concerning auditory processing problems in children as well as adults. However, the focus was either related to the neurological site of functioning felt to be involved with each of the specific APD tasks used *or* to merely describe the specific deficits found on each test in such children. Eventually, tests specifically for use with children were developed.

One of the earliest test batteries was developed by A. Flowers, M. Costello, and V. Small (1970) called the Flowers-

Costello Tests of Central Auditory Abilities. Another test and test battery was also developed and used specifically for children in the early 1970s. This was the Goldman-Fristoe-Woodcock Test of Auditory Discrimination (1970) and the Goldman-Fristoe-Woodcock Auditory Skills Test Battery (1974). A new test focusing on blending sounds into words was developed by Katz. Called the Phonemic Synthesis Test, it focused on assessing this skill in children (1972). A third battery was developed by Jack Willeford from Northern Colorado sometimes called the Willeford Test Battery or the Colorado Test Battery (1977). Thus, assessment of auditory processing in children can be considered to have begun in the 1970s.

In the late 1970s and early 1980s, professionals using Katz's SSW test started to focus its use with children. In the early part of that decade, Lucker (1980, 1981, 1982) described diagnostic application of the SSW test for assessing APD in children. Also, in the early 1980's, Susan and James Jerger developed the Pediatric Speech Intelligibility (PSI) test for use with children as young as preschoolers (1984). In that same decade, Rochelle Cherry (1980) developed a screening test for assessing speech understanding in noise called the Selective Auditory Attention Test or SAAT.

As time went on, tests used initially with adults were normed for use with children and other tests of auditory processing were developed for use with children. Musiek (1983) presented the use of the Dichotic Digit Test with children. Marilyn Pinheiro developed a test using nonspeech tonal patterns sometimes referred to as the Pitch Patterns Test, Frequency Patterns Test, and Pitch (or Frequency) Patterns Perception Test (1977), which was applied with children as well as adults. Later, Musiek, Baran, and Pinhiero (1990) developed a similar task using durations for tones rather than pitch differences (i.e., Durations Patterns Sequence Test) (Musiek, 1994) and he and colleagues described its use in assessing APD (Musiek, Baran, & Pinhiero, 1990).

Another attempt to tax the central auditory system and assess auditory processing skills in children was through the use of time-altered, or compressed speech. Beasley and Freeman (1977) described their Time-Altered Speech test that never really "caught on" as a part of the standard auditory processing test battery. Not until Robert Keith developed the Time Compressed Sentences Test (2002) did time-altered speech become a regular part of the APD battery of tests. However, evaluation of time factors (i.e., temporal processing) was assessed using nonlinguistic materials.

The first test of temporal processing assessment was developed by Sylvia M. Davis and Robert L. McCroskey (1980) called the Wichita Auditory Fusion Test (WAFT). Later (1996) McCroskey revised the test along with Robert W. Keith calling it the Auditory Fusion Test—Revised (AFT-R), which is included by some evaluators in assessing auditory temporal processing in children. More recently, 2002, Keith developed the Random Gap Detection Test based on the WAFT and AFT-R.

With the development of these various tests to assess auditory processing abilities in children, another approach was to develop an entire battery of tests into one assessment that could be used to screen for APD in children. The Willeford Test Battery (1977) was one such attempt, but a more recent attempt was developed by Robert Keith (1986). The SCAN test was originally a screening test that was normed for children 3 years through 11 years of age. The test was then expanded with norms for adolescents and adults (12 years and older), and is widely used today (SCAN-A; 1994). The original SCAN was then revised for children following the SCAN-A (1999) format and is also in wide use today (SCAN-C).

The last of the behavioral tests to be discussed was one developed to help differentiate between children with auditory processing problems and attention deficit disorders (AD/HD). This test used the continuous performance or vigilance test approach that many psychologists use in testing children and adults for AD/HD. The test was developed by Robert Keith and is the Auditory Continuous Performance Test (1994).

Not all attempts to assess auditory processing in children focused on using behavioral measures such as those described above. Electrophysiological measures have been used. Electrophysiological measures for investigating the integrity of the central auditory pathways as an indirect assessment of APD was first used with adults (Musiek, Baran, & Pinheiro, 1994; Schwartz, 1987). However, as cited by Chermak and Musiek (1997), Adrian (1930), Saul and Davis (1932), and Wever and Bray (1930) described the possible applications of using electrophysiological measures to investigate central auditory nervous system functioning. The focus of these measures was, again, on identifying the possible site of lesion or dysfunctioning in the central auditory pathways that could possibly interfere with auditory processing abilities.

Electrophysiological measures were then applied with children (Jerger et al, 1988; Jirsa, 1992; Jirsa & Clontz, 1990; Kraus, McGee, Micco, et al., 1993; Musiek, Baran, & Pinheiro, 1992). However, these measures were found to be of limited value in assessing processing abilities because most children could not sit still long enough to sustain the complete assessments unless they were sedated, and sedation led to an inhibition in the measurement of the higher levels or later latency responses. Thus, research attention turned toward examining what are known as event related and late potential responses such as the P-300 (event related) and Mismatched Negativity (MMN). P-300 results appear to provide some information regarding a child's attention to the auditory stimulus involved as well as discrimination of a change in stimulus (Hall, 1992; Musiek, Baran, & Pinheiro, 1992). MMN results occur when the system identifies or discriminates a change in sound or speech and the MMN can occur without having a subject respond to this change (Kraus, McGee, Ferre, et al., 1993; Musiek et al., 1992). However, only some audiologists have the ability and equipment to measure P-300 and MMN results in children so these electrophysiological measures are not routinely used and their diagnostic significance has not been well established in children of various ages who have APDs.

Of all the electrophysiological tests routinely used to evaluate APD in audiological assessments middle ear immittance measures are likely at the top of the list. One aspect of immittance measures is the measurement of acoustic reflexes, which can provide some information regarding the functioning of the central auditory pathways and may provide further information regarding APD issues in children (Hall, 1985). Currently, it is reasonable to report that electrophysiological measures are not widely used in the routine assessment of auditory processing abilities in children. However, as more sophisticated measurement methods are developed, as more clinically useful protocols are found, and as better understanding of the relationship between electrophysiological measures and behavioral implications related to APD are identified, professionals may see more general clinical use of electrophysiological measures in assessing APD in children.

Defining and Describing APD in Children

If one were to go back into the history of communication disorders in children, one would discover that since the beginning there have been accounts of children who act as if they were deaf or hard-of-hearing, but were found to have normal hearing. That is, children who had "listening" difficulties with or without language deficits (especially expressive language problems). However, it was not until Mykelbust's (1954) description of children with auditory imperception that a "name" or description of children with APD was offered in the literature. As previously stated, Mykelbust identified these children as being unable to "structure the auditory world" (p. 158) and having deficits in dealing with auditory information that led to behavioral and communication problems. Thus, the first description of children with APD was a general notion that they could not successfully manage auditory information.

It was not until 1969 (Chalfant & Scheffelin) that the NIH working group published their report on Central Processing Dysfunctions in Children that included auditory processing as one of the central processing dysfunctions. Thus, the terminology was identified to call APD a central auditory processing dysfunction in children. In their monograph, the working group described children with auditory processing dysfunction as having " . . . hearing acuity within the normal range of hearing, but who have difficulty processing and obtaining meaning from auditory stimuli" (p. 9). The committee further describes some of the tasks on which children with APD would have difficulties. These difficulties include sound localization, auditory discrimination, problems with prosody and the "musical" aspects of spoken language (pitch, rhythm, and melody), difficulties in pulling out the relevant from irrelevant in auditory messages, sound blending/phonemic synthesis, and having difficulties obtaining meaning from sound in general.

It was not until 1977 (Keith) at the Central Auditory Dysfunction symposium in Cincinnati, Ohio that the terms Central Auditory Dysfunction and Auditory-Perceptually-Handicapped Children (Sweitzer, 1977) were used. As time marched on, Central Auditory Dysfunction became Central Auditory Processing Dysfunction, and finally became Central Auditory Processing Disorders or CAPD. However, no consensus or agreement was reached as to the description of what were and were *not* CAPDs in children. Thus, a variety of descriptions and definitions of APD were in use by different professionals in the field. However, all professionals essentially stated that the problems in children with APD (or CAPD as it was called at that time) were due to primary deficits in the children's abilities to obtain meaning from auditory messages not due to hearing loss, cognitive/intellectual deficits, or other *nonauditory* problems.

One of the presenters at the Ohio symposium offered an alternative description of APD. Charlotte Dempsey (1977), citing the research of Paula Tallal (1976), posited an explanation that Tallal and her colleagues hold to this day. That is, Tallal's research indicated that children with APD or what was then called "developmental dysphasia (Dempsey, 1977, p. 293) were unable to discriminate rapid changes in the pitch of tones (i.e., had temporal processing deficits). Thus, Dempsey proposed that APD may be due to a deficit in auditory temporal processing in children. Much of Dempsey's focus, as well as the focus of many of the professionals at the Ohio symposium (Keith, 1977) was on children with language-based learning disabilities. Therefore, the definition of APD at that time could be a disorder in taking in and using auditory information that leads children to have learning disabilities and language disorders.

This new focus on APD was a major theme of Jack Willeford, which was discussed earlier in relation to the development of his test battery for identifying APD in children. In 1985, he and Joan Burleigh published their *Handbook of Central Auditory Processing Disorders in Children*, officially giving the name for the disorder CAPD. They describe CAPD as a specific learning disability, even citing the definition of specific learning disability that was and is still used in education laws (i.e., PL 94-142 passed in 1975 and IDEA passed in 1997 and reauthorized in 2004). That is,

> Specific learning disability" means a disorder in one of more of the basic psychological processes involved in understanding or in using language, spoken or written, which may manifest itself in an imperfect ability to listen, think, speak, read, write, spell, or do mathematical calculations (PL 94-142, Section 121 [a] [5]).

Thus, in the education law, APD is and has always been present, as Willeford and Burleigh point out, as a specific learning disability because APD is a disorder in the psychological processes involved in imperfect listening.

Whether school districts accept or reject the notion of APD as a specific learning disability, not all professionals involved in working with children with these auditory disorders feel that APD is simply an auditory-based learning disability. In 1992, Jack Katz, Nancy Stecker, and Donald Henderson offered the following descriptions of central auditory processing, auditory processing, and auditory perception. They viewed the terms central auditory processing (CAP) and auditory processing (AP) as interchangeable, but feel that auditory perception is not an appropriate term to describe auditory processing. They state that the disorder (called CAPD as well as APD by them with the terms identified as being interchangable) is merely an abnormality in CAP/AP.

According to Katz, Stecker, and Henderson (1992), CAP/AP, " . . . refers to the use we make of the auditory signal" (p. 4). The primary distinction they identify between the terms CAP and AP is that the omission of the "C" (central), ". . . implies that auditory processing involves more than the central system" (p. 4), meaning the central auditory nervous system or the centrally auditory pathways. They go on to state, "This is indeed the case" (p. 4). Thus, they prefer the use of, and do use, AP and APD to describe auditory processing and auditory processing disorders, respectively. Thus, Katz, Stecker, and Henderson broaden the view of auditory processing from the focus on the auditory system only. To summarize their view, these authors wrote that AP is, "what we do with what we hear" (p. 5), a statement that is still in use today.

In contrast to this view of AP and APD as involving more than just the central auditory system, in the same publication (Katz, Stecker, & Henderson, 1992), Frank Musiek and Lloyd Lamb (1992) write,

> Auditory processing involves a complex series of neurophysiological and chemical events that begin in the cochlea and proceed upward, encompassing numerous structures and pathways throughout the brain stem and cerebrum. Descending pathways that run throughout the auditory system enhance processing and, ultimately the interpretation of auditory information (p. 11).

Thus, Musiek and Lamb focus on auditory processing as specific to the central auditory pathways and, thus, APD would then be interpreted as some disorder in the central auditory system. Later, Chermak and Musiek (1997) describe APD as, " . . . a deficit in one or more of the central auditory processes responsible for generating the auditory evoked potentials and the following behaviors . . . ," listing the same behaviors that are in the first ASHA Concensus Statement (1996) describing auditory processing and auditory processing disorders. However, Chermak and Musiek go further to describe auditory processing as involving cognitive processes along with these auditory system specific functions. Thus, a broader view of AP and APD was beginning to emerge.

This broader view with AP described via the various behaviors rather than describing auditory processing itself was not only described by Chermak and Musiek, but is reflected in the first attempt to bring a group of professionals together to come to some consensus regarding what is and what is not AP and APD. This attempt was made by the American Speech-Language-Hearing Association (ASHA) in 1992. ASHA convened a group of professionals including audiologists and speech-language pathologists to form the Task Force on Central Auditory Processing Consensus Development that published (1996) its consensus statement describing auditory processing as:

> Central auditory processes are the auditory system mechanisms and processes responsible for the following behavioral phenomena: sound localization and lateralization; auditory discrimination; auditory pattern recognition; temporal aspects of audition including, temporal resolution, temporal masking, temporal integration, and temporal ordering; auditory performance with competing acoustic signals; and auditory performance with degraded acoustic signals (p. 41).

Review of this description indicates its focus on the auditory system with a definition of auditory processing as being auditory processing. That is, there is no real definition of auditory processing in this definition. As such, it could be considered a description of what may be viewed as ways to investigate auditory processing, (i.e., evaluate the functioning of each of the "behavioral phenomena" stated). That is actually what many professionals did after the consensus report was published.

At about the same time as the publication of the consensus report, Teri James Bellis published her first book on central auditory processing disorders in the educational setting (1996). In her book, Bellis describes auditory processing by citing the ASHA Task Force definition. (It should be stated that Chermak and Musiek [1997] include the ASHA description in their discussion of APD, but move beyond that description to include a discussion of the cognitive aspects that are also involved in auditory processing.) Bellis, however, focuses her discussion of AP and APD on the central auditory system and disorders within that system. This focus on APD as a disorder specific to the auditory system is reflected in Bellis' very popular book, *When the Brain Can't Hear* (2002), a book read by many professionals, educators, and parents of children with APD. Thus, for many, AP and APD is specific to the auditory system.

This focus of AP and APD being specific to the auditory system is highly reflected in the publications of Anthony Cacace and Donald McFarland (1995). These authors argue that AP *must* be described as processes specific to the auditory system, and, thus, APD is a disorder of something specifically happening within the auditory system. The idea of an auditory system specific disorder in describing APD was the focus of the second "consensus statement" published by James Jerger and Frank Musiek (2000). In their article, they describe the outcome from a panel of professionals they brought together who made two presentations on the topic and, then, published their report. The focus of this report seems to summarize a variety of views including: AP and APD are specific to the auditory system, the basis of AP is that it involves those processes that lead to the electrophysiological responses that occur within the central auditory pathways, and that auditory processing is largely related to temporal processing. Thus, ideas proposed by the original ASHA consensus group, those expanded by Chermak and Musiek, the temporal processing focus of Tallal and her colleagues, and the modality specific focus of Cacace and McFarland were brought together into a publication that some identify as the audiologist's position on AP and APD. One other important aspect of the Jerger and Musiek article is that it states that the disorder is best described by dropping the "C" and calling it only APD.

The most recent attempt to come to a fuller understanding of AP and APD was made by a second ASHA Task Force (Working Group on Auditory Processing Disorders, 2005). However, the members of this task force, as well as feedback received from peer reviewers, indicated that we, as audiologists and speech-language pathologists are not in agreement enough to come to a consensus as to what is and what is not

AP and APD. This second ASHA Task Force published its technical report in the spring of 2005 (Working Group on Auditory Processing Disorders).

Some of the outstanding facts presented in the Technical Report are that the "C" of CAPD was felt to be used by many but also *not* used by many regarding auditory processing and auditory processing disorders. Thus, they concluded that the best way to approach AP and APD was to place the "C" (central) in parenthesis calling the disorder (Central) Auditory Processing Disorders or (C)APD. Another focus of the technical report was that the description of (C)APD involved the processes that elicit the electrophysiological activity within the central auditory system. Again, the focus brings us back to a narrow view of auditory processing and its disorders as specific to the auditory system. As written in the report:

> Broadly stated, (Central) Auditory Processing [(C)AP] refers to the efficiency and effectiveness by which the central nervous system (CNS) utilizes auditory information. Narrowly defined, (C)AP refers to the perceptual processing of auditory information in the CNS and the neurobiologic activity that underlies that processing and gives rise to electrophysiological auditory potentials (p. 2).

The description then goes on to describe the same essential behaviors as identified in the 1996 ASHA consensus statement such as localization and auditory discrimination. Based on this description, (C)APD is described as, ". . . difficulties in the perceptual processing of auditory information in the CNS as demonstrated by poor performance in one of more of the above skills" (p. 2). The skills refer to the ones stated in the technical report similar to those identified in the 1996 report.

One important factor brought out in the 2005 Technical Report is that (C)APD is seen as modality specific or specific to the auditory system. The report states, "(C)APD is a deficit in the neural processing of auditory stimuli not due to higher order language, cognitive, or related factors" (p. 2). The report does go on to say that APD can lead to problems in higher order or levels of processing involving language, communication, and learning as well as APD can coexist with other disorders such as AD/HD, language impairment, and learning disabilities. Thus, APD is now being viewed in a similar fashion as described by Chalfant and Scheffelin (1969).

Not all professionals view auditory processing in the ways described above. In the mid 1970s and early 1980s, Norma Rees published articles strongly opposing the view, at that time, that AP and APD involved the perceptual processes involved in taking in and getting auditory information from the outside world to the brain, what has been referred to as a bottom-up process. Rees argued that there are many cognitive and linguistically related processes involved in the processing of auditory information and that one uses what may be referred to as top-down functions in the processing of verbal information. Thus, Rees argued that auditory processing largely involves higher level language and cognitive systems. This approach was picked up by many speech-language pathologists whereas the more narrowly focused auditory system specific/perceptual approach was embraced by many audiologists.

One of the best descriptions of the speech-language pathologist's perspectives on AP and APD is provided by Dorothy Kelly (1995). Kelly cites the 1996 ASHA Task Force definition and description of AP as her definition of AP and describes AP as "what we do with what we hear" as originally defined by Katz and his colleagues. However, Kelly describes the components of "normal" auditory processing involving an intact auditory system (outer, middle, inner ears), an intact central auditory system, a "variety of intact and repeated auditory experiences" (p. 7), and "fundamental cognitive potentials" (p. 7). Thus, in Kelly's description of AP, it involves those higher level cognitive functions along with previous experiences, a new addition to the perspectives professionals have been taking on auditory processing and its disorders.

In further describing AP and, thus, APD as disorders in any one or combination of these skills, Kelly describes the specific skill areas involved with AP as: auditory memory, auditory discrimination, auditory figure-ground, auditory cohesion, and auditory attention. The first three are relatively clear to understand. Auditory cohesion refers to, "The ability to organize, interpret, and process on a higher-order level, wherein information may not be discernable on the surface" (p. 8). Auditory cohesion involves higher level linguistic processes and, thus, her approach to AP and APD does *not* differentiate auditory processes from language processes.

Auditory attention (the fifth skill in Kelly's model) brings up a question that many professionals in the field of APD have discussed. That question is, are we seeing a child with an APD or a child with an attention deficit (such as AD/HD)? As discussed above, one of the specific tests developed for use in the APD test battery by Robert Keith is the Auditory Continuous Performance Test found to be sensitive in differentiating APD from attention problems such as AD/HD (Tillery, 1998, 2001). Keller (1992, 1998) described this differentiation and the importance of differentiating an attention disorder from an APD. Additionally, the treatment for attention disorders and APD are different even if the behaviors observed appear to be the same (Tillery, 1998, 2001). Yet, APD can coexist with an attention disorder.

Another professional who proposes a very different description of AP and APD is Lucker. Lucker (2005) describes auditory processing as those things done by the entire central nervous system when it receives information via the auditory system and gets that information to the brain where it forms meaningful concepts. Lucker states that AP involves four fundamental, interactive, integrated systems including: the auditory system (peripheral and central), the linguistic system, the cognitive-behavioral system, and the sensory system. In his description of AP and APD he also includes prior experiences (similarly found in Kelly's description). Lucker proposes that APD could be due to a deficit in functioning in one or more of these four fundamental systems. Thus, he does not view APD in the relatively narrow sense with which most audiologists approach the disorder, nor in the system-specific focus found in the Jerger and Musiek article or in the 2005 ASHA Technical Report, nor does he view APD with a strong language/cognitive approach as does Kelly, although his view of APD is most in line with Kelly's view.

Treatment for Auditory Processing Disorders in Children

When APD was first identified by Mykelbust and described by Chalfant and Scheffelin, there was little in their discussions of the disorders regarding treatment. Much of the initial focus on APD in the 1960s and 1970s was to identify the disorder and determine whether APD did or did not exist in children. However, once APD was found in a child, what was the treatment?

In reviewing the proceedings of the Ohio symposium (Keith, 1977), 12 professionals presented their opinions and research regarding APD, and 10 of them focus on evaluating APD in children. The first presenter (Duane), discusses the neurological perspectives of APD. The ninth presenter (Richardson) discusses how to explain the APD test results to other professionals. There was no presenter who specifically looked at treatment. Thus, treating auditory processing disorders in children proceeded by professionals doing whatever they felt should be done.

In 1985, Willeford and Burleigh dedicated an entire section of their book to management of auditory processing disorders (Chapter 6). They describe six programs that can be used in treating APD including: Semel Auditory Processing Program, APT: Auditory Perception Training, Auditory Perceptual Training Program, Auditory Discrimination in Depth (ADD), Speech-in-Noise Training, and Phonemic Synthesis Training. Of these programs, the Auditory Discrimination in Depth program remains in widespread use with modifications and updated procedures and materials and has been renamed the Lindamood Phonemic Sequence program of LiPS (www.lindamoodbell.com). Various types of speech-in-noise training have persisted such as the background noise tasks included in some of the Earobics games (www.earobics.com). At the time, a company called Developmental Learning Materials (DLM) produced an entire Auditory Figure-Ground training program that those who still have access to it still use today. Additionally, this same company produced Katz's Phonemic Synthesis Training program that is still in use by those who have the original DLM materials.

In 1985, Willeford and Burleigh also described some of the management strategies or accommodations that could be offered to children with APD. Such accommodations as preferential seating, speaking slowly and clearly, the use of visual aids, and rephrasing/restating verbal messages were part of their recommended management strategies.

Another description of specific training and management techniques was described by Daniel Schneider (1992). He also described the Phonemic Synthesis Training program and the Auditory Discrimination in Depth training, Noise-Desensitization training (i.e., speech-in-noise or auditory figure-ground training), and the use of new technology (at that time), FM systems including personal systems and classroom FM systems (Classroom Sound Reinforcement Systems). What is interesting is that Willeford and Burleigh's and Schneider's recommendations comprise many of the recommendations seen in APD evaluation reports to this day. Thus, little has changed but newer programs and approaches have been developed and described.

Bellis (1996, 2002, 2003) described the approach to managing children with APD that she and her colleague Jeanane Ferre developed (Ferre, 1998). Their recommendations for management do not differ significantly from those presented by Willeford and Burleigh and Schneider. They describe strategies to help children with APD focusing on three factors: enhancing the acoustic signal (i.e., improving the listening environment), teaching the child compensatory strategies (such as, requesting preferential seating, asking people to repeat or rephrase, and asking to reduce the background noise), and remediation activities or what may be referred to as treatment. Many of the treatment strategies are language based and cognitively based. The remediation includes: auditory closure activities, phonemic training activities, prosody and temporal pattern (speech rhythm and temporal processing) activities, and interhemispheric training (verbal-to-motor, motor-to-verbal, and singing) activities.

In 1998, Masters, Stecker, and Katz published their book on APD focusing on, as the book is subtitled, *Mostly Management*. Of the 13 chapters in the book, 10 focus on management and treatment activities and strategies. Included in the book are some newer, still in use, programs such as Fast ForWord (www.fastforword.com) (Cinotti, 1998), memory and attention deficits and strategies (Medwetsky, 1998), Auditory Integration Training or AIT (Yencer, 1998), metacognitive approaches (Chermak, 1998; Chermak & Musiek, 1997), and even applications of APD treatments with children having cochlear implants (Katz, 1998).

In addition to these approaches, some of the professionals writing on APD have presented their own, specific approaches that are based on their models of APD. Stecker (1998) described treatments and management areas specific to the four categories of the Buffalo Model developed by Katz and his colleagues. Chermak and Musiek (1997) describe their perceptual training and metacognitive approaches to treating children with APD. Kelly (1995) describes a variety of language and cognitive/linguistically based treatments for children with APD based on her description of the disorder.

Lucker (2005) combines the management strategies from the past decade along with some of the treatments that have been used over the years as well as some newer treatments, some of which are taken from other disciplines, as well as his focus on metacognitive strategies. His treatments including sound-based interventions (such as using altered and enhanced music and sound in such programs as Tomatis training (www.tomatis.com), Therapeutic Listening (www.vitallinks.com), The Listening Program (www.advancedbrain.com), and Samonas (www.samonas.com). He describes the use of computer programs such as Earobics (www.earobics.com) and Fast ForWord (www.fastforword.com), and Lindamood-Bell programs (www.lindamoodbell.com) such as LiPS and Visualizing and Verbalizing. He also describes some underlying skills that involve auditory/linguistic/cognitive processes.

One of the focuses of the 2005 ASHA Technical Report is a discussion and overview of treatment and management strategies for use with children identified with APD. This section of the technical report includes a variety of treatments that include those already discussed by Bellis, Ferre, Chermak, and Musiek.

The Future for APD

In looking back at the history of auditory processing disorders, we can see where we began and where we are today. We began with professionals from a variety of disciplines identifying children having difficulties dealing with and gaining meaning from auditory information not specifically due to hearing loss alone. This led to the development of tests to evaluate AP in children so that APD could be identified or ruled out. We learned to differentiate between APD and attention problems even developing specific test procedures to aid in this differentiation.

Once we felt we had some satisfactory methods for assessing APD, the field moved toward developing agreement as to what the disorder is, how to evaluate APD, and what to do relative to managing and treating children with APD. To date, we have not reached a consensus as to how we define, describe, evaluate, and manage children with APD problems. However, these children exist and professionals are still assessing and providing treatments for them.

The last aspect of this historical overview has illustrated that professionals have seen the move toward developing management and treatment approaches to help children with APD. One focus has been to borrow from other fields whereas another has been to base the management and treatment relative to the APD-specific approach the professional takes.

What will the future hold for the area of APD? This author feels that the future will see advances in research in areas we have not yet touched upon in the quest to better understand the disorder, identify APD in children, and treat children with APD problems. One area in which future research advances may be seen involves human genetics.

New discoveries in the field of genetics may identify genes that underlie predisposition to APD. Perhaps, as genetic research demonstrates that gene therapy can make positive, predictable changes with APD, there will be treatments in the future incorporating gene therapy to mature or develop neurological factors that may underlie APD.

What about neurobiologic research and neurochemical research? Perhaps, we will learn more about what underlies the neurological factors that lead to APD. Maybe, neurochemical findings will demonstrate neuropharmacologic treatments.

And what about nutritional treatments? Some research has suggested links to neurochemical changes with changes in diet and nutritional supplements. Perhaps a better understanding and more specific information about links between diet, supplements, and APD will be found.

And what about assessment? Research is constantly advancing to examine what *is* and what ***is not*** APD and what factors may underlie APD and how we may identify those factors. Perhaps the future will more clearly illustrate that APD cannot be separated into auditory, language, cognitive, or sensory factors. Perhaps some other, new factors will emerge that describe what underlies APD.

Whatever the future holds, now is an exciting time. APD is being recognized and accepted by more and more individuals, more and more professionals, and more and more school districts. Better methods for evaluation and treatment are being developed. New treatments are being identified as having positive effects in changing the brain and may prove to show positive, long-term effects in improving auditory processing abilities in children with APD. Understanding the past is an important way to grow so that we can move on into the future.

For a further review of the history of developments in the area of APD, the reader is referred to: Baran and Musiek (1991), Hall (1992), Keith and Jerger (1991), and Musiek and Baran (1987).

Summary

This chapter discussed a number of factors related to where the study of APD began and where we are headed in the future, demonstrating that, as far back as the 1950s, APD was a recognized disorder, different from other disorders, but not yet understood or identified as unique. The discussion went on to show how a variety of methods for assessing auditory processing in adults with neurological disorders were applied in assessing children with more functional processing disorders involving auditory information. These early assessment procedures led to the development of specific tests of auditory processing for use with children along with normative data becoming available using the assessment measures originally developed for use with adults.

For years, we have struggled to come to a consensus as to what APDs are and how they shall be assessed and treated. As this chapter has pointed out, we are still at a point where no consensus exists, and various approaches to APD exist with much confusion regarding what professionals mean when they discuss APD, how it is to be assessed, and how it is to be treated.

Regardless of whether we have come to a consensus, research and clinical work with children who have problems receiving information through their auditory systems continues. This research will lead to new developments in the field of APD that may finally allow professionals to come to a consensus so that guidelines can be fostered for assessment and treatment of auditory processing problems in children.

Whatever the future holds, now is an exciting time. APD is being recognized and accepted by more and more people, professionals, and school districts. Better methods for evaluation and treatment are being developed. New treatments are being identified as having positive effects in changing the brain and may prove to show positive, long-term effects in improving auditory processing abilities in children with APD. Understanding the past is an important way to grow so that we can move on into the future.

Key Points Learned

- The first publications describing tests assessing APD including findings and the neurological correlates of these findings in adults were published in the mid-1950s into the 1960s.
- APD in children was first described in the literature in the mid to late 1950s.
- The first symposium dedicated to APD in children was held in the late 1970; proceedings of that conference were published by Keith in 1977. At the symposium, the first description of tests and test findings in children with APD were described as well as some discussion of intervention strategies.
- Interest in APD in children increased during the 1980s, 1990s, into the present millennium.
- The first descriptions of models or approaches to APD were developed including categorical models (Katz's Buffalo Model and Bellis/Ferre Model) during the 1980s and 1990s.
- An argument proposed that APD was not a useful construct was presented by Rees (mid-1970s) and led to a view that APD is really nothing more than a language disorder.
- The first ASHA Committee on Central Auditory Processing Disorders convened and a consensus statement was published in the early to mid-1990s.
- A second consensus statement was published in an article written by Jerger and Musiek (2000) including the use of the term Auditory Processing Disorder (APD) replacing the more commonly used term Central Auditory Processing Disorder (CAPD), but meaning the same thing.
- A second ASHA Committee on APD convened with the publication of their Technical Report including publication of guidelines regarding the Role of the Audiologist in APD Assessment in 2005; including the term central placed in parenthesis to denote that both APD and (C)APD are the same term.
- There is a lack of agreement between professionals regarding how APD is to be described, assessed, and treated.

References

Adrian, E. D. (1930). The activity of the nervous system of the caterpillar. *Journal of Physiology, 30*, 34–36.

American Speech-Language-Hearing Association (ASHA). (1992). *Issues in central auditory processing disorders: A report from the ASHA Ad Hoc Committee on Central Auditory Processing*. Rockville, MD: Author.

American Speech-Language-Hearing Association (ASHA) Task Force on Central Auditory Processing Consensus Development. (1996). Central auditory processing: Current status of research and implications for clinical practice. *American Journal of Audiology, 5*(2), 41–54.

Baran, J. A., & Musiek, F. E. (1991). Behavioral assessment of the central auditory nervous system. In. W. F. Rintelmann (Ed.), *Hearing assessment* (pp. 549–602). Austin, TX: Pro-Ed.

Beasley, D. S., & Freeman, B. A. (1977). Time-altered speech as a measure of central auditory processing. In R. W. Keith (Ed.), *Central auditory dysfunction* (pp. 129–176). New York: Grune & Stratton.

Bellis, T. J. (1996). *Central auditory processing disorders in the educational setting: From science to practice.* San Diego, CA: Singular Publishing Group.

Bellis, T. J. (2002). *When the brain can't hear: Unraveling the mystery of auditory processing disorder*. New York: Pocket Books.

Bellis, T. J. (2003). *Assessment and management of central auditory processing disorders in the educational setting: From science to practice* (2nd ed.). Clifton Park, NY: Thomson Delmar Learning.

Berry, M. F., & Eisenson, J. (1956). *Speech disorders: Principles and practices of therapy*. New York: Appleton-Century-Crofts.

Bocca, E. (1958). Clinical aspects of cortical deafness. *Laryngoscope, 68*, 301–309.

Bocca, E., & Calearo, C. (1963). Clinical aspects of cortical deafness. In, J. Jerger (Ed.), *Modern developments in audiology*. New York: Academic Press.

Bocca, E., Calearo, C., & Cassinari, V. (1954). A new method for testing hearing in temporal lobe tumor. *Acta Otolaryngologica, 44*, 219–221.

Bocca, E., Calearo, C., Cassinari, V., & Migliavacca, F. (1955). Testing "cortical hearing" in temporal lobe tumors. *Acta Otolaryngologica, 42*, 289–304.

Cacace, A., & McFarland, D. (1995). Modality specificity as a criterion for diagnosing central auditory processing disorders. *American Journal of Audiology, 4*, 36–48.

Calero, C., & Lazzaroni, A. (1957). Speech intelligibility in relation to the speech of the message. *Laryngoscope, 67*, 410–419.

Chalfant, J. C., & Scheffelin, M. A. (1969). *Central processing dysfunctions in children: A review of the research*. Bethesda, MD: National Institute of Neurological Diseases and Stroke, National Institutes of Health, U.S. Department of Health, Education, and Welfare, Monograph No. 9.

Chermak, G. D. (1998). Metacognitive approaches to managing central auditory processing disorders. In M. G. Masters, N. A., Stecker, & J. Katz (Eds.), *Central auditory processing disorders: Mostly management* (pp. 49–62). Boston: Allyn & Bacon.

Chermak, G. D., & Musiek, F. E. (1997). *Central auditory processing disorders: New perspectives*. San Diego, CA: Singular Publishing Group,.

Cherry, R. S. (1980). *Selective Auditory Attention Test (SAAT)*. St. Louis, MO: Auditec.

Cinotti, T. M. (1998). The Fast ForWord Program: a clinician's perspective. In M. G. Masters, N. A. Stecker, & J. Katz (Eds.), *Central auditory processing disorders: Mostly management* (pp. 131–150). Boston: Allyn & Bacon.

Davis, S. M., & McCroskey, R. L. (1980). *Wichita Auditory Fusion Test (WAFT)*.

Dempsey, C. (1977). Some thoughts concerning alternative explanations of central auditory test results. In R.W. Keith (Ed.), *Central auditory dysfunction* (pp. 293–318). New York: Grune & Stratton.

Ferre, J. M. (1998). The M3 model for treating central auditory processing disorders. In M. G. Masters, N. A. Stecker, & J. Katz (Eds.), *Central auditory processing disorders: Mostly management* (pp. 103–116). Boston: Allyn & Bacon.

Flowers, A., Costello, M., & Small, V. (1970). *Flowers-Costello Tests of Central Auditory Abilities.* Deerborn, MI: Perceptual Learning Systems.

Goldman, R., Fristoe, M., & Woodcock, R. (1970). *The Goldman-Fristoe-Woodcock Test of Auditory Discrimination.* Circle Pines, MN: American Guidance Service (AGS).

Goldman, R., Fristoe, M., & Woodcock, R. (1974). *The Goldman-Fristoe-Woodcock Auditory Skills Test Battery.* Circle Pines, MN: American Guidance Service (AGS).

Hall, J. W. III. (1985). *The acoustic reflex in central auditory dysfunction.* Baltimore: Williams & Wilkins.

Hall, J. W. III (1992). *Handbook of auditory evoked responses.* Boston: Allyn & Bacon.

Jerger, J., & Jerger, S. (1974). Auditory findings in brain stem disorders. *Archives of Otolaryngology, 99,* 342–351.

Jerger, J., & Jerger, S. (1975). Clinical validity of central auditory tests. *Scandinavian Audiology, 4,* 147–163.

Jerger, J., & Musiek, F. E. (2000). Report of the consensus conference on the diagnosis of auditory processing disorders in school-aged children. *Journal of the American Academy of Audiology, 1,* 467–474.

Jerger, S., & Jerger, J. (1984). *Pediatric Speech Intelligibility Test.* St. Louis, MO: Auditec.

Jerger, S., Johnson, K., & Loiselle, L. (1988). Pediatric central auditory dysfunction: Comparison of children with confirmed lesion versus suspected processing disorders. *American Journal of Otology, 9,* 63–71.

Jirsa, R. E. (1992). The clinical utility of the P3 AERP in children with auditory processing disorders. *Journal of Speech and Hearing Research, 35,* 903–912.

Jirsa, R. E., & Clontz, K. B. (1990). Long latency auditory event-related potentials from children with auditory processing disorders. *Ear and Hearing, 11,* 222–232.

Katz, J. (1962). The use of staggered spondaic words for assessing the integrity of the central auditory system. *Journal of Auditory Research, 2,* 327–337.

Katz, J. (1972). Phonemic synthesis. In E. Lasky & J. Katz (Eds.), *Central auditory processing disorders: Problems of speech, language, and learning.* Baltimore: Williams & Wilkins.

Katz, J. (1998). Central auditory processing and cochlear implant therapy. In M. G. Masters, N. A. Stecker, & J. Katz (Eds.), *Central auditory processing disorders: Mostly management* (pp. 215–232). Boston: Allyn & Bacon.

Katz, J., & Illmer, R. (1972). Auditory perception in children with learning disabilities. In J. Katz (Ed.), *Handbook of clinical audiology.* Baltimore: Williams & Wilkins.

Katz, J., Stecker, N.A., & Henderson, D. (1992). *Central auditory processing: A transdiciplinary approach.* St. Louis, MO: Mosby Year Book.

Keith, R. W. (Ed.). (1977). *Central auditory dysfunction.* New York: Grune & Stratton.

Keith, R. W. (1986). *SCAN: A Screening Test for Auditory Processing Disorders.* San Antonio, TX: Psychological Corporation.

Keith, R. W. (1994). *ACPT: The Auditory Continuous Performance Test.* San Antonio, TX: Psychological Corporation.

Keith, R. W. (1994). *SCAN-A: A Test for Auditory Processing Disorders in Adolescents and Adults.* San Antonio, TX: Psychological Corporation.

Keith, R. W. (1999). *SCAN-C: A Test for Auditory Processing Disorders in Children—Revised.* San Antonio, TX: Psychological Corporation.

Keith, R. W. (2002). *RGDT: The Random Gap Detection Test.* St. Louis, MO: Auditec.

Keith, R. W. (2002). *TCST: The Time Compressed Sentences Test.* St. Louis, MO: Auditec.

Keith, R. W., & Jerger, S. (1991). Central auditory disorders. In J. T. Jacobson & J. L. Northern (Eds.), *Diagnostic audiology* (pp. 235–250). Austin, TX: Pro-Ed.

Keller, W. D. (1992). Auditory processing disorder or attention-deficit disorder? In J. Katz, N. A. Stecker, & D. Henderson (Eds.), *Central auditory processing: A transdisciplinary approach*. St. Louis, MO: Mosby Year Book.

Keller, W. D. (1998). The relationship between attention deficit hyperactivity disorder, central auditory processing disorders, and specific learning disability. In M. G. Masters, N. A. Stecker, & J. Katz (Eds.), *Central auditory processing disorders: Mostly management* (pp. 33–48). Boston: Allyn & Bacon.

Kelly, D. A. (1995). *Central auditory processing disorders: Strategies for use with children and adolescents*. San Antonio, TX: Communication Skill Builders.

Kraus, N., McGee, T. J., Ferre, J., Hoeppner, J., Carrell, T. Sharma, A., & Nicol, T. (1993). Mismatch negativity in the neurophysiologic/behavioral evaluation of auditory processing deficits: A case study. *Ear and Hearing, 14*(4), 223–234.

Kraus, N., McGee, T. J., Micco, A., Sharma, A., Carrell, T., & Nicol, T. (1993). Mismatch negativity in school-age children to speech stimuli that are just perceptibly different. *Electroencephalography and Clinical Neurophysiology, 88*, 123–130.

Lucker, J. R. (1980). Diagnostic significance of the Type A pattern on the Staggered Spondaic Word Test. *Audiology and Hearing Education, 6*(2), 21–23.

Lucker, J. R. (1981). Interpreting SSW results of learning disabled children. *SSW News, 3*, 1–3.

Lucker, J. R. (1982). Diagnostic significance of the Type A pattern on the Staggered Spondaic Word (SSW) Test. In D. Arnst, & J. Katz (Eds.), *Central auditory assessment: The SSW Test—Development and clinical use* (pp. 350–355). San Diego, CA: College-Hill Press.

Lucker, J. R. (2005). Working with children with auditory processing disorders. Self-study continuing education (CEU) program available from http://www.medspdn.com [Audiotape, CD-ROM and VHS video].

Masters, M. G., Stecker, N. A., & Katz, J. (1998). *Central auditory processing disorders: Mostly nanagement*. Boston: Allyn & Bacon

McCroskey, R. L., & Keith, R. W. (1996). *The Auditory Fusion Test—Revised*. St. Louis, MO: Auditec.

Medwetsky, L. (1998). Memory and attention processing deficits: A guide to management strategies. In M. G. Masters, N. A. Stecker, & J. Katz (Eds.), *Central auditory processing disorders: Mostly management* (pp. 63–88). Boston: Allyn & Bacon.

Musiek, F. E. (1983). Assessment of central auditory dysfunction: The Dichotic Digit Test revisited. *Ear and Hearing, 4*, 79–83.

Musiek, F. E. (1994). Frequency (pitch) and duration pattern tests. *Journal of the American Academy of Audiology, 5*, 265–268.

Musiek, F. E., & Baran, J. A. (1987). Central auditory assessment: Thirty years of change and challenge. *Ear and Hearing, 8*(Suppl.), 22–35.

Musiek, F. E., Baran, J. A., & Pinhiero, M. L. (1990). Duration pattern recognition in normal subjects and patients with cerebral and cochlear lesions. *Audiology, 29*, 304–313.

Musiek, F. E., Baran, J. A., & Pinhiero, M. L. (1992). P300 results in patients with lesions of the auditory areas of the cerebrum. *Journal of the American Academy of Audiology, 3*, 5–15.

Musiek, F. E., Baran, J. A., & Pinhiero, M. L. (1994). *Neuroaudiology: Case studies*. San Diego, CA: Singular Publishing Group.

Musiek, F. E., & Lamb, L. (1992). Neuroanatomy and neurophysiology of central auditory processing. In J. Katz, N. A. Stecker, & D. Henderson (Eds.), *Central auditory processing: A transdisciplinary view* (pp. 11–38). St. Louis, MO: Mosby Year Book.

Mykelbust, H. R. (1954). *Auditory disorders in children: A manual for differential diagnosis*. New York: Grune & Stratton.

Pinheiro, M. L. (1977). Test of central auditory function in children with learning disabilities. In R. W. Keith (Ed.), *Central auditory dysfunction* (pp. 223–256). New York: Grune & Stratton.

Rees, N. (1975). Auditory processing factors in language disorders: The view from Procrustes' bed. *Journal of Speech and Hearing Disorders, 38*, 304–315.

Rees, N. (1981). Saying more than we know: Is auditory processing disorder a meaningful concept? In R. W. Keith (Ed.), *Central auditory and language disorders in children.* Houston, TX: College-Hill Press.

Saul. L. J., & Davis, H. (1932). Action currents in the central nervous system: I. Action currents of the auditory tracts. *Archives of Neurology and Psychiatry, 28*, 1104–1116.

Schneider, D. (1992). Audiological management of central auditory processing disorders. In J. Katz, N. A. Stecker, & D. Henderson (Eds.), *Central auditory processing: A transdisciplinary approach* (pp. 161–168). St. Louis, MO: Mosby Year Book.

Schwartz (1987). Neurodiagnostic audiology: Contemporary perspectives. *Ear and Hearing, 8*, 43–48.

Stecker, N. A. (1998). Overview and update of central processing disorders. In M. G. Masters, N. A. Stecker, & J. Katz (Eds.), *Central auditory processing disorders: Mostly management*. Boston: Allyn & Bacon.

Sweitzer, R. S. (1977). Team evaluation of auditory perceptually-handicapped children. In R. W. Keith (Ed.), *Central auditory dysfunction* (pp. 341–360). New York: Grune & Stratton.

Tallal, P. (1976). Auditory perceptual factors in language and learning disabilities. In R. Knights & D. Baker (Eds.), *The neuropsychology of learning disabilities.* Baltimore: University Park Press.

Tillery, K. L. (1998). Central auditory processing assessment and therapeutic strategies for children with attention deficit hyperactivity disorder. In M. G. Masters, N. A. Stecker, & J. Katz (Eds.), *Central auditory processing disorders: Mostly management* (pp. 175–194). Boston: Allyn & Bacon.

Tillery, K. L. (2001). The relationship of learning, attention deficits, and auditory processing disorders. *NCAPD Newsletter.* Available on-line at http://www.ncapd.org.

Wepman, J. (1958) *Wepman Auditory Discrimination Test.* Available on-line at: http://www.listen.org/pages/listening_tests_from_Listening_Instructor_Manual.html

Wepman, J. (1973). *Wepman Auditory Discrimination Test—Revised.* Available on-line at: http://www.listen.org/pages/listening_tests_from_Listening_Instructor_Manual.html

Wever, E. G., & Bray, C. W. (1930). Auditory nerve impulses. *Science, 71*, 215.

Willeford, J. A. (1977). Assessing central auditory behavior in children: A test battery approach. In R. W. Keith (Ed.), *Central auditory dysfunction*. New York: Grune & Stratton.

Willeford, J. A., & Burleigh, J. M. (1985). *Handbook of central auditory processing disorders in children*. New York: Grune & Stratton.

Working Group on Auditory Processing Disorders. (2005). *(Central) auditory processing disorders: Technical report.* Rockville, MD: American Speech-Language-Hearing Association (ASHA)

Yencer, K. A. (1998). Is auditory integration training an effective treatment for children with central auditory processing disorders? In M. G. Masters, N. A. Stecker, & J. Katz (Eds.), *Central auditory processing disorders: Mostly management* (pp. 151–174). Boston: Allyn & Bacon.

2

Central Auditory Processing Disorders

Definition, Description, and Behaviors

Donna Geffner

Overview

This chapter reviews the definition of auditory processing and auditory processing disorders and describes the behaviors that are inherent within the classification. The formal definitions from the ASHA Technical Report of 2005 and the Task Force Consensus Report 1996 are provided, along with the American Academy of Audiology's adoption of the Bruton Consensus Conference. The controversy regarding whether central auditory processing disorder is modality-specific or multimodality is addressed. Behaviors identifying an auditory processing problem are described with particular emphasis on how it affects the child's performance in the classroom. Clinical observations of behaviors and symptoms that serve as a red flag to the classroom teacher, parent, and health care professional are highlighted in the hope that such individuals will be alert to identifying these children so they may be properly evaluated and treated. The comorbidity with attention deficit/hyperactivity disorder (AD/HD), its similarities and differences, along with other disorders such as learning and language impairment are explored. Furthermore, possible causes and predisposing factors that lead to an auditory processing deficit are discussed. Unfortunately, the direct cause(s) are not known, but conditions that are associated with or may be considered the underlying event(s) or precipitating factors that predispose one to having an auditory processing disorder ([C]APD) are presented.

What Is Auditory Processing?

Central auditory processing is the efficiency and effectiveness by which the central nervous system utilizes auditory information. It encompasses the perceptible processing of auditory information in the central nervous system and the neurobiologic activity that underlies that processing and gives rise to electrophysiologic auditory potentials. This definition was provided by the ASHA Technical Report (2005), after an extensive study by its Working Group on Central Auditory Processing. (C)APD, as it has been called, is a deficit in the neural processing of auditory stimuli that is not due to higher order language, cognitive, or related factors (ASHA, 1996, 2005). This is important as many families attribute (C)APD to autism and receptive language impairments. There is a distinction to be made among these disorders. Children and adults are a heterogeneous group of people who have difficulty using the auditory information to communicate and learn (Jerger & Musiek, 2000). There is a set of problems that occur in different and difficult listening conditions, with a deficiency in processing the auditory input as the listening environment becomes more unfavorable. We often see the individual struggling with "listening" and understanding of speech, resulting in difficulty using and understanding language and learning. CAPD may lead to difficulties in higher order language learning and communication, but it is not the result of these disorders.

Children and adults with (C)APD present with a pattern of difficulties and poor performance in one or more of the following skills (ASHA, 2005):

Sound Localization and Lateralization—the ability to know where sound has occurred in space. Localization is the ability to identify the source of sound.

Auditory Discrimination—the ability to distinguish one sound from another.

Auditory Pattern Recognition—the ability to determine similarities and differences in patterns of sounds

Temporal Aspects of Audition—the ability to process acoustic stimuli over time, including:

Temporal masking—the potential to mask (muffle or obliterate) weaker phonemes after (backward) or before (forward) stronger phonemes. The ability of one sound to mask another that precedes or follows it.

Temporal resolution—the perception of fast changing signals

Temporal integration—the ability to integrate acoustic energy in brief sounds and add up information over time or duration. The ability to sequence sounds, integrate a sequence of sounds and process stimuli over time by both ears.

Temporal ordering—the ability to process durational patterns in sequence and perceive a sequence of sounds (Rawool, 2006).

Auditory Performance Decrements with Competing Acoustic Signals—the ability to perceive speech or other sounds when another signal is present. Such a signal may be noise or another speech signal

Auditory Performance Decrements with Degraded Acoustic Signals—the ability to perceive a signal in which some information is missing, such as parts of the sound spectrum, high or low frequencies extracted, or the sound is compressed in time.

If one could put the definition into laymen's terms so that parents understand it, it would be safe to describe APD in the words of Jack Katz. It is "what we do with what we hear" (Lasky & Katz, 1983). Dr. Katz, in a personal communication, answered a client's inquiry who questioned the author about the existence of central auditory processing by saying, "What do you think the enormous auditory system is used for?"

Regardless of which definition you ascribe to, there are approximately 3 to 5% of school-age children with an (C)APD (Chermak & Musiek, 1997). Depending upon the research, Katz found a prevalence of 20% (2005) and DiMaggio and Geffner (2003) found a prevalence of 12%. (C)APD is not limited to children only. It is prevalent in adults and more pronounced in people over the age of 60.

Functional Definition

Often youngsters in the classroom are sending signals that raise a "Red flag" to the teacher that that they are not "getting the message." Functionally, one then can define (C)APD as a disorder in the ability to take in the spoken message, make it meaningful, and interpret the message. Does that go beyond the auditory system, to some degree, since it involves an understanding of language and an ability to process a mes-sage that is linguistic in content? Some think so, but the auditory system starts the input for the process to begin. Thus, the support for a multimodality function.

Audiologist's Definition

Audiologists generally agree that (C)APD exists; however, there is disagreement about whether it is a purely central, part of a multimodality deficit, or a more sensory modality-specific auditory deficit. The current thinking is that CAP encompasses the entire auditory system and its related processes. This is particularly relevant in regard to the child with a hearing loss or a conductive loss that precludes the organ from hearing clearly. The interference from the conductive block interferes with the clarity of the message. We know that for those with longstanding otitis media, there is a higher risk of a speech discrimination loss and a degradation of signal clarity as one gets older due to the deprivation effect of occluding the conductive pathway (Rubin et al., 1997).

However, there is an opposing point of view that has challenged the validity of (C)APD. The authors, in a very comprehensive review of the literature, argue its existence on the basis of it being a modality-specific disorder (Cacace & McFarland, 1998). Cacace and McFarland (1995) have argued that the primary deficit in (C)APD should be manifested in tasks that require the processing of acoustic information, where it should not be apparent or manifested to a lesser extent when similar types of information are presented to other modalities. They emphasize that (C)APD should be distinguished from cognitive, language-based, and polysensory and attentional problems, in which modality-specific perceptual dysfunctions are not expected. Their review of the literature did not reveal the modality-specific nature of auditory-based learning problems, largely due to the "inclusive" framework used in the evaluation of (C)APD. This "inclusive" framework holds that performance on auditory tests alone provides enough evidence to diagnose (C)APD. The risk, according to these authors, is that individuals with problems that are not of a unimodal nature, or a perceptual nature, can be misdiagnosed. They support testing that allows for differentiation between auditory perceptual deficits from those with nonperceptual deficits, limiting tasks in the cognitive, motor, memory, and attention realm (Cacace & McFarland, 2006). Thus the modality-specific nature should be what is ultimately evaluated.

Cacace and McFarland ascribe to the American Academy of Audiology's definition that was an outgrowth of the Bruton Consensus Conference (Jerger & Musiek, 2000, p. 468) that states [C]APD is a modality-specific perceptual dysfunction not due to peripheral hearing loss. Another definition that is more expansive is that espoused by Masters, Stecker, and Katz, (1998), which states an auditory processing disorder is a physical hearing impairment that affects the development of the integrated processes of language (listening and speaking) and literacy (reading and writing). If problems occur when recognizing the sound system of language then there will be problems when the child matches sounds to letters, a skill underlying the basis for reading and writing. Such problems lead to comprehension problems and poor academic performance (ASHA, 1996). The current ASHA Technical Report (2005) supports the multisensory model and concludes that ". . . any definition that specifies complete modality-specificity as a diagnostic criterion is neurophysiologically untenable. Instead our definition and conceptualization of (C)APD must be consistent with the manner in which auditory and related processing occurs in the CNS" (central nervous system) (ASHA, 2005, p. 2).

Not only are definitions variable, often resulting in misdiagnoses, the very existence of (C)APD has been challenged by speech-language pathologists who have ascribed a child's inability to process phonemes, blend sounds, and understand that letters have sounds, to be a function of language and reading, separate from auditory neural substrates. The controversy as to whether phonologic processing is an auditory skill or a linguistic skill remains unresolved. The Technical Report is clear on its exclusion. "Although abilities such as phonological awareness, attention to and memory for auditory information, auditory synthesis, comprehension and interpretation of auditorily presented information, and similar skills may be reliant on or associated with intact central auditory function, they are considered higher order cognitive–communicative and/or language-related functions and, thus, are not included in the definition of (C)APD" (ASHA, 2005, p 2).

However, today with electrophysiologic methods, sensory areas can be identified by their modality-specific responsiveness and auditory-specific areas beyond Heschl's gyrus (Kaas & Hackett, 2000). Modality-specific activation in humans using imaging techniques such as positron emission tomography (PET), and functional magnetic resonance imaging (fMRI) (Warren & Griffiths, 2003) reveal possible streams of processing for identification of auditory stimuli. Historically, the presence of (C)APD was based on a pathologic model and the pathology of the auditory cortex. Today, we have additional evidence to support other models and provide additional information regarding sensitivity and specificity.

Behaviors Associated with APD

It is well established that children with (C)APD exhibit the following behaviors as originally delineated by Robert Keith (1994, 2000):

- Poor listening skills
- Difficulty leaning through the auditory modality
- Difficulty following auditory instructions
- Short-term memory span deficiencies
- Difficulty understanding in the presence of background noise
- Frequently asking "What?" or saying "huh?"
- Misunderstanding what is said to them or "mishearing" the word or message.
- Difficulty understanding speech when it is muffled or distorted
- Requesting information to be repeated
- Poor auditory attention—unable to stay focused on an auditory event and experiences fatigue after a period of "intense listening"
- Easily distracted, especially in background noise—hearing the background more prominently than others—thus interfering with the foreground message
- Deficits with auditory integration for sound blending, auditory

closure task, phonologic awareness, and phonic skills

Weak auditory memory span for commands and sequences—one often forgets the last part of the sequence or forgets the first part, soon after it is spoken

Delayed response or slow speed of response to verbal stimuli

Reduced tolerance to loud noise and sensitivity to noise

Heightened sensitivity or better-than-normal thresholds-hypersensitivity

Poor speech recognition in noise

Figure-ground deficits

Problems understanding rapid speech

Problems with spelling, reading, and academics

Although the above symptoms are present in a group of individuals with (C)APD, they do not have to exist in totality. In addition, other concomitant problems may arise like a reading disorder, behavior disorder, and an expressive and receptive language disorder. There is a great deal of overlap of symptoms due to the presence of other disorders such as AD/HD, learning disabilities, and language disabilities and the polyperceptual nature of them.

Comorbidities

In a research study conducted by DiMaggio and Geffner (2003), the files of 425 students, aged 7 through 14, diagnosed with (C)APD were studied to determine the presence of comorbid conditions. Each student was diagnosed as having an auditory processing disorder based on two measures (SCAN-C and SSW) in addition to having poor speech in noise scores. For each of the children, a thorough study of his or her history was conducted which included birth history, health history, parental history, history of otitis media in childhood, reading scores, presence of AD/HD. In some cases where AD/HD was not formally diagnosed, the parent was asked to complete a questionnaire (McCarney, 1995) to determine if the child was at risk for having AD/HD.

The results were quite astounding in that there was an unusually high prevalence of AD/HD among this population. In fact, 31% of the children were diagnosed medically as having AD/HD, whereas 53% were suspected as having the disorder by virtue of the responses on the questionnaire. Thus, for 84% of the population, behaviors consistent with AD/HD were present. Whether all the suspected children would meet the criteria for identification remains a question; nevertheless, their behaviors mirrored the disorder. The study further revealed that 83% of the population had a speech and language disorder, whereas 47% had a reading disorder, that is, they were reading at least one grade below grade level. Interestingly there were a number of neurobiological conditions that arose when the intake histories were studied. Namely, there was a high propensity for birth mothers to have complications during pregnancy (gestational diabetes), or to have been smokers. There were neurological insults at birth such as the umbilical cord tied around the neck, loss of oxygen at birth, trauma to the mother, or precipitous birth. Reading disorders had a high prevalence rate. Among the children, only 27% did not have any problem with reading. The 73% did have problems with nearly twice as many boys having more difficulty than girls (48% to 25%).The prevalence of otitis media with effusion was nearly 50% in the population and that would include those parents who knew their child had an ear infection. Many youngsters go undiagnosed as long as they are asymptomatic; thus, there were probably more children at risk for this condition. Nevertheless, in the general population, it is not unusual to see infants and young children at risk for early otitis media with effusion, approximately 50%. So our data are not out of the ordinary or different from what would be expected in a normal population for the age group studied. However, we now know that such conditions put the child at risk for future processing delays. What we do not know yet is the true prevalence of concomitant disorders such as AD/HD, given the difficulty in arriving at a diagnosis and the overlap of symptoms.

As indicated in the above list of symptoms, some youngsters display a hypersensitivity to sounds. In a study that investigated comfort levels and tolerance levels of hearing (Geffner, Lucker, & Koch, 1996; Lucker, Geffner, & Koch, 1996), children with (C)APD and AD/HD were shown to have statistically lower levels of comfort and tolerance, by about 8 dB HL. This is consistent with parental report that their child does not like to attend a birthday party or the circus because the noise is too loud, or the fire engine is too loud. It should be noted here that the children were dually diagnosed.

Given the difficulties with receiving language and understanding the spoken message, there are often complications that implicate receptive language. Such deficits are seen when the youngster is asked to interpret, infer, and make predictions about the language presented to him or her. The youngster is often at a loss when expected to understand humor, a joke, sarcasm, puns, and nuances of the spoken message. After all, if he or she can't get the whole message, then the superlinguistic aspects of it will surely not be interpreted accurately. Thus, there is need to assess the child's understanding of superlinguistic content. It would be of value to acknowledge that this population is at risk for having a higher language level disorder affecting the superlinguistic components such as nonliteral language, inferential language, ambiguous language, and failure to interpret the (implied) message, or understand figures of speech. Often the youngster is very "literal" in his or her thoughts and is unable to "see the forest from the trees. " It is not unusual to see these children responding "very literally" with no interpretation of the message. As an example:

> Robert's mom thought that her son was too literal and told him that he needed to "broaden his horizons". The next day, Robert came home from school and proudly announced to his mom that he joined the sailing club. When his mother asked him "Why?" he replied "You wanted me to broaden my horizon, so I joined the sailing club to sail the ocean."

This difficulty with figures of speech and expressions are often found when testing these children using measures of nonliteral language. Such a discussion regarding their language competence will ensue in a subsequent chapter. These patterns are typically seen as well in children with AD/HD.

How Can a Differential Diagnosis Be Made Between AD/HD and CAPD?

For one, the child with AD/HD needs to be diagnosed medically in order to be managed. A medical diagnosis is needed in some states with or without a psychological assessment to diagnose AD/HD.

Children with AD/HD have either a hyperactivity, an inattentiveness, or a combination of the two. Depending on the type, the following behaviors will be seen.

For the *inattentive* type, the child will exhibit difficulty staying focused, or fail to give close attention to detail, make careless mistakes in schoolwork, homework or other activities, appear not to listen, be unable to follow through on instructions, or finish schoolwork or chores. Organization will be difficult and as a result there will be procrastination, delay, and reluctance to engage in tasks that require sustained mental effort. The child will lose things or forget to have those items needed to do a task, such as homework. The child will be easily distracted throughout the day and be forgetful about daily activities, so reminding is needed. Here is where the confusion arises. The parent often remarks how she or he has to tell the child to do something several times before he or she responds or has to repeat directions many times before the child "gets it." Thus the confusion about whether it is an auditory processing deficit, as opposed to an attentional deficit.

If the child is *hyperactive*, the teacher will see the child fidget with hands or feet or squirm in the chair, leave the seat, or run about. This child will have difficulty playing with others and playing quietly, as he or she is often too noisy and plays loudly. This child will have problems engaging in leisure activities, appear to be always on the go, and can talk excessively. Impulsive children will blurt out the answer in class, have trouble waiting their turn and interrupt others, or burst into a room when others are talking.

There is the *combined type* of AD/HD, which encompasses both the inattentive form and the hyperactive/impulsive form.

The reader needs to remember that to diagnose AD/HD, the symptoms need to be present for at least six or more of the behaviors delineated by the *DSM-4 Manual*, exist for longer than 6 months, and appear before the age of 7. Individuals with AD/HD are susceptible to having attentional problems that affect academic careers, school performance, and life.

Differential diagnosis should involve the following:

Questionnaires to determine the presence of AD/HD-like symptoms and its frequency and intensity.

Clinical interviews and observations done in the home and at school since two environments need to be investigated. It is clear that youngsters may perform better in one setting than another, depending on the level of distractions present.

Continuous performance measures can be used to obtain a more objective evaluation. On these tests (CPT, Conners, 1995) and IVA, (Integrated Visual and Auditory Continuous Performance Test, Sanford & Turner, 1995), the youngster is asked to remain vigilant to a screen that projects visual images to which he or she must respond in a given period of time. Results are interpreted based on norms for errors and response time. For a more descriptive analysis of test measures, the reader is referred to Geffner, (2005).

The diagnosis of AD/HD, the term currently in use by the American Psychiatric Association (APA) and the *Diagnostic and Statistical Manual* (DSM-IV, 1994), is made when the behaviors are seen across the three domains (inattention, hyperactivity, impulsivity) with symptom onset before age 7, lasting for longer than 6 months and occurring across two settings (home, school, playground). It is seen as a neurobiological disorder that is heritable and involves neurochemical and neurobiological functions affecting the neurotransmitters in the brain.

Keep in mind that children with AD/HD are not always discovered if they are inattentive in the early grades. However, as the work gets harder, when organization skills are called into action, and note-taking demands are made, the youngster reveals, as his grades fail, that he has been daydreaming in class. For the hyperactive child, the diagnosis is easier in that he or she is more obvious and more difficult to manage. Thus, diagnosis is often made earlier in the child's academic life.

What Is the Difference Between AD/HD and CAPD?

It is clear that many of the behaviors seen in AD/HD and CAPD overlap. For instance, the child with AD/HD often demonstrates inconsistencies in response to auditory stimuli, has reduced attention span, easily fatigues, is distracted to auditory (and visual) stimuli, needs information to be repeated, has difficulty remembering days of the week, phone numbers, addresses, and has trouble listening in the presence of noise. The similarities are remarkable. For the CAPD child, such behaviors have been cited as hyperactive, inattentive, trouble following directions, short memory span, and difficulty listening in noise (Chermak & Musiek, 1997). There may be some validity to the notion that children classified as having CAPD may, in fact, have some form of AD/HD. However, for AD/HD, there is a behavioral aspect, namely, problems with self-regulation (Barkley, 1997) and inhibition. To test only the auditory modality—as a deficit specific function without looking at other modalities, according to Cacace and McFarland (2006), results in incomplete assessment and a diagnosis that is indeterminable.

In an attempt to differentiate between CAPD and AD/HD, Chermak, Tucker, and Seikel, (2002) questioned a group of audiologists and pediatricians to determine those symptoms endorsed by audiologists as belonging to CAPD, distinct from those attributed to AD/HD as determined by pediatricians. They concluded based on symptoms and conceptual distinctions, that they are two distinct entities. The differences cited were that for AD/HD-I pediatricians marked inattentiveness and academic difficulties as 2 SD above the mean whereas audiologists for (C)APD ranked poor listening skills and asking for repetition 2 SD above the mean. Six of the 15 behaviors that were ranked were common to both groups, and 9 were different (Chermak et al., 2002). Similarities included academic difficulties, distraction, poor listening skills, asking for things to be repeated, auditory divided attention deficit, and difficulty hearing noise. Ultimately, the respondents saw similarities, but the prominence was different, in that the children with AD/HD clearly had the behavioral manifestations whereas the CAPD children had the auditory manifestations. The difference in the use of medication and behavioral management thereby served to separate the two groups.

Results indicated that, in spite of marked differences in pediatricians' and audiologists' rankings (100 in each group), there was considerable overlap across the disorders. The reasoning presented for the differences was due to the different sources at the root of similar behaviors, that is, for AD/HD-inattentive, cognitive disorders involve disorganization and executive function, whereas in (C)APD, the difficulties stem from a perceptual disorder causing deficits in processing information through the auditory channel. One can conceptualize differences between (C)APD and AD/HD as presented in Table 2–1.

Differences between (C)APD and AD/HD can be further delineated as cited in the literature by Chermak and Musiek (1997); Chermak, Hall, and Musiek (1999); and Geffner, (2005) as presented in Table 2–2.

When McFarland and Cacace (2003) re-examined the total data of Chermak et al. (2002), they, to the contrary, found similarities and overlap. They pointed out that Chermak et al. (2002) dealt with conceptual overlap and did not address the diagnostic overlap issue. Because there is no set agreement

Table 2–1. When Is It (C)APD or AD/HD?

CAPD	AD/HD
Difficulty hearing in background noise	Inattentive
Difficulty following directions	Distracted
Poor listening skills	Hyperactive
Academic difficulties	Fidgety/restless
Poor auditory association	Hasty/impulsive
Input disorder	Interruptive/intrusive
Executive function disorder is secondary	Output disorder
Mishears words	Blurts out answers
Attention deficits are secondary	Management includes meds
Top-down processing	Bottom-up processing

Table 2–2. Differences Between AD/HD and CAPD

AD/HD	CAPD
Prevalence is 5–10% in school-age population	Prevalence 2–3%, as much as 20%
2–4% prevalence in adult	Prevalence in older adults 10–20%; 70% in over 60 year olds
4:1 male-female ratio	2:1 male-female ratio
Must be manifested in at least two settings	Measured by a battery of standardized audiological tests administered under acoustically controlled environment
Output disorder	Input disorder
Must be present before the age of 7	Should evaluate following auditory maturation at age 7
Attention deficits are primary and global	Executive dysfunction is secondary source of listening problems
Selective attention	Attention deficits are secondary to auditory perceptual deficits
Executive dysfunction	Difficulty organizing, monitoring, and understanding acoustic signals
Excessive talking, interruptive, poor topic maintenance	Receptive language problems and word-retrieval problems
Difficulty producing coherent extended discourse	Difficulty with metacognitive language
Diagnosis is based on observational criteria	Difficulty organizing thoughts
Defined as a cluster of behaviors	Based on a series of audiologic tests
Management includes medication	Management includes signal enhancement, modification of environment
Executive control strategy training	Executive strategies/Learning strategies
Social-pragmatic skills training	May need social skills training
Contingency management system	
learning strategies	

about the conceptualization of either (C)APD and AD/HD, the difference remains questionable. If a CAPD is diagnosed based on performance on an auditory stimuli test, then underlying mechanisms are not addressed. Historically, the definition has been based on auditory behaviors and performance on auditory-specific tests, rather than on auditory perceptual processes. According to Cacace and McFarland (2006), defining CAPD in terms of whatever the specific auditory tests measure does not provide a definition that can be usefully generalized to practical situations. As there is a recognized overlap of CAPD and knowing that AD/HD is a "polysensory" dysfunction in the frontal cortex and basal ganglia, given the localization that is shared, it is hard to argue that AD/HD is specific to encoding information in the auditory sensory modality. Thus, it is not yet clear what the perceptual and construct validity of CAPD is in children with learning and behavioral problems. To resolve this issue, tests specific to AD/HD and not sensitive to other comorbid disorders need to be developed (Cacace & McFarland, 2006).

How Does a Child with CAPD Behave in the Classroom?

It is generally understood that children diagnosed with CAPD are at risk for attentional, memory, language, and learning disabilities which will affect his or her ability to perform in the classroom.

There are general red flags that alert a teacher to the possibility that a child has a CAPD. As a result of these comorbidities, there is often frustration and low self-esteem. It is not unlikely that the child will have difficulty making friends and sustaining friendships. Depending upon the child's level of language sophistication, the understanding of nuance, tone of voice, and nonverbal cuing reduce his or her ability to be accepted by the peer group. Parents frequently report that the child is unable to get the message, or participate with his or her peers, as he or she misses the joke or the pun. The child may experience inconsistent ability to perform tasks, or feel fatigued after a day of "heavy listening." The child will experience difficulties with comprehension, especially if the aural information is presented in less than ideal acoustic conditions. Noisy classrooms, filled with too many children, in a room that is not insulated from outside noise or interferences are deadly grounds for such children. They will be easily distracted, miss the main message, and do the wrong assignment for which they will be penalized. Many of these children fail to ask for help or repetition for fear that everyone will think they are "stupid." They fail to "self-advocate," that is, to ask for clarification and reduced speed of speaking. Often, if the teacher is a rapid talker, it will be difficult to understand him or her. Pausing is needed and time for breaks from listening to digest the information presented auditorily are necessary for this child.

Teachers need to be sensitive to the child's weaknesses and realize that repetition and, better yet, clarification are needed. The child is often too fearful to ask the teacher to repeat. The teacher is often the first person to pick up on the child's deficiencies. He or she plays an essential role in getting the child evaluated and altering the listening environment in the classroom to accommodate the child's needs.

What Are the RED FLAGS?

- *A child who is doing poorly in reading and writing, spelling*

- *A child who does not pay attention or is daydreaming during class*
- *A child who is having problems learning a foreign language*
- *A child who can learn through the auditory channel but does better with visual stimuli*
- *A child who cannot write from dictation*
- *A child who "mishears" words*
- *A child who doesn't participate in class discussions*
- *A child who misunderstood homework assignments or fails to follow directions*
- *A child who cannot tolerate a noisy room or who is fidgety in loud/noisy places such as the cafeteria, gym, playground.*
- *A child who has trouble understanding stories read aloud.*
- *A child who takes notes that are cryptic and insignificant.*
- *A child who does not get the salient points or relevant facts*
- *A child who has trouble depicting directions that are embedded in other information*
- *A child who has trouble with math word problems*
- *A child who appears to have a latency of response or a delayed response to a question*

There are other symptoms, but these are the most common. The reader is cautioned about selecting only those children at risk. It is important to be vigilant for older students who may have done well academically in earlier grades, but with the increase in workload, these deficits begin to surface more readily. It is usually by third grade that such children become more apparent. What is most unfortunate is the report of an unsuspecting teacher that presumes the student is not trying hard enough or is just "lazy."

Here again, the child who is struggling to follow directions and pass a spelling test may also be experiencing a learning disability and/or an attention deficit hyperactivity disorder. There are often multiple neurosensory factors interacting.

It is not too early to identify preschoolers who may be at risk for a CAPD. In fact, were there to be a measure for early identification, these children stand the best chance of remediation given their neuroplastic auditory systems.

Early Childhood Indicators

The "at risk" behaviors for young children include poor rhyming skills, or inability to follow songs and melodies, inattention to the speaker or ignoring the speaker when engaged in other activities, sensitivity to sound or noise, and difficulty with complex directions. There are language indicators as well such as difficulty formulating a sentence, searching for words, and trouble remembering simple commands. Their inability to exercise good pragmatic skills is often a predictor of later language and social problems. Their inability to rhyme or match sounds to letters is a precursor to a reading disability. Thus, early signs are useful for identification and remediation.

Formal testing for CAPD has been suggested at age 7 because of neuromaturational development of the auditory system. However, with test norms available for younger children (i.e., SSW, Katz, 1986; CID Auditory Test W-22, Katz, 1997; SCAN-C, Keith, 2000; Phonemic Synthesis Picture Test, Katz, 2000; CTOPP, Wagner, Torgesen, &

Rashotte, 1999; SAAT, Cherry, 1980), these youngsters can at least be identified as being "at risk" for an auditory processing disorder and be eligible for Response to Intervention (RTI). Surely in the hands of an audiologist trained to deliver and interpret the test battery, results will be favorable for identifying these children for early intervention. According to the ASHA Scope of Practice (ASHA, 2004), the audiologist is and should be responsible for testing and diagnosing (CAPD). The speech-language pathologist has a role to play in identification, screening, and treatment (ASHA, Scope of Practice, 2001). With a team of professionals, young children can receive early input and training to reduce the impact of an auditory processing disorder.

For these children, modifications and management are needed. Curriculum needs to be modified, pacing of the teacher's speech may be necessary, along with breaks, and other accommodations such as reduced speed, supplemental notes, and directions read and repeated. Future chapters address these suggestions and modifications.

Causes and Predisposing Factors

It is generally accepted that certain predisposing factors contribute to CAPD, such as chronic otitis media, inheritable factors, auditory neuropathy, and environmental influences. An early history of chronic otitis media with effusion (OME) is associated with higher incidence of learning disabilities, language deficits, and attention disorders (Haggard & Hughes, 1991).

Chronic suppurative otitis media is an inflammation of the middle ear accompanied by pus that persists for more than 3 months. The child who has experienced recurrent ear infections along with persistent middle ear effusion appears to be at greatest risk. The research suggests that the severe otitis population is more apt to have language and learning problems by school age. In a study involving children with AD/HD (Hagerman & Falkenstein, 1987) 94% of children diagnosed with AD/HD and medicated with psychostimulants experienced three or more episodes of chronic otitis media and 69% had more than 10 episodes of chronic otitis media. Fifty percent of children who experienced school failure but were not hyperactive had three or more episodes.

Darling and Sedgwick (2003) found a correlation between otitis media and subsequent auditory difficulties (APD). However, many factors contributed to the extent of the auditory deficit. The study compared 20 individuals with normal hearing and no history of OM and 20 individuals (ages 18–30) with normal hearing and a self-proclaimed childhood history of recurrent OM. The SCAN-A (Keith, 1994), Test for Auditory Processing Disorders in Adolescents and Adults, was used to obtain the data. The results of the total test standard score of the SCAN-A suggested that adults with childhood history of OM had a higher incidence of signs of (C)APD than individuals with no significant childhood history of OM. These adults had more difficulty with auditory closure, listening in the presence of background noise, and with binaural integration tasks. Keller (1998) found an increased incidence of otitis media in children with (C)APD, resulting in frequent absences from school, leaving them to play "catch-up" in their academic work. Other researchers found children having difficulty extracting signals from background noise even with normal postoperative hearing sensitivity (Bellis, 2003; Pillsbury, Grose, & Hall, 1991). Possible explanations were that there was abnormal development of brainstem auditory structures responsible for binaural processing, inadequate mapping of stimulus, or an inability of the CANS to process cues for signal detection, or extract the signal from the noise.

Children with a history of OME have been shown to have abnormally reduced masking level differences (MLDs) with such a reduction continuing even after tube placement. This results in reduced ability to extract signals from noise. MLD is the perception of signals in noise. When the phase of the marker is changed in relation to the signal phase, it is easier to detect the signal than when they are both in phase (Rawool, 2006). Auditory brainstem interwave intervals were found to be abnormal in the ear with the OME suggesting a physiologic impact on the auditory system resulting from early deprivation. The MLD at 500 Hz was reduced as compared to adults, increasing as a function of age. Pillsbury, Grose, and Hall (1991) found children with a history of OME demonstrated reduced MLDs and greater variability than did the control children. The MLD abnormality continued to be present in 64% of the children even after insertion of pressure equalization tubes (PE tubes).

Hall, Grose, and Pillsbury (1995) studied the long-term effects of OME on MLD performance longitudinally and found abnormalities in MLD continued up to 2 years following medical intervention. Even 2 years postsurgery, some children continued to have reduced MLDs. Their results suggested that there was a slow recovery of binaural function over a long period of time in children with a history of OME. Other studies reveal degradation of localization skills and lateralization abilities (Hausler, Colburn, & Marr, 1983), and abnormalities in binaural processing even when hearing returns to normal thresholds.

In a study by Keogh et al.(2005) conducted in Australia, groups of 484 school-age children with and without a history of OM were compared in their ability to understand everyday speech in noise, using the Queensland Understanding of Everyday Speech Test (UQUEST). Children selected were native to Australia, English-speaking with normal hearing and no reported physical or behavioral impairments. There were three groups selected according to number of episodes of OM since birth, Group 1 had fewer than 4 episodes and served as the control; Group 2 (MILD) had 4 to 9 episodes; and Group 3 (moderate-severe) had 10 or more. Results showed no significant differences in mean speech scores across the grades and noise conditions. The children with a history of OM performed equally well when compared to controls, but exhibited a large range of abilities in speech comprehension. The mean scores for the three groups for the more difficult noise condition were poorer than for the easier noise condition. Although their scores were similar across the noise conditions, it was postulated that it might have been the level at which the speech words were presented that obviated the difference. When a lower presentation level was used, children with a history of OM performed significantly worse than their OM-free counterparts. The individual differences noted were ascertained to be due to the fact that some individuals are more affected by OM than others, either due to their early occurrence, extended duration, or recurrent nature of the disease (Gravel & Ellis, 1995). Thus, children as a group may perform as well as OM-free children in speech understanding, but some children may experience great difficulty, particularly when the noise condition worsens. The younger children seemed to perform more poorly, which may suggest that as children age, they are better able to adapt.

Other studies of children with OM indicate impairments in phonological skills (Rubin et al., 1997).

- Children with history of OM fail to follow instructions or comprehend conversations (Haggard & Smith, 1997).
- There is a body of research to support the concept that children with a history of early otitis media demonstrate auditory processing deficits in receiving information in background competition, as well as demonstrate behavioral, attentional, and learning challenges in the classroom (Gravel & Wallace, 1992, 1995).
- It is generally understood that children with a history of otitis media with effusion may exhibit long-term difficulty with binaural interaction, localization, speech in noise clarity. and comprehension, possibly due to the sensory deprivation that results from the long-standing condition that compromises the conductive system from transmitting sound accurately to the upper auditory pathways.
- Reorganization has been observed in auditory brainstem structures following auditory deprivation (Gabriele et al., 2000), resulting in neurochemical and structural changes. Furthermore, deprivation beyond the developmental years can have an impact on the brainstem auditory processing.
- It is theorized that auditory deprivation from OME can result in morphologic changes within the central auditory nervous system (CANS), leaving a compromised auditory processing ability. The corollary is true in that stimulation of the auditory system can result in improved auditory processing abilities. Stimulation and experience activates and strengthens the auditory pathways, whereas those pathways that are unstimulated atrophy (Aoki & Siekeitz, 1988).

Other predisposing factors or causes remain unresolved, but CAPD has been associated with other impairments such as Alzheimer's disease, learning disabilities, multiple sclerosis, traumatic brain injury, and psychiatric disorders (Chermak & Musiek, 1997). Those with known lesions or pathologies of the central nervous system pathways, such as aphasia and TBI, or with neuromaturational or neuromorphological disorders are more susceptible, such as children with developmental language delays, dyslexia, and learning disabilities. The majority of pediatric CAPD, according to Musiek et al. (1990) is probably a result of a neuromorphological disorder and to a lesser extent due to a maturational delay, or neurological disorder (Musiek et al., 1985). Recent research supports the presence of heterectopias in the left temporal lobe in Heschl's gyrus and the planum temporale that are viewed under contrast spectrography. Further interhemispheric connectivity via the corpus callosum may be impaired due to loss of fibers (Bellis, 2003). For a review of comorbidities, the reader is referred to Chapter 3.

Summary

This chapter focused on the definition and variations of definitions as proposed and accepted by different professional organizations. Central Auditory Processing (CAP) refers to the perceptual processing of auditory information in the central nervous system and the neurobiological activity that underlies that processing and gives rise to electrophysiologic auditory potentials. The various behaviors associated with auditory processing were delineated. Operative definitions and symptomatology associated with (central) auditory processing disorders were provided as they present themselves in the classroom and in other environments. Red flags for the classroom teacher were listed to enable the teacher to identify those youngsters at risk for CAPD. The difference and similarities between CAPD and AD/HD along with other comorbid conditions were highlighted. The controversy surrounding the operative definition of CAPD was discussed presenting the views of Cacace and McFarland against those of Musiek, Chermak, and Jerger. The causative factors reduced to relational predisposing factors include otitis media with effusion, neuromaturational delay, and neurological disorders of the central auditory nervous system. Other conditions such as learning disabilities, cognitive, and neurological disorders often co-occur. However, even though these conditions may coexist, they are not the result of CAPD, nor are children with autism or with spoken language disorders the result of having a deficit in the central auditory nervous system, but rather possess a more global, higher function disorder. The effect of chronic otitis media and data supporting the deprivation effect on the auditory processing mechanism were presented. Greater explanations of comorbid conditions are presented in future chapters.

Key Points Learned

- The definition according to the ASHA Technical Report states that CAPD refers to the efficiency and effectiveness by which the central auditory nervous system utilizes auditory information (ASHA, 2005).

- There are a number of behaviors that encompass auditory processing: sound localization and lateralization, auditory discrimination, auditory pattern recognition, temporal aspects of audition (temporal integration, temporal discrimination, temporal ordering, temporal masking), auditory performance in competing acoustic conditions, auditory performance with degraded acoustic signals (ASHA, 1996, 2005).
- CAPD is a deficit in neural processing of auditory stimuli that is not due to higher order language, cognitive or related factors, but can lead to language, learning, and communication difficulties.
- CAPD can coexist with other disorders such as AD/HD, learning disabilities and language impairment.
- Key behaviors that are seen in youngsters with CAPD include: trouble following directions, trouble listening in the background of noise, or trouble filling in the missing sounds, sensitivity to loud sounds, trouble locating the source of sound, asking"what?"or huh?, mishearing words or misinterpreting messages, delayed responding to an oral question.
- The predisposing factors for CAPD include otitis media with effusion, neuromaturational delay, neurological insult to the central auditory nervous system, and any pathology that could affect the central auditory nervous system. CAPD and AD/HD share similar behaviors but CAPD is sensory specific and AD/HD is behavioral in nature affecting self regulation and executive functions. Chronic otitis media with effusion can lead to deprivation causing decreased ability to discriminate sounds in the background of noise, to localize sounds, and perform auditory/listening tasks in the classroom. Children with a history of long standing otitis media in early childhood are at risk for having CAPD.
- Because of the multimodality nature of processing in the CNS, the construct of CAPD as a modality-specific function is neurophysiologically unsound. Rather, individuals with CPD exhibit sensory processing deficits that are more pronounced in the auditory modality, but not necessarily exclusive to it.

References

American Psychiatric Association. (1994). *Diagnostic and Statistical Manual of Mental Disorders, 4th edition (DSM-IV).* Washington, DC: Author..

American Speech-Language-Hearing Association. (1996). *Central auditory processing: Task Force on Central Auditory Processing Consensus Development.* Rockville, MD: Author.

American Speech-Language-Hearing Association. (2001). *Scope of practice in speech-language pathology.* Rockville, MD: Author.

American Speech-Language-Hearing Association. (2004). *Scope of practice in audiology.* Rockville, MD: Author.

American Speech-Language Hearing Association. (2005). *(Central) auditory processing disorders, Technical report: Working Group on Auditory Processing Disorders.* Rockville, MD: Author.

Aoki, C., & Siekevitz, P. (1988). Plasticity in brain development. *Scientific American, 259,* 56–64.

Barkley, R. (1997) Behavioral inhibition, sustained attention, and executive functions: Constructing a unifying theory of ADHD. *Psychological Bulletin, 121,* 65–94.

Bellis, T. J. (2003). *Assessment and management of central auditory processing disorders in the educational setting: From science to practice* (2nd ed.). Clifton Park, NY: Delmar Learning.

Cacace, A. T., & McFarland, D. J. (1995). Modality specificity as a criterion for diagnosing central auditory processing disorders. *American Journal of Audiology, 4,* 36–48

Cacace, A. T., & McFarland, D. J. (1998). Central auditory processing disorder in school-aged children: A critical review. *Journal of Speech, Language, and Hearing Research, 41,* 355–373.

Cacace, A. T., & McFarland, D. J. (2006). Delineating auditory processing disorder (APD) and attention-deficit hyperactivity disorder (AD/HD): A conceptual, theoretical, and practical framework. In T. K. Parthasarathy (Ed.), *An introduction to auditory processing disorders in children* (pp. 39–61). Mahwah, NJ: Lawrence Erlbaum Associates.

Chermak, G. D., Hall, J. W., & Musiek, F. E. (1999). Differential diagnosis and management of central auditory processing disorders and attention deficit hyperactivity disorder. *Journal of the American Academy of Audiology, 10*(6), 289–303.

Chermak, G. D., & Musiek, F. E. (1997). *Central auditory processing disorders: New perspectives.* San Diego, CA: Singular Publishing Group.

Chermak, G. D., & Musiek, F. E. (2002). Auditory training: Principles and approaches for remediating and managing auditory processing disorders. *Seminars in Hearing, 23*(4), 297–308.

Chermak, G. D., Tucker, E., & Seikel, J. A. (2002). Behavioral characteristics of auditory processing disorder and attention-deficit hyperactivity disorder: Predominantly inattentive type. *Journal of the American Academy of Audiology, 13,* 332–338.

Cherry, R. (1980). *Selective Auditory Attention Test.* St. Louis, MO: Auditec of St. Louis.

Conners, C. K. (1995). *Conners' Continuous Performance Test.* North Tonawanda, NY: Multi-Health Systems.

Darling, R. M., & Sedgwick, R. M. (2003, April). *Signs of auditory processing disorders in adults with a childhood history of otitis media.* Paper presented at the annual; meeting of the American Academy of Audiology, San Antonio, TX.

DiMaggio, C., & Geffner, D. (2003). *Prevalence of AD/HD, speech and language delay, reading difficulties and familial factors associated with CAPD in children.* Paper presented at the annual convention of the American Academy of Audiology, Salt Lake City, UT.

Gabriele, M. L., Brunso-Bechtold, J. K., & Henkel, C. K. (2000). Plasticity in the development of afferent patterns in the inferior colliculus of the rat after unilateral cochlear ablation. *Journal of Neuroscience, 21*, 6939–6949.

Geffner, D. (2005). *Attention-deficit/hyperactivity disorder: What professionals need to know.* Eau Claire, WI: Thinking Publications.

Geffner, D., Lucker, J., & Koch, W. (1996) Evaluation and auditory discrimination in children with ADD and without ADD. *Child Psychiatry and Human Development, 26*(3), 169–180.

Gravel, J. S., & Ellis, M. A. (1995). The auditory consequences of otitis media: The audiogram and beyond. *Seminars in Hearing, 16*, 44–59.

Gravel, J. S., & Wallace, I. F. (1992). Listening and language at four years of age: Effects of early otitis media. *Journal of Speech and Hearing Research, 35*, 588–595.

Gravel, J. S., & Wallace, I. F. (1995). Early otitis media, auditory abilities, and educational risk. *American Journal of Speech-Language Pathology, 4*(3), 89–94.

Haggard, M. P., & Hughes, E. A. (1991). *Screening children's hearing: A review of the literature and implications of otitis media.* London: HMSO.

Haggard, M. P., & Smith, S. C. (1997). *Correlated improvements in subjective and objective outcomes in otitis media with effusion.* Paper presented at the Third Extraordinary Symposium on Recent Advances in Otitis Media, Copenhagen, Denmark.

Haggerman, R. J., & Falkenstien, A. R. (1987). An association between recurrent otitis media and later hyperactivity. *Clinical Pediatrics, 26*, 253–257.

Hall, J. W., Grose, J. H., & Pillsbury, H. C. (1995). Predicting binaural hearing after stapedectomy from pre-surgery results. *Archives of Otolaryngology-Head and Neck Surgery, 116*, 946–950.

Hausler, R., Colburn, H. S., & Marr, E. (1983). Sound localization in subjects with impaired hearing. *Acta Otolaryngology* (Suppl. 400), Monograph.

Jerger, J., & Musiek, F. (2000). Report of the consensus conference on the diagnosis of auditory processing disorders in school-aged children. *Journal of the American Academy of Audiology, 11*, 467–474.

Kaas, J. H., & Hackett, T. A. (2000). Subdivisions of auditory cortex and processing streams in primates. *Proceedings of the National Academy of Sciences, 97*, 11793–11799.

Katz, J. (1986). *The Staggered Spondaic Word Test.* Vancouver, WA: Precision Acoustics.

Katz, J. (1997). *CID Auditory Test W-22.* Vancouver, WA: Precision Acoustics.

Katz, J. (2000). *Phonemic Synthesis Picture Test.* Vancouver, WA: Precision Acoustics.

Katz, J. (2005, May). *Central auditory processing disorders: Identification and management.* Presentation to the Long Island Hearing Council at St. John's University, Queens, NY.

Keith, R. W. (1994). *SCAN-A: A Test for Auditory Processing Disorders in Adolescents and Adults.* San Antonio, TX: The Psychological Corporation.

Keith, R. W. (2000). *SCAN-C: Test for Auditory Processing Disorders in Children.* San Antonio, TX: The Psychological Corporation.

Keller, W. D. (1998). The relationship between attention deficit hyperactivity disorder, central auditory processing disorders, and specific learning disability. In M. G. Masters, N. A. Stecker, & J. Katz. (Eds.), *Central auditory processing disorder: Mostly management* (pp. 33–48). Boston: Allyn & Bacon.

Keogh, T., Kei, J., Driscoll, C., Cahill, L., Hoffman, A., Wilce, E., Kondamuri, P., & Marinac, J. (2005). Measuring the ability of school children with a history of otitis media to understand everyday speech. *Journal of the American Academy of Audiology, 16*, 301–311.

Lasky, E., & Katz, J. (1983). *Central auditory processing disorders: Problems of speech, language, and learning.* University Park, MD: University Park Press.

Lucker, J., Geffner, D., & Koch, W. (1996). Perception of loudness in children with

ADD and without ADD. *Child Psychiatry and Human Development* 26(3), 181–190.

Masters, M., Stecker, N., & Katz, J. (1998). *Central auditory processing disorders: Mostly management*. Boston: Allyn & Bacon.

McCarney, S. B. (1995). *Attention Deficit Disorders Evaluation Scale* (2nd ed.). Columbia, MI: Hawthorne Educational Services.

McFarland, D. J., & Cacace, A. T. (2003). Potential problems in the differential diagnosis of (central) auditory processing disorder (CAPD or APD) and attention-deficit hyperactivity disorder. *Audiology, 36*, 249–260.

Musiek, F. E., Baran, J. A., & Pinheiro, M. L. (1990). Duration pattern recognition in normal subjects and in patients with cerebral and cochlear lesions. *Audiology, 29*, 304–313.

Musiek, F. E., Gollegly, K., Kibbe, K., & Reeves, A. (1985). Electrophysiologic and behavioral auditory findings in multiple sclerosis. *American Journal of Otology, 10*, 343–350.

Pillsbury, H. C., Grose, J. H., & Hall, J. W. (1991). Otitis media with effusion in children. *Archives of Otolaryngology, 6*, 90–119.

Rawool, V. W. (2006). A temporal processing primer, Part 1: Defining key concepts in temporal processing. *Hearing Review, 16*, 30–34.

Rubin, R. J., Wallace, I. F., & Gravel, J. S. (1997). Long term communication deficiencies in children with otitis media during their first year of life. *Acta Otolaryngology, 117*, 206–207.

Sanford, J. A., & Turner, A. (1995). *Intermediate Visual and Auditory Continuous Performance Test*. Richmond, VA: BrainTrain.

Wagner, R. Torgesen, J., & Rashotte, C. (1999). *Comprehensive Test of Phonological Processing*. Austin, TX: Pro-Ed.

Warren, J. D., & Griffiths, T. D. (2003). Distinct mechanisms for processing spatial sequences and pitch sequences in the human brain. *Journal of Neuroscience, 23*, 5799–5804.

Resources

http://www.add.org—National Attention Deficit Disorder (ADDA)

http://www.chadd.org—Children and Adults with AD/HD

http://www.interdys.org—The International Dyslexia Association

http://www.ldaamerica.org—Learning Disabilities Association of America

http://www.ncapd.org—National Coalition on Auditory Processing Disorders, Inc.

Special Education, Disability, Health Issues

http://www.aap.org—American Academy of Pediatrics

http://www.aacap.org—American Academy of Child and Adult Psychiatry

http://www.healthlaw.org—National Health Law Program

http://www.dssc.org/frc—Federal Resource Center for Special Education

http://www.ldonline.org—Learning Disabilities Online

http://www.cec.sped.org—Council for Exceptional Children

http://www.nasponline.org—National Association of School Psychologists

http://www.dredf.org—Disability Rights Education Defense Fund http://www.copaa.net—Council of Parent Attorneys and Advocates

http://www.protectionandadvo cacy.com—National Association of Protection and Advocacy

http://www.nichcy.org—National Information Clearing House on Children and Youth

http://www.specialeducationmuck-raker.com—Dee Alpert, Publisher

http://www.wrightslaw.com—Web site of Peter W. D. Wright and Pamela Darr Wright dedicated to special education legislation and law.

http://www.webmd.com—WebMD and WebMD Health

http://www.ericec.org—ERIC Clearinghouse on Disabilities and Gifted Children

ADHD Support and Advocacy Groups

American Academy of Audiology
11730 Plaza America Drive,
Suite 300
Reston, VA 20190
Phone: 800-AAA-2336;
703-790-8466
Web site: http://www.audiology.org

American Academy of Pediatrics
141 Northeast Point Boulevard
Elk Grove Village, IL 60007-1098
Phone: 847-434-4000
Fax: 847-343-8000
Web site: http://www.aap.org

American Speech-Language-Hearing Association
10801 Rockville Pike
Rockville, MD 20852
Phone : 800-638-8255
Web site: http://actioncenter@asha.org
http://www.asha.org

American Psychiatric Association
1000 Wilson Boulevard, Suite 1825
Arlington, VA. 22209-3901
Phone: 703-907-7300
Web sites: http://apa@psych.org
http://www.psych.org

American Psychological Association
750 First Street NE
Washington, DC 20002-4242
Phone: 800-374-2721; 202-336-5500.
TDD/TTY: 202-336-6123
Web site: http://www.apa.org

Attention Deficit Disorders Association (ADDA)
P.O. Box 543
Pottstown, PA 19464
Phone: 484-945-2101
Fax: 610-970-7520
E-mail: mail@add.org
Web site: http://www.add.org

Attention Deficit Disorders Association of Parents and Professionals Together (ADDAPPT)
P.O. Box 293
Oak Forest, IL 60452
Phone : 708-614-7012
E-mail: president@adappt.org
Website: http://www.adappt.org

Children and Adults with Attention Deficit Disorder (CHADD)
National Headquarters
8181 Professional Place, Suite 201
Landover, MD 20785
Phone: 301-306-7070; 800-233-4050
Web site: http://national@chadd.org
http://www.chadd.org

Council for Exceptional Children
1110 North Glebe Road,
Suite 300
Arlington, VA 22201-5704

Phone: 888-232-7733; 703-620-3660
TDD/TTY: 866-915-5000
Fax: 703-264-9494
Web site: http://www.cec.sped.org

International Dyslexia Association, Inc.
40 York Road, 4th floor
Baltimore, MD 21204
Phone: 410-296-0232; 800-ABCD-123
Fax: 410-321-5069
Web site: http://www.interdys.org

Learning Disabilities Association of America
4156 Library Road
Pittsburg, PA 15234
Phone: 412-341-1515
Fax: 412-344-0224
Web site: http://www.ldanatl.org

National Information Center for Handicapped Children and Youth
New center called the National Dissemination Center for Children with Disabilities
P.O. Box 1492
Washington, DC 20013
Phone & TTD/TTY: 703-893-6061; 800-695-0285
Fax: 202-884-8441
E-mail: nichcy@aed.org
Web site: http://www.nichcy.org

3

Comorbidity of APD with Other "Look-Alikes"

Patricia McAleer Hamaguchi
Yvette N. Tazeau

Overview

The processing of spoken language requires the auditory and linguistic system to function within a complex framework of cognition, attention, and motivation. When there is a breakdown within any of these associated systems, the result can often mimic the outward appearance of an Auditory Processing Disorder (APD). Likewise, the child with deficits in these areas *may* have APD. APD can also sometimes be a comorbid condition in those with neurobiological disorders, an umbrella term which refers to organic brain disorders that result in deficits affecting the thought process, emotions, or relating (Batshaw, 2002). Regarding terminology, readers will see the terms neurobiological, neuropsychiatric, and neurodevelopmental in related texts and scientific articles. Current knowledge about psychiatric conditions with neurological correlates affirms a biological basis, hence the term neurobiological and, when established in early childhood, a developmental trajectory is anticipated (e.g., Asperger's Disorder).

Psychiatric conditions with neurological correlates affect one in every five children in the United States (U.S. Public Health Service, 2000). This chapter reviews select disorders including Attention-Deficit/Hyperactivity Disorders (ADHDs),

Learning Disabilities including Reading and Written Expression Disorders, as well as Nonverbal Learning Disorder (NVLD), neurobiological disorders such as anxiety disorders (including Selective Mutism and Obsessive-Compulsive Disorder/OCD) and depressive disorders such as Depression and Bipolar Disorder, as well as Tourette's Disorder, Asperger's Disorder, and Sensory Integration Dysfunction (SID).

Making matters even more complex, APD can also co-occur with these disorders, making the process of identifying APD all the more difficult, especially when a client has an involved clinical history and presentation. For a recent review of the relationship of general communication disorders to neurobiological disorders see Hamaguchi (2006), "Neurobiological Disorders: Information for the SLP & Audiologist." Our goal for this chapter is to provide practical information, useful to practitioners in differentiating APD from the "look-alikes."

Introduction

As medical professionals often say, "When you hear hoof-beats, you can't just think of horses." This axiom needs to hold true for the professions of speech and language and audiology as well. Of course, we have all had the term "differential diagnosis" drummed into our heads since graduate school. Intellectually, we know that we need to do more than administer standardized tests, score them, and make recommendations. We know how important it is to look at the "whole" person and carefully put the diagnostic pieces together. Why is this child having difficulty communicating? Listening? Following directions? Looking confused or disinterested during conversations?

Attention Deficit Hyperactivity Disorders (ADHDs)

Like many disorders, attention-deficit/hyperactivity disorder (ADHD) is a syndrome, that is, a cluster of symptoms. ADHD is not one condition, but actually can be of three different types: Predominantly Inattentive, Predominantly Hyperactive-Impulsive, and Combined Type; the latter is a combination of the first two types. Children who have ADHD can be inattentive, hyperactive, and impulsive. In order to be properly diagnosed as having ADHD, children (before the age of 7) must demonstrate symptoms at a level of causing impairment in two or more settings (e.g., at home and at school).

The cognitive skills generally associated with the frontal lobe of the brain are the skills for which individuals with ADHD usually have deficits and are known as executive function skills. Executive function skills include attention (including divided attention), concentration, memory, information processing, reasoning, problem solving, tracking abilities, set shifting, initiation, planning, and insight (Lezak, Howieson, & Loring, 2004).

The proper diagnosis of ADHD is still a complex task in that many of the inappropriate behaviors observed also can be representative of other emotional or physical illnesses (Barkley, 2000; Root & Resnick, 2003). Recognizing this challenge for a proper diagnosis, the American Academy of Pediatrics (2000) has stipulated that pediatricians use behavior rating scales to help determine the presence of symptoms in more than just one setting (i.e., the home, school, or clinician's office). In the case of ADHD, and in order to avoid a potential misdiagnosis, here the adage might well be, "When you hear hoofbeats don't necessarily think it's zebras, it might well be only horses!"

Features of ADHD to Consider When Testing for APD

From outward appearances, someone with an ADHD condition may appear to be quite similar to another with APD. To complicate matters, those with ADHDs including inattentive, hyperactive, and combined forms, may have a coexisting APD (Geffner, 2005; Riccio, 2005). Great care must be given during the assessment process to ensure that the child's difficulty in responding to auditory stimuli is not strictly due to inattention. Keep in mind the following confounding issues for those individuals with ADHD.

Attending Issues

Individuals with ADHD have difficulty attending not only to auditory tasks, but to any structured task that requires prolonged and sustained attention, such as completing a worksheet or homework (video games and TV seem to be an exception to this rule, however). The neural processing of incoming auditory information of the central nervous system does not seem to be affected. With the individuals with ADHD, there is a systemic and physiological difficulty with attention, whereas with APD it is a deficit of the auditory pathway itself. A child with only an auditory processing disorder typically should attend normally to visual or hands-on tasks, such as worksheets, presuming the content is at the child's academic level. Therefore, if one of the primary, presenting complaints is that the child "doesn't get homework done," it would not support a suspicion of APD unless the homework is related to specific deficits (e.g., phonemic awareness) that are associated with APD. It is more likely that the child is having difficulty physically sitting down, getting organized, and keeping his or her mind on the task at hand. If the clinician suspects a pervasive problem with attending, a referral for an attention-deficit/hyperactivity Disorders assessment should be made before finalizing an APD diagnosis.

For individuals with APD, we would expect to see a decrease in attending during auditory-only activities, such as a lecture in the classroom. We often see a marked decrease in attending when the auditory modality is overloaded and fatigued, typically after a high-demand listening task. Many individuals report a gradual diminishment in auditory focus as the morning turns into the afternoon.

Ritalin Will Help Individuals With ADHD, But Not APD

A double-blind, placebo controlled study with a large group of children with both APD and ADHD (Tillery, Katz, & Keller, 2000) found there was notable improvement in auditory attention (as tested by Keith's Auditory Continuous Performance Test) when children took their routine dosage of Ritalin, but not for performance on APD assessment measures. Therefore, whenever possible, it is recommended that children with ADHD take their medication before the administration of the test battery because we know that inattention can have a negative impact on any kind of standardized testing that requires sustained focus.

Interrupting Behaviors

A child with ADHD may frequently interrupt the test prompts with comments, observations, and an inability to sufficiently attend to the testing task. The clinician should note these qualitative observations when determining whether the child's performance is in fact an "input" disorder of the auditory channel, difficulty focusing on the auditory stimuli, or in some cases, both. We would not expect to see interrupting behaviors as a feature of APD.

Overattention and "Mis-attention" Issues

It is often thought that one of the primary distinguishing features of ADHD is the lack of an "attending filter," which means individuals with ADHD give equal importance to all incoming stimuli: visual, auditory, and tactile. The weakness in the executive function system results in difficulty tuning in to just one thing, so students attend to the chirping bird outside the window with the same degree of attention as to the teacher speaking in the classroom. Individuals with ADHD may attend to the wrong things or irrelevant stimuli, such as the pattern on their shirt or a scab on their forearm. In these cases, this "mis-attention" is to the exclusion of things to which they should be attending.

Those with APD also may have difficulty "hearing" with background noise, but it is due to a deficit in the auditory pathways and a function of the acoustic environment. They don't turn their attention to the background noise, such as the child with ADHD, but it adds further distortion and impedes the acoustic signal that may be already compromised. The linguistic content they extract from the acoustic signal can be confusing for them, and so there is less payoff for them to "tune in."

Patterns of Performance on Standardized APD Tests

Typically, a child who presents with an ADHD diagnosis and who does not have APD should perform within normal limits on all audiological tests. Tests that require sustained attention, such as the Auditory Continuous Performance Test, may likely be poorer. However, when the ADHD disorder is not medicated and yet is severe enough, it is possible that one might find abnormal scores across the board on all testing tasks, whether auditory in nature or not, simply because the child is not able to sustain attention on these kinds of tasks. In the case of a child with an APD, we would expect to find some variability between subtests and some predictable strengths and weaknesses, depending on the nature of the presenting complaints. One would not expect to see depressed scores across the board on all testing tasks.

Case Study

"Carlos," 8 years old, was brought for a comprehensive assessment for APD. He was a third-generation Mexican-American boy whose family had only spoken English for the past two generations. His mother reported that he had difficulty "following conversations" and "following directions." Although he was bright, it took extraordinary measures to get him to complete written tasks at school or at home. He would often forget what to do and struggled to follow along with the teacher's lectures. His classroom teacher suspected a possible auditory processing disorder since another child she had in class with APD seemed quite similar.

During the speech-language assessment and the audiological assessment, Carlos was quite animated. He was obviously bright and had much to say about the things he saw in the office, as well as anecdotes he shared that popped into his mind during testing tasks. This would cause Carlos to focus more on what he was thinking about than to attend to the question he had just heard. After he finished interrupting, he would forget the test question. Because, technically, the testing stimuli could not be repeated, Carlos' scores were fairly low on many of the auditory-language tests, including serial memory tasks and auditory comprehension of directions and stories. His ability to sequence and retell stories with age-appropriate cohesion and reference points was weak. On the audiology assessment, Carlos' scores ranged from low-average to above-average on all the subtests, but no scores were in the disordered range.

Carlos presented with fairly typical behaviors and test results for a child with ADHD, not APD. His spelling difficulties were related to his visual memory and not a function of auditory discrimination deficits. His distractibility was not limited to auditory tasks, but across the board and during all tasks that required sustained attention, including homework and worksheets at school. Carlos' weak performance during the story-retelling tasks pointed to a fairly predictable difficulty with sequencing and organization, often associated with poor executive function. Carlos was referred to an ADHD specialist who worked with the classroom teacher so that the tasks and teaching methods were more appropriate for Carlos, including giving him fewer (but well-chosen) written tasks, task organizers, walk-around breaks, and cues to help him stay on task.

Learning Disabilities

The learning disabilities selected for review in this chapter as "look-alikes" include Reading Disorder, Disorder of Written Expression, and Nonverbal Learning Disorder (NVLD). Public Law 108-446, the Individuals with Disabilities Education Improvement Act of 2004, states that a "specific learning disability means a disorder in one or more of the basic psychological processes involved in understanding or in using language, spoken or written, which disorder may manifest itself in the imperfect ability to listen, think, read, write, spell, or do mathematical calculators" (*Federal Register*, December 3, 2004).

Assessed through psychoeducational or neuropsychological testing (Braaten & Felopulos, 2004), specific learning disabilities of Reading Disorder, Disorder of Written Expression, and Mathematics Disorder can be evaluated. Woodrich and Schmitt (2006) include these disorders, along with specific language impairments, as information-processing-related conditions.

Researchers dating back to the 1960s began to identify the deficits that characterize Nonverbal Learning Disorder/NVLD (Stewart, 2002). Although not a formally recognized diagnosis by the American Psychiatric Association, NVLD is often diagnosed as a Learning Disorder Not Otherwise Specified.

Reading and Written Language Disorders

In the case of reading disorders, marked impairment is observed in the development of word recognition and reading comprehension (Feifer & De Fina, 2000). Omissions, distortions, and substitutions of words are characteristic of the oral reading of individuals diagnosed with a Reading Disorder. Regarding writing disorders, there is marked impairment in the ability to compose written texts often characterized by spelling errors, grammatical or punctuation errors within sentences, or poor paragraph organization (Feifer & De Fina, 2002).

Features of Reading and Written Language Disorders to Consider When Testing for APD

A comprehensive assessment for auditory processing disorders should note the client's reading (decoding, as well as comprehension) and writing skills. As described in Chapter 9 (Auditory Processing Versus Literacy), certain reading and spelling error patterns are associated with APD, but weak reading and writing skills are not, in and of themselves, a necessary feature of an APD. Due to space constraints, the following are but a few of the error patterns that one can expect to uncover during the assessment process. Clinicians are urged to become more familiar with reading and written language disorders by further research and reading (Ciocci, 2002; King, 2003). The following are symptoms that often mimic those caused by an APD:

Decoding Error Pattern

George thought about taking the bus to Philadelphia. When 10-year-old Sue read that sentence, this is how it sounded, "Ge-or-gee th-ou-guh-ht abo-utt tacking the boos to puh-hill-a-delp-hi-a." Her painstaking production made it nearly impossible for her to blend the words or even monitor her productions to see if they made sense in that context. She was simply just trying to "get through it." However, Sue is doing a good job matching the letters she is reading to their corresponding phonetic sound. She is also doing well to sequence the sounds in the same order as the words on the page. But Sue is still "reading" sound-by-sound and not visually recognizing regular and irregular spelling patterns.

At her age, these common words ("thought") and spelling patterns ("taking" instead of "tacking," "bus" instead of "boos") should be read as a whole and not require a sound-by-sound breakdown, as one would expect to see in a new reader. This kind of error pattern would be indicative of a weakness in this skill, which directly correlates to slow reading fluency. When reading decoding is this poor, it nearly always compromises reading comprehension, especially if auditory closure is poor. When the decoding demands are reduced by dropping down to a simpler reading level, there should be a simultaneous increase in reading comprehension because Sue would be able to focus more on the content than on the process itself. Because she is struggling to blend sounds, this error pattern should alert the clinician to examine Sue's phonemic awareness, specifically in the area of sound blending. Can Sue auditorily blend a series of sounds ('c-a-t') and recognize it as a word ("cat")? If Sue is presenting with other behaviors that are associated with APD, additional testing for APD should be administered to rule out APD.

George thought about taking the bus to Philadelphia. When 10-year-old Anna read the same sentence, quite fluently, it was heard as: "Judge though abbot taking the bus to Philadelphia." In fact, she didn't even pause for the period that followed the sentence and continued to move through the rest of the story in a similar vein, with little intonation or reaction to the other punctuation. Anna's errors show us that she is not processing what she is reading, and certainly not visualizing the words themselves. She is adding and taking away letters. The words are a meaningless string of letters on a page, connected to no real thoughts. Because of this, she is unaware of her decoding errors, and thus, makes no attempt to trouble-shoot a production that doesn't make sense in that context.

Anna is demonstrating a poor use of metacognitive skills, as she is somewhat passive in the reading process and is not attempting to extract any meaning from it. Likewise, her difficulty with prosodic perception in reading may be rooted in poor temporal patterning (both humming and labeling of pitch/duration) and should be ruled out. Since Anna is not visualizing what she is reading, it also would be helpful to assess how well she comprehends (and visualizes) when the information is read to her. A treatment program for Anna would need to address metacognition, visualization, and spelling pattern recognition.

Spelling Error Patterns

"tome iz a ruf kat but I lik im," translated, this means, "Tommy is a rough cat, but I like him." Looking closely at what is written, one can see that the letters written on the page are actually quite phonetic. In this particular case, the child is hearing the correct sequence of sounds, matching the phonetic sounds to the letters that represent them, and marking word boundaries correctly. In an older child, this error pattern would suggest difficulty with visual memory for sight words and irregular spelling patterns. In a kindergarten or first grade child, writing phonetically is sometimes referred to as "invented spelling," and would be a normal first step in the writing process.

"Temeen as ravgat bat I luk hem." Translated, this also means, "Tommy is a rough cat, but I like him." Although this spelling pattern may be within normal limits for a child in kindergarten, by second and third grade this sample would be of concern. Spelling errors of this nature, which persist beyond the early primary years, may be due to an underlying weakness in auditory discrimination. We often find there is difficulty "hearing" vowel sounds as well as word boundaries, which may be indicative of weak phonemic awareness and metalinguistic skills. Does the child have difficulty with interhemispheric tasks, which might explain difficulty with sound-symbol association skills? This kind of a spelling pattern would raise a concern that there is an underlying auditory disorder that may be contributing to these difficulties and should be further investigated.

Reading Comprehension Error Patterns

In the decoding section above, we met "Anna" who was reading, but not making any connection to what the words meant, substituting words with similar phonemic shapes, and fluently reading along but with no sense of what she was reading. This problem is even more apparent when children substitute nonsense words for real words and don't pause to consider the fact that what they are reading makes no sense. In this case, we would not be surprised to find that Anna's reading comprehension scores were very low. She is not visualizing or processing what she reads.

From a differential diagnosis perspective, it would be helpful to see how Anna performs when the information is read to her. Does she have a global difficulty comprehending language or is it limited to the written form only? Are there auditory closure weaknesses that make it difficult for her to "fill-in-the-blank" with words that would make sense in that context? From a metacognitive point of view, why isn't Anna stopping and questioning herself when it is apparent that the sentence doesn't make sense?

Another type of common reading comprehension problem is found specifically in those children who are beginning readers or are poor decoders. They pour their mental energy into the decoding process and struggle to "multitask" by decoding and processing the meaning of the words at the same time. In these cases, one might find that if the passages are read to the child, their comprehension scores will fall into the normal or higher range. Therefore, by improving the decoding fluency, one would expect the reading comprehension score to improve accordingly.

For some children, the "gestalt" of a reading passage is easy to ascertain. They understand the key points and the main idea, but when queried, forget little details, such as characters' names or which day an event took place. In this case, it may be helpful to do testing in the area of auditory memory. If there are associated deficits in this area, teaching the child to use metamemory and key-word strategies may improve this weakness.

As children move into the upper elementary school years, we often find a group of children who decode quite fluently, and who previously scored within the normal limits on reading comprehension tests. However, at this level, the demands of the written material require a deeper analysis of the author's intent, symbolism, idiomatic language, sarcasm, perspective-taking, interpretation, dialogue written in local dialect, higher level vocabulary, and more. It requires more than a regurgitation of facts, which can be easily culled from scanning back into the story. Those with underlying weak language or cognitive foundations often will find this level of comprehension particularly challenging. They may need to reread passages before they can really understand it or they miss the point of the passage entirely. However, if we find a pattern of right-hemisphere weaknesses, (left-ear deficits, poor temporal patterning performance, etc.) we may find associated auditory deficits as well.

There is another group of children who are proficient decoders and can even retell the events of a given passage, with accuracy. Their comments and observations about the story tell us they are certainly visualizing what they read and are processing it. However, when asked higher level questions ("How would you compare the way the mother reacted to the crisis to the way the father reacted?"), their responses are off the mark ("I think the mother was really angry.") Close, but not correct. In these cases, the underlying issue is often a result of difficulty with question interpretation and/or difficulty with the expressive language skills that are needed to adequately answer them. It is important for the clinician to determine whether the weakness is in the content, question format, expressive language requirement, or a combination.

Written Language Error Patterns

> "Frank," said his mother, "was tall."
>
> Frank said his mother was tall.
>
> Frank said, "His mother was tall!"

Each of these three sentences contains the same words, but with the proper punctuation, the meaning of each changes. To read and write them correctly, one must not only understand the written punctuation marks, but also "hear" the pauses and intonation patterns in the spoken sentences. For students who struggle with this, on an audiological assessment, the pitch-pattern test may reflect difficulty with prosody comprehension.

Children who consistently report they "can't hear" the difference between a question and statement and thus misuse the punctuation marks for these, should also have audiological tests that target right-hemisphere dysfunction included in their battery.

Case Study

"Brian," a 9-year-old boy, was brought for a speech-language-auditory skills assessment due to concerns about a possible auditory processing disorder. As a young child, Brian had frequent ear infections and allergies. He had some mild articulation delays, which at this point had been resolved. He had been identified as having a learning disability by his school's IEP team but his parents felt there might be an underlying auditory issue that was further impacting him. Brian's primary symptoms were difficulty with "hearing" how words were put together, which resulted in very poor word attack skills. In addition, his punctuation, spelling, and grammar skills were poor. Brian could not discriminate between similar sounding vowels (e.g., short *e, i, u*) and even some consonants (e.g., *f/th, m/n/*) and so it was very difficult to solidify a consistent letter-sound relationship. Brian had a core of sight words he had memorized. In this case, there were no associated concerns about Brian's comprehension and use of language, auditory memory, or vocabulary and his scores in those areas were at or above average.

The audiological assessment showed low-average to normal scores across the board, revealing no significant deficits in any area. However, on the speech-language assessment, Brian's scores on all phonemic awareness tasks, including phoneme segmentation and auditory discrimination, were significantly below average.

A plan was put into place which included a systematic approach to learning how phonemes were formed and ordered within words. Auditory discrimination training helped facilitate improved letter-sound learning and carried over into decoding and encoding tasks. Brian's teacher sought to enhance the signal-to-noise ratio so Brian could hear the acoustic features of the phonemes with increased accuracy. The speech-language pathologist and the resource teacher put greater emphasis on phonemic awareness, helping Brian to isolate initial, final, and medial sounds, find rhyming patterns, and identify the number of phonemes and syllables within a word. Lastly, phonemic synthesis training helped Brian learn to segment and synthesize phonemes auditorily, which laid the foundation for him to carry this over into his reading and spelling. Just 3 months after an intensive program was initiated, Brian began to learn to read!

Nonverbal Learning Disorder (NVLD)

Individuals with Nonverbal Learning Disorder (NVLD) have higher functioning for language tasks and comparatively lower functioning for visual-perceptual tasks. When assessed with standardized psychological tests of intellectual functioning, they often demonstrate a statistically significant difference between their verbal and visual-spatial skills. Educational testing of these students often highlights difficulties for mathematics. These children also have difficulty reading social situations, tend to be solitary, are anxious in social situations, try to avoid situations that produce anxiety, and have a poor sense of time. Among the areas of difficulties, they struggle to send or receive nonverbal cues, "dyssemia," which is an area often targeted for treatment (Nowicki & Duke, 1992). Children with NVLD also have poor initiative, poor self-organization, poor follow-through, and their speed for writing can be slow. They can appear attention disordered, experience difficulty dealing with novel or complex situations (adaptability), can appear impulsive, have difficulty in using information to self-correct their own behavior, and may present with some oppositionality.

According to the work of Rourke (1989), children with NVLD have many auditory strengths including perception, attention, and memory. Other neuropsychological assets include good verbal reception, repetition, storage, associations, output (volume), and good phonology. However, areas of difficulty often include oral-motor praxis and the suprasegmental and pragmatic aspects of language function: interpreting the nuances of prosody, facial affect, humor, nonliteral language, and the use of gestures. Therefore, although accompanying verbal directions with gestures may ordinarily increase the likelihood of a message being processed in a typical child, for these children, it adds another layer of confusion. Because their visual-perceptual skills are often weak, there are some who believe this weakness can contribute to a diminished ability to conceptualize more complex oral and written language structures with adequate speed and accuracy. That is, while rote auditory information is easily repeated back, the weak visualizing component may interfere with the content being processed. Additionally, these children often "miss the point" of a conversation due to their overattention to unimportant details. It is no wonder that children with NVLD are often referred for an auditory processing disorder assessment.

Neurobiological Disorders

The National Institute of Mental Health (NIMH) deemed the 1990s the "Decade of the Brain" ushering in a programmatic effort to fund the study of the human brain. Much of the research from that effort has gone a long way toward confirming the biological and neurological bases of psychiatric conditions that we know as neurobiological/neurodevelopmental disorders. Codified for identification in the *Diagnostic and Statistical Manual of Mental Disorders, Fourth Edition, Text Revision* (DSM-IV-TR: American Psychiatric Association, 2000) there are literally hundreds of disorders. This chapter focuses on a select group of these disorders chosen, in part, for their developmental presence in early childhood.

Anxiety Disorders, Including Selective Mutism, and Obsessive-Compulsive Disorder (OCD)

Conditions within the realm of anxiety disorders include Generalized Anxiety Disorders (GAD), Panic Disorder, specific phobias, Obsessive-Compulsive Disorder (OCD), Social Phobia, Separation Anxiety Disorder, Selective Mutism, Acute Stress Disorder, and Posttraumatic Stress Disorder (PTSD). Relevant to all these conditions is the basic sensation of apprehension felt by the client.

Sometimes the source of the apprehension is not readily known but in other cases it can be related to actual threats or merely perceived threats.

Anxiety is known to be partially inherited. Beyond inheritance, the factors that can contribute to anxiety in children include stressful life events, family interaction patterns, and child-rearing practices (Rapee, Spence, Cobham, & Wignall, 2000). Selective Mutism is a phobia-based condition and is characterized by a fear of being heard in select situations such as public ones (McHolm, Cunningham, & Vanier, 2005). For children, this usually means fear of speaking at school. Obsessive-Compulsive Disorder (OCD) is typified by repetitive, intrusive thoughts, images, or impulses (obsessions). The repetitive behaviors or mental activities (compulsions) used are to lessen the anxiety, distress, and tension often associated with obsessions (Chansky, 2000).

Depression and Bipolar Disorder

Depression falls along a continuum and the disorders include Dysthymic Disorder and Major Depressive Disorder. These mood disorders are characterized by sad feelings, a lack of interest and/or pleasure in activities, low energy, changes in eating and sleeping patterns, problems for concentration and thinking, and in some cases thoughts of death and dying (Barnard, 2003; McClure, Kubiszyn, & Kaslow, 2002). Although we think of a withdrawal from life's activities when adults are depressed, children who are depressed can also appear as agitated, irritable, and aggressive.

Bipolar Disorder is another mood disorder with several criteria sets for diagnosis; however, the common feature to all six of the different types is manic symptoms. Severe mood fluctuations in a given day or over many days, uncontrolled outbursts, reckless behavior, pressured speech, racing thoughts, and even psychotic symptoms such as delusions and hallucinations can characterize the condition (Birmaher, 2004).

Tourette's Disorder

Tourette's Disorder (also known as Tourette Syndrome or "TS") is a tic disorder. A tic is a sudden, rapid, recurrent, nonrhythmic, stereotyped motor movement or vocalization. Tourette's Disorder involves multiple motor tics and one or more vocal tics (Brill, 2002). A motor tic can be eye-blinking, squinting, nose twitches, tongue protrusion, shoulder shrugging, arm jerking, leg kicking, and abdominal contractions. A vocal tic can include sniffing, snorting, throat clearing, coughing, and gulping. Tics can be complex. Examples of complex motor tics include smelling and licking things, touching parts of body, and abnormalities of gait. Examples of complex vocal tics include whistling, making animal sounds, and belching.

Psychotherapeutic Treatment

Treatment for the neurobiological/neuropsychiatric disorders identified in childhood includes an evaluation as to the suitability for use of a psychotropic medication. Given their specialized training, child psychiatrists are often in the best position to determine if a child can tolerate a stimulant, antidepress-sant, antianxiety, antipsychotic, mood stabilizing, or other psychotropic medication for management of symptoms. Child psychiatrists play a key role in administering appropriate psychotropic medications for children, in monitoring for side effects, and making adjustments to dosage, time of administration, use of certain types/classes of drugs, and trying other brands when necessary.

As summarized in a recent overview (Tazeau, 2006), the role of psychotropics notwithstanding, research points to the efficacy of the *combination* of psychotropic medication and psychotherapeutic treatments for common psychological problems including anxiety disorders such as school refusal, panic disorders, Selective Mutism, phobias, OCD; depressive disorders, impulse control disorders such as tics, Tourette's, trichotillomania (hair-pulling); interpersonal problems, social problems, and health and pain management conditions. Particularly strong is the research indicating the efficacy of psychotropic medication and Cognitive-Behavioral Therapy (CBT) for both anxiety and mood disorders (Antonuccio, Danton, & DeNelsky, 1995; Compton, McKnight, & March, 2004; Friedman et al., 2004). CBT and the closely related Habit Reversal Therapy (HRT) for impulse and tic disorders are evidence-based, clinical treatment interventions (Christophersen & Mortweet, 2001). CBT is a cohesive, rational intervention that focuses on the relationship between what the child thinks (cognitions), what the child feels (emotions), and what the child does (behaviors). As a scientifically testable model, CBT provides both the rationale for the therapeutic intervention and determines the focus and nature of the treatment.

Cognitive-Behavioral Therapy is objective and structured and, as a process, begins with an assessment, then problem formulation, followed by intervention, monitoring, and evaluation of progress. It is time limited in that it usually requires 15 to 20 weekly sessions (at a rate of one visit per week, it is approximately a 4- to 5-month commitment). Its "here-and-now" focus on current problems and difficulties emphasizes the creation and implementation of adaptive ways of coping. CBT is a skills-based approach by which the child learns problem-solving and alternative patterns of thinking and behavior (Stallard, 2002). It is a brief therapy model which fosters independence in children in that they learn skills, strategies, and techniques to make them self-sufficient to cope with their conditions. The child is encouraged to actively question and challenge some of his or her assumptions and beliefs about the psychiatric condition and associated behaviors and to experiment with the skills, strategies, and techniques taught by the clinician and "coached" at home by his or her parents. CBT is based on a collaborative model wherein the psychotherapist partners with the child, and caregivers also help form the team. When working with children, the team can and should include other professionals such as classroom teachers, daycare providers, physicians such as psychiatrists and pediatricians, and other treating clinicians such as speech and language therapists, occupational therapists, educational therapists, and so forth.

CBT is a treatment approach also favored by many clinicians who work with children and families from ethnically and racially diverse backgrounds (Organista, Chun, & Marin, 1998). Studies of ethnic/racial minority groups in the United States, such as African-Americans, Asians, and Hispanics, highlight their sociocultural values of interdependence and collectivism and focus on activities and relationships. CBT's team approach for children and use of activities and tasks to practice outside the psychotherapy session resonate with participants. For many recent immigrants and/or low-income groups who face "survival" situations, CBT is most relevant because of its short-term, directive, problem-solving style (Satterfield, 2002).

CBT-based techniques are many and a CBT approach for any given neuropsychiatric condition can include: thought monitoring, identification of cognitive/thinking distortions, learning new cognitive skills, monitoring and managing feelings and emotional reactions, role playing, role modeling, rehearsal, reinforcement and reward schedules, home-based assignments and tasks, relaxation techniques such as controlled, deep breathing, imagining calming pictures/imagery, and muscle relaxation, graduated exposure and shaping (i.e., step-by-step and hierarchical mastery), response prevention, flooding, systematic desensitization, contingency management, and relapse prevention.

When properly adapted for the child's chronological, mental, and developmental ages and when other caregivers are incorporated as "coaches" in the treatment planning and intervention, CBT is a powerful tool for children and their families and an empowering source of control for children whose lives are affected by neuropsychiatric disorders. Resources for clinicians and families regarding the select disorders described in this chapter include Web sites listed at the end of this chapter as well as the books listed in the References section of this chapter.

Features of Neurobiological Disorders to Consider When Testing for APD

Presently, there are no statistics or research to document the percentage of those who have both neurobiological and Auditory Processing Disorders. Literature on these disorders frequently cite comorbidity (Riccio, 2005), but the authors are typically medical professionals or psychologists who may place all spoken language processing weaknesses into the category of "Auditory Processing Disorders." That said, clinical experience, an understanding of the underlying physiology, and anecdotal reports do make one suspect that this population is particularly susceptible to having a greater than normal incidence of APD.

Neurobiological disorders can be present in someone with an accompanying speech, language, or auditory disorder, or it can merely mimic one. It therefore becomes imperative that we as clinicians become skilled in recognizing these symptoms and make the necessary referral to the professionals who can best treat them. The following are features that often mimic those caused by an APD.

Slow Rise Time

A slow "rise" time (response time) to auditory input is associated with a variety of neurobiological disorders. There are many causes, including preoccupation with other internal or external conflicts, medications that globally "dull" the speed of cognition, and associated attention span and executive function disorders.

Difficulty Following Directions

For those with anxiety disorders, other fear/worry thoughts may so overwhelm the person that he or she cannot focus on what is being said. There may be a continual inner dialogue that literally crowds out the ability to receive or process any complex incoming verbal stimuli. (What if I have to go to the bathroom? Who is that other person in the room? Will they be able to hear my answers? What if I get it wrong?) Or the individual gets so bogged down with their fear of making a mistake that they simply don't attempt the task or respond (avoiding raising their hand in school or will say, "I don't know" even if they do know the answer). This can often create a diagnostic dilemma because, with this population, we may not be sure that the responses we receive on standardized tests are, in fact, reliable, particularly if the disorder is exacerbated by the testing process itself. Children may continually ask, "Was that right?" They become so consumed with their performance that they may be off-task during the presentation of the next test prompt and unable to process the stimulus.

Children with OCD may have trouble following directions for other reasons. They may not be acting out of fear (as does the anxious child) but out of a deep need for rules, routines, consistency, "fairness," and not wanting to make mistakes. If the instruction requires them to do something they would ordinarily not do, such as hanging their coat in a different spot, sitting somewhere else, crossing out an error to edit it, lining up out of the usual order, and so forth, it can be so discomforting that the child may not be able to bring him- or herself to do it. When substitute teachers or modified school days require changes in routine, the child may be very irritable and upset for what seems no apparent reason.

When someone with OCD is mentally perseverating on something such as needing to count to 100, not stepping on cracks, or repeating the words to the Pledge of Allegiance over and over in his or her mind, they may not be able to process what is being heard until the "required" OCD task is completed (although some people have an uncanny ability to do both!). You can sometimes see the person's mouth slightly moving, even though no sound is heard, particularly if the child is aware of the inappropriateness of saying something aloud. Trying to follow directions while performing obsessive rituals is extremely difficult to do.

In addition, the child with OCD may also struggle with things that seem "dirty" or "germy" such as using a public restroom or doing arts and crafts projects that require getting his or her hands dirty. Even though they know what to do, they may not be able to follow the direction. This issue is not due to a difficulty with comprehension, despite their reluctance or resistance in completing the required action.

Those with Tourette's Disorder may be asked to do certain things, such as refrain from making noises, saying repetitive phrases, or touching certain things. Although they may wish to comply with these directions, their disorder may, in fact, make that nearly impossible. What further complicates the picture is that, at times, there is a brief amount of time under which the behaviors can be controlled, leading teachers or adults to draw the erroneous conclusion that the behaviors are able to be controlled for longer periods of time.

Difficulty Processing Spoken/Written Language

People who are preoccupied with fears or worries (anxiety disorders) or obsessions and/or compulsions (OCD) may have difficulty attending to, and processing, what they read or hear during an acute episode, which can last for minutes, days, or longer. There is often an accompanying, perseverative internal dialogue that loops inside the person's mind, crowding out incoming messages and causing difficulty attending to any other complex linguistic input. The fluctuating nature of these disorders requires serious detective work, as their performance is quite variable according to the situation, person, and place. It is particularly tricky to determine this in younger children who are not yet able to articulate what is happening inside their mind. We also often see this phenomenon in those with Pervasive Developmental Disorders (e.g., autism).

For this reason, a low score on a receptive language standardized test may or may not be reliable if the child's responses are impacted by an acute exacerbation of these underlying disorders. In other words, the question we may be asking might be, "Tell me how a cow and a horse are the same or different" but the child may be literally "listening" to perseverative internal thoughts at the same time. A poor verbal response may have nothing to do with the child's lack of knowledge of the salient features of a cow and horse, but a reflection of the struggle to tune out their inner competing thoughts, whether it is of an anxious or obsessive nature.

Interrupting behaviors, that is, "cutting-off" the other speaker before the message has even been received, is characteristic of those with ADHD, anxiety, and Asperger's Disorder, as well as those in the manic phase of a bipolar episode. For these people, the thoughts keep flowing and it is difficult for them to suppress the thoughts, or even process what someone else is saying.

When in the midst of an acute depressive episode, all cognitive tasks are slowed down. Processing spoken or written language is often painstaking and confusing. In teasing out whether or not the presenting complaints are due to a depressive component, it is important to note the onset of the presenting symptoms. Since we expect processing disorders to be somewhat constant throughout childhood, a referral for APD testing in an adolescent who is only recently coping with these issues should raise a very big red flag.

Individuals with Tourette's Disorder may be attempting to suppress tics, particularly in a situation out of their ordinary comfort zone, such as in a formal testing situation, with an unfamiliar clinician. Their performance may vary greatly from day to day and situation to situation. By expending mental concentration on suppressing the tics, it may be difficult for them to completely tune in to any higher level linguistic tasks, and therefore the reliability of standardized scores should be carefully considered.

Lastly, many individuals with neurobiological disorders may be taking one or more psychotropic medications to control their symptoms. Often, these medications can have a sedative effect, sometimes directly correlated to the time of day during which they are taken (Wilens, 2001). The resulting "sluggishness" can often mimic symptoms of APD. The person may use coping strategies by saying, "What?" in order to hear the auditory input again and buy a little more time; however, this is not due to a deficit in the auditory pathways.

Case Study

"Thuy," age 12, was a second-generation Vietnamese-American girl who grew up speaking only English. She was brought for a speech-language assessment by her mother to determine if the problems she was having were due to an underlying auditory processing disorder or perhaps a receptive language disorder. The main concerns described by her mother, as well as her teacher, were difficulties with "following directions" and "following conversations." She was already diagnosed with ADHD and had a history of speech-language delay as a preschooler. She was described as being "difficult" in terms of her behavior. At times, she was impulsive and would repeatedly do something (e.g., hit the wall while walking down a corridor) even though she was expressly forbidden to do so. She often said and did "odd" things around her peers, or simply became withdrawn.

It was suggested to her mother by a friend that perhaps intense auditory therapy might help alleviate some of these issues. It was also suggested by other professionals (including the family physician) that perhaps she was somewhere on the autism spectrum, and this might explain her perseverative behaviors and, at times, her repetitive use of certain words and phrases, often blurted out of any appropriate context (e.g., "Pirate Patch on the job! Pirate Patch on the job!"). This was an easy conclusion to draw, since she also had a history of hyperacusis and other sensory issues, including tactile and smell hypersensitivities, as well as some weak social skills. Thuy was reported to have allergies, as she tended to clear her throat frequently and snort and sniff throughout the day. Prior to being examined by an audiologist, it was felt that getting a thorough speech-language-auditory evaluation would help determine if there were associated auditory and language deficits.

Thuy had been receiving speech-language services by a school-based SLP, as well as a private SLP. When her mother was asked about the child's treatment for ADHD, she said that Thuy had taken Ritalin for about 3 months but it was stopped when she developed rather obvious facial tics and blinking. The mother was asked if she had ever noticed the tics before and she said the tics did happen from time to time, but it was "nonstop" once she was taking the psychostimulant, Ritalin. The medication also seemed to make her "allergies" much worse. (Note to reader:

The use of stimulants, such as Ritalin, can greatly exacerbate an underlying Tourette's Disorder condition, which can manifest itself as blinking, facial tics, as well as throat clearing, snorting, and sniffing and which are often mistaken for allergies.)

Thuy was given a standard speech-language-auditory assessment. She had some weakness in the auditory memory of serial words, and difficulty with using language during narrative tasks. Her sequencing, cohesion, and word retrieval seemed weak during open-ended language tasks, but not so much as to be considered "disordered." At times, she appeared to present with a "cluttering" style of speech delivery—somewhat staccato, lots of stops and starts, whole-word repetitions, and fast overall rate. Yet, her ability to follow oral directions, as well as listen to stories, answer questions, and participate in a typical conversation, were all fine. Reading and spelling were above age level. Receptive vocabulary was at the 91st percentile on the Peabody Picture Vocabulary Test III. She denied having difficulty "hearing" the teacher, and her phonemic awareness skills were superb.

Thuy was always moving, so her eye contact was not as strong as that of a typical child, but she did "check in" with the examiner from time to time through eye contact. Her affect and prosody were fairly typical. She laughed at the examiner's jokes and even made some, too. She had friends and liked to do things that girls her age like to do. These strengths did not seem to fit the autism spectrum diagnosis that was being considered. Her performance on this assessment also did not point to an auditory processing disorder, and subsequent testing by an audiologist supported this fact.

Thuy spoke about school and was asked about how she follows directions at school. She described how much she wanted to be a "good girl" and how hard she tries, but how difficult it is for her. She was asked about why she had been merely sitting there lately, not writing anything, when the teacher had already asked her to do the first two rows on a math page. After some hemming and hawing, she shared that she had lost her green pencil and she simply could *not* write with the yellow one that the teacher had given her. As it was already suspected that Tourette's Disorder may be playing a role and knowing that there is a high correlation between Tourette's Disorder and OCD, this explanation of an OCD behavior was not too hard to believe. Thuy's mother was apprised of Thuy's concerns and, for diagnostic purposes, several green pencils were provided to Thuy to use at school to see if the problem of "difficulty following directions" would improve with the introduction of the green pencil. It did, instantly!

A discussion ensued about the issues surrounding her difficulties for "following directions" in the hallway (obsession to hit each brick on the wall going to the bathroom) and how distracted she apparently was in the afternoon. She said she could not bring herself to use the public bathroom, because she had seen a spider on the floor once. By midafternoon, she was absolutely restless and not able to think of anything else except keeping herself from wetting her pants. The dilemma was solved by having Thuy use the bathroom in the nurse's office, which was sparkling clean.

When Thuy was trying to suppress other tics, such as saying socially inappropriate things, it made it very difficult for her to focus on what her communicative partner was saying. The squirming and stress made it nearly impossible for her to stay still and maintain eye contact. Once she began a new psychotropic medication regimen and Cognitive-Behavioral Therapy (CBT), she was able to put more mental energy into what was happening around her and less energy into suppressing her urges, tics, and obsessions. About 4 to 6 months after beginning these treatments, Thuy's difficulties with following directions, participating in conversations, and "inappropriate behavior" were all significantly improved.

Asperger's Disorder

Asperger's Disorder is classified as a Pervasive Developmental Disorder (PDD) according to the psychiatric coding of diagnoses (DSM-IV-TR: American Psychiatric Association, 2000). In contrast to children with other PDDs (e.g., Autistic Disorder), those diagnosed with Asperger's Disorder do not demonstrate significant delays for aspects of language such as language acquisition and spontaneous language. However, they do have similar challenges for reciprocal social interaction and demonstrate patterns of restricted interests and repetitive behaviors.

The term "High-Functioning Autism" is often referenced in the same breath with Asperger's Disorder, and is frequently a source of confusion for parents of newly diagnosed children (Ozonoff, Dawson, & McPartland, 2002). "High-Functioning Autism" is not a formal, clinical diagnosis, rather it is a phrase for describing children who are formally diagnosed with Autistic Disorder but who represent the 30% or so who do not have Intelligence Quotient (IQ) scores in the Mental Retardation range (i.e., 70 or below). Treatment options for those with Asperger's Disorder vary by the child's age and severity of symptoms (Ozonoff, Dawson, & McPartland, 2002).

Those diagnosed with Asperger's Disorder develop an expanse of receptive and expressive language; however, their ability to use it appropriately within the context of reciprocal social interactions is often limited. Despite the sheer volume of language output, they struggle with reading nonverbal cues, comprehending humor, and nonliteral language. Their prosody is often flat or atypical. Although often thought of as being "peculiar" or eccentric, those with Asperger's Disorder sometimes are quite gifted, and although awkward, generally do seek social interaction.

Children with Asperger's Disorder will sometimes describe auditory sensitivities (e.g., a ticking clock) that become so bothersome that they are not able to attend to more important stimuli, such as someone talking. (See Sensory Integration Dysfunction below.) It is easy to see how this, coupled with other suprasegmental processing deficits, could mimic the symptoms of an auditory processing deficit.

Sensory Integration Dysfunction

Sensory integration is the organizing of the senses for functional use (Ayres,

2000). A child's basic awareness of his or her body and the surrounding world is integration. The senses must work together and for most children this happens naturally. Information from the visual, auditory, tactile (touch), vestibular (movement sense), and proprioceptive (muscle and joint) systems must all come together to help a child learn to perform common tasks such as sitting, jumping rope, balancing, paying attention in class, copying an assignment, or reading a book. Dysfunction in sensory integration is when the information from the senses gets jumbled, lost, or processed incorrectly (Kranowitz, 1998).

As we have said about the other disorders in this chapter, the differential diagnosis for Sensory Integration Dysfunction (SID) can be difficult. Children with dysfunction in the sensory system can appear hyperactive or with low energy, have poor attention spans, and have difficulty with fine and/or gross motor function (Smith & Gouze, 2004). Children faced with the challenges of sensory problems can become tense, unhappy, or act out inappropriately. Solutions for children with sensory processing problems are outlined by the specialty of occupational therapy.

Although often first identified by school psychologists or clinical neuropsychologists, Sensory Integration Dysfunction is typically best confirmed through an occupational therapist (OT). The auditory features of this disorder are identified by the OT through anecdotal report, including behaviors such as:

- Hypo- or hypersensitivity to loud or unexpected noises
- Difficulty tuning in to auditory stimuli
- Holding hands over ears to show discomfort with auditory input.

Although these symptoms are categorized as auditory in nature, the OT does not conduct actual audiological testing to determine the etiology of the behaviors. It is felt that the auditory sensory issues are a part of a larger constellation of sensory symptoms that make up the features of a child with SID. The role of hyperacusis, discomfort with certain environmental sounds or overreaction to sudden or loud sounds, in the diagnosis of APD is not clear. Although hyperacusis is often associated with individuals on the spectrum of Pervasive Developmental Disorders (e.g., autism), there is sometimes a report by the client or parent of fairly extreme reactions to sounds of everyday objects by those with APD, too. Aside from anecdotal report, we presently have no objective way of measuring how hypo- or hypersensitive a child's reaction to auditory input may be except through audiometric threshold levels which fall below average or 0 dB HL.

The occupational therapist seeks to stimulate the inner ear and auditory sensory input through activities that stimulate the vestibular system (such as with swinging) and the cochlea. They may sometimes suggest auditory integration training (AIT) programs, including commercially produced CDs with acoustically enhanced or modified music. The efficacy of these programs remains unclear, with most pre-post comparisons consisting of anecdotal listings of a wide range of symptoms and the parent/client's perceived changes in those areas.

The American Speech-Language-Hearing Association (2004) has issued a position on auditory integration training that cites a lack of empirical evidence on its efficacy and advises its members to refrain from recommending or administering AIT until such time that the clinical benefit of such can be better documented through peer-reviewed research. However, there continues to be a group of practitioners in the speech-audiology field who advocate for the inclusion of therapeutic listening programs, such as Tomatis, as part of a comprehensive APD intervention program. As of this writing, additional research is expected to become available that may offer another perspective on this intervention and its application within the APD population. The American Speech-Language-Hearing Association supports further research in this area. Perhaps its position would be reconsidered should the data support its efficacy.

Overlapping Conditions

The comorbidity of these select disorders, Attention-Deficit/Hyperactivity Disorders (ADHDs), learning disabilities (including Non-Verbal Learning Disorder/NVLD), and Asperger's Disorder is substantial (Kutscher, 2005). For example, 30 to 70% of children and adolescents with anxiety disorders have a depressive disorder and up to 25% can meet criteria for ADHD. In Tourette's Disorder, multiple tics are frequently found together with other problems such as ADHD, OCD, bipolar disorder, and schizophrenia. Other disorders that often occur with Pervasive Developmental Disorders (e.g., Asperger's Disorder) include anxiety disorders, ADHD, depression, and Tourette's Disorder. Up to a quarter of children with ADHD have associated mood symptoms, another quarter have an associated anxiety disorder, and up to 40% have learning disabilities (Jensen, 2000).

An appropriate review of the neurological correlates of these disorders would merit a separate chapter, although it may suffice to say that the neurology of many of these disorders frequently implicates the frontal lobe of the brain. The frontal lobe (located in the forehead area) is the area of the brain responsible for higher cognitive functions, including executive functions, and these involve problem solving, spontaneity, memory, language, motivation, judgment, impulse control, and social and sexual behavior.

Summary

The diagnostic process requires one not only to examine the results of commercially produced standardized tests, but also to employ keen observational skills that look at presenting symptoms and behaviors. In this chapter, we have outlined for the reader a host of conditions which in some cases overlap with Auditory Processing Disorders, whereas in others, merely imitate it. It is imperative that any professional who works in the diagnostic field (speech-language pathologists, audiologists, resource consultants, psychologists, etc.) become familiar with the features of these disorders and the differential diagnostic process that is required to properly treat them. By learning to recognize these comorbid conditions, it is hoped that no child or adult will struggle needlessly or waste valuable time in treatments that do not address their underlying disorders. By having the most appropriate professionals and interventions, individuals with APD can look forward to living a happy and productive life.

Key Points Learned

- Neurobiological disorders are highly comorbid and can include the following conditions: Attention-Deficit/Hyperactivity Disorders, Learning Disorders (including for reading, written language, and Non-Verbal Learning Disorder), anxiety disorders (such as Selective Mutism and Obsessive-Compulsive Disorder), mood disorders including Depression and Bipolar Disorder, Tourette's Disorder, Asperger's Disorder, and Sensory Integration Dysfunction.
- Referral to an appropriate professional such as a psychiatrist and/or clinical psychologist is indicated to facilitate an appropriate intervention plan when features of these disorders have an adverse impact on the quality of an individual's life.
- Features of these disorders frequently mimic the behavioral symptoms often associated with Auditory Processing Disorders.
- Some symptoms associated with learning disabilities such as Reading Disorders and Written Language Disorders can be indicative of Auditory Processing Disorders.
- A careful analysis of the reading or writing patterns can help the clinician determine whether or not there is a need for further testing for APD.

References

American Academy of Pediatrics. (2000). Clinical practice guideline: Diagnosis and evaluation of the child with Attention-Deficit/Hyperactivity Disorder. *Pediatrics, 105*, 1158–1170.

American Psychiatric Association. (2000). *Diagnostic and statistical manual of mental disorders* (text revision, 4th ed.). Washington, DC: Author.

American Speech-Language Hearing Association. (2004). Auditory integration training. *Asha*, (Suppl. 24), 1–7.

Antonuccio, D. O., Danton, W. G., & DeNelsky, G. Y. (1995). Psychotherapy versus medication for depression: Challenging the conventional wisdom with data. *Professional Psychology: Research and Practice, 26*, 574–585.

Ayres, A. J. (2000). *Sensory integration and the child.* Los Angeles: Western Psychological Services.

Barkley, R. A. (2000). *Taking charge of ADHD: The complete, authoritative guide for parents.* New York: Guilford.

Barnard, M. U. (2003). *Helping your depressed child: A step-by-step guide for parents.* Oakland, CA: New Harbinger

Batshaw, M. L. (2002). *Children with disabilities* (5th ed.). Baltimore: Paul H. Brookes.

Birmaher, B. (2004). *New hope for children and teens with bipolar disorder.* New York: Three Rivers.

Braaten, E., & Felopulos, G. (2004). *Straight talk about psychological testing for kids.* New York: Guilford.

Brill, M. T. (2002). *Tourette syndrome.* Brookfield, CT: The Millbook Press.

Chansky, T. (2000). *Freeing your child from obsessive-compulsive disorder.* New York: Three Rivers.

Christophersen, E. R., & Mortweet, S. L. (Eds.). (2001). *Treatments that work with children: Empirically supported strategies for managing childhood problems.* Washington, DC: American Psychological Association.

Ciocci, S. R. (2002). *Auditory processing disorders: An overview* (ERIC Digest, ED474303). Arlington, VA: ERIC Clearing-house on Disabilities and Gifted Education.

Compton, S. N., McKnight, C. D., & March, J. S. (2004). Combining medication and psychosocial treatments: An evidence-based medicine approach. In T. L. Morris & J. S. March (Eds.), *Anxiety disorders in children and adolescents* (2nd ed.). New York: Guilford.

Federal Register. (2004, December 3). Public Law 108-446 (Reauthorization of the Individuals with Disabilities Act. Vol. 29, No. 232.

Feifer, S. G., & De Fina, P. A. (2000). *The neuropsychology of reading disorders: Diagnosis and intervention workbook.* Middeltown, MD: School Neuropsych Press.

Feifer, S. G., & De Fina, P. A. (2002). *The neuropsychology of written language disorders: Diagnosis and intervention.* Middletown, MD: School Neuropsych Press.

Friedman, M. A., Detweiler-Bedell, J., Leventhal, H. E., Horne, R., Keitner, G. I., & Miller, I. W. (2004). Combined psychotherapy and pharmacotherapy for the treatment of major depressive disorder. *Clinical Psychology: Science and Practice, 11*, 47–68.

Geffner, D. (2005). *Attention-deficit/hyperactivity disorder: What professionals need to know.* Eau Claire, WI: Thinking Publications.

Hamaguchi, P. (2006). Neurobiological disorders: information for the SLP & audiologist. *California Speech-Language Hearing Association (CSHA) Magazine, 36*, 12–13, 24–25, 31.

Jensen, E. (2000). *Different brains, different learners: How to reach the hard to reach.* San Diego, CA: The Brain Store.

King, W. M. (2003). Comorbid auditory processing disorder in developmental dyslexia. *Ear and Hearing, 24*, 448–456.

Kranowitz, C. S. (1998). *The out-of-sync child: Recognizing and coping with sensory integration dysfunction.* New York: Perigee.

Kutscher, M. (2005). *Kids in the mix of ADHD, LD, Asperger's, Tourette's, bipolar and more!* London, UK: Jessica Kingsley Publishers.

Lezak, M. D., Howieson, D. B., & Loring, D. W. (2004). *Neuropsychological assessment.* New York: Oxford University Press.

McClure, E. B., Kubiszyn, T., & Kaslow, N. J. (2002). Advances in the diagnosis and treatment of childhood mood disorders. *Professional Psychology: Research and Practice, 33*, 125–134.

McHolm, A. E., Cunningham, C. E., & Vanier, M. K. (2005). *Helping your child with selective mutism: Practical steps to overcome a fear of speaking.* Oakland, CA: New Harbinger.

Nowicki, S., & Duke, M. P. (1992). *Helping the child who doesn't fit in.* Atlanta, GA: Peachtree.

Organista, P. B., Chun, K. M., & Marin, G. (Eds.). (1998). *Readings in ethnic psychology.* New York: Routledge.

Ozonoff, S., Dawson, G., & McPartland, J. (2002). *A parent's guide to Asperger's syndrome & high-functioning autism: How to meet the challenges and help your child thrive.* New York: Guilford.

Rapee, R. M., Spence, S. H., Cobham, V., & Wignall, A. (2000). *Helping your anxious child: A step-by-step guide for parents.* Oakland, CA: New Harbinger.

Riccio, C. A. (2005). Auditory processing measure: Correlation with neuropsychological measures of attention, memory, and behavior. *Child Neuropsychology, 11,* 363–372.

Root, R. W., & Resnick, R. J. (2003). An update on the diagnosis and treatment of attention-deficit/hyperactivity disorder in children. *Professional Psychology: Research and Practice, 34,* 34–41.

Rourke, B. P. (1989). *Nonverbal learning disabilities: The syndrome and the model.* New York: Guilford Press.

Satterfield, J. J. (2002). Culturally sensitive cognitive-behavioral therapy for depression with low-income and minority clients. In F. W. Kaslow & T. Patterson (Eds.), *Comprehensive handbook of psychotherapy: Cognitive-behavioral approaches* (Vol. 2). Hoboken, NJ: John Wiley & Sons.

Smith, K., & Gouze, K. (2004). *The sensory-sensitive child.* New York: Harper Resource.

Stallard, P. (2002). *Think good-feel good: A cognitive behaviour therapy workbook for children and young people.* West Sussex, England: John Wiley & Sons.

Stewart, K. (2002). *Helping a child with nonverbal learning disorder or Asperger's syndrome.* Oakland, CA: New Harbinger.

Tazeau, Y. N. (2006). Neuropsychiatric disorders in childhood. *California Speech-Language-Hearing Association (CSHA) Magazine, 36,* 5–7, 15.

Tillery, K. M., Katz, J., & Keller, W. D. (2000). Effects of methylphenidate (Ritalin) on auditory performance in children with attention and auditory processing disorders. *Journal of Speech, Language and Hearing Research, 43,* 893–901.

U.S. Public Health Services. (2000). *Report on the Surgeon General's conference on children's mental health: A national action agenda.* Washington, DC: U.S. Government Printing Office.

Wilens, T. (2001). *Straight talk about psychiatric medications for kids.* New York: Guilford.

Woodrich, D. J., & Schmitt, A. J. (2006) *Patterns of learning disorders: Working systematically from assessment to intervention.* New York: Guilford.

Internet Resources

Anxiety Disorders Association of America
http://www.adaa.org

Asperger Syndrome Coalition of the United States
http://www.asperger.org

Child and Adolescent Bipolar Foundation
http://www.bpkids.org

Children and Adults with Attention-Deficit/Hyperactivity Disorder
http://www.chadd.org

Learning Disabilities Association of America
http://www.ldanatl.org

Learning Disabilities Online
http://www.ldonline.org

National Information Center for Children and Youth with Disabilities
http://www.nichy.org

National Institute of Mental Health
http://www.nimh.nih.gov

National Mental Health Association
http://www.nmha.org

NLD Line (Nonverbal Learning Disability)
http://www.nldline.com

Obsessive-Compulsive Foundation
http://www.ocfoundation.org

Tourette Syndrome Association
http://www.tsa-usa.org

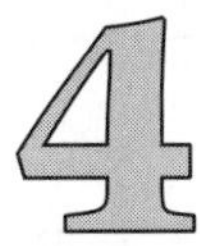

Audiologic Assessment of (C)APD

Marni L. Johnson
Teri James Bellis
Cassie Billiet

Overview

This chapter addresses audiologic assessment and diagnosis of (C)APD. Specifically, categories of behavioral test tools for the diagnosis of (C)APD are described, including the types of auditory processes assessed by each. Furthermore, interpretation of central auditory test results are discussed with an eye toward determination of presence and nature of disorder and relationship of auditory test findings to functional behavioral sequelae for purposes of developing individualized, deficit-specific management and treatment plans. In addition, the current definition and conceptualizations of (C)APD are reviewed, as are methods of screening for (C)APD and scopes of practice of the speech-language pathologist and audiologist in the assessment and diagnosis of (C)APD.

Introduction

In recent years, the term *(central) auditory processing disorder* ([C]APD) has been used increasingly to describe numerous auditory difficulties experienced by both children and adults, and public awareness of this disorder has risen dramatically. Those working in the professions of audiology, speech-language pathology, education, psychology, and related fields have seen a concomitant surge in the number of requests for information and clinical services related to the assessment and treatment of (C)APD. To properly address these inquiries, it is important for professionals to understand the basic principles underlying central auditory processing and its disorders.

This chapter focuses on the audiologic assessment of (C)APD. However, background knowledge is necessary to understand fully the assessment and diagnostic process. Therefore, this chapter begins with an overview of the current conceptualizations of (central) auditory processing and its disorders. Although previous chapters discussed the definition, description, and behaviors of (C)APD, these topics are reviewed briefly here due to their importance in understanding the audiologic assessment and diagnosis of (C)APD. The roles of audiologists, speech-language pathologists, and related professionals in the assessment, diagnosis, and management of individuals with (C)APD also are discussed.

The issue of terminology related to this topic has been a controversial one within the field of communication disorders for quite some time. Following the Bruton conference of 2000, Jerger and Musiek (2000) suggested use of the term *auditory processing disorder* (APD) in place of the previously used term *central auditory processing disorder* (CAPD). However, the 2005 technical report and position statement set forth by the American Speech-Language-Hearing Association's Working Group on Auditory Processing Disorders use the term *(central) auditory processing disorder ([C]APD)* to acknowledge the key role of the central auditory nervous system in these disorders (ASHA, 2005a, 2005b). To ensure consistency with the most recent literature, (C)APD is used throughout this chapter; however, readers should keep in mind that CAPD, APD, and (C)APD are all considered synonymous terms.

Current Conceptualizations of (Central) Auditory Processing and Its Disorders

The definition of (central) auditory processing ([C]AP) has evolved since its concepts were first introduced in the 1950s (Myklebust, 1954). (C)AP is currently defined as the "perceptual processing of auditory information in the central nervous system (CNS) and the neurobiological activity that underlies that processing and gives rise to the electrophysiological auditory potentials" (ASHA, 2005a, p. 2). (C)AP involves the auditory mechanisms responsible for auditory discrimination, sound localization and lateralization, temporal aspects of audition, and auditory performance with degraded and/or competing acoustic signals (ASHA, 1996. 2005a, 2005b; Bellis, 2003a; Chermak & Musiek, 1997).

Information processing theory shapes our current conceptualization of (C)AP and its disorders. This theory describes the way information is processed via distributed and parallel networks with significant contributions from both bottom-up and top-down factors (Massaro, 1975). **Bottom-up or data-driven factors** are those that pertain to the incoming acoustic signal as well as to the integrity of the central auditory pathways. **Top-down or concept-driven factors** are those that relate to higher order central resources such as cognition, attention, and language and their role in the processing of auditory information. When we consider the complexity of the human brain and the fact that very few, if any, regions of the brain are dedicated entirely to a single modality, it becomes clear that (C)AP involves much more than simply the hierarchical relay of acoustic features from the ear to the cortex. Instead, when discussing (C)AP, we must acknowledge the importance of both the basic neural representation of the fundamental characteristics of the acoustic signal throughout the central auditory pathways as well as higher order functions such as attention, memory, experience, linguistic competence, executive function, and metacognition, all of which affect the basic sensory percept and, thus, the ability to process auditorily presented information.

It is true that higher order cognitive and language processing problems may lead to difficulties with auditory tasks (e.g., problems comprehending spoken language, other "listening" difficulties). However, by definition, a (central) auditory processing disorder **([C]APD) is a deficit in the neural processing of auditory information that *cannot be attributed to* higher order disorders** including those related to learning, attention, memory, cognitive-communicative and/or language-related skills (ASHA, 2005a, 2005b). Therefore, although (C)APD may coexist with higher order deficits (e.g., attention deficit disorder [ADHD], learning disability, language impairment), it is not the *result* of these disorders (ASHA, 2005a, 2005b; Bellis, 2002a, 2003a). **The terms *auditory processing, language processing,* and *cognitive processing* are not synonymous**, although disorders in any of these areas may manifest themselves in similar overt behaviors. Thus, although a child with, for example, autism or mental retardation may have difficulty following verbal directions or comprehending spoken language, it is likely that his or her auditory difficulties are due to this higher order, more global disorder rather than to a specific deficit in the central auditory pathways, per se. In these cases, per current definitions of (C)APD, it would be inappropriate to apply the diagnostic label of (C)APD (ASHA, 2005a; Bellis, 2002a, 2003a).

Because (C)APD is an auditory disorder, it should manifest itself primarily, if not entirely, in the auditory modality. It should be noted, however, that the complex nature of neural organization and information processing in the brain renders the requirement of complete modality-specificity—that is, the demonstration of a deficit in the central auditory system and nowhere else—as a necessary criterion for diagnosis of (C)APD incompatible with the underlying science (ASHA, 2005a, 2005b; Bellis, 2003a; Musiek, Bellis, & Chermak, 2005). The organization of the CNS underlies the oft-reported comorbidity of (C)APD with disorders such as ADHD, learning disorder, and language disability. The task of those involved in assessment and diagnosis, then, becomes one of disentangling the central auditory factors from the other presenting disorders for purposes of accurate differential diagnosis and deficit-specific intervention.

In short, (C)APD is currently conceptualized as dysfunction in the central auditory nervous system (CANS) that leads to a deficit in one or more basic auditory mechanisms or functions. As such, **to diagnose (C)APD, one must demonstrate the presence of dysfunction in the central auditory pathways using tools developed for that purpose.** Although (C)APD may lead to or be associated with deficits in phonological processing, language, attention to and memory for auditory information, auditory comprehension, and similar skills, these are considered higher order cognitive/communicative functions and are excluded from current definitions of (C)APD (ASHA 2005a, 2005b).

Scopes of Practice in the Assessment and Diagnosis of (C)APD

At this point it becomes **important to differentiate between the terms *assessment* and *diagnosis*.** *Assessment* involves the process of collecting data or gathering evidence in order to determine an individual's functional areas of strength and weakness. Assessment may include both formal and informal procedures. In contrast, *diagnosis* refers to the identification and categorization of a specific impairment or dysfunction. This involves determining both the presence and nature of the disorder using diagnostic tools developed specifically for that purpose. Because (C)APD is an auditory disorder, **the diagnosis of (C)APD is the responsibility of the audiologist** (ASHA, 2004a, 2005a, 2005b). Assessment, on the other hand, requires a multidisciplinary approach in order to delineate fully the functional deficits of the individual with a suspected (C)APD. (C)AP represents an interconnection among many disciplines; therefore, a multidisciplinary approach is critical to the assessment, differential diagnosis, and treatment of (C)APD (ASHA, 2005a, 2005b).

The role of the SLP specifically is to collaborate with the audiologist and other professionals in the assessment and treatment of (C)APD (ASHA, 2004b, 2005a, 2005b). **SLPs are "uniquely qualified to delineate the cognitive-communicative and/or other speech-language factors that may be associated with (C)APD"** (ASHA, 2005b, p. 1). For example, individuals with language disorders, phonological processing disorders, or similar higher order cognitive/communicative or speech-language disorders may exhibit behavioral symptoms that mimic those of (C)APD. Similarly, (C)APD may lead to or be associated with difficulties in language, learning, and phonological processing; however, this is not always the case. Ultimately, the diagnosis will determine directly the intervention and treatment that is indicated in a given case. Therefore, it is important that the SLP work closely with the audiologist and others involved in the multidisciplinary team to achieve accurate differential diagnosis of these disorders for the purpose of designing an individualized, deficit-specific intervention plan.

When an individual presents with listening, language, learning, or related difficulties, **(C)AP assessment should not be a starting point in the diagnostic process.** Instead, the patient's overall level of functioning should be explored using a multidisciplinary team approach that allows information to be gathered that will reflect the individual's functional abilities and overall strengths and weaknesses across many different areas. The team often will include, but not be limited to, the audiologist, SLP, special education and classroom teachers, psychologist, parents, physician, and any additional persons significant in the individual's life. A team approach is particularly essential when working with pediatric patients because parents and school personnel ultimately will be responsible for managing the child's listening difficulties (Bellis, 2002a, 2003a).

In conclusion, (C)APD diagnosis falls squarely under the scope of practice of the audiologist. Nevertheless, the SLP is a critical team player in the overall assessment of individuals suspected of (C)APD for purposes of differential diagnosis as well as for the development and implementation of comprehensive treatment plans for children and adults with (C)APD and concomitant cognitive/communicative and/or language-related difficulties.

Screening for (C)APD

The purpose of (C)AP screening is to obtain preliminary information about an individual's auditory functional abilities to determine whether there is a need for further comprehensive diagnostic testing (Bellis, 2003a; ASHA, 2005a). Screening for (C)APD may involve functional observation of listening behaviors, behavioral checklists and questionnaires, or specific screening tools (ASHA 2005a; Bellis, 2002a, 2003a; Jerger & Musiek, 2000; Musiek, Gollegly, Lamb, & Lamb, 1990). Regardless of which screening measure is employed, **it is important to obtain information about an individual's auditory behaviors, listening skills, communication, and function across all disciplines** (Bellis, 2002a, 2003a). A second goal of (C)AP screening is to reduce the number of inappropriate referrals of individuals with higher order global deficits who are erroneously suspected of having a (C)APD. When an effective screening procedure is in place, overall costs are reduced, valuable time is saved, and the efficiency of identification and rehabilitation of (C)APD is improved.

There are several checklists and questionnaires currently available that may be used to screen for (C)APD. However, many of the behaviors addressed in these tools are not specific to (C)APD and encompass a variety of higher order cognitive and language skills. Nonetheless, these questionnaires can provide valuable information regarding auditory function in a variety of situations (e.g., listening in background noise, following-directions, and understanding rapid or distorted speech) (Jerger & Musiek, 2000). A list of commonly used checklists and questionnaires is provided in Table 4–1. In addition, the topic of checklists and questionnaires, as well as speech and language tools for assessing individuals suspected of (C)APD, are discussed more fully in Chapter 7 of this book.

Table 4–1. Selected Behavioral Checklists and Questionnaires Useful for (C)APD Screening

Children's Auditory Performance Scale (CHAPS) (Smoski, Brunt, & Tannahill, 1998)
Fisher Auditory Processing Checklist (Fisher, 1985)
The Children's Home Inventory of Listening Difficulties (CHILD) (Anderson & Smaldino, 2000)
Screening Instrument for Targeting Educational Risk (SIFTER) (Anderson & Matkin, 1996)
Listening Inventory for Education (LIFE) (Anderson & Smaldino, 1998)

During the screening process, each member of the multidisciplinary team should be responsible for gathering information in his or her area of expertise. Cognitive and psycho-educational testing to delineate cognitive and academic strengths and weaknesses, speech and language testing to assess receptive and expressive abilities, audiologic testing to rule out hearing loss as a contributing factor, medical evaluation to rule out or treat any confounding disorders (e.g., ADHD), and any other related assessments all should be completed during the screening process. **Primary deficits in language, cognition, and attention as well as other higher order global deficits need to be identified or ruled out as significant contributing factors to an individual's listening difficulties as it is possible that deficits in these areas may preclude central auditory testing** (Bellis, 2003a). For the most part, these evaluations typically are completed as part of a multidisciplinary team evaluation or child study process when a child presents with difficulties in the educational setting; for adults, many of these evaluations may be waived.

The determination of the need to refer an individual for comprehensive (C)AP diagnostic testing should be based on the information gathered during the screening process. Although many screening methods for (C)APD have been proposed, Bellis (2002a, 2003a) suggests a comprehensive team approach that addresses four primary questions. These are:

1. **Are the current evaluations sufficient in scope?** It important to be sure that the information gathered from members of the multidisciplinary team is complete. The information should provide a picture of auditory strengths and weaknesses across disciplines in order to address the presenting difficulties of the whole individual. For children suspected of (C)APD, information obtained should address, at minimum, cognitive and speech-language function; academic strengths and weak-

nesses; and, when indicated, any potentially confounding issues such as attention-related disorders, pertinent otological, neurological, or other medical history, and others.

2. **Is there a likelihood that (C)APD is present?** After key information has been gathered, the information obtained is analyzed for general patterns that emerge across disciplines that suggest the likelihood of a central auditory deficit. Reviewing the multidisciplinary information also is important for determining whether a higher order global deficit is present (e.g., mental retardation, autism, significant ADHD) that may better account for the individual's difficulties.
3. **Is the individual capable of undergoing central auditory diagnostic testing?** Most diagnostic behavioral tests used to diagnose (C)APD require a child to be 7 to 8 years of age and are of highly questionable reliability in younger children. Furthermore, central auditory testing requires that individuals be able to attend to and understand the task and to repeat sentences, words, and groups of numbers. In addition, although there exist some diagnostic tests of central auditory function that are relatively resistant to mild-to-moderate hearing loss, a significant peripheral hearing loss may preclude diagnostic testing for (C)APD.
4. **Will results of a (C)AP evaluation add to the current management of the individual's difficulties?** It is important to consider the current management and/or compensatory strategies utilized by the individual suspected of having (C)APD. If a diagnosis of (C)APD is made, further recommendations should provide functional benefit to the individual. However, if the individual is already receiving appropriate intervention and is progressing at a satisfactory pace, adding the label of (C)APD may not be necessary. In these cases, it may be preferable to the referring source to proceed with the status quo and reconsider central auditory evaluation at a later date.

Bellis (2002a, 2003a) suggests that, if the answer to all four of the above questions is "yes," then a referral for comprehensive (C)AP diagnostic testing is warranted.

Finally, it is critical to emphasize that **informal assessments and screening tools** including checklists; questionnaires; and cognitive or speech-language measures of spoken language processing, comprehension, phonological awareness, and similar abilities, while providing important information regarding a child's functioning in the real world, **should never be used for diagnostic purposes.** Although there currently is no universally accepted screening method for (C)APD, the multidisciplinary approach described above may lead to a more holistic view of the individual's functional abilities and, ultimately, to a more ecologically valid intervention plan that addresses the individual's specific functional difficulties in those cases in which a diagnosis of (C)APD is eventually obtained (Bellis, 2002a, 2002b, 2003a).

Diagnostic Testing for (C)APD

Once it has been determined through the screening process that there is a need for further testing, specific diagnostic tests can be performed to determine whether a (C)APD is present and to describe its parameters. ASHA (2005a) suggests that the tests used to diagnose (C)APD should meet accepted scientific and psychometric standards, should control as much as possible for confounding factors such as memory and attention, and should be appropriate to the individual being tested. Central auditory testing should be performed in a sound-treated booth by an audiologist who is qualified and competent in the area of (C)APD. It should be noted that not all audiologists have the knowledge base necessary to perform and interpret diagnostic tests of central auditory function. As such, **the knowledge and skills necessary to provide the best quality services in (central) auditory processing may require significant additional training and education beyond what is typically received in audiology professional preparation programs** (ASHA, 2005a, 2005b).

During the diagnostic evaluation, an in-depth case history should be taken in order to obtain additional information that may complement the multidisciplinary information reviewed previously during the screening process. Following the case history, the diagnostic evaluation takes place. On the day of testing, it is important that any medication prescribed for disorders (e.g., ADHD) or other medical conditions (e.g., depression) be taken as recommended by the prescribing physician. This will reduce confounding factors associated with these conditions that may adversely affect diagnostic test results. Once testing is complete, diagnostic test findings as well as treatment and management recommendations should be discussed with the patient, his or her family, and other members of the multidisciplinary team when applicable.

The Diagnostic Test Battery

The audiologist is uniquely qualified to select, administer, and interpret the central auditory diagnostic test battery. A test battery approach is essential for comprehensive assessment of (C)AP. There are a number of tests available for use in diagnosing (C)APD; however, no one test battery will be appropriate for every situation. Diagnostic testing for (C)AP should not be test driven. Rather, the tests should be chosen on a case-by-case basis according to the presenting complaints and other information that was obtained during the case history and screening process. Special consideration needs to be given to several factors including the patient's chronological and developmental age, cognitive capacity, linguistic experience, attention, memory, fatigue, and motivation as these factors will influence the types of tests selected, an individual's performance on certain tests, and the interpretation of test results (ASHA, 2005a).

As (C)APD is defined as a disorder in the CANS, **it is critical that diagnostic tests be selected tests that have been shown to be valid for dysfunction of the CANS.** That is, the tests used to diagnose (C)APD should be both sensitive (e.g., detect the presence of a disorder when it is indeed present) and specific (e.g., do not detect the presence of a disorder when it is absent) to CANS dysfunction. Therefore, audiologists must be familiar with the literature regarding the validity of currently available (C)AP tests and use this information when selecting their test batteries.

The tests selected should include both verbal and nonverbal stimuli, and should examine multiple levels and/or neuroanatomical regions of the CANS as well as different auditory processes. Most test batteries for (C)APD diagnosis provide information regarding integrity of left-, right-, and interhemispheric central auditory regions, as well as brainstem function. (C)APD is a heterogeneous disorder; therefore, it is important to examine a variety of processes in the CANS to understand each individual's specific deficits and how they relate to functional difficulties in real-world listening, learning, and communication situations. This ultimately will lead to individualized treatment and management strategies. **The importance of accurate and comprehensive diagnosis to the development of appropriate intervention goals cannot be overstated.**

Categories of Central Auditory Diagnostic Tests

Both behavioral and electrophysiological test measures may be used to diagnose (C)APD. Although electrophysiological tests play an important role in objectively demonstrating the presence of abnormal neurophysiologic representation of sound throughout the CANS (from brainstem to cortex), and also may have utility for early indication of treatment efficacy, the utility of electrophysiological tests in driving treatment and management goals is questionable. Furthermore, electrophysiological findings may be normal in many cases of (C)APD and the equipment needed for such tests may not be available in schools or other settings in which (C)APD diagnostic testing takes place. For these reasons, this chapter focuses on the categories of behavioral central auditory tests that are used most commonly in clinical practice and that provide the most useful information for the development of deficit-specific intervention programs. Nonetheless, electrophysiological measures may be useful as a cross-check of behavioral test results, if a neurological disorder is suspected, and in cases where behavioral assessment of central auditory function is not possible (ASHA, 2005a).

Behavioral tests most commonly used by audiologists to diagnose (C)APD can be divided into five categories: Dichotic speech tests, monaural low-redundancy speech tests, auditory temporal processing and patterning tests, binaural interaction tests, and auditory discrimination tests. **It is important to note that tests of phonological awareness, phonemic synthesis, auditory comprehension, and language are not diagnostic tests of (C)APD** (ASHA 2005a; Bellis, 2003a; Chermak & Musiek, 1997). A brief description of these test categories and the processes assessed by each is provided below.

Dichotic Speech Tests

Dichotic listening refers to an auditory stimulation condition in which two different stimuli, one to each ear, are presented simultaneously. Dichotic listening skills play an important role in situations in which auditory distractions are present such as hearing speech in the presence of background noise. Dichotic speech tests vary in terms of the stimuli presented, level of difficulty, task required, and linguistic loading. Depending on the task required of the listener, dichotic speech tests may assess the process of ***binaural integration*****, which involves reporting the stimuli presented to both ears, or *binaural separation*, which involves report of the stimuli presented to the target ear only while ignoring the competition in the contralateral ear.** Dichotic speech tests have been found to be sensitive to brainstem, cortical, and corpus callosum dysfunction. Dichotic speech tests commonly used clinically include, but are not limited to, Dichotic Digits (Musiek, 1983), Competing Sentences Test (Willeford & Burleigh, 1994), Dichotic Consonant-Vowels (CVs) (Berlin, Lowe-Bell, Jannetta, & Kline, 1972), and the Staggered Spondaic Word Test (SSW) (Katz, 1962).

Monaural Low-Redundancy Speech Tests

Monaural low-redundancy speech tests assess the ability to **fill in the missing components of a degraded signal, a process referred to as *auditory closure*.** Monaural low-redundancy speech tests can detect dysfunction of the brainstem as well as cortical regions, and are particularly sensitive to dysfunction of the primary auditory cortex. Examples of monaural low-redundancy speech tests in common clinical use include Low-Pass Filtered Speech (Willeford, 1977; *Tonal and speech materials for auditory perceptual assessment*, 1998; Wilson & Mueller, 1984), Time Compressed Speech with and without reverberation, (Fairbanks, Everitt, & Jaeger, 1954; *Tonal and speech materials*, 1998; Wilson & Mueller, 1984), and the Synthetic Sentence Identification Test with Ipsilateral Competing Message (SSI-ICM) (Jerger & Jerger, 1974).

Auditory Temporal Processing and Patterning Tests

Auditory temporal processing and patterning tests use nonspeech stimuli to **evaluate a variety of auditory processes including temporal resolution, temporal ordering, frequency and duration discrimination, and linguistic labeling.** Temporal, or timing-related, aspects of auditory function are critical to virtually all tasks requiring auditory processing, and they involve the ability to analyze acoustic events over time. For example, discrimination between two speech sounds that have rapidly changing spectrotemporal acoustic features requires precise temporal resolution. The perception of prosodic aspects of speech reliant on rhythm, stress, and intonation requires intact temporal processing and patterning abilities. Depending on the task, auditory temporal processing and patterning tests have been shown to be sensitive to cortical and corpus callosum dysfunction. Commercially available tests of auditory temporal processing and patterning at the time of this writing include the Random Gap Detection Test-Revised (Keith, 2000), Frequency Patterns Test (Pinheiro & Ptacek, 1971), and Duration Patterns Test (Pinheiro & Musiek, 1985). Additional temporal processing tests that involve gap detection, auditory fusion, backward and forward masking, and similar skills can be administered using specialized equipment, as well; however, there is a need for additional commercially available tests of temporal processing for common clinical use.

Binaural Interaction Tests

Tests of binaural interaction assess **binaural processes that are dependent on intensity, timing, or related differences between ears.** For the most part, these processes are mediated by central auditory brainstem structures. Although some commercially available tests of binaural interaction exist, their poor sensitivity to anything other than gross brainstem dysfunction suggests that they may be of limited clinical utility (e.g., Bellis, 2003a; Lynn & Gilroy, 1975). One exception to this is the masking level difference (MLD), which assesses the effects of interaural phase relationships on binaural processing at the brainstem level. However, at the present time, special equipment is needed for administration of tonal MLDs; therefore, although these are a useful adjunct to the audiologist's test battery, they are seldom used by most clinical audiologists testing for (C)APD. Electrophysiologic measures of brainstem function via the auditory brainstem response (ABR) also are very useful in assessing integrity of brainstem auditory pathways.

Auditory Discrimination Tests

Auditory discrimination tests assess **the ability to distinguish between similarly sounding acoustic stimuli.** As such, auditory discrimination is another skill that factors into virtually every test of central auditory function. Auditory discrimination difficulties can be verbal as in speech sound discrimination or nonverbal such as detecting subtle differences in frequency, duration, or intensity. Tasks of phoneme discrimination; frequency, intensity, or duration discrimination thresholds or *difference limens*; and psychophysical tuning curves can be used to assess auditory discrimination abilities. Once again, however, there is a paucity of commercially available, acoustically controlled tests of auditory discrimination that meet accepted psychometric standards at the present time, and most require specialized equipment. Speech and language test tools that assess speech-sound discrimination may provide important information in this area; however, it should be remembered that these are not diagnostic tools for (C)APD.

The categories of behavioral central auditory tests discussed in this section, and the processes assessed by each, are summarized in Table 4–2.

Interpretation of Central Auditory Diagnostic Test Results

Results of diagnostic tests of central auditory function can be interpreted using several approaches, each of which may fulfill a different goal or purpose. If the goal of testing is simply to determine whether a (C)APD is present, then test results should meet specified diagnostic criteria. If the goal is to identify the nature of the (C)APD, then additional analysis and identification

Table 4–2. Categories of Diagnostic Tests of Central Auditory Function

Category	Process(es) Assessed
Dichotic Speech Tests	Binaural Separation; Binaural Integration
Monaural Low-Redundancy Speech Tests	Monaural Separation/Closure
Auditory Temporal Processing and Patterning Tests	Temporal Resolution; Nonspeech-Sound Discrimination; Temporal Ordering
Binaural Interaction Tests	Binaural Interaction
Auditory Discrimination Tests	Speech and/or Nonspeech Discrimination

of deficient auditory processes should occur. Finally, if the goal includes differential diagnosis and determination of the relationship between auditory deficits observed and functional difficulties in everyday communicative situations, an analysis of intertest patterns across both central auditory and multidisciplinary tests is critical. Typically, a combined approach is recommended, involving all of these levels of test-battery interpretation, as this will help to ensure appropriate and accurate differential diagnosis while, at the same time, providing a wealth of information that will be useful for the development of individualized, deficit-specific, ecologically valid intervention plans. This section briefly explores each of these methods or levels of test battery interpretation; for a more in-depth discussion of test battery interpretation, readers are referred to Bellis (2003a).

Determination of Presence of Disorder

Absolute, or norm-referenced, interpretation involves comparing the performance of the person being tested against age-specific normative values. It is important to recognize that, due to maturation within the CANS, normative values will differ depending upon the specific test administered, the patient's age, and—in many cases—the ear (right or left). For example, during many types of dichotic speech testing, it is normal for young children to have a significant difference between right- and left-ear performance, with left ear worse than right. This difference, or *right-ear advantage,* decreases with increasing age. **Typically, diagnosis of (C)APD requires performance greater than two standard deviations below the mean on two or more central auditory diagnostic tests** (ASHA, 2005a; Chermak & Musiek, 1997). A deficit greater than three standard deviations below the mean on one test, combined with significant functional difficulty in the process assessed by that test, also may lead to a diagnosis of (C)APD; however, caution should be exercised when applying the label of (C)APD when a deficit is observed on only one test (ASHA, 2005a; Bellis, 2003a).

A caveat is in order here. **Individuals may perform poorly on tests of central auditory function for reasons other than (C)APD.** These reasons can include failure to understand the directions, attention difficulties, lack of motivation, global cognitive or language problems, and many others. Therefore, it is critical that intra- and intertest comparisons also be made to ensure that a pattern is observed across test results consistent with the underlying neuroscience. **When inconsistency is seen across test results (e.g., a left-ear deficit on one dichotic speech test accompanied by a right-ear deficit on another, poor performance on all test measures, poor test-retest reliability), factors other than (C)APD should be suspected.** Because the test battery is chosen to assess various regions/levels of the CANS and various auditory processes, poor performance on all tests administered argues for a more global cognitive or related deficit, or poor overall motivation or attention difficulties, rather than dysfunction in a particular CANS region.

Process-Based Interpretation

Once a (C)APD has been identified, it is important to delineate the specific auditory process or processes that are found to be areas of deficit for the individual. **This will determine the types of auditory training activities that will be indicated to remediate the disorder.** Thus, for example, if speech-sound discrimination and temporal resolution are at issue, then temporal processing training and phoneme discrimination activities will be indicated. If the individual exhibits difficulties with binaural separation or integration, dichotic listening training may be an appropriate means of remediating the deficit. The processes assessed by each of the various behavioral categories of central auditory function tests were presented in Table 4–2.

Differential Diagnosis and Functional Deficit Profiling

Simply identifying the presence of disorder and the nature of the auditory deficits present is extremely useful for the development of a deficit-specific intervention plan. However, in most cases, further interpretation that takes into account the multidisciplinary information obtained during the screening and case history process is necessary both to determine how the auditory deficits observed relate to reported real-world functional difficulties and to differentiate the auditory element from other confounding disorders that may have similar or overlapping functional symptoms. One way of doing this is via subprofiling methods, or functional deficit profiling.

(C)APD is a heterogeneous disorder. Thus, it can take many forms, each of which typically produces distinct patterns across central auditory test performance and leads to or is associated with different functional sequelae. These patterns have been recognized and developed into functional deficit profiling models (Bellis 1996; 2002a, 2002b, 2003a; Bellis & Ferre, 1999; Ferre, 1997; Katz, 1992). These subprofiling models recognize the heterogeneous nature of (C)APD and draw upon the neuropsychology, cognitive science, auditory neuroscience, and other literature to differentiate among the various types of (C)APD; the associated sites of dysfunction in the CANS; and the possible language, learning, and communication areas that are most likely affected with each. It is important to emphasize that a good subprofiling model is dynamic and, thus, reflects evolving scientific and theoretical constructs, particularly as it relates to current understanding of the underlying neuroscience (Bellis, 2003a). It should be noted that, at the present time, no subprofiling model of (C)APD has been universally accepted and continuing research is underway to verify their utility in (C)APD diagnosis.

Subprofiling methods should be viewed as guides to assist professionals in differentiating (C)APD from higher order more global disorders and for relating central auditory deficit areas to reported difficulties in the classroom, workplace, home, and other communication or learning environments. In particular, these models are useful in developing ecologically valid, individualized intervention plans that address the particular difficulties exhibited by the person in question. **They should not be considered "cookie-cutter" approaches to (C)APD diagnosis and treatment**, as no subprofiling model can capture accurately the complexity and heterogeneity of this disorder, and each individual with (C)APD likely will present with difficulties that are unique to his or her own bottom-up and top-down abilities and life situations (Bellis, 2002a, 2002b, 2003a).

One method of functional deficit profiling that has been proposed in recent years is the Bellis/Ferre Model (Bellis, 1996, 2002a, 2002b, 2003a; Bellis & Ferre, 1999; Ferre, 1997). This model draws upon patterns of central auditory test findings and muldisciplinary functional sequelae that are well established in the auditory neuroscience, neuropsychology, and related literature for purposes of delineating three primary subtypes of (C)APD reflecting dysfunction in left-, right-, and interhemispheric CANS regions. Because this model is a dynamic one, and is modified as new understandings and conceptualizations of central auditory function are reached, it has evolved over the past decade or so. At present, the Bellis/Ferre Model describes three primary profiles of (C)APD: Auditory Decoding Deficit, Prosodic Deficit, and Integration Deficit. Each of these profiles are discussed briefly below. For a more detailed description of diagnostic indicators, symptoms, and treatment/management, readers are referred to Bellis (2002a, b; 2003a), and Bellis and Ferre (1999). Additional information regarding specific management and treatment strategies for individuals with (C)APD also can be found in subsequent chapters of this book.

Auditory Decoding Deficit. Individuals with Auditory Decoding Deficit exhibit a **left-hemisphere, likely primary auditory cortex, pattern of findings on central auditory testing.** Most commonly observed are bilateral and/or right-ear deficits on dichotic speech tasks and tests of monaural low-redundancy speech. Speech-sound discrimination, fine-grained temporal resolution tasks, and other auditory skills reliant on intact processing in primary auditory cortex often are affected, as well. Many individuals with Auditory Decoding Deficit also exhibit reduced middle latency and/or cortical electrophysiological responses recorded over left-hemisphere electrode sites, especially in response to speech stimuli. These individuals typically complain of speech-in-noise difficulties, and frequently "mis-hear" auditorily presented information and do better when visual or multimodal augmentations are employed. Reading and spelling difficulties involving phonological decoding (or word attack) skills also may be noted, as may speech production errors involving substitution of similar-sounding phonemes, especially stop consonants. Treatment for Auditory Decoding Deficit often includes but is not limited to auditory closure skills, speech-sound discrimination and fine-grained temporal processes, and enhancement of the acoustic signal (including assistive listening devices when appropriate).

Prosodic Deficit. Also referred to as "right-hemisphere (C)APD," Prosodic Deficit **reflects dysfunction in the right hemisphere.** As such, central auditory testing reveals a pattern of left-ear deficit on dichotic speech tasks as well as deficits on temporal patterning tests in both labeling and humming conditions. Additional right-hemisphere findings may be noted, including poor nonspeech-sound discrimination deficits. Typically, performance on tests of monaural low-redundancy speech, fine-grained temporal processing, speech-sound discrimination skills, and similar abilities is intact. Reduced electrophysiological responses may be noted over right-hemisphere electrode recording sites. Listening difficulties exhibited by individuals with Prosodic Deficit often consist of difficulty appreciating prosodic elements of speech, including rhythm, stress, and intonation cues. As a result, individuals with Prosodic Deficit may misinterpret the communicative intent of the communication. Associated symptoms of Prosodic Deficit may include poor automatic (sight-word) reading and spelling skills, deficits in mathematics calculation, visual-spatial difficulties, and monotonic speech production. It is important to note that these associated symptoms, with the exception of monotonic speech production, are not *caused by* the central auditory deficit, but likely reflect shared neuroanatomical substrates in the right hemisphere. Direct remediation for Prosodic Deficit typically addresses nonspeech discrimination, prosody training, and temporal patterning training, with acoustic signal clarity being less critical.

Integration Deficit. Inefficient interhemispheric transfer of auditory information via the corpus callosum is the presumed underlying cause of Integration Deficit, which yields a classic pattern on tests of central auditory function consisting of a left-ear deficit on dichotic speech tests and a deficit on temporal patterning tests in the linguistic labeling condition only. Performance on other central auditory tests may be within normal limits, as may electrophysiological responses. The primary functional complaint associated with Integration Deficit is difficulty hearing speech in noise, and localization difficulties also may be seen. Associated difficulties may be noted with any task that requires interhemispheric cooperation. As such, individuals with Integration Deficit may exhibit mild difficulties with bimanual and/or bipedal skills, problems with sound-symbol association required for reading and spelling, and difficulty linking prosodic and linguistic elements of speech to comprehend subtle communication forms such as sarcasm. Treatment for Integration Deficit usually includes enhancements of acoustic signal clarity, dichotic listening training, and interhemispheric exercises. On a related note, Integration Deficit often is seen both in children with delayed neuromaturation as well as in aging adults (Bellis, 2002a, 2003b; Bellis, Nicol, & Kraus, 2000; Bellis & Wilber, 2000; Musiek, Gollegly, & Baran, 1984) due to the changes occurring in the corpus callosum during these time periods in the life span.

The initial iterations of the Bellis/Ferre Model (Bellis, 1996; Bellis, 2002a, 2003a; Ferre, 1997) included two additional secondary subprofiles, Associative Deficit and Output-Organization Deficit that appeared to reflect the auditory difficulties seen in primary language and attention disorders. However, **given the evolving conceptualization of (C)APD as an auditory deficit that is not due to higher order language, attention, or related disorders, these profiles now are excluded from the Bellis/Ferre Model as they are inconsistent with current definitions of (C)APD.** Finally, it should be noted that it is not uncommon to see an individual who exhibits two overlapping profiles that involve adjacent brain areas (e.g., left- and interhemispheric deficit or right- and interhemispheric deficit) due to the close proximity of these structures. However, **an individual who performs poorly on all tests administered and, thereby, exhibits deficits in all brain regions would, by definition, be presenting with a global cognitive or related issue and, as such, the diagnostic label of (C)APD would be inappropriate.**

A brief summary of the three primary subprofiles of the Bellis/Ferre Model of (C)APD and sequelae associated with each is provided in Table 4–3.

Communication of Test Results

An audiologist qualified and knowledgeable in the area of (C)APD is responsible for making a proper diagnosis that will ultimately drive treatment and management endeavors. A comprehensive report should be written by the audiologist and distributed to the patient as well as to other professionals. Typically, the report should delineate the case history, diagnostic tests employed, and results of the central auditory diagnostic battery. Impressions that describe the individual's (C)APD and how it may relate to his or her functional listening and related difficulties should be included. Finally, the report should clearly describe a comprehensive intervention plan that includes individualized environmental modifications and compensatory strategies, as well as direct remediation activities. It is important for speech-language pathologists to understand the link between the patient's behavioral test results and their functional deficits. This knowledge is necessary to understand the rationale behind deficit-specific interventions as speech-language pathologists often have an intimate role in executing treatment and management plans for individual's with (C)APD.

Table 4–3. Bellis/Ferre Subprofiles of (C)APD

Subprofile	Key Diagnostic Central Auditory Findings	Commonly Seen Associated Sequelae	Presumed Site of Dysfunction
Auditory Decoding Deficit	Bilateral or right-ear deficit on dichotic speech and monaural low-redundancy tests; poor temporal resolution and speech-sound discrimination.	Difficulty hearing in noise; "mis-hears" frequently; spelling and reading errors involving phonologic decoding; may exhibit phonologic errors that are nondevelopmental and include substitutions of similar-sounding phonemes.	Left hemisphere, primary auditory cortex
Prosodic Deficit	Left-ear deficit on dichotic speech tests; deficit on temporal patterning tests in both the linguistic labeling and humming conditions; poor nonspeech-sound discrimination skills	Difficulty perceiving rhythm, stress, and intonational cues that convey communicative intent; reading and spelling difficulties involving automatic or sight-word skills; may be a monotonic reader or speaker; may exhibit other right-hemisphere sequelae such as math calculation and visual-spatial difficulties that are not related causally to the auditory deficit. Acoustic clarity less critical.	Right hemisphere
Integration Deficit	Left-ear deficit on dichotic speech tests; deficits on temporal patterning tests in the linguistic labeling condition only.	Significant difficulty hearing in noise; may exhibit difficulties in other areas requiring interhemispheric communication, including linking prosodic and linguistic elements of speech, mild bimanual or bipedal difficulties, and sound-symbol association difficulties in reading or spelling.	Corpus callosum

Summary

In conclusion, assessment for (C)APD requires a multidisciplinary approach; however, the actual diagnosis of (C)APD falls under the scope of practice of the audiologist. SLPs play a key role in the assessment, differential diagnosis, and treatment of (C)APD. Although informal assessments such as questionnaires and checklists, as well as measures of language processing and other skills, will provide important information about the individual's real-world functioning, they are not diagnostic tests of (C)APD. During diagnostic testing for (C)APD, it is important that audiologists determine the nature and possible site of dysfunction within the CANS to develop an appropriate deficit-specific intervention plan for the individual. The diagnosis will determine directly the appropriate means of managing and treating the disorder. As our knowledge of (C)APD continues to grow, so will the need for additional reliable and valid screening and diagnostic test tools.

Key Points Learned

- Current conceptualizations of (C)APD emphasize that it is a disorder of the CANS that is not due to higher order language, cognitive, or related deficit.
- SLPs and other professionals play critical roles in the assessment and management/treatment of patients with (C)APD; however, audiologists are responsible for the diagnosis of (C)APD via the administration and interpretation of specific tests of central auditory function.
- Screening for (C)APD should be a multidisciplinary endeavor and should provide guidance as to the need for further comprehensive diagnostic testing. Screening tools should never be used for diagnostic purposes.
- Diagnostic testing for (C)APD should employ a test-battery approach that assesses various auditory processes and levels/regions of the CANS. Only tools that have been shown to be sensitive to CANS dysfunction should be used for diagnosis of (C)APD.
- Diagnostic central auditory testing should provide information regarding the presence and nature of the disorder, the ways in which the auditory deficits relate to the individual's functional complaints, and the appropriate means of managing and treating the individual's disorder. Accurate diagnosis is critical to the development of individualized, deficit-specific intervention plans.

References

American Speech-Language Hearing Association. (1996). Central auditory processing: Current status of research and implications for clinical practice. *American Journal of Audiology, 5*, 41–54.

American Speech-Language Hearing Association. (2004a). Scope of practice in audiology. *ASHA* (Suppl. 24).

American Speech-Language Hearing Association. (2004b). *Preferred practice patterns for the profession of speech-language pathology.* Available at: http://www.asha.org/members/deskref-journals/deskref/default

American Speech-Language Hearing Association. (2005a). *(Central) auditory processing disorders* [Technical report]. Available at: http://www.asha.org/members/deskref-journals/deskref/default.

American Speech-Language Hearing Association. (2005b). *(Central) auditory processing disorders—The role of the audiologist* [Position statement]. Available at: http://www.asha.org/members/deskref-journals/deskref/default.

Anderson, K., & Matkin, N. H. (1996). *Screening instrument for targeting educational risk (S.I.F.T.E.R.).* Tampa, FL: Educational Audiology Association.

Anderson, K., & Smaldino, J. J. (1998). *Children's home inventory of listening difficulties (C.H.I.L.D.).* Tampa, FL: Educational Audiology Association.

Anderson, K., & Smaldino, J. J. (2000). *Listening inventory for education (L.I.F.E.).* Tampa, FL: Educational Audiology Association.

Bellis, T. J. (1996). *Assessment and management of central auditory processing disorders in the educational setting: From Science to practice.* San Diego, CA: Singular Publishing Group.

Bellis, T. J. (2002a). *When the brain can't hear: Unraveling the mystery of auditory processing disorder.* New York: Pocket Books.

Bellis, T. J. (2002b). Developing deficit-specific intervention plans for individuals with auditory processing disorders. *Seminars in Hearing, 23*, 287–295.

Bellis, T. J. (2003a). *Assessment and management of central auditory processing disorders in the educational setting: From Science to practice* (2nd ed.). Clifton Park, NY: Thomson Learning.

Bellis, T. J. (2003b). Auditory processing disorders: It's not just kids who have them. *The Hearing Journal*, 56, 10–20.

Bellis, T. J., & Ferre, J. M. (1999). Multidimensional approach to the differential diagnosis of central auditory processing disorders in children. *Journal of the American Academy of Audiology, 10*, 319–328.

Bellis, T. J., Nicol, T., & Kraus, N. (2000). Aging affects hemispheric asymmetry in the neural representation of speech sounds. *Journal of Neuroscience, 20*, 791–797.

Bellis, T. J., & Wilber, L. A. (2001). Effects of aging and gender on interhemispheric function. *Journal of Speech, Language and Hearing Research, 44*, 246–263.

Berlin, C. I., Lowe-Bell, S. S., Jannetta, P. J., & Kline, D. G. (1972). Central auditory deficits after temporal lobectomy. *Archives of Otolaryngology, 96*, 4–10.

Chermak, G. D., & Musiek, F. E. (1997). *Central auditory processing disorders: New perspectives.* San Diego, CA: Singular Publishing Group.

Fairbanks, G., Everitt, W., & Jaeger, R. (1954). Methods for time or frequency compression-expansion of speech. *Trans IRE-PGA, AU-2*, 7–12.

Ferre, J. M. (1997). *Processing power: A guide to CAPD assessment and management.* San Antonio, TX: Communication Skill Builders.

Fisher, L. I. (1985). Learning disabilities and auditory processing. In R. J. Van Hattum (Ed.), *Administration of speech-language services in the schools* (pp. 231–292). San Diego, CA: College-Hill Press.

Jerger, J., & Jerger, S. W. (1974). Auditory findings in brainstem disorders. *Archives of Otolaryngology, 99*, 342–349.

Jerger, J., & Musiek, F. (2000). Report of the consensus conference on the diagnosis of auditory processing disorders in school-aged children. *Journal of the American Academy of Audiology, 11*, 467–474.

Katz, J. (1962). The use of staggered spondaic words for assessing the integrity of the central auditory nervous system. *Journal of Auditory Research, 2*, 327–337.

Katz, J. (1992). Classification of auditory processing disorders. In J. Katz, N. Stecker, & D. Henderson (Eds.), *Central auditory processing: A transdisciplinary view* (pp. 81–91). St. Louis, MO: Mosby Year Book.

Keith, R. W. (2000). *Random Gap Detection Test.* St. Louis, MO: Auditec.

Lynn, F. E., & Gilroy, J. (1975). Effects of brain lesions on the perception of monotic and dichotic speech stimuli. In M. D. Sullivan (Ed.), *Central auditory processing disorders* (pp. 47–83). Omaha, NE: Proceedings of the Conference at University of Nebraska Medical Center.

Massaro, D. W. (1975). *Understanding language: An information-processing analysis of speech perception, reading, and psycholinguistics.* New York: Academic Press.

Musiek, F. E. (1983). Assessment of central auditory dysfunction: The Dichotic Digits Test revisited. *Ear and Hearing, 4*, 79–83.

Musiek, F. E., Bellis, T. J., & Chermak, G. D. (2005). Nonmodularity of the central auditory nervous system (CANS): Implications for central auditory processing disorder. *American Journal of Audiology, 14*, 128–138.

Musiek, F. E., Gollegly, K. M., & Baran, J. A. (1984). Myelination of the corpus callosum and auditory processing problems in children: Theoretical and clinical correlates. *Seminars in Hearing, 5*, 231–241.

Musiek, F. E., Gollegly, K. M., Lamb, L. E., & Lamb, P. (1990). Selected issues in screening for central auditory processing dysfunction. *Seminars in Hearing, 11*, 372–384.

Mykelbust, H. R. (1954). *Auditory disorders in children: A manual for differential diagnosis:* New York: Grune & Stratton.

Pinheiro, M. L., & Musiek, F. E. (1985). Sequencing and temporal ordering in the auditory system. In M. L. Pinheiro & F. E. Musiek (Eds.), *Assessment of central auditory dysfunction: Foundations and clinical correlates* (pp. 219–238). Baltimore: Williams & Wilkins.

Pinheiro, M. L., & Ptacek, P. H. (1971). Reversals in the perception of noise and tone patterns. *Journal of the Acoustical Society of America, 49*, 1778–1782.

Smoski, W. J., Brunt, M. A., & Tannahill, J. C. (1998). *Children's auditory performance scale.* Tampa, FL: Educational Audiology Association.

Tonal and speech materials for auditory perceptual assessment, disc 2.0. (1998). Long Beach, CA: Research and Development Service, Veterans' Administration Central Office.

Willeford, J. (1977). Assessing central auditory behavior in children: A test battery approach. In R. W. Keith (Ed.), *Central auditory dysfunction* (pp. 43–72). New York: Grune & Stratton.

Willeford, J. A., & Burleigh, J. M. (1994). Sentence procedures in central testing. In J. Katz (Ed.), *Handbook of clinical audiology* (4th ed., pp. 256–268). Baltimore: Williams & Wilkins.

Wilson, L., & Mueller, H. G. (1984). Performance of normal hearing individuals on Auditec filtered speech tests. *Asha, 27*, 189.

5

Auditory Processing in Individuals with Auditory Neuropathy/Dys-synchrony

Gary Rance

Overview

Auditory neuropathy/dys-synchrony (AN/AD) type hearing loss forms a subset of the population of children and adults with auditory processing disorders. Affected patients fit the CAPD definition produced by the American Speech-Language-Hearing Association insofar as they show severe deficits in auditory discrimination, sound localization/lateralization, temporal aspects of audition, and auditory performance in competing signals (ASHA, 2005a, 2005b). Different models of information analysis have been discussed in the auditory processing literature. AN/AD patients fit the "bottom-up" model in that they show evidence of neural disruption in the auditory brainstem and beyond.

Auditory neuropathy/dys-synchrony patients differ from the broader population of CAPD in two important respects. First, unlike the majority of CAPD patients who show normal or only mildly disrupted electrophysiological potentials, AN/AD subjects show clear evidence of neural transmission disorder presenting with either absent or barely recognizable ABR waveforms. Second, this group of subjects typically present with significant hearing loss (in addition to their central processing difficulties). As such, discussion of auditory processing in subjects with AN/AD in this chapter is considered in relation to both normally hearing listeners and subjects with equivalent degrees of cochlear (sensorineural) hearing loss.

Introduction

Auditory neuropathy/dys-synchrony is a form of hearing impairment in which cochlear function appears normal but afferent neural activity in the auditory nerve and central auditory pathways is disordered (Berlin et al., 2001; Starr et al., 1996). This chapter summarizes the clinical profile for affected individuals and outlines the pattern of auditory processing deficits typically associated with the condition.

The Auditory Neuropathy/ Dys-synchrony Result Pattern

The clinical findings that distinguish AN/AD from "sensorineural" type hearing loss are the demonstration of preneural cochlear activity, in conjunction with an inability to record evoked neural activity from the auditory pathway. Cochlear outer hair cell function in such cases is reflected by the presence of otoacoustic emission (OAE) responses (the acoustic byproduct of the active mechanical processes of the cochlea [Kemp, 1978]) and cochlear microphonic (CM) responses (the receptor potentials produced by the polarization and depolarization of the cochlear outer hair cells [Dallos & Cheatham, 1976]). The auditory pathway disorder is suggested by the absence (or severe distortion) of electrical potentials from the auditory nerve (compound action potential) and auditory brainstem (ABR).

Figure 5–1 shows an example of the typical electrophysiological result pattern for a subject with AN/AD type hearing loss. The top tracing shows no ABR waveform to acoustic clicks presented at 100 dB nHL. Response absence to clicks at this level in a subject with peripheral (sensorineural or mixed) hearing loss would suggest that the stimulus was not loud enough to elicit electrical activity in the auditory pathway and would be indicative of at least a severe/profound loss in the mid-to-high frequency range (Rance et al., 1998). An ear with hearing loss of this degree would typically, however, show no response from the cochlear hair cells and yet this subject demonstrates clear CM potentials to unipolar stimuli (middle tracings). (Note the change in phase of the response as the stimulus polarity changes from rarefaction to compression indicating that the response is preneural and not part of the neural waveform.) Hence, it is the inconsistency between preneural and neural findings that is indicative of auditory pathway disorder in this case.

Disruption of the ABR in ears with AN/AD type hearing loss is thought to be the result of either a paucity of neural elements available to contribute to the response, or a disruption of the integrity of the neural activity (Rance, 2005). In the former case, the electrical signal produced by the auditory brainstem may simply be too small to be detected by scalp-sited recording electrodes distant from the generators in the auditory brainstem. In the latter, the auditory brainstem response may be unrecognizable due not to a lack of neural activity, but to a compromise of the temporal integrity of that activity (Berlin et al., 2001). Precise neural synchrony is required for the successful recording of the ABR as response extraction from within the overall EEG is typically based upon signal averaging processes which combine responses

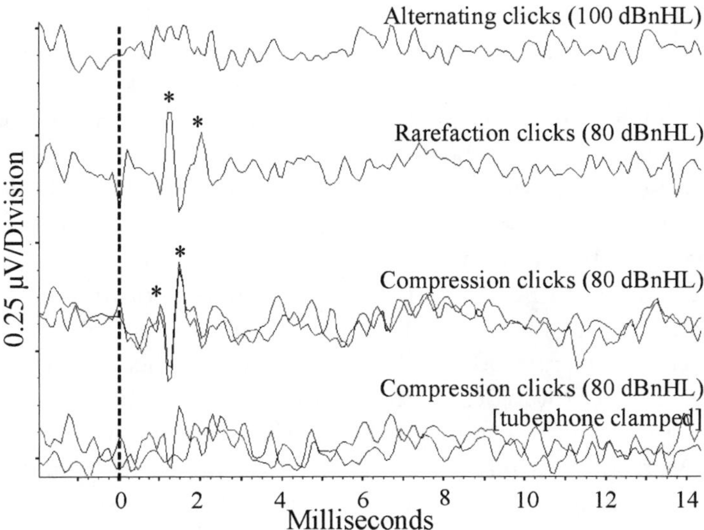

Figure 5–1. Averaged EEG tracings for a 2-month-old subject. The dashed line represents the point at which the stimulus was generated (at the transducer). The top tracing shows no recordable potentials to alternating acoustic clicks presented at 100 dB nHL. The middle tracings show repeatable cochlear microphonic responses but absent ABRs to unipolar stimuli at 80 dB nHL. Asterisks denote the positive peaks in the CM waveform. The bottom tracings were obtained to compression clicks presented with the tubephone clamped.

from individual stimuli to reduce random background activity (Clarke et al., 1961). As "dys-synchrony" or variation in the timing of neural firing of only a fraction of a millisecond is sufficient to disrupt recording of the averaged ABR waveform, it has been postulated that temporal inconsistency may be a factor in ears with the AN/AD result pattern (Kraus et al., 2000; Michalewski et al., 2005; Rance et al., 2004; Starr et al., 1991).

Despite the absence of auditory brainstem responses in affected ears, sound information can be transmitted through the auditory pathway. Many subjects, for example, can detect sounds at normal or near normal levels (Rance et al., 1999; Sininger & Oba, 2001). Furthermore, cortical auditory evoked potentials (in particular the N_1-P_2 waveform complex) which are thought to provide physiologic evidence of the perception of stimuli at the cortical level (Stapells, 2002) are identifiable in many AN/AD subjects (Kraus et al., 2000; Michalewski et al., 2005; Rance et al., 2002).

Mechanisms

A number of mechanisms that could produce the AN/AD result profile have been identified. Some possible sites of lesion include the cochlear inner hair cells, the synapse between these cells and Type 1 auditory nerve fibers and the auditory nerve itself (Amatuzzi et al., 2001; Rapin & Gravel, 2003, 2006; Starr et al., 1996).

Specific damage to the cochlear inner hair cells (IHC) could result in the decrement of the auditory brainstem response with preservation of preneural (outer hair cell) responses. The commonly held notion that the outer hair cells are particularly vulnerable to cochlear insult and that OHC loss occurs before IHC for most cochlear pathologies argues against the possibility of measuring OAE and CM responses in ears with significant IHC damage. There is, however, evidence from a range of animal models suggesting that certain types of cochlear insult (notably those caused by prolonged hypoxia) can have a greater effect on inner than outer hair cell survival (Billet et al., 1989; Bohne, 1976; Shirane & Harrison, 1987). In human subjects a large body of temporal bone work has failed to show specific IHC loss, but one study (Amatuzzi et al., 2001) has identified three babies from a group of NICU nonsurvivors with this result pattern.

A disorder affecting the synapse between cochlear IHCs and Type 1 auditory nerve fibres may also produce the AN/AD result pattern (Starr et al., 1991). Mechanisms by which synaptic disruption might occur in the auditory pathway are yet to be determined, but genetic dysfunction involving the otoferlin (OTOF) protein which affects neurotransmitter release and which has been found in the IHCs, has been identified in subjects with the AN/AD result pattern (Varga et al., 2003).

As the term "auditory neuropathy" suggests, the site of lesion in many affected patients is thought to be the nerve itself. Thirty to 40% of all AN/AD cases, and approximately 80% of all subjects with symptom onset above the age of 15 years, in fact, present with generalized neuropathic conditions and show a range of nonauditory symptoms including muscle weakness and atrophy, sensory loss, paresthesia (unusual sensations), and dysesthesia (discomfort). The site of the disorder affecting the auditory neural pathway may be the myelin sheath, the neuron, or a combination of both.

Myelin serves as an electrical insulator in the central nervous system. Demyelination results in delays in excitation, reductions in the velocity of action potential propagation, and an increase in conduction vulnerability (McDonald & Sears, 1970; Rasminsky & Sears, 1972). Fibers that are myelinated to differing degrees will, therefore, conduct neural signals at different speeds. Hence, the synchrony of discharges can be disrupted and processes dependent on temporal precision (such as the recording of ABRs) would be affected.

Loss of axons can occur as a result of specific disease processes or in conjunction with demyelinating conditions (Rapin & Gravel, 2003). An axonal neuropathy in the auditory pathway might not necessarily affect the timing of neural discharges, but would reduce the number of neural elements available to contribute to the overall response and might reduce the amplitude of the scalp-recorded ABR to the point where it is indistinguishable from the overall EEG.

Clinical Profile

Prevalence. The prevalence of auditory neuropathy/dys-synchrony in adult populations is difficult to determine. This is primarily because the physiologic test techniques that identify the condition (ABR/CM/OAE) are not routinely undertaken unless there are specific clinical indicators for retrocochlear abnormality such as asymmetric hearing or unusually poor speech perception. Pediatric populations, on the other hand, do routinely undergo these assessments in both newborn screening and diagnostic contexts, and the findings from this group suggest that AN/AD is a relatively high-incidence condition, particularly among babies who have had a difficult neonatal course. Data collected in our laboratory over a 5-year period (1991–1996), for example, found that 0.23% or 1 in every 423 subjects with risk factors for hearing loss presented with the AN/AD result pattern (Rance et al., 1999). Furthermore, a number of more recent studies have indicated that AN/AD-type loss accounts for a significant proportion (5–10%) of all permanent hearing loss in children (for a review see Rance, 2005).

Etiology. Although auditory neuropathy/dys-synchrony can occur in the absence of obvious health problems, the majority of reported cases (>70%) have presented with specific medical risk factors (Sininger & Oba, 2001). A number of different etiologies have been linked with the condition. These include transient neonatal insults (in particular involving anoxia and hyperbilirubinemia), infectious processes (such as mumps and meningitis) and genetic abnormalities (including mutations of several genes [OTOF, PMP22, MP2, NDGRGI] important for peripheral nerve function). (For reviews see Rance, 2005; Rapin & Gravel, 2003; Starr et al., 2003.)

Behavioral Audiogram. Hearing threshold levels in individuals with AN/AD vary across the audiometric range. Despite the fact that all affected subjects show absent or severely distorted auditory brainstem potentials, behavioral detection thresholds in both adult and pediatric populations are reasonably evenly distributed and range from normal to profound levels (Rance et al., 1999; Siniger & Oba, 2001). Interestingly, auditory perceptual ability (in particular the perception of speech information) is not strongly correlated with the behavioral audiogram in the AN/AD population (Rance et al., 2002; Zeng et al., 2001).

Speech Perception. Difficulties with speech understanding are a consistently reported feature of AN/AD type hearing loss. Most affected adults report perceptual deficits far greater than would be predicted from their audiometric results (Starr et al., 1996; Starr et al., 2000; Zeng et al., 2001). A high proportion of children with AN/AD also show only limited capacity to understand speech, even in favorable (quiet) listening conditions. Figure 5–2 shows open-set speech perception scores plotted against average hearing level for all of the children presented in the literature thus far. As can be seen from these data, approximately 50% of cases show perceptual ability poorer than the expected minimum for sensorineural hearing loss of equivalent degree.

In addition to these perceptual limitations in quiet, speech understanding in noise is also a particular problem for listeners with AN/AD type hearing loss. This may in some cases reflect the fact that their perceptual ability is so poor to begin with that any loss of

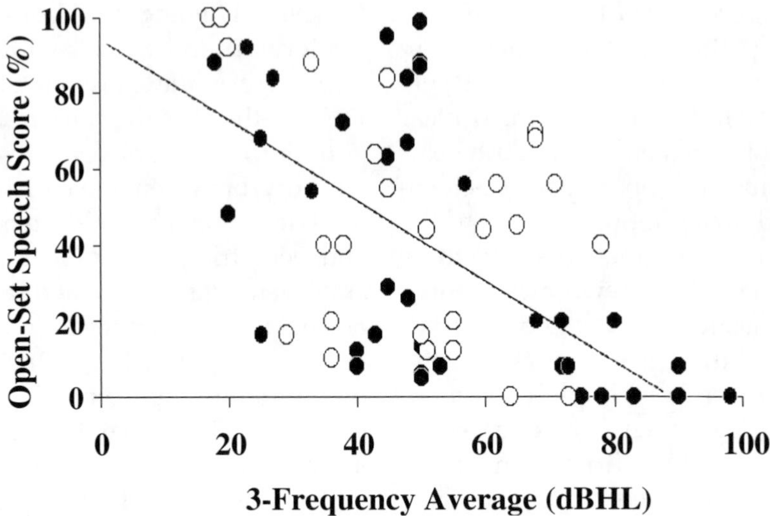

Figure 5–2. Open-set speech perception score/average hearing level comparisons for 76 children with AN/AD type hearing loss. The filled data points represent findings from open-set word tests and the open points show open-set sentence test results. The dashed line represents the minimum expected score for ears with sensorineural hearing loss (Yellin et al., 1989). Data for this meta-analysis were obtained from the following studies: Berlin et al. (1996); Konradsson (1996); Lee et al. (2001); Michalewski et al. (2005); Miyamoto et al. (1999); Picton et al. (1998); Rance et al. (2004); Sininger et al., (1995); Starr et al. (1991); Starr et al. (1998); Zeng et al. (2005); and Zeng and Liu (2006).

information in noise has a dramatic effect on overall speech understanding. However, a number of studies have presented subjects who could score at 100% on speech perception tasks in quiet, but who showed little or no perceptual ability even in relatively low levels of background noise (Kraus et al., 2000; Shallop, 2002).

Auditory Processing

The fact that understanding of speech is severely disrupted by auditory neuropathy/dys-synchrony despite adequate detection of sound (in many cases) suggests that signal distortion is the limiting factor to perceptual ability. In these subjects, who all show evidence of neural code disruption, it is useful to consider the "building-blocks" of auditory perception and how these basic processes are affected by AN/AD. Various perceptual abilities that underpin the perception of complex auditory signals (including speech) have been studied in subjects with normal acuity and subjects with sensorineural hearing loss. Some of these include: frequency resolution, intensity-related perception, temporal processing, and frequency discrimination.

Frequency Resolution

Frequency resolution is the ability of the auditory system to separate components in a complex sound. For example, to identify or "resolve" the formant peaks in a vowel sound. Spectral processing of this sort occurs at the level of the cochlea and is mediated by the active processes of the outer hair cells which amplify and sharpen the peaks of basilar membrane movement (Yates et al., 1992). As outer hair cell function (reflected by the presence of OAE and/or CM responses) is "normal" in ears with AN/AD type hearing loss, it is not surprising to find that frequency resolution measured both physiologically (through the generation of OAE suppression tuning curves [Abdala et al., 2000]), and psychophysically (Cacace et al., 1983; Rance et al., 2004) have been normal in most reported cases.

Intensity-Related Perception

Discrimination of intensity cues also appears to be normal in subjects with AN/AD. Zeng et al. (2005), in their recent study found, that intensity difference limen (the smallest perceivable level difference between stimuli) for a group of AN/AD subjects were similar to those obtained for a normally hearing control group. Subjects in both groups, for example, were able to consistently detect intensity differences of as little as 2 to 3 dB when stimuli were presented at reasonable sensation levels (≅ 50 dB). Furthermore, these authors also found that binaural intensity processing was normal in their cohort of AN/AD subjects. In this case, the sound lateralization percepts produced by the simultaneous presentation of stimuli at different levels in each ear were equivalent for the normal and AN/AD test groups (Zeng et al., 2005).

Processing of Temporal Cues

Apart from a reduction in signal audibility, disruption of timing-related information is the major way in which auditory perception is affected in subjects with AN/AD type hearing loss. Profound deficits have been reported in this population for a range of monaural and binaural processing abilities.

Temporal Resolution

Temporal resolution is the ability to perceive changes in auditory signals over time. The limit of the auditory system's ability to accurately encode or "resolve" rapid stimulus changes has most commonly been measured using "gap detection" tasks where the shortest detectable silent period in a burst of noise is determined. Gap detection ability in subjects with AN/AD type hearing loss is significantly poorer than for normally hearing listeners (Michalewski et al., 2005; Starr et al., 1991; Zeng et al., 1999; Zeng et al., 2005). Where normal subjects can typically perceive gaps of less than 5 msec (in stimuli presented at reasonable sensation levels), individuals with AN/AD typically require silent periods of 20 msec or more.

Temporal resolution can also be assessed by determining a subject's "temporal modulation transfer function (TMTF)" which measures their ability to detect sinusoidal amplitude fluctuations (at different modulation rates) in the level of a steady-state signal. (See

Case Study later in this chapter.) TMTF findings for AN/AD patients have been variable, but have typically shown an impaired capacity to detect amplitude changes (Rance et al., 2004; Zeng et al., 1999; Zeng et al., 2005). Extreme cases have even shown an inability to detect 100% amplitude changes for modulation rates in excess of 100 Hz (Rance et al., 2004). Overall, TMTF findings indicate that individuals with AN/AD struggle to track fast and even relatively slow (<10 Hz) amplitude envelope changes over time.

Forward and Backward Masking

Impaired processing abilities in AN/AD patients have also been demonstrated in temporal masking studies (Kraus et al., 2000; Zeng et al., 2005). Forward and backward masking experiments examining the detection of brief tones in the proximity of masking stimuli, have suggested that short signals within approximately 100 msec of a masker are more difficult for AN/AD listeners to perceive. Normally hearing subjects, in contrast, show only limited masking effects when the target is beyond approximately 10 to 20 msec of the masker (Zeng et al., 2005). As such, AN/AD patients show a reduced capacity to separate sounds that occur successively.

Binaural Temporal Processing

As well as demonstrating monaural temporal processing limitations, AN/AD patients also show an impaired ability to integrate binaural temporal cues. Abnormal Masking Level Difference (MLD) results, for example, are a consistently reported finding (Berlin et al., 1993; Hood et al., 1999; Starr et al., 1991; Starr et al., 1996). MLD assessment measures the release from masking obtained when a signal or noise is presented out of phase with a competing signal in the contralateral ear. Normally hearing subjects typically show a masking level difference (with dichotic phase inversion) of approximately 10 dB indicating that phase information from each ear has been accurately represented at the level of the lower brainstem (Licklider, 1948). AN/AD subjects, in contrast, typically show no masking release suggesting an inability to accurately combine the neural code from each ear.

Localization based upon binaural timing cues is also impaired in AN/AD patients. Despite the fact that affected individuals can use interaural intensity differences to make lateralization judgments (Zeng et al., 2005) a number of studies have found that even gross timing differences (between ears) are not interpreted as changes in sound direction (Starr et al., 1991; Kaga et al., 1996; Zeng et al., 2005). Zeng et al. (2005), for example, found that in their normally hearing cohort, interaural timing differences of <0.2 msec resulted in a consistent change in perceived stimulus position whereas their AN/AD subjects showed no perceptual shift even with interaural differences of 0.5 msec.

Frequency Discrimination

Frequency discrimination is the ability to perceive changes in the pitch of a single stimulus over time, or across individual stimuli. High-frequency discrimination (≥4 kHz) is thought to be dependent upon the spatial excitation arrangement along the basilar membrane (Sek & Moore, 1995). Discrimination of lower frequency sounds is similarly influenced by this tonotopic cochlear representation, but is also enhanced by temporal information (Sek & Moore, 1995). In particular it has been hypothesized that "phase locking" (where neural firing patterns reflect the stimulus waveform) can fine-tune discrimination in this frequency range. (Neural refractory limitations prevent phase locking for high-frequency signals.) Phase locking requires a high degree of temporal precision and so, not surprisingly, individuals with AN/AD type hearing loss show an inability to use these cues and demonstrate severely impaired frequency discrimination ability (Rance et al., 2004; Zeng et al., 2005). Elevated frequency difference limen have been reported for AN/AD subjects at all frequencies in the audiometric range, but low-frequency perception is most affected, typically showing difference limen more than 10 times greater than those of normally hearing subjects.

Temporal Processing and Neural Conduction Disorder

The precise mechanisms by which temporal cues are disrupted in the auditory pathway of AN/AD patients are unclear. As mentioned previously, the absence or severe distortion of the auditory brainstem response does, however, point to a dys-synchrony of neural firing in the peripheral auditory system. The degree to which neural precision is affected in individual cases is difficult to determine and may vary significantly across the AN/AD population. Disruption of averaged potentials from the brainstem would suggest a temporal distortion of at least 0.5 msec (Kraus et al., 2000; Sininger et al., 1995) and some patients, perhaps those with only mildly depressed psychophysics results and reasonable speech perception (see Figure 5–2), may suffer a temporal disruption close to this limit. On the other hand, some psychophysics results (such as the TMTF findings which in some cases reveal an inability to accurately encode even slow [≤10 Hz] amplitude changes), suggest neural disruptions of the order of tens of milliseconds.

Temporal Processing and Speech Perception

The specific effects of temporal processing deficits in subjects with AN/AD type hearing loss on speech perception are yet to be fully considered. Kraus et al. (2000) have suggested that an inability to detect brief gaps in the speech signal affects the perception of brief vowel features such as third formant onset frequency. One might also expect consonant place of articulation cues based upon subtle voice onset time differences to be similarly affected. A compromised ability to perceive overall amplitude envelope cues (as suggested by the TMTF findings) might also be expected to have a negative impact on speech understanding (Shannon et al., 1995; Turner et al., 1995). Furthermore, an impaired ability to separate sounds occurring successively (as indicated by the forward and backward masking studies) may produce excessive intraspeech masking effects where louder speech elements (such as vowels) could mask out brief consonant information.

Whatever the specific effects, it is clear that temporal processing deficits in subjects with AN/AD do limit overall speech understanding. In studies involving both adults (Zeng et al., 1999) and children (Rance et al., 2004) the degree of temporal processing disruption has been strongly correlated with speech perception performance. As such, these populations resemble other subject groups (including elderly listeners, children with learning disorders, and patients with multiple sclerosis) in which temporal processing disorders have been linked with speech understanding deficits (Gordon-Salant & Fitzgibbons, 1993; Kraus et al., 1996; Levine et al., 1993; Tallal, 1981; Wright et al., 1997).

Case Study

To illustrate the pattern and severity of the perceptual difficulties associated with auditory neuropathy/dyssynchrony type hearing loss, findings for a "typical" child are presented. Subject X is a 9-year-old girl who was born at 32 weeks gestation weighing 2.1 kg. Despite her prematurity she showed no neonatal risk factors for permanent hearing loss apart from hyperbilirubinemia (Peak SBR: 420 µmol/L). Click-ABR assessment carried out at 2 months (corrected age) revealed the AN/AD result pattern with absent ABRs at maximum presentation levels but clear cochlear microphonic potentials to unipolar clicks at 80 dB nHL (see Figure 5–1). Transient otoacoustic emission responses were also present bilaterally.

This child was not immediately provided with amplification (as it is not possible to predict the audiogram of babies with AN/AD type hearing loss from evoked potential findings) but was subsequently fit with behind-the-ear hearing aids at 6 months of age when conditioned audiometric testing revealed symmetric mild/moderate hearing loss (Figure 5–3). The hearing aids were fit to match the audiometric configuration and afforded Subject X complete access to the speech spectrum at normal levels.

Apart from her hearing-related difficulties, Subject X has shown a reasonably normal developmental course. She met all of her physical milestones at the expected times. A Kaufman Brief Intelligence Test conducted at 7 years of age also demonstrated age-appropriate (nonverbal) cognitive development.

Subject X attended an early intervention center from the age of 3 months where her family was supported in their desire to pursue an oral-aural communication strategy. She was sub-

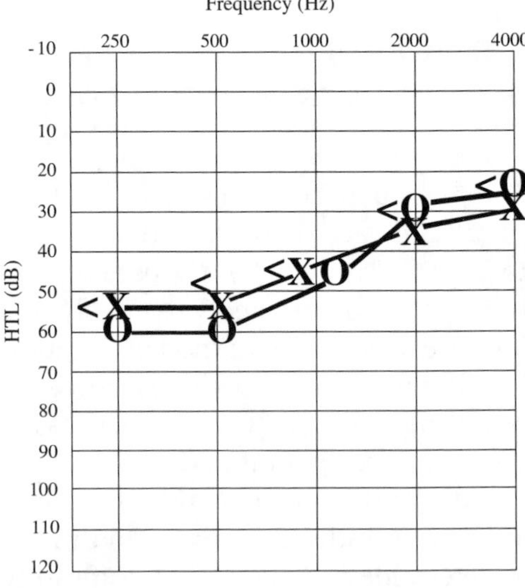

Figure 5–3. Behavioral audiogram for Subject X.

sequently integrated into her local (mainstream) primary school with visiting teacher support. Her overall speech and language development has been delayed (relative to normally hearing children) but is similar to that of her peers with sensorineural hearing loss. Subject X's Language Quotient (LQ) score on the Peabody Picture Vocabulary Test, for example, indicated that her word comprehension is developing at about 60% of the normal rate. Similar results are common for children with congenital sensorineural loss in the mild-severe range (Blamey et al., 2001).

Speech perception ability in quiet listening conditions for Subject X was also broadly consistent with that of her peers with sensorineural hearing loss. As can be seen in Figure 5–4, her open-set word score (69%) was somewhat lower than those of an age-matched group of sensorineural children, but was still within the range expected for permanent SN-loss of moderate degree.

Listening in noise, however, has been a consistent problem for Subject X. Although she does wear an RF-device at school to improve her signal-to-noise ratio, both she and her teachers report extreme difficulties in understanding speech in the classroom environment. Figure 5–5 shows the effects of a competing signal on her perceptual ability. As can be seen in the performance functions for the hearing-impaired control children, background noise impairs perception in subjects with sensorineural hearing loss more than it does individuals with normal

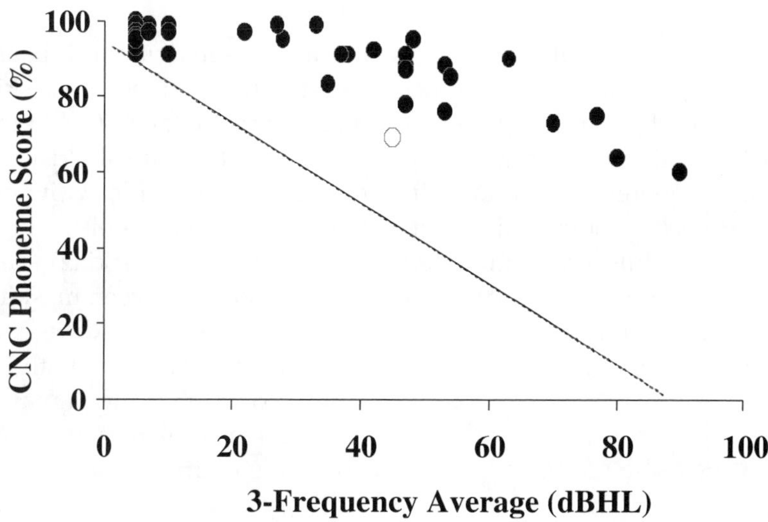

Figure 5–4. Open-set speech perception score/average hearing level comparisons for a group of subjects aged 5 to 12 years at assessment. Filled data points represent the findings for 25 normally hearing children and 20 children with sensorineural hearing loss (Rance et al., in press). The unfilled data point shows the CNC phoneme score obtained for Subject X. The dashed line represents the minimum expected score for ears with sensorineural hearing loss (Yellin et al., 1989).

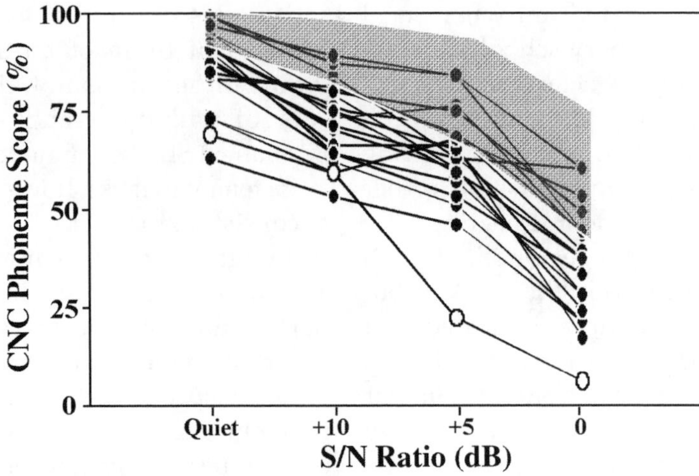

Figure 5–5. Open-set speech perception score plotted as a function of signal-to-noise ratio. The shaded area represents the performance range (mean ± 2 SD) for a group of normally hearing subjects (*n* = 25). Functions with filled datapoints show the findings for 20 children with sensorineural hearing loss (Rance et al., in press). Results obtained for Subject X are represented by unfilled data points.

hearing. (Regression analysis in this study showed significantly steeper functions for the SN subject group [Rance et al, in press].) The findings for Subject X, were however, poorer again and indicate that at speech-to-noise ratios typically endured by children in untreated classroom environments (0–3 dB) this child's perceptual ability was negligible (Crandell & Smaldino, 2000).

Psychophysical Profile

Frequency resolution, as discussed previously in this chapter is often normal in individuals with AN/AD-type hearing loss. Figure 5–6 shows findings from a masking experiment that measured spectral resolution and (indirectly) auditory filter width, in children with normal hearing (3-frequency average ≤15 dB HL) and children with mild/moderate sensorineural hearing loss using a notched noise masking technique (Rance et al., 2004). In this procedure, detection threshold for a 1-kHz tone is established in white noise, and then again in white noise with a 500-Hz notch (centered at 1 kHz). The threshold difference between masking conditions (the masking difference level) provides an estimate of the subject's ability to resolve the signal in noise. (Greater release from masking in the notched condition indicates a narrower auditory filter.) As can be seen in Figure 5–6, frequency resolution in the subjects with SN hearing impairment was significantly reduced, presumably as a result of a loss of outer hair cell function and, hence, disruption of the "active process" (Sellick et al., 1982). Similar frequency resolution results have been reported in other studies involving both adults and children

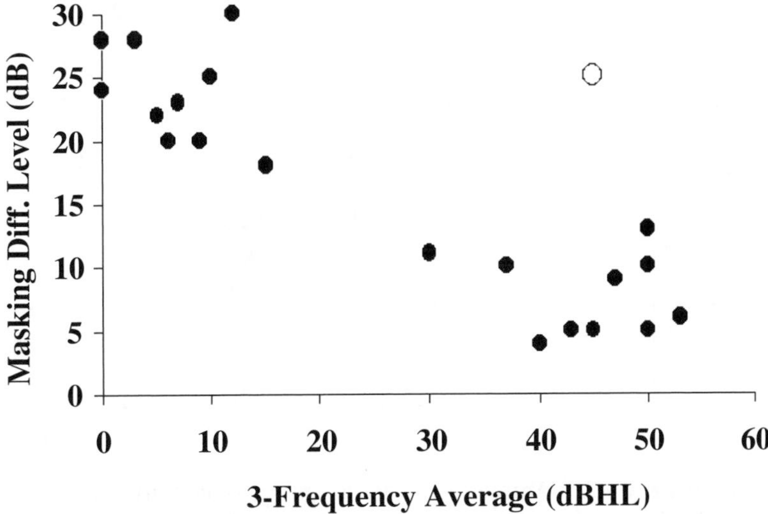

Figure 5–6. White/notched noise masker difference levels for subjects with normal hearing (3-frequency average ≤15 dB HL) and children with sensorineural hearing loss of mild-moderate degree (three-frequency average 30–55 dB HL). (Rance et al., 2004). Masking difference level for Subject X is represented by the unfilled data point.

with sensorineural loss (for a review, see Moore, 1995). Subject X, in contrast, showed evidence of normal frequency resolution, consistent with the presence of normal cochlear mechanics.

An estimate of temporal resolution ability was obtained for Subject X by measuring a temporal modulation transfer function (Figure 5–7). This example demonstrates the common finding that temporal processing is relatively unaffected by sensorineural hearing loss. Other studies have shown similar results (provided the stimuli can be presented at a sufficient sensation level) for temporal resolution measured in both TMTF (Moore, 1995, 1996) and gap detection (Florentine & Buus, 1984; Nelson & Thomas, 1997) experiments. Results for Subject X, in contrast, show a severely impaired awareness of amplitude changes, and hence suggest impaired temporal processing capacity. Her inability to detect high-rate modulation in particular, suggest that dys-synchrony in the auditory pathway may have degraded the encoding of rapidly occurring amplitude fluctuations. At the 150-Hz modulation rate for example, Subject X could only perceive amplitude changes of 0 dB (or 100%).

Subjects X's ability to detect pitch changes was measured for low- and high-pitch stimuli. Her discrimination limen for 500-Hz and 4-kHz tones are shown along with those of control subjects with normal hearing and sensorineural hearing loss (Figures 5–8A and 5–8B). Of note in these data is the high degree of precision shown by the normal listeners. At the 500-Hz test frequency, for example, subjects could typically hear a pitch difference between stimuli only 4 Hz apart (i.e., between 500 Hz and 504 Hz). Similarly, at 4 kHz the normal subjects could in most cases

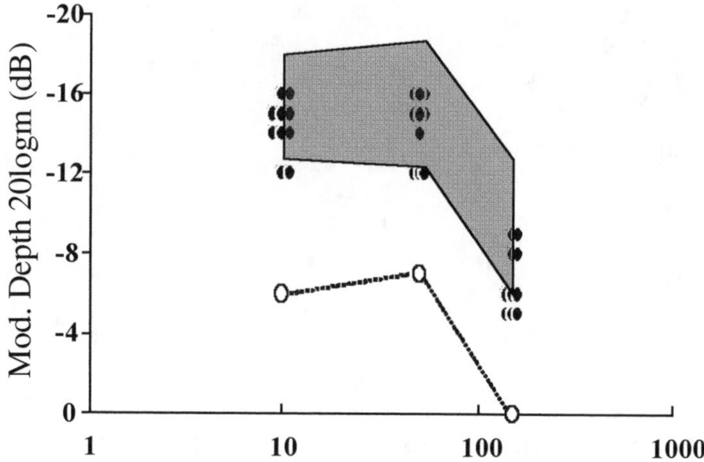

Figure 5–7. Amplitude modulation detection thresholds plotted as a function of modulation rate. The shaded area represents the performance range for a group of normally hearing children (n = 10). Filled data points show the findings for 10 children with sensorineural hearing loss of mild-moderate degree (Rance et al., 2004). Unfilled circles represent the findings for Subject X.

detect a difference of 40 Hz or only 1% of the target frequency. Children with sensorineural hearing loss were mildly impaired in their ability to discriminate both low- and high-frequency signals. This finding is consistent with other studies that have shown degradation of frequency discrimination ability with cochlear damage (Freyman & Nelson, 1986; Moore & Peters, 1992). Frequency discrimination for Subject X was poorer than that of the normal cohort and that of subjects with equivalent degrees of sensorineural loss at both test frequencies. This was particularly the case for the 500-Hz tone where her difference limen (75 Hz) was approximately 4 times the SN-group mean. As Subject X shows normal frequency resolution, it seems likely that her significant discrimination deficits are the result of an impaired ability to use temporal (phase locking) cues.

In summary, the findings presented in this case study demonstrate that the perceptual profile typical of subjects with auditory neuropathy/dys-synchrony is quite different from that seen for sensorineural hearing loss. Subjects in the latter group, as a result of their abnormal cochlear function, show impaired frequency resolution and frequency discrimination but normal temporal processing. Individuals with AN/AD, on the other hand, typically present with normal cochlear processing and hence normal frequency resolution, but as a consequence of their neural transmission deficiencies, show severe disruption of timing cues. Both types of hearing loss affect speech understanding (although probably in different ways) and both result in difficulties in background noise, but overall the perceptual disruption caused by auditory neuropathy/dys-synchrony is far more pronounced.

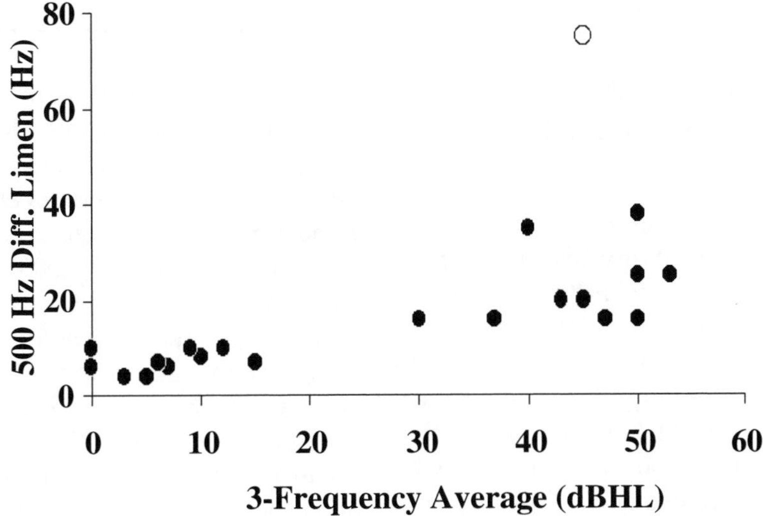

A

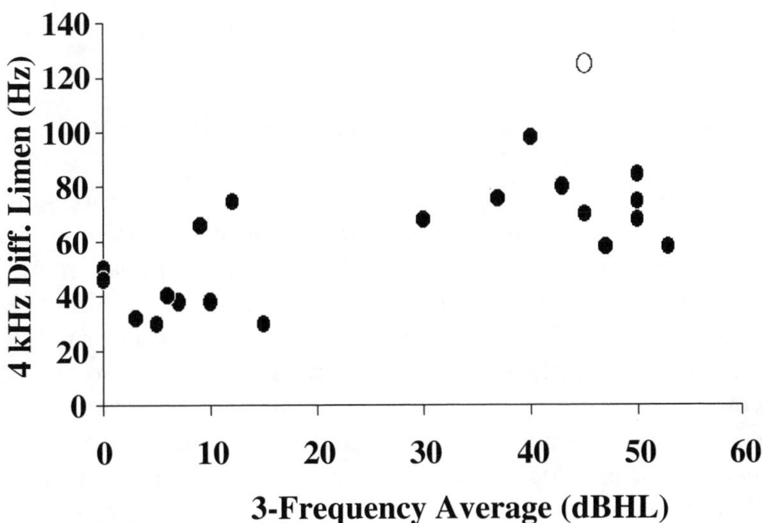

B

Figure 5–8. A. Frequency discrimination limen for a 500-Hz target stimulus plotted as a function of three-frequency average hearing level in subjects with normal hearing (*n* = 10) and sensorineural hearing loss (*n* = 10) (Rance et al., 2004). The unfilled data point shows the difference limen for Subject X. **B.** Frequency discrimination limen for a 4-kHz target stimulus plotted as a function of three-frequency average hearing level in subjects with normal hearing (*n* = 10) and sensorineural hearing loss (*n* = 10) (Rance et al., 2004). The unfilled data point shows the difference limen for Subject X.

Management of AN/AD Type Hearing Loss

As the pattern of perceptual deficits in auditory neuropathy/dys-synchrony type hearing loss is fundamentally different from that associated with sensorineural loss, different management approaches are required. The application of AN/AD-specific habilitation strategies in this population is yet to be thoroughly investigated. Optimization of the input provided to affected ears has, however, been considered.

Amplification

The provision of hearing aids to AN/AD patients (particularly children) has been a controversial issue. There are two main arguments against amplification in this population. The first is that high-level inputs may damage the cochleae in these ears with normal outer hair cell function. The second is that conventional amplification will not overcome the temporal distortion introduced into the system by the auditory pathway disorder. That is, the listener will be presented with a louder, but equally disrupted, signal. The potential benefit offered by amplification relates to the subjects' access to sound. As many affected individuals have significantly elevated hearing thresholds, they simply cannot detect speech and other signals at normal levels.

Conventional amplification outcomes in patients with AN/AD have been mixed. Some children (perhaps those with lesser degrees of temporal disruption) have responded well to hearing aids and have shown aided speech perception abilities consistent with their sensorineural counterparts (Rance et al., 2002). In many youngsters and almost all affected adults, however, conventional amplification has been of little or no benefit (Rance et al., 2005; Starr et al., 1996). As a result, amplification systems employing signal-processing strategies designed to target the particular processing deficits associated with AN/AD have been considered (Zeng et al., 2001). For example, processing algorithms that accentuate temporal and/or amplitude differences or transpose spectral information into the high-frequency region where temporal (phase locking) cues are less of an issue may, in the future, improve outcomes in some cases.

Cochlear Implants

Cochlear implantation is currently the intervention option of choice for AN/AD patients with severe auditory processing difficulties. Almost all reported cases have shown normal device function, significant perceptual benefits, and speech perception performance levels consistent with their implanted sensorineural peers (Madden et al., 2002; Mason et al., 2003; 2001; Shallop, 2002; Trautwein et al., 2001; Zeng & Liu, 2006). These findings may seem counterintuitive for a group of subjects with evidence of auditory pathway disorder, and yet of the more than 100 reported subjects, only a handful have shown poor outcomes (Miyamoto et al., 1999; Rance et al., 1999). The ways in which perception is improved by the cochlear implant in ears with AN/AD is currently under investigation. Interestingly, most implanted subjects show recordable ABRs to electrical stimulation (where previously, to acoustic stimulation, they had not). This suggests either an increase in the number of neural elements contributing to the ABR (perhaps as a result of bypassing a cochlear abnormality when stimulating the spiral ganglion directly) or an improvement in the synchrony of neural firing in the brainstem (perhaps reflecting the fact that the electrical stimuli produced by cochlear implants are presented in the form of discrete pulses rather than analog signals). Whatever the explanation, it would seem that cochlear implants offer a means of reducing the perceptual challenges posed by AN/AD type hearing loss.

Summary

Auditory neuropathy/dys-synchrony is a clear example of a "bottom-up" type processing disorder. Affected individuals show physiologic evidence of neural transmission disorder in the auditory brainstem, which results in a unique pattern of perceptual deficits and appears to resolve (at least to the point where ABRs are recordable) when the stimulus mode changes from an acoustic signal passed through the peripheral auditory system to electrical stimulation presented directly to the auditory neural pathway.

Key Points Learned

- Auditory neuropathy/dys-synchrony is a disorder affecting transmission of afferent neural signals in the auditory brainstem (and beyond).
- Subjects with this condition show electrophysiological evidence (absent or distorted ABR waveforms) of auditory pathway disorder.
- Affected children and adults typically demonstrate a range of perceptual deficits related to the disruption of timing cues.
- Speech understanding in quiet, and particularly in background noise, can be severely compromised by AN/AD type hearing loss.

References

Abdala, C., Sininger, Y. S., & Starr, A. (2000). Distortion product otoacoustic emission suppression in subjects with auditory neuropathy. *Ear and Hearing, 21*, 542–553.

Amatuzzi, M. G., Northrop, C., Liberman, C., Thornton, A., Halpin, C., Herrmann, B., et al. (2001). Selective inner hair cell loss in premature infants and cochlear pathological patterns from neonatal intensive care unit autopsies. *Archives of Otolaryngology-Head and Neck Surgery, 127*, 629–636.

American Speech-Language-Hearing Association. (2005a). *(Central) auditory processing disorders* [Technical report]. Rockville, MD: Author.

American Speech-Language-Hearing Association. (2005b). *(Central) auditory processing disorders—The role of the audiologist* [Position statement]. Rockville, MD: Author.

Berlin, C. I., Hood, L. J., Cecola, R. P., Jackson, D. F. & Szabo, P. (1993). Does Type I afferent neuron dysfunction reveal itself through lack of efferent suppression? *Hearing Research, 65*, 40–50.

Berlin, C. I., Hood, L. J., Hurley, M. S., & Wen, H. (1996). Hearing aids: only for hearing impaired patients with abnormal otoacoustic emissions. In C. I. Berlin (Ed.), *Hair cells and hearing aids* (pp. 99–111). San Diego, CA: Singular Publishing Group.

Berlin, C. I., Hood, L. J., & Rose, K. (2001). On renaming auditory neuropathy as auditory dys-synchrony. *Audiology Today, 13*, 15–17.

Billet, T. E., Thorne, P. R., & Gavin, J. B. (1989). The nature and progression of injury in the organ of Corti during ischemia. *Hearing Research, 41*, 189–198.

Blamey, P. J., Sarant, J. Z., Paatsch, L. E., Barry, J. G., Bow, C. P., Wales, R. J., et al. (2001). Relationships among speech perception, production, language, hearing loss, and age in children with impaired hearing. *Journal of Speech, Language and Hearing Research, 44*, 264–285.

Bohne, B.A. (1976). Mechanisms of noise damage in the inner ear. In D. Henderson, R. P. Hamernick, D. S. Dosanjh, & J. H. Mills (Eds.), *Effects of noise on hearing* (pp. 41–68). New York: Raven.

Cacace, A. T., Satya-Murti, S., & Grimes, C. T. (1983). Frequency selectivity and temporal processing in Friedreich's ataxia. *Annals Otology, Rhinology and Laryngology, 92*, 276–280.

Clarke, W. A., Goldstein, M. H., Brown, R. M., Molnar, C. E., O'Brien, D. F., & Zeiman, H. E. (1961). The average response computer (ARC): A digital device for computing averages and amplitudes and time histograms of electrophysiological responses. *Transactions of IRE, 8*, 46–51.

Crandell, C. C., & Smaldino, J. J. (2000). Classroom acoustics for children with normal hearing and with hearing impairment. *Language Speech and Hearing Services in Schools, 31*, 362–370.

Dallos, P., & Cheatham, M. A. (1976). Production of cochlear potentials by inner and outer hair cells. *Journal of the Acoustical Society of America, 60*, 510–512.

Florentine, M., & Buus, S. (1984). Temporal gap detection in sensorineural and simulated hearing impairments. *Journal of Speech and Hearing Research, 27*, 449–455.

Freyman, R. L., & Nelson, D. A (1986). Frequency discrimination as a function of tonal duration and excitation-pattern slopes in normal and hearing-impaired listeners. *Journal of the Acoustical Society of America, 79*, 1034–1044.

Gordon-Salant, S., & Fitzgibbons, P. J. (1993). Temporal factors and speech recognition performance in young and elderly listeners. *Journal of Speech Hearing Research, 36*, 1276–1285.

Hood, L. J. (1999). A review of objective methods of evaluating neural pathways. *Laryngoscope, 109*, 1745–1748.

Kaga, K., Nakamura, M., Shinogami, M, Tsuzuku, T., Yamada, K. & Shindo, M. (1996). Auditory nerve disease of both ears revealed by auditory brainstem responses, electrocochleography and otoacoustic emissions. *Scandinavian Audiology, 25*, 233–238.

Kemp, D. T. (1978). Stimulated acoustic emission from the human auditory system. *Journal of the Acoustical Society of America, 64*, 1386–1391.

Konradsson, K. S. (1996). Bilaterally presented otoacoustic emissions in four children with profound idiopathic unilateral hearing loss. *Audiology, 35*, 217–227.

Kraus, N., Bradlow, A. R., Cheatham, J., Cunningham, C. D., King, D. B., Koch, T. G., et al. (2000). Consequences of neural asynchrony: A case of auditory neuropathy. *Journal of Association of Research in Otolaryngology, 1*(1), 33–45.

Kraus, N., McGee, T. J., Carrell, T. D., Zecker, S.G., Nicol, T. G., & Koch, D. B. (1996). Auditory neurophysiologic responses and discrimination deficits in children with learning problems. *Science, 273*, 971–973.

Lee, J. S. M., McPherson, B., Yuen K. C. P., & Wong, L. L. N. (2001). Screening for auditory neuropathy in a school for hearing impaired children. *International Journal of Paediatric Otorhinolaryngology, 61*, 39–46.

Levine, R. A., Gardner, J. C., Fullerton, B. C., Stufflebeam, S. M., Carlisle, E. W., Furst, M., et al. (1993). Effects of multiple sclerosis brainstem lesions on sound lateralization and brainstem auditory evoked potentials. *Hearing Research, 68*, 73–88.

Licklider, J. C. R. (1948). The influence of interaural phase relation upon the masking of speech by white noise. *Journal of the Acoustical Society of America, 20*, 150–159.

Madden, C., Rutter, M., Hilbert, L., Greinwald, J., & Choo, D. (2002). Clinical and audiological features in auditory neuropathy. *Archives of Otolaryngology-Head and Neck Surgery, 128*, 1026–1030.

Mason, J. C., De Michele, A., Stevens, C., Ruth, R. & Hashisaki, G. (2003). Cochlear implantation in patients with auditory neuropathy of varied etiologies. *Laryngoscope, 113*(1), 45–49.

McDonald, W. I., & Sears, T. A. (1970). The effects of experimental demyelination on conduction in the central nervous system. *Brain, 93*, 583–598.

Michalewski, H. J., Starr, A., Nguyen, T. T., Kong, Y-Y., & Zeng, F- G. (2005). Auditory temporal processes in normal-hearing individuals and in patients with auditory neuropathy. *Clinical Neurophysiology, 116*, 669–680.

Miyamoto, R. T., Iler Kirk, K., Renshaw, J., & Hussain, D. (1999). Cochlear implantation in auditory neuropathy. *Laryngoscope, 109*, 181–185.

Moore, B. C. J. (1995). Speech perception in people with cochlear damage. In *Perceptual consequences of cochlear damage* (Chapter 7, pp. 147–172). Oxford: Oxford University Press.

Moore, B. C. J. (1996). Perceptual consequences of cochlear hearing loss and their implications for the design of hearing aids. *Ear and Hearing, 17*, 133–160.

Moore, B. C. J., & Peters, R. W. (1992). Pitch discrimination and phase sensitivity in young and elderly subjects and its relationship to frequency selectivity. *Journal of the Acoustical Society of Am*erica, *91*, 2881–2893.

Nelson, P. B., & Thomas, S. D (1997). Gap detection as a function of stimulus loudness for listeners with and without hearing loss. *Journal of Speech and Language Hearing Research, 40*, 1397–1394.

Picton, T. W., Durieux-Smith, A., Champagne, S. C., Whittingham, J., Moran, L. M., Giguere, C., et al. (1998). Objective evaluation of aided thresholds using auditory steady-state responses. *Journal of the American Academy of Audio*logy, *9*, 315–331.

Rance, G. (2005). Auditory neuropathy/dys-synchrony and it's perceptual consequences. *Trends in Amplification, 9*(1), 1–43.

Rance, G., Barker, E., Mok, M., Dowell, R., Rincon, A., & Garratt, R. (in press). Speech perception in noise for children with auditory neuropathy/dys-synchrony type hearing loss. *Ear and Hearing.*

Rance, G., Beer, D. E., Cone-Wesson, B., Shepherd R. K., Dowell, R. C., King, A. K., et al. (1999). Clinical findings for a group of infants and young children with auditory neuropathy. *Ear and Hearing, 20*, 238–252.

Rance, G., Cone-Wesson, B., Wunderlich, J., & Dowell, R. C. (2002). Speech perception and cortical event related potentials in children with auditory neuropathy. *Ear and Hearing, 23*, 239–253.

Rance, G., Dowell, R. C., Rickards, F. W., Beer, D. E., & Clark, G. M. (1998). Steady-state evoked potential and behavioural hearing thresholds in a group of children with absent click-evoked auditory brainstem response. *Ear and Hearing, 19,* 48–61.

Rance, G., McKay, C., & Grayden, D. (2004). Perceptual characterisation of children with auditory neuropathy. *Ear* and *Hearing, 25,* 34–46.

Rapin, I., & Gravel, J. (2003). "Auditory neuropathy": physiologic and pathologic evidence calls for more diagnostic specificity. *International Journal of Pediatric Otorhinolaryngology, 67,* 707–728.

Rapin, I., & Gravel, J. (2006). Auditory neuropathy: A biologically inappropriate label unless acoustic nerve involvement is documented. *Journal of American Academy of Audiology,* 17, 147–150.

Rasminsky, M., & Sears, T. A. (1972). Internodal conduction in undissected demyelinated nerve fibres. *Journal of Physiology, 227,* 323–350.

Sek, A., & Moore, B. C. J. (1995). Frequency discrimination as a function of frequency, measured in several ways. *Journal of Acoustical Society of America, 97,* 2479–2486.

Sellick, P. M., Patuzzi, R., & Johnstone, B. M. (1982). Measurement of basilar membrane motion in the guinea pig using the Mossbauer technique. *Journal of Acoustical Society of America, 72,* 131–141.

Shallop, J. K. (2002). Auditory neuropathy/dys-synchrony in adults and children. *Seminar in Hearing, 23*(3), 215–223.

Shannon, R. V., Zeng, F.- G., & Kamath, V. (1995). Speech recognition with primarily temporal cues. *Science, 270,* 303–304.

Shirane, M., & Harrison, R. V. (1987). The effects of hypoxia on sensory cells of the cochlea. *Scanning Microscopy, 1,* 1175–1183.

Sininger, Y. S., Hood, L. J., Starr, A., Berlin, C. I., & Picton, T. W. (1995). Hearing loss due to auditory neuropathy. *Audiology Today, 7,* 10–13.

Sininger, Y. S., & Oba, S. (2001). Patients with auditory neuropathy: Who are they and what can they hear? In Y. S. Sininger & A. Starr (Eds.), *Auditory neuropathy* (pp. 37–50). San Diego, CA: Singular Publishing Group.

Stapells, D. R. (2002). Cortical event-related potentials to auditory stimuli. In J. Katz (Ed.), *Handbook of clinical audiology*. Baltimore: Lippincott Williams & Wilkins.

Starr, A., McPherson, D., Patterson, J., Don, M., Luxford, W., Shannon, R., et al. (1991). Absence of both auditory evoked potentials and auditory percepts dependent on timing cues. *Brain, 114,* 1157–1180.

Starr, A., Michalewski, H. J., Zeng, F.- G., Fujikawa-Brooks, S., Linthicum, F., Kim, C. S., et al. (2003). Pathology and physiology of auditory neuropathy with a novel mutation in the *MPZ* gene. *Brain, 126,* 1604–1619.

Starr, A., Picton, T. W., Sininger, Y. S., Hood, L. J., & Berlin, C. I. (1996). Auditory Neuropathy. *Brain, 119*(3), 741–753.

Starr, A., Sininger, Y. S., & Pratt, H. (2000). The varieties of auditory neuropathy. *Journal of Basic and Clinical Physiology and Pharmacology, 11*(3), 215–230.

Starr, A., Sininger, Y. S., Winter, M., Derebery, M. J., Oba, S., & Michalewski, H. J. (1998). Transient deafness due to temperature-sensitive auditory neuropathy. *Ear and Hearing, 19,* 169–179.

Tallal, P. (1981). Language disabilities in children: perceptual correlates. *International Journal of Pediatric Otorhinolaryngology,* 3, 1–3.

Trautwein, P., Shallop J., Fabry, L., & Friedman, R. (2001). Cochlear implantation of patients with auditory neuropathy. In Y. S. Sininger & A. Starr (Eds.), *Auditory neuropathy* (pp. 203–232). San Diego, CA: Singular Publishing Group.

Turner, C. W., Souza, P. E., & Forget, L. N. (1995). Use of temporal envelope cues in speech recognition by normal and hearing-impaired listeners. *Journal of Acoustical Society of America, 97,* 2568–2576.

Varga, R., Kelley, P. M., Keats, B. J., Starr, A., Leal, S. M., Cohn, E., et al. (2003). Nonsyndromic recessive auditory neuropathy is the result of mutations in the otoferlin (OTOF) gene. *Journal of Medical Genetics, 40*, 45–50.

Wright, B. A., Lombardino, L. J., King, W. M, Puranik, C. S., Leonard, C. M., & Merzenich, M. M. (1997). Deficits in auditory temporal and spectral resolution in language-impaired children. *Nature. 387*, 176–178.

Yates, G. K., Johnstone, B. M., Patuzzi, R. B., & Robertson, D. (1992). Mechanical preprocessing in the mammalian cochlea. *Trends in Neuroscience, 15*, 57–61.

Zeng, F.- G., Kong, Y.,-Y., Michaelewski, H. J., & Starr, A. (2005). Perceptual consequences of disrupted auditory nerve activity. *Journal of Neurophysiology, 93*, 3050–3063.

Zeng, F.- G. & Liu, S. (2006). Speech perception in individuals with auditory neuropathy. *Journal of Speech Language and Hearing Research, 49*, 36.

Zeng, F.- G., Oba, S., Garde, S., Sininger, Y., & Starr, A. (1999). Temporal and speech processing deficits in auditory neuropathy. *NeuroReport, 10*(16), 3429–3435.

Zeng, F.- G., Oba, S., & Starr, A. (2001). Supra threshold processing deficits due to desynchronous neural activities in auditory neuropathy. In D. J. Breebaart, A. J. M. Houstma, A. Kohlrausch, V. F. Prijs, & R. Schoonhoven (Eds.), *Physiological and psychophysical bases of auditory function* (pp. 365–372). Maastricht, Netherlands: Shaker Publishing BV.

6

Temporal Processing in the Auditory System

Vishakha Waman Rawool

Overview

Investigators have used a variety of approaches to understand the ability of the human auditory system to process auditory stimuli over time. In this chapter, approaches used for measuring temporal resolution, temporal asynchrony, temporal separation, temporal ordering, temporal masking, and temporal integration are described. In addition, comprehension of various forms of temporally degraded speech and various approaches used in measuring binaural temporal processing abilities are also reviewed. It should be noted that there is some overlap in the underlying abilities across these various approaches. However, separate contemplation of these approaches is likely to be helpful in understanding temporal processing and thus comprehending the associated scientific and clinical literature. This chapter includes descriptions of procedures that are used for assessing temporal processing abilities in research laboratories and the procedures that are available for clinical use.

Introduction

Temporal processing refers to the processing of acoustic stimuli over time. This type of processing is very important for us to be able to understand speech in quiet and in background noise, as speech stimuli and other background sounds vary over time. Speech and hearing professionals need to be familiar with the various aspects of temporal processing for two reasons. First, some children with auditory processing problems have difficulty in processing auditory stimuli over time. Such difficulties can hinder the acquisition of speech, language, and reading. Secondly, older individuals can also have temporal processing deficits, which can affect their ability to understand speech or to benefit from speech and language therapy in the presence of aphasia or Alzheimer's disease or to benefit from amplification in the presence of hearing loss (Rawool, 2006a).

Temporal Resolution

In measuring temporal resolution, the lower limit to the ability of the human auditory system to resolve time is assessed. Temporal resolution can be measured in a variety of ways.

Gap Detection Threshold

This is the measurement of the minimum time gap necessary to detect that the gap is present. Without the presence of a minimum time gap, the two stimuli occurring before and after the gap are perceived as one stimulus. When stimuli are presented near auditory thresholds, larger gaps are necessary for detecting gaps compared to when stimuli are presented at comfortable listening levels.

Within-Channel Gap Detection Threshold

This is the minimum gap necessary to detect gaps between sounds that are similar in spectrum. (Hirsh 1959; Purcell et al., 2004).

Across-Channel Gap Detection Threshold

This is the minimum gap necessary to detect gaps between sounds that are spectrally dissimilar (e.g., tone and noise) or sounds that are presented to two ears (Heinrich, Alain, & Schneider, 2004; Hirsh, 1959).

Individuals with compromised central auditory nervous systems need larger gaps to detect gaps (Bamiou et al., 2006; Musiek et al., 2005). They may have difficulty in processing rapidly occurring elements in speech. Fast speech has smaller gaps and poor temporal resolution can make it difficult to detect the small gaps and cause difficulty in keeping sounds apart from each other. Gap detection thresholds also appear to be related to speech perception in noise (Glasberg & Moore, 1989). Real-life background sounds often fluctuate in intensity, allowing extraction of useful information from the signal of interest during the softer levels of background noise. The poor gap detection in some individuals may not allow them to take advantage of the gaps in background noise.

Three commercially available tests (Auditory Fusion Test—Revised, Random Gap Detection Test, Gaps-in-Noise) can be used for estimating approximate gap-detection thresholds. All of these measures incorporate a practice test, which allows familiarization of the test material. They all are administered at comfortable listening levels, as temporal resolution tends to be poorer at softer levels. However, when obtaining ear-specific data, care should be taken to keep the presentation level below the levels at which crossover of the stimuli to the other ear is possible. Children often have very good bone conduction sensitivity (–10 dB HL or better thresholds), which may allow crossover of signals at levels as low as 25 to 30 dB HL (Snyder, 1973), as the possibility of cross-over is greater for broadband stimuli such as noise. The Auditory Fusion Test—Revised (AFT-R) was developed by McCrosky and Keith (1996). The test consists of pairs of tonal bursts, which are varied in frequency from 250 to 4000 Hz. The bursts are presented with the gaps between the pairs of bursts or interpulse intervals (IPIs) increasing in duration from 0, 2, 5, 10, 15, 20, 25, 30, and 40 ms (ascending) and then decreasing in duration from 40 msec to 0 ms (descending). The listener's task is to judge whether a single sound ("1") was audible or two sounds ("2") were audible. When the listener perceives the gap between the two pulses, the pulses are identified as two pulses. On the other hand, the perception of the tonal pair as a single sound image suggests that the gap between the pair was not perceived. On the ascending trial, the auditory fusion point is identified as that IPI which yields the last "1" response before the "2" responses. On the descending trial, it is that IPI that yields the first of two consecutive "1" responses. The average of the ascending and descending auditory fusion points is the auditory fusion threshold for that frequency or mode (right ear or left ear or binaural). If the listener judged all pairs as single sounds up to the IPI of 40 msec, subtest 3 or the expanded test can be administered in which the IPIs are varied from 40 ms to 100 ms in 10-msec steps and two additional pairs are presented with IPIs of 200 and 300 msec. Normative data for the auditory fusion points are provided on the back of the test form for age groups varying from 3 to 70 years. Although the test does not directly measure gap-detection thresholds, approximate gap-detection thresholds can be estimated as average of the minimal IPIs where the response "2" occurred on the ascending and descending trials.

The Random Gap Detection Test (RGDT) (Keith, 2000) is a less time consuming (10 minutes) version of the Auditory Fusion Test—Revised described above. The RGDT includes pairs of clicks (1 ms white noise) and tonal bursts (duration 15 ms, 1.5 msec rise-fall time) with frequencies ranging from 500 to 4000 Hz. The interpulse intervals or gaps are varied from 0, 2, 5, 10, 15, 20, 25, 30, 35, and 40 msec in a random order. The listener's task is to verbally or manually (fingers) indicate if "1" or "2" sounds were perceived. The approximate gap-detection threshold can be estimated from this test by determining the smallest interpulse interval, or gap, at which the listener perceives two stimuli. There is an expanded version available called RGDT-EXP which includes gaps with additional interpulse intervals up to 300 msec.

The Gaps-in-Noise (GIN) test was developed by Musiek et al. (2005). It consists of a series of 6-sec segments of broad-band noise and 0 to 3 gaps are embedded within each segment. The gaps vary in duration from 2, 3, 4, 5, 6, 8, 10, 12, 15, and 20 msec. The approximate gap-detection threshold is defined as the shortest gap duration which is correctly identified at least four out of six times. The percentage of correct responses out of the total 60 gaps can also be calculated.

Chermak and Lee (2005) compared the above three tests in a group of 10 normal children ranging in age from 7 to 11 years. The GIN test required 20 minutes for administration, which is longer than the 10 to 16 minutes required for other tests. However, the GIN test also yielded the smallest range and standard deviations, and thus may provide better specificity.

Detection of Temporal Modulation

Temporal modulation refers to a change in the stimulus over time. For example, a stimulus can change in amplitude over time (amplitude modulation). The characteristics of a modulating signal can be described with reference to modulation depth and modulation rate. Modulation depth refers to the degree of change. For example, if the amplitude of the signal changes over time from very high amplitude to very low amplitude, then the signal is considered to have greater modulation depth. Modulation rate refers to the speed with which the change occurs. For example, if the amplitude of the signal changes vary frequently over time, the modulation rate is considered to be high. We need to have a minimum modulation depth to detect that a stimulus is modulated in some way. For signals with a high modulation rate, the modulation depth needs to be greater to detect that the signal is modulated (Lorenzi et al., 2001; Viemeister, 1979).

Individuals with poor abilities to detect temporal modulations may have difficulty in processing speech because many consonants have rapid intensity changes or amplitude modulations that must be perceived correctly for accurate recognition of the consonants. In addition, as stated before, normal individuals are able to take advantage of the fluctuations that occur in background noise that make it easier to listen to speech occurrences during the dips or softer levels in the noise. Individuals with poor abilities to detect temporal modulations of background noise may not be able to take advantage of the dips in noise to improve speech recognition in background noise.

Duration Discrimination

This is the minimum difference in duration necessary to perceive that two otherwise identical stimuli are different in duration (Hellstrom & Rammsayer, 2004). Note that such duration discrimination is affected by temporal integration, which can make the sound with longer duration sound louder for stimuli that are shorter than about 200 to 300 msec. For tonal stimuli, duration discrimination can also be affected by changes in the frequency composition of the signal with changes in duration.

Duration discrimination is very important for accurate speech recognition. For example, the differentiation between unvoiced and voiced consonants partially depends on the duration of the vowel preceding the consonant. The duration is longer for voiced consonants than that for unvoiced consonants. Also, fricatives can be differentiated from affricates based on the difference in the duration of the fricative noises associated with these sounds (Dorman, Raphael, & Isenberg, 1980).

Gap-Duration Discrimination

This is the minimum difference in the duration of two gaps that is necessary to perceive that the two gaps are different in duration. The two gaps can be created by using acoustic markers (e.g., brief tones) at the beginning and at the end of the gap. One of the gaps serves as the standard gap. The duration of the second gap is varied to determine the minimum difference in gap duration necessary to detect that the two gaps differ in duration.

Gap-duration discrimination is important for discriminating fricatives and affricates, for identifying the presence or absence of a stop consonant in a consonant cluster, for detecting voicing of a stop consonant in word-medial position, and for discriminating between single and double stop consonants (Dorman, Raphael, & Liberman, 1979).

Temporal Asynchrony

In a temporal asynchrony task, the temporal alignment of one or more of the frequency bands of two complex stimuli differs and the listener is expected to differentiate between the two stimuli.

Temporal Asynchrony Detection Threshold

Thresholds can be measured for detecting asynchrony among complex signals composed of many sinusoidal components (Zera & Green, 1993a, 1995). The components either form a harmonic series and/or are uniformly spaced on a logarithmic frequency scale. In the standard synchronous stimulus, all components start and stop synchronously. In the comparison stimulus, asynchrony is created by starting (onset asynchrony) or stopping (offset asynchrony) only one or certain components slightly before or after the other components in the complex (Figure 6–1). The listener's task is to discriminate between the standard and the comparison stimulus. The asynchrony in turning the components "on" or "off" is varied. Thresholds for detecting onset asynchrony in harmonic signals generally are better than those required for detecting offset asynchrony.

Temporal Asynchrony Discrimination

In this case, a standard asynchronous stimulus is created by linearly delaying successive components of a complex stimulus. Another asynchronous comparison stimulus is created by altering the temporal position of a single component in the complex relative to its temporal position in the standard stimulus (Zera & Green, 1993b). The listener's task is to discriminate between the standard and the comparison stimulus.

Detection and discrimination of temporal asynchrony is important for understanding speech in background noise or where more than one speaker

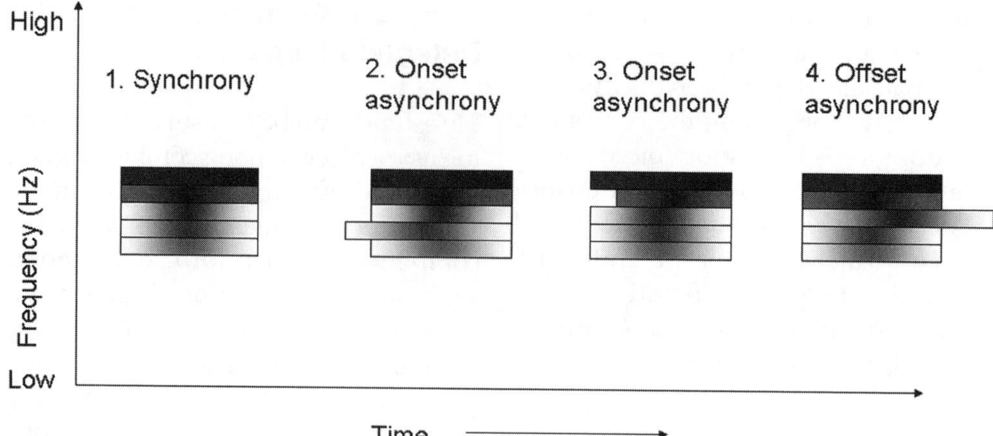

Figure 6–1. Illustration of temporal asynchrony tasks. The first illustration demonstrates a complex synchronous stimulus. The second and third illustrations show onset asynchrony in which one of the frequency bands begins earlier or later than the rest of the frequency bands. The fourth illustration shows offset asynchrony as one of the frequency bands ends later in time.

is speaking at the same time. The rapid sequence of sounds in such environments is not always perceived as a coherent whole. The sounds may actually be divided into different groups according to their general attributes such as loudness, perceived location, pitch, closeness to each other, or temporal synchrony of different frequency bands, and so forth. The different frequency components from a particular sound source tend to start and finish together. Thus, if the different frequency bands start together or have onset synchrony, they are detected as part of the same sound source; otherwise, they are perceived as separate auditory streams. The ability to detect and discriminate temporal synchrony allows us to concentrate on the signal of interest (e.g., a single speaker) while ignoring the signals that are not of interest (e.g., background music or other speakers speaking in the background).

Temporal Separation

In a temporal separation task, two sounds, tone A and tone B, that are different in some dimension (level, temporal modulation pattern, frequency, etc.) are presented in an alternating fashion to the ear. Both sounds are turned on and off in such a way, that when the first sound is off, the second sound is on and when the first sound is on, the second sound is off. The listener's task is to judge whether two separate sound sources are occurring simultaneously or there is just one sound, which is fluctuating in some way. For example, Tone A can be fixed in frequency at 250 Hz. Tone B can be started with a frequency well above or below that of tone A, and then its frequency can be swept toward that of tone A so that the frequency separation between the two tones decreases (Figure 6–2) in an expo-

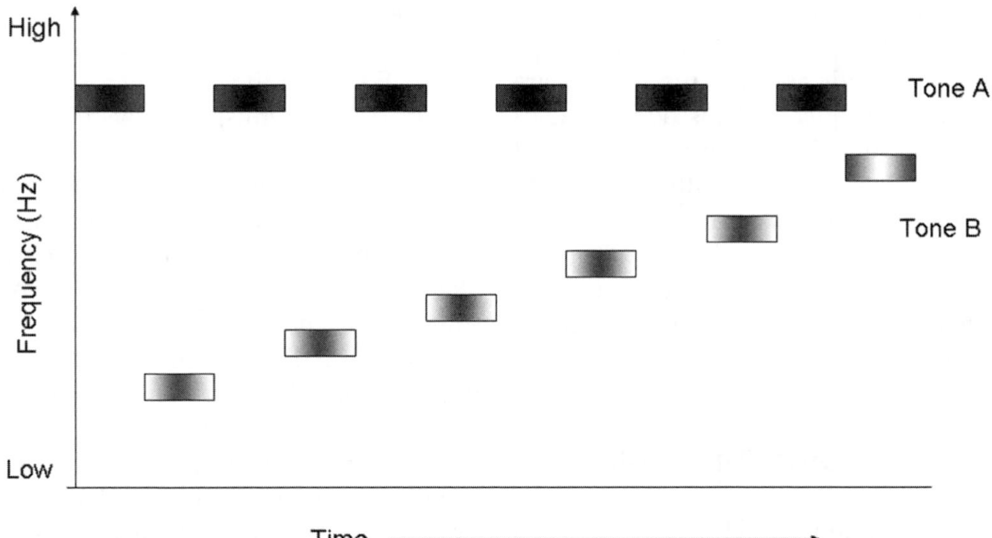

Figure 6–2. Illustration of the temporal separation task. Tone B is lower in frequency than tone A. The two tones alternate in time. At the beginning of the task two auditory streams will be perceived by the listener. The frequency of Tone B is then changed so that the tone becomes closer in frequency to Tone A. The listener's task is to report when a change from two auditory streams to one auditory stream is perceived.

nential manner. Listeners are expected to indicate when they could no longer perceive tones A and B as two separate streams, but perceived a single stream with a "gallop" rhythm. This is called the fission boundary (Rose & Moore, 1997).

Stream Fusion

Under certain stimulus conditions the two alternating sounds appear as one source. This is referred to as stream fusion.

Stream Segregation or Separation

Under other stimulus conditions, the two sounds are perceived as two separate sounds that are occurring at the same time. For example, if the sounds differ in frequency, the individual does not perceive the sounds as a sound from a single source, which is alternating in pitch. Instead, the listener perceives two coexisting sounds. This is referred to as stream segregation.

Most acoustic environments have sounds that come from several coexisting sound sources. Our ability to segregate the sound streams from each source can help us in focusing on the signal of interest (e.g., music in the background of noise).

Temporal Ordering

Temporal ordering refers to our ability to accurately perceive the *sequence* of sounds. Most acoustic stimuli in nature follow one another. In speech, sounds appear in sequence with minimum gaps across sounds and, in music, notes are played in sequence. Thus, accurate temporal order judgment in the presence of minimal gaps across different sounds is necessary for accurate perception of speech. Otherwise, a child may say "aks" instead of "ask" or "nam" instead of "man." Temporal ordering can be viewed and measured in two ways.

Temporal Order Threshold

This is the minimum time gap between sound sequences necessary to correctly perceive the order of incoming stimuli (e.g., click-tone). This time gap is generally larger (15–20 msec) than the gap necessary to just perceive that there is a gap (2 msec) between two sounds (Hirsh, 1959). Furthermore, the minimum gaps necessary for accurate temporal order judgments increases with the number of stimuli in the sequence of items. For example, the necessary gap is smaller when the order of only two stimuli is to be judged compared to when there are three stimuli in the sequence. Individuals who need larger time gaps to accurately judge sound sequences may have difficulty understanding rapid speech. Patients with injuries to the left cerebral hemispheres need larger gaps for accurate perception of temporal order (Efron, 1963; Swisher & Hirsh, 1972).

Temporal Order Judgment

We can measure the ability of individuals to correctly order sound sequences after providing sufficient gaps between the sound sequences (Musiek, 1994; Warren, Obusek, Farmer, & Warren, 1969). Some individuals with hemispheric or interhemispheric dysfunction may have difficulty in ordering sound sequences even after sufficient time gaps are provided between sounds (Bamiou et al., 2006; Musiek, Baran, & Pinheiro, 1990; Musiek & Pinheiro, 1987). For example, if the sound sequence consists of variations in pitch; low-low-high; the individuals may respond back an incorrect sequence such as high-low-high. Sound sequences that vary in duration or intensity (Pinheiro & Ptacek, 1971) also can be used in such tasks. It should be noted that temporal order judgment tasks are partially dependent on good short-term memory.

Two temporal order judgment tests called Frequency Pattern Test and Duration Pattern Test are available for clinical use. Before administering the tests, clinicians should ensure that the individual has understood the instructions, by using visual cues or gestures if necessary.

The Frequency Pattern Test consists of 60 segments with three 200-msec tones in each segment, with a rise-fall time of 10 msec. The tones are separated from each other by a silent interval of 150 msec. The low tone has a frequency of 880 Hz and the high tone has a frequency of 1122 Hz. These two frequencies are perceived as being equally loud; thus, listeners are forced to listen to the differences in pitch. The listener's task is to identify each pattern verbally (e.g. high, low, low) and/or through humming. The test scores are expressed in terms of the percentage of correctly identified patterns.

The Duration Pattern Test is similar to the Frequency Pattern Test except for the fact that the listener identifies the pattern by specifying the duration of the tones (e.g. short, long, long). Each tone has the same frequency of 1000 Hz, but the duration can be either long (500 msec) or short (250 msec). The tones are separated from each other by a 300 msec silent interval.

Temporal Pattern Discrimination

In this task, the ability of the individual to detect differences between two patterns is assessed. For example, the standard sound sequence may consist of 10 tones with durations of 40 msec. In the comparison stimulus the duration of one of the tones can be varied to determine the smallest change in duration that leads to the perception of a temporal pattern that is different from the pattern of the standard stimulus (Espinoza-Varas & Watson, 1986). The task can be varied by asking listeners to detect changes in the frequency instead of duration of brief (40 to 50 msec) components of word-length (400–500 msec) tonal sequences.

Temporal Masking

Temporal masking refers to the ability of one sound (masker) to mask another sound (probe) that precedes and/or follows it (Elliott, 1962; Hartley & Moore, 2002). The shift in the threshold of the probe signal or the amount of masking produced by the masker is determined while adjusting the time interval between the probe and the masker. The amount of masking reduces with increase in the time interval between the probe and the masker. Several other parameters of the masker such as level, duration, and frequency composition also have an effect on the amount of temporal masking. For example, more masking occurs when the frequency of the probe is similar to the frequency of the masker. Temporal masking can be considered in three ways:

1. *Forward masking:* The masker is presented and following a brief time-delay the signal is presented. Thus the masker can be considered as "moving" forward in time to mask the signal.
2. *Backward masking:* In this case the masker follows the signal after a brief time interval. Thus the masker can be viewed as moving backward in time to mask the signal.
3. *Combined backward and forward masking:* The signal is separated briefly in time by a masker that precedes it and another masker that follows it.

Abnormally large temporal masking from adjacent sounds can affect perception of speech. More specifically, forward masking effects appear to play a role in the perception of speech in quiet (Dreschler & Plomp, 1985). In average conversational speech, the intensity of sounds can vary by about 30 dB. If an individual demonstrates abnormally large forward masking, this may result in frequent masking of a weaker sound when it is followed by a relatively intense sound (backward masking). Children with specific language impairment show more backward masking than children with no such impairments

(Wright et al., 1997). It should be noted that abnormally large temporal masking also can affect temporal separation or the ability to perceive two alternating sound sources as two sound streams because the sound from one source may mask the sound from another source occurring earlier or later in time.

Temporal Integration or Temporal Summation

Temporal integration or summation refers to the assumed ability of the auditory system to add up information over time or over duration up to a critical duration. Normal temporal summation can provide important cues for duration discrimination for very short sounds. As stated before, duration discrimination is important for normal speech perception. In addition, individuals with temporal lobe pathologies have difficulty in detecting sounds of very short duration (1 msec) and thus their thresholds are elevated for such brief sounds (Baru & Karaseva, 1972). Temporal summation can be measured by presenting auditory stimuli near thresholds or above thresholds. It can be measured subjectively using behavioral thresholds or objectively using acoustic reflex thresholds.

Temporal Summation at Thresholds

Temporal Summation at Threshold Due to Increase in Stimulus Duration

In this case the thresholds improved due to an increase in the duration of the stimulus (Pedersen & Salomon, 1977). As an example of this phenomenon, if an individual has a threshold of 15 dB for a stimulus lasting 20 msec, the threshold may be 5 dB for a stimulus that is 200 msec long. In this example, the threshold improved by 10 dB due to an increase in the duration of the stimulus. Thus, the auditory system appears to operate as an energy detector. A certain amount of energy is needed to detect the sound. This energy may be achieved by using higher intensity over a shorter duration or lower intensity over a longer duration. The ear appears to integrate energy over an integration time frame of about 200 msec. Thus, auditory thresholds do not improve much with increase in stimulus duration beyond 200 msec. In fact, if the stimulus duration is too long (e.g., 2 minutes), the thresholds can become worse and this phenomenon is referred to as adaptation.

Some commercially available audiometers allow changes in the duration of tones. Thus, the thresholds can be measured by varying the duration of the tones to obtain a temporal integration function. A more time-saving approach may be to measure the thresholds for brief tonal duration (20 msec) and for long stimulus duration (500 msec) and then to compare the difference between the two thresholds with age-appropriate norms.

Temporal Summation at Threshold Due to Increase in Stimulus Rate

In this case, the auditory thresholds improve due to increase in stimulus rates (Beattie & Rochverger, 2001; Garner, 1947). This is partially due to the fact that, at higher rates, more stimuli are presented within a shorter period. Thus, the energy is added over time.

However, at very low rates (1 to 4/sec), thresholds may also improve due to more opportunities to detect the stimulus at higher rates (Garner, 1947). In other words, when stimuli are presented at a rate of 4 per second, the number of opportunities to detect the stimulus is higher than when stimuli are presented at a rate of 1 per second.

Temporal Summation of Loudness at Suprathreshold Levels

Improvement in Perceived Loudness Due to Increase in the Duration of Suprathreshold Stimuli

When two equally intense stimuli of differing durations are compared, the stimulus with longer duration is perceived as being louder due to the fact that there is more energy in the long-duration stimulus (Buus, Florentine, & Poulsen, 1999; Miller, 1948).

Increase in the Perceived Loudness of Suprathreshold Stimuli with Increases in Stimulus Rate

When two equally intense stimuli of differing stimulus rates are compared, the stimulus with higher rate sounds louder (Darling & Price, 1989).

Temporal Summation in Acoustic Reflex Thresholds

Stimulus-Duration Induced Improvement of Acoustic Reflex Thresholds

This is the improvement in acoustic reflex thresholds apparent with increase in the duration of stimuli (Moller, 1962; Cacace, Margolis, & Relkin, 1991).

Rate-Induced Facilitation of Acoustic Reflex Thresholds

This is the improvement in acoustic reflex thresholds apparent with increase in the stimulus rate (Fielding & Rawool, 2002; Johnsen & Terkildsen, 1980; Rawool, 1995). The rate-induced facilitation is reduced in older individuals probably due to slower processing which may lead to lack of processing of some of the stimuli at higher rates (Rawool, 1996).

Temporally Degraded Speech

Investigators have used a variety of approaches to alter normal speech in the temporal dimension. Temporally altered speech can stress the processing ability of the auditory system in a variety of ways and can reveal deficits in temporal processing.

Rapid Speech

Asking someone to speak at a relatively rapid rate produces this type of speech. TV and radio-news announcers often speak at relatively faster rates. Some individuals process speech at a slower rate and thus may have difficulty in processing rapid speech.

Time-Compressed Speech

In this case, tiny segments are removed from the spoken message (words or sentences) and the remaining elements are moved closer together. The amount of compression is described by the compression rate (e.g., 60%), which refers to the amount of time occupied by the compressed signal, compared to that occupied by the original uncompressed signal (100%). The resultant speech sounds similar to rapid speech and thus, as can be expected, individuals with slower processing speed have more difficulty in recognizing time-compressed speech. At the rate of 60% compression, individuals with diffused temporal lobe lesions (Kurdziel, Noffsinger, & Olsen, 1976) show poorer performance than normal individuals. Older individuals also have more difficulty in recognizing time-compressed speech even in the presence of normal hearing. It should be noted that comprehension of compressed speech might also require the ability to fill in the missing or removed segments (closure).

Time-compressed monosyllabic words are available on a CD titled *Tonal and Speech Materials for Auditory Perceptual Assessment* (1992). The test includes NU-6 monosyllabic words that are compressed at two compression rates, 45% and 65%. Time-compressed sentences are available on a test developed by Keith (2002) and is designed for children between the ages of 6 and 11 years. The sentences are compressed at the rate of 40% and 60%. Uncompressed sentences are available for practice and for obtaining baseline scores. McCroskey (1984) developed the Wichita Auditory Processing Test (WAPT), which includes time-altered sentences at the compression ratios of 100% (uncompressed), 200% (expanded), 70% (compressed), and 130% (expanded). Ten sentences are presented at each compression rate and the child is expected to point to the appropriate picture. Normative data are provided for different age groups at each of the compression rates.

Reverberant Speech

This is another form of temporal waveform distortion due to the smearing of the original signal by reflections of the original signal from surrounding surfaces. Individuals with temporal processing difficulties may have increased difficulty in understanding reverberant speech.

Speech with Temporal Asynchrony

The pattern of energy in different frequency regions in normal speech is precisely timed with the periodic action of the vocal folds or the fundamental frequency of the speaker's voice. Temporal asynchrony in speech can be created by misaligning some frequency bands (e.g., 12.5 to 100 msec) in the temporal domain compared to other frequency bands. Healy and Bacon (2002) suggested that reverberation times for low frequencies can be longer than high-frequency sounds as low-frequency sounds are absorbed less efficiently. Thus, low-frequency components can persist longer in a reverberant field than high-frequency components, which can make the indirect signals asynchronous. This suggests that poor tolerance for temporal asynchrony in some individuals can contribute to difficulty in perceiving speech in reverberant environments.

Speech Mixed with Other Competing Signals such as Cafeteria Noise

When speech is mixed with other competing signals, the temporal waveform of the speech signal can get masked by other signals or some individuals may have difficulty in separating the source signal from the background noise. Several tests are available for assessing speech recognition in the presence of competing signals.

Temporally Jittered Speech

In this case, the sequence of amplitude values in the sound file is changed by shifting them slightly earlier or later in the sequence. This type of speech attempts to simulate neural asynchrony or the inability of auditory neurons to fire in a synchronous manner to a single phase of the stimuli referred to as phase-locking (Miranda & Pichora-Fuller, 2002).

Binaural Temporal Processing

This type of processing requires the processing of stimuli over time by both ears. For this type of processing to occur, stimuli presented to two ears must be compared at some central location in the auditory system.

Between-Ears (Across Channel) Gap Detection

This is the ability to detect gaps between sounds that are being presented to two ears. The Binaural Fusion Test developed by Musiek (Chermak & Lee, 2005) requires listeners to attend to pairs of noise bursts that are presented sequentially to each ear and are separated by gaps or interpulse intervals (IPIs) that vary randomly from 0 to 100 msec with a smallest step-size of 5 msec. The ear that receives the first noise burst is also randomized to minimize guessing. The listener is required to respond by indicating whether "1" or "2" noise-bursts were heard. Chermak and Lee (2005) compared the performance on the binaural fusion test with other monaural measures of gap detection in young children. They reported similar performance on monaural and across-ear measures of gap detection and attributed the similarity to the relatively large step-size used in the BFT. However, they measured the binaural fusion threshold as the shortest IPI where the perception of "1" noise-burst was reported which as expected was 0 msec for most of their 10 subjects. Perhaps the minimum IPI which yields the "2" response may provide better estimation of the gap detection thresholds for appropriate comparisons across the different tasks. In addition, the tests were administered either at 50 dB SL with reference to the pure tone average or at 55 dB HL. At such high presentation levels, the monaural performance may not be ear-specific due to crossover of stimuli, because children have very good bone conduction sensitivity. Furthermore, the across-ears performance may not be truly across ears since both ears may get stimulated through the entire presentation sequence. As stated previously, crossover is possible in young children at 30 dB HL assuming bone conduction thresholds of

−10 dB HL and interaural attenuation of 40 dB.

Between-Ears Temporal Order Judgment

This is the ability to correctly judge the order of sounds being presented at two ears.

Dichotic Temporal Masking

This is similar to the forward and/or backward masking described earlier except that the probe signal is presented to one ear and the masking signal is presented to the other ear.

Precedence Effect or the Principle of the First Wavefront

A signal that precedes any other signals (e.g., echos or reverberation) in time dominates our perception of the sound (Yost & Soderquist, 1984). In other words, the auditory system suppresses signals that occur within about 40 msec after the earlier arriving sound, provided that the later occurring signals are quieter than the original signal. The precedent effect helps us in locating sounds in reverberant fields. If an individual has poor ability to fuse direct sounds with the early reflections of that sound, the listener may have difficulty in recognizing speech in reverberant environments (Roberts, Koehnke, & Besing, 2003). The performance on precedence effect localization tasks is correlated with speech recognition in the presence of a competing message (Cranford & Romereim, 1992).

Sound Localization

Our ability to determine the direction of sound is partially dependent on the differences in the arrival in time of the sound at the two ears. For example, we perceive the sound as coming from the left side if the sound arrives sooner at the left ear when compared to the right ear. Our ability to encode such interaural time differences diminishes with increasing frequency. However, the localization of complex sounds is also dependent on temporal cues. Temporal cues are available at high frequencies in such sounds due to the interaural delays in the amplitude envelopes of these sounds.

Interaural Time Difference (ITD) Discrimination

Interaural time difference refers to the difference in arrival of the sound at two ears. In an ITD discrimination task the test stimulus differs from the standard stimulus in interaural delay (Koehnke, Culotta, Hawley, & Colburn, 1995).

Time-Intensity Trade

The lateralized image of a signal arriving earlier in time at one ear can be brought back to a center location by making the later arriving signal louder. If a signal is presented earlier to the left ear as compared to the right ear, the sound image is perceived in the left ear. This effect can be canceled by making the late-arriving sound to the right ear louder than that presented to the left ear. Thus, in this case, the advantage of the earlier arriving signal can be canceled by making the sound louder in the other ear (Moushegian & Jeffress, 1959).

Masking Level Difference

The perception of signals (tonal or speech) in noise can be improved by changing the phase of the masker in relation to the signal at the two ears. For example, it is easier to detect a signal presented in phase at the two ears in the presence of noise that is presented out of phase at the two ears compared to the condition where both the signal and the noise are presented in phase at both ears (Hirsh, 1948). This is likely to occur because of the fact that, when both the signal and noise are presented in phase to the two ears, the signal and noise images both occur at a central location in the head. When the noise is out of phase, the noise image shifts to the ear that has the 0 degree phase, whereas the image of the signal that is in phase remains at the center of the head. This separation of the noise and signal can allow easier detection of the signal when the noise or the signal is out-of-phase. Children with suspected auditory processing deficits can yield significantly lower MLDs for tones (Sweetow & Redell, 1978). Abnormal MLDs for tonal stimuli have also been reported in patients with multiple sclerosis (Hendler, Squires, & Emmerich, 1990; Noffsinger, Olsen, Carhart, Hart, & Sahagal, 1972; Olsen & Noffsinger, 1976).

Some commercially available audiometers allow the measurement of masking level difference for tonal stimuli. In most cases the MLDs are measured for the frequency of 500 Hz, in the presence of a noise that is presented at 45 to 65 dB EM or effective masking. (Effective masking refers to the amount of threshold shift relative to 0 dB HL. For example, 45 dB EM noise shifts all thresholds below 45 dB HL to 45 dB HL. Masking noise on most audiometers is calibrated in EM for easier clinical use.) The thresholds are determined in two conditions: (1) both the signal and the noise are presented in phase to the two ears and (2) either the signal or the noise is presented out of phase at the two ears. The MLD is the difference between these two thresholds. Thus if the threshold is 45 dB HL for the in-phase condition and it is 35 dB HL for the out-of-phase condition, then the size of the MLD in this case is 10 dB HL.

MLDs for speech can be determined by using the CD titled *Tonal and Speech Materials for Auditory Perceptual Assessment* (1998). On this CD, spondee words are recorded after 500 msec of the initiation of a noise burst. In the out-of-phase condition, the spondees are presented out-of-phase to the two ears and the noise is presented in phase to the two ears at a level of 65 or 85 dB SPL. The MLD for speech is generally smaller than that obtained for 500 Hz tones.

Improvement in Binaural Speech Perception Due to Spatial Separation of Speech and Noise Sources

As stated earlier, a signal presented on the left side arrives earlier to the left side compared to the right side and this cue partially helps the listener in recognizing that the signal is being presented to the left ear. Such interaural time difference cues are especially important for the correct localization of signals containing low-frequency information. Thus, if both speech and a competing signal (e.g., babble) are presented from a source in front of the listener, both the speech-image and the babble-image are perceived at a central location. If the babble is then moved to one or the other side of the listener, then the image of the babble moves to one or the other side, allowing better perception of the speech signal that is presented in front of the listener. This is referred to as spatial advantage and is related to effective use of the detection of interaural time and intensity difference cues by the listener to understand speech in competing signals.

The Listening in Spatialized Noise test (LISN) allows the assessment of the use of spatial advantage to understand speech in competing babble. It is designed to simulate a three-dimensional auditory environment under headphones. The listener is required to follow the story presented by a target talker arriving at 0°, in the presence of distracting sentences spoken by the same talker or spoken by two different talkers arriving from either 0° or 90°. For example, the distracting sentences can be presented at 40 dB HL. The level of the target talker is then adjusted adaptively to find the minimum level where the listener can "just understand" the story. While listening to the target story in the presence of distracting sentences from two different talkers at 0°, the listener must rely on the temporal asynchrony between the target and the competing talkers to focus on the target talker; no such cues are available when the target story and competing sentences are spoken by the same talker and both are presented at 0° azimuth. However, when the story is presented at 0° azimuth in the presence of distracting sentences from the same talker presented at 90° azimuth, the listener can use spatial cues and thus can understand the story at softer levels. If the distracting sentences from different talkers are presented at 90° azimuth, the listener can use both spatial and temporal asynchrony cues to understand the target story. Children with auditory processing disorders show less spatial advantage on such a task than age-matched controls (Cameron, Dillon & Newall, 2006a, 2006b, 2006c).

Rapidly Alternating Speech

In this case separate segments (e.g., 300 msec long) of a sentence are alternated between the two ears (Willeford, 1977). Ideally, for such a task to be sensitive to auditory processing deficits, if the listener could hear segments that are supposed to be presented only to the left or only to the right ear, the segments should not be intelligible. Under such circumstance, the alternating segments presented to the two ears will have to be combined effectively by the listener for accurate perception of the spoken message.

Summary

Temporal processing of acoustic stimuli can be viewed in a variety of ways. Several measures of temporal processing have been used in laboratory and clinical settings. The temporal processing measures that are available for clinical use vary in sensitivity and specificity. Some of the measures are also affected by hearing loss as reviewed in Rawool (2006b, 2006c). For appropriate use of these measures, clinicians should be experienced in administering the tests and interpreting the data. Also, to the best extent possible, clinicians should establish their own norms appropriate for the clinical population they normally encounter. When an individual is identified as having a temporal processing deficit, appropriate intervention strategies should be used, some of which are reviewed in Rawool (2006d).

Key Points Learned

- Auditory temporal processing refers to the processing of acoustic stimuli by the auditory system.
- Auditory temporal processing can be viewed in various ways including temporal resolution, temporal asynchrony, temporal separation, temporal ordering, temporal masking, and temporal summation.
- Temporal resolution refers to the lower limit to the ability of the human auditory system to resolve time. It can be measured by using the following tasks: gap detection, temporal modulation detection, duration discrimination, and gap-duration discrimination.
- In a temporal asynchrony task, the temporal alignment of some of the frequency bands of two complex stimuli differs and the listener is expected to differentiate between the two stimuli.
- In a temporal separation task, two sounds, tone A and tone B that are different in some dimension (level, temporal modulation pattern, frequency, etc.) are presented in an alternating fashion to the ear. The listener's task is to judge whether there are two separate sound sources that are occurring simultaneously (stream separation) or there is just one sound (stream fusion), which is fluctuating in some way.
- Temporal ordering refers to our ability to accurately perceive the *sequence* of sounds.
- Temporal masking refers to the ability of one sound (masker) to mask another sound (probe) that precedes and/or follows it.
- Temporal integration or summation refers to the assumed ability of the auditory system to add up information over time or over duration up to a critical duration.

- Binaural temporal processing requires the processing of stimuli over time by both ears. For this type of processing to occur, stimuli presented to the two ears must be compared at some central location in the auditory system.
- Normal speech can be altered in the temporal dimension in a variety of ways. Such temporally altered speech can stress the processing ability of the auditory system and can reveal deficits in temporal processing.
- In evaluating ear-specific temporal processing deficits, the stimuli must be presented at sufficient levels as some temporal processing tasks yield poorer performance near threshold levels. However, the stimulus levels should be low enough to minimize crossover of stimuli to the other ear or contribution of the contra lateral ear to the performance of the test ear. The same precaution is necessary in evaluating binaural temporal processing abilities.
- Poor temporal processing abilities can affect speech perception in quiet and in the presence of background noise and reverberation. Early detection and intervention for temporal processing deficits can be expected to prevent or minimize speech and language delays or difficulties in processing speech in complex backgrounds such as noisy and reverberant classrooms.

References

Bamiou, D-E., Musiek, F. E., Stow, I., Stevens, J., Cipolotti, L., Brown, M. M., & Luxon, L. M. (2006). Auditory temporal processing deficits in patients with insular stroke. *Neurology, 67*, 614–619.

Baru, A., & Karaseva, T. (1972). *The brain and hearing: Hearing disturbances associated with local brain lesions.* New York: Consultation Bureau.

Beattie, R. C., & Rochverger, I. (2001). Normative behavioral thresholds for short tone-bursts. *Journal of the American Academy of Audiology, 12*(9), 453–461.

Buus, S., Florentine, M., & Poulsen, T. (1999). Temporal integration of loudness in listeners with hearing losses of primarily cochlear origin. *Journal of the Acoustical Society of America, 105*, 3464–3480.

Cacace, A. T., Margolis, R. H., & Relkin, E. M. (1991). Threshold and suprathreshold temporal integration effects in the crossed and uncrossed human acoustic stapedius reflex. *Journal of the Acoustical Society of America, 89*, 1255–1261.

Cameron, S., Dillon, H., & Newall, P. (2006a). Development and evaluation of the listening in spatialized noise test. *Ear and Hearing, 27*, 30–42.

Cameron, S., Dillon, H., & Newall, P. (2006b). The Listening in Spatialized Noise Test: Normative data for children. *International Journal of Audiology, 45*, 99–108.

Cameron, S., Dillon, H., & Newall, P. (2006c). Listening in Spatialized Noise Test: An auditory processing disorder study. *Journal of the American Academy of Audiology, 17*, 306–320.

Chermak, G. D., & Lee, J. (2005). Comparison of children's performance on four tests of temporal resolution. *Journal of the American Academy of Audiology, 16*, 554–563.

Cranford, J. L., & Romereim, B. (1992). Precedence effect and speech understanding in elderly listeners. *Journal of the American Academy of Audiology, 3*, 405–409.

Darling, R. M., & Price, L. L. (1989). Temporal summation of repetitive click stimuli. *Ear and Hearing, 10*, 173–177.

Dorman, M. F., Raphael, L. J., & Isenberg, D. (1980). Acoustic cues for a fricative and affricate contrast in word-final position. *Journal of Phonetics, 4*, 397–406.

Dorman, M. F., Raphael, L. J., & Liberman, A. M. (1979). Some experiments on the sound of silence in phonetic perception. *Journal of the Acoustical Society of America, 65*(6), 1518–1532.

Dresschler, W. A., & Plomp, R. (1985). Relations between psychophysical data and speech perception in hearing impaired subjects. II. *Journal of the Acoustical Society of America, 78*, 1261–1270.

Efron, R. (1963). Temporal perception, aphasia and déjà vu. *Brain, 86*, 403–424.

Elliott, L. L. (1962). Backward and forward masking of probe tones of different frequencies. *Journal of the Acoustical Society of America, 34*, 1116–1117.

Espinoza-Varas, B., & Watson, C. S. (1986). Temporal discrimination for single components of nonspeech auditory patterns. *Journal of the Acoustical Society of America, 80*, 1685–1694.

Fielding, E. D., & Rawool, V. W. (2002). Acoustic reflex thresholds at varying click rates in children. *International Journal of Pediatric Otorhinolaryngology, 63*, 243–252.

Garner, W. R. (1947). Auditory thresholds of short tones as a function of repetition rates. *Journal of the Acoustical Society of America, 19*, 600–608.

Glasberg, B. R., & Moore, B. C. (1989). Psychoacoustic abilities of subjects with unilateral and bilateral cochlear hearing impairments and their relationship to the ability to understand speech. *Scandinavian Audiology Supplement, 32*, 1–25.

Hartley, D. E. H., & Moore, D. R. (2002). Auditory processing efficiency deficits in children with developmental language impairments. *Journal of the Acoustical Society of America, 112*, 2962–2966.

Healy, E. W., & Bacon, S. P. (2002). Across frequency comparison of temporal speech information by listeners with normal and impaired hearing. *Journal of Speech, Language and Hearing Research, 45*, 1262–1275.

Heinrich, A., Alain, C., & Schneider, B. A. (2004). Within- and between-channel gap detection in the human auditory cortex. *NeuroReport, 15*, 2051–2056.

Hellstrom, A., & Rammsayer, T. H. (2004). Effects of time-order, interstimulus interval, and feedback in duration discrimination of noise bursts in the 50- and 1000-ms ranges. *Acta Psychologica (Amsterdam), 116*, 1–20.

Hendler, T., Squires, N. K., & Emmerich, D. S. (1990). Psychophysical measures of central auditory dysfunction in multiple sclerosis: Neurophysiological and neuroanatomical correlates. *Ear and Hearing, 11*, 403–416.

Hirsh, I. J. (1948). The influence of interaural phase on interaural summation and inhibition. *Journal of the Acoustical Society of America, 20*, 536–544.

Hirsh, I. J. (1959). Auditory perception of temporal order. *Journal of the Acoustical Society of America, 31*, 759–767.

Johnsen, N. J., & Terkildsen, K. (1980). The normal middle ear reflex thresholds towards white noise and acoustic clicks in young adults. *Scandinavian Audiology, 9*, 131–135.

Keith, R. W. (2000). *Random Gap Detection Test.* St. Louis, MO: Auditec.

Keith, R. W. (2002). *Time Compressed Sentence Test. Examiner's manual.* St. Louis, MO: Auditec.

Koehnke, J., Culotta, C. P., Hawley, M. L., & Colburn, H. S. (1995). Effects of reference interaural time and intensity differences on binaural performance in listeners with normal and impaired hearing. *Ear and Hearing, 16*(4), 331–353.

Kurdziel, S., Noffsinger, D., & Olsen, W. (1976). Performance by cortical lesion patients on 40% and 60% time-compression materials. *Journal of the American Auditory Society, 2*, 3–7.

Lorenzi, C., Simpson, M. I., Millman, R. E., Griffiths, T. D., Woods, W. P., Rees, A., & Green, G. G. (2001). Second-order modulation detection thresholds for pure-tone and narrow-band noise carriers. *Journal of the Acoustical Society of America, 110*(5 Pt. 1), 2470–2478.

McCroksy, R. (1984). *Wichita Auditory Processing Test: User's manual.* Tulsa, OK: Modern Education Corp.

McCrosky, R. & Keith, R. W. (1996). *Auditory Fusion Test—Revised.* St. Louis, MO: Auditec.

Miller, G. A. (1948). The perception of short bursts of noise. *Journal of the Acoustical Society of America, 20*, 160–170.

Miranda, T. T., & Pichora-Fuller, M. K. (2002). Temporally jittered speech produces performance intensity, phonetically balanced rollover in young normal-hearing listeners. *Journal of the American Academy of Audiology, 13*, 50–58.

Moller, A. R. (1962). Acoustic reflex in man. *Journal of the Acoustical Society of America, 34*(9B), 1524–1534.

Moushegian, G., & Jeffress, L. A. (1959). Role of interaural time and intensity differences in the lateralization of low-frequency tones. *Journal of the Acoustical Society of America, 31*, 1441–1445.

Musiek, F. E. (1994). Frequency (pitch) and duration pattern tests. *Journal of the American Academy of Audiology, 5*, 265–268.

Musiek, F., Baran, J., & Pinheiro, M. (1990). Duration pattern recognition in normal subjects and patients with cerebral and cochlear lesions. *Audiology, 29*, 304–313.

Musiek, F., & Pinheiro, M. (1987). Frequency patterns in cochlear, brainstem and cerebral lesions. *Audiology, 26*, 78–88.

Musiek, F., Shinn, J., Jirsa, R., Bamiou, D., Baran, J., & Zaiden, E. (2005). The GIN (Gaps-in-Noise) Test performance in subjects with central auditory nervous system involvement. *Ear and Hearing, 26*, 608–618.

Noffsinger, D., Olsen, W. O., Carhart, R., Hart, C. W., & Sahagal, V. (1972). Auditory and vestibular aberrations in multiple sclerosis. *Acta Otolaryngologica Supplement, 303*, 1–63.

Olsen, W. O., & Noffsinger, D. (1976). Masking level differences for cochlear and brainstem lesions. *Annals of Otology, Rhinology and Laryngology, 85*, 820–825.

Pedersen, C. B., & Salomon, G. (1977). Temporal integration of acoustic energy. *Acta Otolaryngologica, 83*(5–6), 417–423.

Pinheiro M. L., & Ptacek, P. H. (1971). Reversals in the perception of noise and tone patterns. *Journal of the Acoustical Society of America, 49*(6.2), 1778–1782.

Purcell, D. W., John, S. M., Schneider, B. A., & Picton, T. W. (2004). Human temporal auditory acuity as assessed by envelope following responses. *Journal of the Acoustical Society of America, 116*, 3581–3593.

Rawool, V. W. (1995). Ipsilateral acoustic reflex thresholds at varying click rates in humans. *Scandinavian Audiology, 24*(3), 199–205.

Rawool, V. W. (1996). Effect of aging on the click-rate induced facilitation of acoustic reflex thresholds. *Journal of Gerontology A: Biological Sciences & Medical Sciences, 51*, B124–B531.

Rawool, V. W. (2006a). A temporal processing primer. Part 1. Defining key concepts in temporal processing. *Hearing Review, 13*(5), 30–34.

Rawool, V. W. (2006b). The effects of hearing loss on temporal processing. Part 2:

Looking beyond simple audition. *Hearing Review, 13*(6), 30, 32, 34.

Rawool, V. W. (2006c). The effects of hearing loss on temporal processing. Part 3: Addressing temporal processing deficits through amplification strategies. *Hearing Review, 13*(7), 30, 35, 36, 38.

Rawool, V. W. (2006d). The effects of hearing loss on temporal processing. Part 4: Addressing temporal processing deficits via ALDs, environmental modifications, and training. *Hearing Review, 13*(8), 42, 44, 46, 48, 50.

Roberts, R. A., Koehnke, J., & Besing, J. (2003). Effects of noise and reverberation on the precedence effect in listeners with normal hearing and impaired hearing. *American Journal of Audiology, 12*(2), 96–105.

Rose, M. M., & Moore, B. C. (1997). Perceptual grouping of tone sequences by normally hearing and hearing-impaired listeners. *Journal of the Acoustical Society of America, 102*(3), 1768–1778.

Snyder, J. M. (1973). Interaural attenuation characteristics in audiometry. *Laryngoscope, 83*, 1847–1855.

Sweetow, R. W., & Redell, R. C. (1978). The use of masking level difference in the identification of children with perceptual problems. *Journal of the American Auditory Society, 4*, 52–56.

Swisher, L., & Hirsh, I. (1972). Brain damage and the ordering of two temporally successive stimuli. *Neuropsychologia, 10*, 137–152.

Tonal and speech materials for auditory perceptual assessment. (1992). Long Beach, CA: Research and Development Service, Veterans' Administration Central Office.

Tonal and speech materials for auditory perceptual assessment [Compact disc 2.0]. (1998). Department of Veterans Affairs. Mountain Home, TN: VA Medical Center.

Viemeister, N. F., (1979). Temporal modulation transfer functions based upon modulation thresholds. *Journal of the Acoustical Society of America, 66*, 1364–1380.

Warren, R. M., Obusek, C. J., Farmer, R. M., & Warren, R. P. (1969). Auditory sequence: confusion of patterns other than speech or music. *Science, 164*(879), 586–587.

Willeford, J. (1977). Assessing central auditory behavior in children: A test battery approach. In R. Keith (Ed.), *Central auditory dysfunction* (pp. 43–72). New York: Grune & Stratton.

Wright, B., Lombardino, L., King, W., Puranik, C., Leonard, C., & Merzenich, M. (1997). Deficits in auditory temporal and spectral resolution in language-impaired children. *Nature, 387*, 176–178.

Yost, W. A., & Soderquist, D. R. (1984). Precedence effect: revisited. *Journal of the Acoustical Society of America, 76*(5), 1377–1383.

Zera, J., & Green, D. M. (1993a) Detecting temporal onset and offset asynchrony in multicomponent complexes. *Journal of the Acoustical Society of America, 93*(2), 1038–1052.

Zera, J., & Green, D. M. (1993b). Detecting temporal asynchrony with asynchronous standards. *Journal of the Acoustical Society of America, 93*(3), 1571–1579.

Zera, J., & Green, D. M. (1995). Effect of signal component phase on asynchrony discrimination. *Journal of the Acoustical Society of America, 98*(2 Pt. 1), 817–827.

7

The Speech-Language Pathologist's Assessment of Auditory Processing Disorders

Deborah Ross-Swain

Overview

The role of the speech-language pathologist in the assessment and treatment of auditory processing disorders (APD) continues to expand as our professions work to provide a collaborative and effective means to diagnose and treat this ever growing area of interest. According to the American Speech-Language and Hearing Association's Scope of Practice (ASHA, 2005) the diagnosis of auditory processing disorders is the role of the audiologist. Because there may be some areas in the United States that do not have trained audiologists in the assessment and diagnosis of APD, parents and educators refer clients or students to the speech-language pathologist for testing to assess the processes that are often associated with APDs and request specific recommendations for further assessment, management, and treatment if deemed necessary. This chapter is designed to assist speech-language pathologists in making decisions regarding the use of screeners as well as selecting appropriate standardized batteries that will provide information relative to a client/student's processing of auditory input. As we know, test scores alone do not "diagnose" disorders, but rather the addition of qualitative analysis of scores provide more in-depth information concerning the meaning of test scores. This chapter provides guidelines for interpreting what the test scores may mean in terms of a child's *functional* ability with regard to listening, communicating, and learning.

Introduction

Auditory processing skills provide the foundation for listening, communicating, and learning. Deficits with auditory processing typically present in problems with academic and/or curricular achievement and success. Parents and educators want to know "What is going on with my child?" or "Who can tell me what is wrong and why my child struggles in learning?" Often it is the speech-language pathologist who is expected to answer these questions, as this profession is mandated in public school districts.

We have come to realize that just being able to "hear" a spoken message is not enough to properly listen, communicate, and learn (Geffner & Ross-Swain, 2006). A simple hearing test cannot and does not indicate whether a person has difficulty listening, in particular, in difficult listening conditions. Auditory processing is not a singular skill, but rather an integration of skills that are basic to the listening, communicating, and learning process (CSHA Task Force Document, 2004). The auditory system is complex encompassing skills of sound awareness, attention to the message, auditory discrimination, localization of sound, auditory figure-ground discrimination, and auditory closure (Chermak, 2001; Ross-Swain & Long, 2004). In addition, higher order functions such as auditory synthesis and integration, auditory cohesion, and auditory memory are reliant on an intact auditory processing system (Geffner & Ross-Swain, 2006). Often, when an individual is experiencing problems with auditory processing, a number of *auditory problem behaviors* may be present (Fahey, 2000; Keith, 2000), such as those listed in Table 7–1. In addition, individuals with weak auditory processing skills often demonstrate the *language problem behaviors* listed in Table 7–2 (Geffner & Ross-Swain, 2006).

Ideally, assessment of auditory processing skills involves a team of professionals that include an audiologist, speech-language pathologist, educator, psychologist, social worker, parents, and physician (Bellis, 2003). However, in most educational settings assembling the "ideal" team is not possible because of fiscal and time restrictions as well as having a limited number of professionals trained in assessing auditory processing skills. Many school districts do not have an audiologist employed in their setting, nor one who works contractually. Most, however, employ a speech-language pathologist, school nurse, and school psychologist who can perform appropriate testing to provide information regarding cogni-

Table 7–1. Auditory Problem Behaviors

• Frequently says "huh?" or "what?" • Misunderstands or misinterprets what is being said • Needs information to be repeated or rephrased • Is easily distracted by noise • Has difficulty following conversations or discussions • Has difficulty following spoken directions • Has difficulty listening in the presence of background noise	• Confuses words that sound alike—"mishears" • Has poor short-term memory • Inability to retain information • Has difficulty localizing sound sources • Has difficulty discriminating among sounds • Has trouble blending sounds to form words

Table 7–2. Language Problem Behaviors

• Difficulty "getting to the point" in conversation • Difficulty organizing and expressing thoughts • Difficulty "getting started" with open-ended questions • Uses vague language • Difficulty knowing what to say	• Difficulty reading and responding to social cues • Experiences word-finding problems • Difficulty remembering lengthy directions • Has pronounced differences between measures of verbal and performance abilities

tion, hearing acuity, speech-language skill abilities, and the auditory processing of spoken language.

Finally, not every child who demonstrates *auditory problem behaviors* should be scheduled for a thorough auditory processing skills assessment by the speech-language pathologist. Bellis (2003) reports that the term *central auditory processing disorder* has become a catch-all phrase, often used inappropriately, to explain a wide variety of learning and attention problems. Therefore, screening for auditory processing skill weaknesses would be a practical first step to help identify conditions that may require medical attention, foster increased educators' and parents' awareness of APD, reduce the shopping around associated with attempts to determine the cause of a particular child's listening and learning difficulties, and minimize psychological factors on the part of the child arising from anxiety, stress, and fear of the unknown. Such actions allow for insightful educational planning based upon the individual child's auditory strengths and weaknesses (Musiek, Gollegly, Lamb, & Lamb, 1990). In addition, screening for CAPD also would reduce time and cost investments on the part of the special education team by reducing the number of overreferrals for comprehensive CAPD evaluation and other diagnostic assessments, and helping to provide direction to special educators, speech-language pathologists, rehabilitative audiologists, and other professionals entrusted with the task of developing a remediation program to help manage children's disorders in the most efficient way possible (Bellis, 2003).

Assessment, therefore, by the speech-language pathologist is just that. The speech-language pathologist *assesses* the various skills of auditory processing that include auditory perception and discrimination and auditory/speech perception under degraded listening conditions. *Auditory-language* processing skills assessed by the speech-language pathologist include auditory association/receptive vocabulary, auditory memory, phonemic awareness, auditory closure, auditory cohesion, and auditory comprehension (California Speech-Language-Hearing Association, CSHA Task Force Document, 2004). Further assessment of language skill weaknesses often coexisting with APD include assessing expressive vocabulary, word retrieval, syntax, and grammar, even nonliteral language as well as narrative language. It is essential to recognize how the different categories of testing by the speech-language pathologist contribute to the multidimensional aspects of auditory processing skills (e.g., auditory, linguistic, and cognitive). Additionally, assessment of *behaviors* that tend to typify children with auditory processing disorder is helpful to capture information that standardized testing is insensitive to measure.

The APD assessment process begins with screening, followed by a thorough assessment, as deemed necessary. The results of the evaluation will guide intervention recommendations for remediation and management.

Screening Tests for the Speech-Language Pathologist

Before a formal testing battery is initiated, the speech-language pathologist should examine qualitatively the presenting symptoms, behaviors, history, and other academic issues which may point to a possible APD. The following is necessary and relevant information that should be obtained and reviewed before screening and/or testing (CSHA Task Force Document, 2004, p. 7):

1. Referral source and reason for the referral
2. A thorough client history and/or parent interview to gather background information such as:
   a. Family history
   b. Pregnancy and delivery history
   c. Postnatal history
   d. Adoption history
   e. Infancy and childhood history
   f. Developmental milestones
   g. Health history, including otologic history or middle ear fluid and allergies

h. Auditory development history
i. Visual development history
j. Motor and sensory developmental history
k. Social and behavioral developmental history
l. Speech and language developmental history
m. Previous evaluations and treatment with results
n. Educational history
o. School/educational issues
p. Behavior
q. Parent expectations
r. Classroom and social observations

3. Behavioral Survey
   a. Attending and focusing during auditory tasks
   b. Requests for frequent repetition or clarification of input information
   c. Misinterpretation of what is said
   d. Lack of response to name when called
   e. Processes better in quiet environment
   f. Learns poorly through lecture-style teaching
   g. Is easily distracted, primarily by noise
   h. Sensitive to loud noises

A qualitative analysis of this information can direct decision-making relative to screening versus a comprehensive evaluation. This information can be obtained through the development of a thorough parent questionnaire that can minimize the time needed for parent interview. However, when deciding to begin with a screening for auditory processing skill weaknesses versus a comprehensive assessment, some factors should be considered. A key factor in considering tools for screening is the time involved in administration. As a general rule of thumb, the time involved in gathering preliminary information, with respect to any team member, should not exceed the time needed for comprehensive central auditory assessment (Bellis, 2003).

There are two standardized instruments for screening auditory processing skills that may be used by the speech-language pathologist. They are The Listening Inventory (Geffner & Ross-Swain, 2006) and the SCAN-C: A Test for Auditory Processing Disorders in Children—Revised (Keith, 2000).

The Listening Inventory (TLI) is a validated criterion referenced instrument and was developed to serve as an initial screener for speech-language pathologists, teachers, special educators, and audiologists to identify children (especially those in kindergarten and early primary grades) who may be at risk for having APD. TLI identifies individuals who may be at risk for a listening disorder, to confirm that further evaluation should be made, or to help differentiate a listening/auditory disorder from among other coexisting conditions. TLI *is especially useful in the identification of children in the early grades to maximize the effects of early intervention* (Geffner & Ross-Swain, 2006).

TLI assesses specific behaviors (in 6 categories) that can be associated with auditory processing skill weaknesses. The categories include Linguistic Organization (LO), Decoding and Language Mechanics (DL), Attention and Organization (AO), Sensory-Motor (SM), Social and Behavioral Skills (SB), and Auditory Processes (AP). TLI captures and quantifies specific behaviors that are typically reported anecdotally. Heretofore, there have been no validated instruments designed specifically to screen children for *listening* disabilities and to assist in differentiating that disorder from among others. It has been noted that individuals with (C)APD may also experience language and academic difficulties, as well as have a higher likelihood of behavioral, emotional, and social difficulties (ASHA, 2005). TLI is useful for Response to Intervention (RTI)'s current goals.

TLI can assist professionals in determining which children should be assessed further for (C)APD by utilizing input from several knowledgeable sources (i.e., parents, teachers, speech-language pathologists, psychologists, and school nurses). Another intention of TLI is to identify children for whom formal testing is not yet warranted, but who exhibit "at risk" behaviors and for whom therapeutic intervention may be implemented. Auditory processing skills have been associated recently with emergent literacy (Moncrief & Musiek, 2002); thus, early recognition of these deficit areas may improve later academic performance.

The SCAN-C Test for Auditory Processing Disorder in Children—Revised (Keith, 2000) was designed to be administered by speech-language pathologists, audiologists, neuropsychologists, and other professionals (e.g., special educators knowledgeable in the administration and interpretation of tests designed for special education programs for children with learning or processing problems (Keith, 2000).

The SCAN-C consists of four subtests chosen to obtain information about areas that have been demonstrated to be among those most relevant to understanding auditory processing abilities. The four subtests include: Subtest 1: Filtered Words; Subtest 2: Auditory Figure-Ground; Subtest 3: Competing Words; and Subtest 4: Competing Sentences. A description of each subtest follows:

Subtest 1: Filtered Words—The Filtered Words subtest enables the examiner to assess a child's ability to understand distorted speech. Results of research using such tasks indicates that children with APD have difficulty understanding distorted speech and often exhibit receptive language with poor auditory closure (Keith, 2000).

Subtest 2: Auditory Figure-Ground—The Auditory Figure-Ground subtest enables the examiner to assess the child's ability to understand speech in the presence of background noise. Difficulty in understanding speech in the presence of background noise is a frequent complaint of individuals with auditory processing difficulties (Keith, 2000). These children are unable to completely comprehend auditory input in noisy situations, reverberant rooms, and in other unfavorable listening conditions. Poor performance on such tasks may also indicate a delay in development of the auditory system (Mueller & Bright, 1994).

Subtest 3: Competing Words—The Competing Words subtest enables the examiner to assess the child's ability to understand competing speech signals, sometimes referred to as binaural separation (BS). The Competing Words subtest is a dichotic task that is used to assess function of neurological pathways of the auditory system. Poor overall performance may indicate a developmental delay in maturation, underlying neurological disorganization, or damage to auditory pathways (Keith, 2000).

Subtest 4: Competing Sentences—The Competing Sentences subtest is a binaural summation task procedure. It is used to determine levels of auditory maturation, hemispheric dominance for language, and identify disordered or damaged central auditory pathways.

The combination of The Listening Inventory and SCAN-C comprise an excellent screening battery providing both qualitative and quantitative information that can be used to determine the need for a more comprehensive battery for assessing auditory processing skills and a referral to an audiologist, if needed.

Other Nonstandardized Screening Inventories

There are several nonstandardized behavioral questionnaires and checklists that are designed to provide qualitative information relative to a child's functioning in a variety of environments and situations. These inventories include:

1. Children's Auditory Performance Scale (CHAPS) (Smoski, Brunt, & Tannahill, 1992).
2. Children's Home Inventory of Listening Difficulties (CHILD) (Anderson & Smaldino, 2000)
3. Fisher's Auditory Problems Checklist (Fisher, 1976)
4. Listening Inventory for Education (LIFE) (Anderson & Smaldino, 1998)
5. Screening Instrument for Targeting Educational Risk (SIFTER.) (Anderson & Markin, 1989)

The majority of these inventories may be purchased from the Educational Audiology Association in Tampa, Florida.

Observation of Classroom and Nonclassroom Behavior

Bellis (2003) reported that it should be emphasized that **the value of simple, old-fashioned behavioral observation in both classroom and nonclassroom environments should not be underestimated.** These types of observations enable the clinician to glean information that standardized testing cannot provide because test items may not be sensitive enough. Observations should target *listening* behaviors that may or may not be affecting a child's ability to listen for learning purposes. Suggested behaviors warranting observation are listed in Table 7–3.

This list of behaviors is not intended to be exhaustive, but rather to provide clinicians with general suggestions when observing a child who may be experiencing auditory processing skill weaknesses. Answers to these questions provide important information relative to a child's functional ability in the classroom and may assist in differentiating among auditory process-

Table 7–3. Behaviors Warranting Observation

• Is the child able to follow age level appropriate instructions? • What does the child do when he/she can't follow instructions? • Does the child "tune out" or daydream and under what conditions? • Can the child follow and participate in discussions? • Is the child easily distractible? What distracts the child? • Does the child need to have verbal directions repeated or rephrased? • What happens to the child's listening ability when there is competing noise? • Is the child able to complete work independently? How much support is needed for the child to complete tasks that are intended to be performed independently? • Does the child appear to fatigue from listening? What happens when the child fatigues? • Is the child able to consistently and successfully perform routine classroom procedures? • Does the child listen better earlier in the day than later in the day? • Does the child appear to forget what has just been said? • Does the child appear to have a short attention span? • What are the acoustic conditions of the classroom that may be contributing to the child's listening ability?

ing skill weaknesses, attention deficit hyperactive disorder (ADHD), or other deficits that may be coexisting or interfering with the effective processing of input information.

Suggested Speech-Language Battery for Assessing Auditory Processing Skills

Once a screening of auditory processing skill weaknesses has been performed and the results indicate the need for comprehensive testing, the speech-language pathologist is faced with many decisions, primarily, what to assess and how best to assess to gain both qualitative and quantitative information relative to auditory processing skills. The clinician is urged to remember that the purpose of assessment is to *assess* and measure (or quantify) specific auditory processing skills. Auditory processing is not a *singular* skill ability, but rather relies on a constellation of auditory functions/skills that are basic to the listening and communication process. The boundaries of each are not well defined but rather are interdependent (Chermak & Musiek, 1997). Therefore, when selecting specific standardized batteries for the assessment process the clinician must keep in mind that there is not *one* specific battery that can assess all of the auditory processing skills. Rather, the clinician should consider a variety of tests that can best measure the many and relevant auditory processing skills in order to provide parents, teachers and other professionals with necessary information to direct decision-making about therapeutic interventions, educational placement, and environmental modifications.

There may be instances where novice parents or other professionals (including speech-language pathologists) interpret the findings of the assessment by the speech-language pathologist as being a diagnosis for APD. Keep in mind that the information that the speech-language pathologist is providing is not a diagnosis but rather a reporting of auditory processing skill weaknesses that impact language, cognition, and memory.

The following standardized tests represent suggested batteries that measure abilities in each of the areas of auditory perception and discrimination, auditory association/receptive vocabulary, auditory memory, phonemic awareness, auditory closure, auditory comprehension, auditory cohesion, and auditory/speech perception under degraded listening conditions. It is worthy to note that there may be other instruments not mentioned that are appropriate and others will be developed but this list constitutes what has been determined to be useful and familiar to practicing clinicians. Although the list is not exhaustive (e.g., listing every test battery) it is intended to provide the speech-language pathologist with guidance when selecting tests needed for a comprehensive battery. However, not unlike other speech-language assessments, the clinician is cautioned to use judgment when selecting tests that measure skill abilities in those areas in which presenting symptoms have been identified. The tests listed under the specific auditory processing skills are arranged in alphabetical order. In some cases, these tests measure auditory-language abilities. It is often difficult to separate auditory-only components from the auditory-language components.

Tests for Assessing Skills of Auditory Perception and Discrimination

1. The Goldman-Fristoe-Woodcock Test of Auditory Discrimination: Quiet Subtest and Selective Attention (Goldman, Fristoe, & Woodcock 2000)
2. The Lindamood Auditory Conceptualization Test—Third Edition (LAC-3; Lindamood & Lindamood, 2004)
3. The Test of Auditory Processing Skills—Third Edition (TAPS-3; Martin & Brownell, 2005)
4. The Test of Language Development—Third Edition (TOLD-P:3; Newcomer & Hammill, 1997)
5. Wepman's Auditory Discrimination Test (Wepman & Reynolds, 1997)

Tests for Assessing Skills of Auditory Association/Receptive Vocabulary

1. The Comprehensive Receptive and Expressive Vocabulary Test—Revised (CREVT-2; Wallace & Hammill, 2002)

2. The Clinical Evaluation of Language Function—Fourth Edition (CELF-4; Semel et al., 2003)
3. The Comprehensive Assessment of Spoken Language (CASL; Carrow-Woolfolk, 1994)
4. The Peabody Picture Vocabulary Test (PPVT; Dunn & Dunn, 1997)
5. The Receptive One-Word Picture Vocabulary Test (ROWPVT; Brownell, 2000)
6. The Test of Language Development—Third Edition (TOLD-P:3) Subtest 1

Tests for Assessing Skills of Auditory Memory

1. The Auditory Processing Abilities Test (APAT; Ross-Swain & Long, 2004) (Subtests 2, 6, and 9)
2. Clinical Evaluation of Language Fundamentals—Fourth Edition (CELF-4) (Subtests of Understanding Concepts and Following Directions; Number Repetition; and Familiar Sequences, Recalling Sentences)
3. The Comprehensive Test of Phonological Processing (CTOPP): Subtest III (Wagner et al., 1999)
4. The Test of Language Development-Primary—Third Edition (TOLD-P:3): Subtest V
5. The Token Test for Children—Second Edition (TTFC-2) (McGhee, Ehrer, & DiSimoni, 1978)
6. The Test of Auditory Processing Skills—Third Edition (TAPS-3): Subtests of Number Memory Forward; Number Memory Reversed; Word Memory and Sentence Memory
7. Wepman's Auditory Memory Battery (Wepman & Morency, 1985)
8. The Wide Range Assessment of Memory and Learning—Second Edition (WRAML-2; Sheslow & Adams, 2003)

Tests for Assessing Skills of Phonemic Awareness

1. The Auditory Processing Abilities Test (APAT): Subtest 1
2. The Clinical Evaluation of Language Fundamentals—Fourth Edition (CELF-4): Subtest of Phonological Awareness
3. The Comprehensive Test of Phonological Processing (CTOPP): Subtests 1, 2, 8, 10, 11, and 12
4. The Lindamood Auditory Conceptualization Test—Third Edition (LAC-3)
5. The Phonological Awareness Test (PAT)
6. The Test of Language Development—Primary—Third Edition (TOLD-P:3)
7. The Test of Auditory Processing Skills—Third Edition (TAPS-3): Subtests of Phonological Segmentation and Phonological Blending
8. The Phonemic Synthesis Test (Katz & Fletcher, 1982)

Tests for Assessing Skills of Auditory Closure

1. The Comprehensive Assessment of Spoken Language (CASL): Subtest of Meaning from Context
2. Test of Language Competence (TLC): Subtest 3 (Wiig & Secord, 1989)
3. SCAN-C: Subtest 1

Tests for Assessing Skills of Auditory Comprehension and Auditory Cohesion

1. The Auditory Processing Abilities Test (APAT): Subtests 7, 8, and 10
2. The Clinical Evaluation of Language Fundamentals—Fourth Edition (CELF-4): Subtests of Linguistic Concepts, Sentence Structure, Understanding Concepts and Following Directions, and Understanding Spoken Paragraphs
3. The Comprehensive Assessment of Spoken Language (CASL): Subtests of Sentence Comprehension, Paragraph Comprehension, Nonliteral Language, Ambiguous Sentences, and Inference
4. The Listening Test (Barrett et al., 1992)
5. The Test of Auditory Processing Skills—Third Edition (TAPS-3): Subtests of Auditory Comprehension and Auditory Reasoning
6. The Test of Language Competence (TLC): Subtests 1 and 4
7. The Token Test for Children—Second Edition (TTFC; DiSimoni, 1978)
8. The Wide Range Assessment of Memory and Learning—Second Edition (WRAML-2): Subtests 1 and 6

Tests for Assessing Skills of Expressive Vocabulary

1. The Comprehensive Receptive and Expressive Vocabulary Test (CREVT)
2. The Clinical Evaluation of Language Fundamentals—Fourth Edition (CELF-4): Subtest of Expressive Vocabulary and Word Definitions
3. The Detroit Test of Learning Abilities—Fourth Edition (DTLA-4): Subtest of Story Construction
4. The Illinois Test of Psycholinguistic Abilities—Third Edition (ITPA-3): Subtest 3 (Hammill et al., 2001)
5. The Expressive One-Word Picture Vocabulary Test (EOWPVT; Brownell et al., 2000)
6. The Test of Language Development—Primary—Third Edition (TOLD-P:3): Subtest 3
7. The Expressive Vocabulary Test (EVT; Williams, 1997)

Tests for Assessing Skills of Word Retrieval

1. The Clinical Evaluation of Language Fundamentals—Fourth Edition (CELF-4): Subtests of Word Associations and Rapid Automatic Naming
2. The Comprehensive Assessment of Spoken Language (CASL): Subtests of Antonyms, Synonyms, and Sentence Completion
3. The Comprehensive Test of Phonological Processing (CTOPP): Subtests IV, VI, VII, and IX
4. The Illinois Test of Psycholinguistic Abilities—Third Edition (ITPA-3): Subtest 1
5. The Test of Language Development—Primary—Third Edition (TOLD-P:3): Subtests II and VI
6. The Test of Word Finding—Second Edition (TOWF-2; German, 1999)
7. The Boston Naming Test

Testing for Assessing Skills of Auditory/Speech Perception Under Degraded Listening Conditions

1. The Goldman-Fristoe-Woodcock Test of Auditory Discrimination (GFWTAD): Selective Attention Subtest
2. SCAN-C or SCAN-A
3. Test of Auditory Processing Skills—Third Edition (TAPS-3): Auditory Figure-Ground Subtest

Interpretation of Testing Results

Interpretation of auditory processing assessment results may be undertaken with a variety of goals in mind and, depending on the desired outcome, the interpretation process may be involved and lengthy, or quick and simple (Bellis, 2003). Careful interpretation of testing results can provide useful information relative to a child's strengths and weaknesses as well as making clinical decisions about treatment intervention and management (Geffner & Ross-Swain, 2006; Ross-Swain & Long, 2004). Too often clinicians forget that "tests don't diagnose, people do" and base their diagnoses and/or recommendations exclusively on test scores or results. Test results are merely observations that provide quantitative and qualitative data. They report a performance level at a given time within a specific context. However, they do not reveal to the clinician/examiner why a child performed as he or she did.

The speech-language pathologist should be extremely cautious and vigilant to avoid drawing conclusions or using test scores without consideration of the child's other speech-language, psychological, behavioral, and/or motor issues which may adversely affect the validity of the test scores (Bellis, 2003; CSHA, 2004). When selecting tests for assessing auditory processing skills the clinician should use batteries that would require output modalities that are not influenced by the child's other skill weaknesses whenever possible. For example, a child with expressive language deficits may have difficulty responding to auditory comprehension or memory tasks requiring lengthy verbal responses. That is, their responses on the auditory tasks that result in errors may be errors due to expressive language deficits and have nothing to do with auditory memory or comprehension.

Pitfalls in Testing

A typical auditory memory task is one that requires a child to repeat sentences of increasing length and complexity. If a child experiences expressive language deficits that affect age-level appropriate use of vocabulary, syntax and morphology error responses may occur. If the clinician were to ignore these underlying weaknesses, a low score could be interpreted as a weak auditory memory. It is necessary to be aware of any expressive language weaknesses that may confound results. When reporting findings the clinician must reveal the confounding effects of expressive language (or other) deficits on the immediate memory testing results.

1. Another typical measure of auditory memory requires a child to repeat a series of single words of increasing length. If a child is experiencing deficits with auditory discrimination and "mishears" a word or words, most certainly error responses will occur that are not reflecting a weak auditory memory but weaknesses with discrimination that are affecting his or her performance on this task. For example, if a child is asked to repeat "box nail pen" and responds with "fox mail pan" it will be scored as an error response, but the clinician should have information regarding a child's auditory discrimination skills to correctly interpret the results.
2. Many tests assessing auditory processing skills require that a child follow directions of increasing length and complexity that incorporate temporal and spatial concepts. A child's low score on such subtests could be a result of being unfamiliar with these concepts and being unable to accurately perform the task. For example if a child is asked to "put an X in the lower right-hand corner" a child may not know what "lower" or "right" means, thus failing the task.
3. Auditory latency (slow processing speed) is often observed in children with auditory processing skill weaknesses. Slow processing speed can result in errors with even simple auditory processing tasks. The clinician should be vigilant in making clinical interpretations about the effects of processing delays on a child's overall processing. For example, delays may occur because a child is working overtime to understand what has been said because he or she has "misheard" as a result of an auditory discrimination deficit. Or a child may have an auditory association weakness that may result in slow processing. Finally, if a child experiences auditory fatigue as a result of ongoing listening and processing or "working overtime" to listen, processing delays may occur. It is incumbent upon the clinician to observe and report these behaviors and include them when interpreting testing results.

Any number of factors can occur that can affect test results and should be noted so as to be considered when interpreting test results. Some of these factors may include that the child: is tired from lack of sleep; is hungry; has middle ear fluid related to a recent cold or ear infection; is taking medication; may not be feeling well; or is required to sit and attend for a time that exceeds his or her tolerance. Bellis (2003) states that APD is a heterogeneous disorder; therefore, it is not possible to address all possible combinations of findings for interpretation purposes. The remainder of this chapter offers guidelines for interpretation of test results used by the speech-language pathologist when assessing auditory processing skills.

Because children with auditory processing skill weaknesses typically experience problems with learning, the interpretation of the test results should answer the questions: (1) "What are the effects of the auditory processing skill weaknesses on his or her learning success?" and (2) "What can be done about it?"

Guidelines for Interpretation of Test Results

The "data" to be analyzed and interpreted when assessing auditory processing skills would include: client history, behavioral observations, relevant information from teachers, psychologists, physicians, and other professionals involved in the care of the child, results from hearing testing, results from auditory processing skills screening and results from the comprehensive assessment of auditory processing skills. The purpose of data analysis and interpretation typically include:

1. Identifying the presence or absence of auditory processing skill weaknesses;
2. Identifying specific auditory processing skill weaknesses (e.g., auditory discrimination, auditory memory, etc.);
3. Determining the effects of the identified skill weaknesses on specific learning processes (e.g., reading, spelling, following directions, understanding spoken language, etc.);
4. Determining which treatment interventions and/or management processes would be beneficial for the child; and
5. Sharing the results with other professionals involved in the educational and remedial care of the child.

Identifying the Presence of Auditory Processing Skill Weaknesses

Most clinicians use test scores to determine if an auditory processing problem may be present. That is, they are looking at the quantitative data. However, many professionals would agree that examining both quantitative and qualitative data will provide maximal information when determining if an auditory processing problem is present. Test scores can be deceiving when used as a solitary index for measure. Qualitative data refers to "how" a child finally got to his or her response, behaviors observed during testing, functional abilities in the classroom, and information reported by parents and teachers.

The problem facing professionals is determining when auditory processing skill weaknesses are really a problem or not. Bellis (2003) suggests that the decision of whether an auditory processing problem is present will depend on many factors but stresses that the most important is the criterion for abnormal performance chosen by the clinician, such as a lax or strict criterion. The most common criterion used to determine eligibility references standard deviations. That is, depending upon policies of different setting (e.g., schools, clinics, etc.) two or three standard deviations below the mean will serve as a measure for meeting diagnostic criteria.

Overall, Bellis (2003) advocates for a lax criterion for interpretation in which an abnormal finding on any given test tool, *combined with significant educational and behavioral findings,* may be considered as evidence of CAPD.

However, **typically, the diagnosis of (C)APD requires performance greater than two standard deviations below the mean on two or more central auditory diagnostic tests**. A deficit greater than three standard deviations below the mean on one test, combined with significant functional difficulty in the process assessed by that test, also may lead to a diagnosis of (C)APD; however, caution is suggested when a deficit is observed on only one test (ASHA, 2005a; Bellis, 2003a; Bellis, 2007, see Chapter 4).

The role of the speech-language pathologist, once testing has been performed, is not to diagnose, but to determine if there are auditory processing skill weaknesses present and to assist in determining how these weaknesses are affecting the child's listening, communicating, and learning abilities.

Identifying Specific Auditory Processing Skill Weaknesses

A comprehensive standardized assessment battery should examine a number of auditory processing skills, some of which could be considered embedded in language skills. These skills that are assessed would include: auditory perception and discrimination, auditory closure, auditory memory, auditory association, auditory comprehension, auditory cohesion, and phonemic awareness. All test batteries yield raw scores, standard scores, and percentile rankings. Some provide age-level equivalents as well. Depending on the criterion that is used for identifying "a real problem" the quantitative data that results from the testing will identify which specific auditory processing skills are deemed impaired, which auditory processing skills are weak, but not considered to be impaired, and which auditory processing skills are within the average range.

Scoring systems used on standardized measures by speech-language pathologists are quantitative in nature. Typical scoring systems are plus/minus or a system that assigns a numerical score depending upon the response that is elicited. A drawback to this type of scoring system is that it does not capture qualitative information (behaviors that may result from an auditory processing problem). For example, if a child experiences difficulty with immediate memory skills but frequently requests repetition of stimulus items throughout testing, scoring an accurate response would preclude the child's weaknesses leading to inaccurate results. This may be a child who, in the classroom, has difficulty following directions, frequently needs to have instructions repeated, or often says "what?" The risk may be that the quantitative and qualitative data conflict.

Dr. Bruce Porch (1981) introduced a multidimensional scoring system designed to describe response behaviors when testing aphasic adults. The scoring system had five basic dimensions that are very useful when implemented in administering testing to assess auditory processing skills: accuracy, responsiveness, completeness, promptness, and efficiency. All of these dimensions are applicable when describing response behaviors of children with auditory processing skill weaknesses. When analyzing results with this type of scoring system the clinician can determine the percentage of the time a child shows delays, requires repetition or cues, is incomplete, and so on. This qualitative data is then included in a summary report that *interprets* testing results.

Therefore, clinicians are reminded that, if possible, descriptive scoring systems can be extremely beneficial in describing response behaviors that affect a child's overall processing and learning abilities, that is, a scoring system that could assist the clinician to record and measure delayed responses, repetitions of task instructions or stimulus items, and self-corrected errors. This type of scoring system enables the clinician to note behavior patterns such as tuning in and out, a "slow rise time," or fatigue, thus offering valuable information to parents, teachers, and other educators involved in the child's care.

Determining the Effects of the Identified Auditory Processing Skill Weaknesses on Specific Learning Processes

Children who have difficulty with listening tend to have difficulty with learning. It is helpful to remember that when children learn to listen then they can listen to learn. Gillet (1993), reports that the auditory modality is of prime importance in the school environment, especially reading, language development, and comprehension, communication, and in the general learning process, (i.e., the acquisition and processing of incoming information). The typical school environment places significant emphasis on learning through the auditory modality, especially as the child progresses to higher grades (Gillet, 1993). A child who has auditory processing skill weaknesses and is having difficulty with overall learning, may be the child in the classroom who has difficulty understanding spoken directions, following age-level-appropriate multistep directions, tunes out or daydreams, is having difficulty learning to read and spell, difficulty understanding age-level-appropriate concepts through the auditory modality, and/or saying "I didn't hear you," despite manifesting proper attention.

Effective analysis and interpretation of the results of the comprehensive assessment of auditory processing skills by the speech-language pathologist can be extremely helpful in providing an explanation to parents and teachers regarding the effects of auditory processing skill weaknesses on a child's learning. For example, if testing indicates that a child is having difficulty with auditory discrimination, this may provide an explanation as to why the child has difficulty understanding directions. In addition, problems with discrimination may result in a child "stopping" the listening process to try to figure out what was being said (e.g., was that "get the comb" or "get the cone") and/or not hearing the remainder of the direction or instruction. This child, too, may spend a great deal of time "working overtime" to listen in order to figure out what is being said. Fatigue can result, leading to "tuning out." Problems with discrimination may result in a number of behaviors that require careful interpretation. Problems with discrimination can result in difficulty following directions that, at times, appear to be weaknesses with auditory memory. However, careful analysis and interpretation of testing can assist in "sorting out" what is more likely the actual cause of a child's difficulty with following directions.

If testing indicates difficulty with auditory memory skills then the child may have difficulty following age-level-appropriate multistep directions or comprehending paragraph material. Furthermore, the child will process the information that his or her auditory memory will allow and then lose information that surpasses his or her capacity. The child may then begin to process additional input information that may not be related to the information that was presented initially. This child, like the child with auditory discrimination problems, may be "working overtime" to understand or make sense out of fragmented pieces of input that do not relate to one another. In other words, he or she is attempting to make sense out of nonsense.

Processing delays pose additional problems for the child with auditory processing skill weaknesses. Behaviorally, these children may have difficulty following directions, comprehending spoken information, daydreaming, and/or tuning out. Yes, these behaviors certainly interfere with learning (e.g., parents and teachers often say "If he would listen then he could follow directions" or "If he would pay attention he could listen better," etc.); however, delays with processing speed often prevent children from processing at the same rate as the speaker is speaking. So, they only get part of what is being said and not the entire spoken message. The effects of processing delays should be differentiated between similar effects that are a result of auditory discrimination or immediate auditory memory deficits.

Mastery of reading and spelling skills requires prior mastery of specific auditory processing/phonemic awareness skills. Gillet (1993) reports that the child with auditory processing problems may be affected in the area of reading and spelling in the following ways: (a) difficulty hearing the similarities in initial and final sounds in words; (b) difficulty hearing adjacent sounds in consonant blends; (c) difficulty discriminating short vowel sounds; (d) difficulty rhyming; (e) difficulty breaking a word into syllables or individual sounds (phoneme analysis); (f) difficulty retaining each of the sounds or syllables; (g) difficulty blending sounds together as a whole, even though the individual sounds are known; (h) difficulty remembering the sound of a letter or how to say a word, even though the meaning may be known; (i) difficulty imprecisely relating the auditory symbol with the visual symbol; (j) may substitute words when reading aloud; and/or (k) may distort the pronunciation of multisyllable words as there is difficulty in sequencing sounds.

The relationship of reading problems to auditory processing skill weaknesses needs further analysis. Possible questions to answer would include: (1) What are the effects of poor auditory discrimination on a child's reading skills?; (2) What are the effects of immediate memory on a child's reading skills?; (3) What are the effects of auditory association on a child's reading skills; and (4) What are the effects of processing speed and/or fatigue on the child's reading skills?

Another concern is the difference between weak versus disordered skills. The results of testing may not provide the clinician with a clear-cut answer. Sometimes it may be necessary to treat the symptoms, if they are weak. For children who have poor compensatory or coping strategies or other issues (e.g., low frustration tolerance, difficulty working independently, etc.) or if they score in the 12th to 20th percentiles on subtests assessing specific auditory processes, they can experience problems, especially if they are in a high-performing school or there is a discrepancy among their other abilities. So, a child may have weaknesses but not a definitive diagnosis of an auditory processing disorder. Nevertheless, specific intervention is needed to develop strategies or techniques that can improve his or her functional abilities in a learning or listening environment.

Careful analysis and interpretation of comprehensive auditory processing assessment results administered by the speech-language pathologist can provide valuable information to parents, teachers, and other educators involved in a child's care offering an explanation as to why a child performs a certain way in different listening and learning situations. Too often, reports that are prepared summarizing testing results only report quantitative data without an interpretation of what test scores mean. Test scores do not interpret nor explain a child's functional ability. It is the careful and vigilant interpretation of the testing results and observed behaviors that provides necessary and useful information.

Determining Which Treatment Interventions and/or Management Processes Would Be Beneficial

Most of the children who are experiencing auditory processing skill weaknesses that affect their communication and learning skills typically have a classification as speech-language impaired and have an Individual Educational Plan (IEP) in place. Therefore, there will be a team of educators and professionals involved in making recommendations for remedial or management interventions. The team may consist of the child's teacher, the speech-language pathologist, the psychologist, the audiologist (if possible), the school nurse, a resource specialist, and parents. The role of the speech pathologist and audiologist is to present and discuss the effects of a child's auditory processing skill weakness on his or her overall learning, resulting in recommendations for interventions that are available for remediating specific auditory skill weaknesses (remediation processes and programs are discussed in Section II of this text). Additional recommendations would include environmental modifications that can assist a child in enhancing his or her listening skills both at home and at school (see Chapter 10).

Currently, there is not a national educational policy about assessment and intervention for auditory processing problems in the public schools. Rather, individual school districts determine how children with auditory processing skill weaknesses will be managed in their special education programs. However, the results of comprehensive assessment of auditory processing skills should be performed and reported relative to their impact on a child's listening, communication, and learning skills.

Sharing the Results with Other Professionals Involved in the Educational and Remedial Care of the Child

The results of a comprehensive auditory processing skills assessment yield important information that may be relevant to a child's educational placement, special education services, psychological status, and therapeutic interventions. Testing results should be shared with appropriate and responsible professionals eligible to receive such information. Hammill et al. (2001) report that the clinician should consider the following three points when sharing the findings of testing:

1. A thorough understanding of the purposes, content, and construction of the batteries used in the assessment prior to any presentation. When presenting the results of testing to those professionals who may be unfamiliar with the test instruments it is necessary to describe each battery with regard to normative statistics, reliability, and validity.
2. Explanation of test scores should always be accompanied by a personal interpretation from the clinician regarding (a) meaning; (b) possible alternative interpretations; (c) reports of other diagnostic assessments and how they relate to the findings of the current assessment; (d) integration of other information and data sources (e.g., classroom observations; teacher observations; parent observations, etc.); (e) suggestions for instructional or remedial changes; and (f) recommendations for further testing by other professionals. All of these appropriate points should be presented and discussed prior to making final recommendations to parents and other professionals involved in the child's care.
3. Every effort should be made to translate the testing results into language that is familiar to the person with whom the information is being shared. The language that is used in speech-language reports is often unfamiliar to other professionals. Whenever possible that language should be defined to enhance the understanding of the reader or listener. Clinicians should refrain from using professional jargon. Test analysis and interpretation require that the clinician examine the data both quantitatively and qualitatively. There is no preferred method or one method that is better than another. However, the clinician should examine the data from as many perspectives as possible (Bellis, 2003).

Bellis (2003) states that the results of testing should be related to the academic, communicative, and behavioral characteristics of the individual child so that a multidisciplinary management program that will address the child's functional difficulties may be developed.

Summary

The speech-language pathologist plays an integral role in assessing skills of auditory processing for purposes of identifying areas of weakness, determining how these areas of weakness may be affecting the child's functional abilities in the classroom, determining which intervention programs or processes may be effective in remediating areas of weakness, and sharing the results with other professionals.

Although the diagnosis of APD is the role and responsibility of the audiologist, the speech-language pathologist can add important information related to auditory processing skill weaknesses and their effects on listening, language, communicating, and learning. There are a number of standardized instruments designed to screen for APDs that can be used in decision making for further testing. The appropriate selection and use of standardized tests by the speech-language pathologist can offer specific information relative to a child's skills of auditory perception and discrimination, auditory memory, auditory closure, auditory association, auditory comprehension, and auditory cohesion. A qualitative and quantitative analysis and interpretation of this information can offer understanding and explanation of a child's functional abilities with regard to listening, communication, and learning behaviors and skills. Working in a multidisciplinary collaborative model the speech-language pathologist's finding is not intended to replace the testing of other professionals but rather to provide additional information to add to the overall picture and assist in critical decisions about educational placement and therapeutic interventions.

Key Points Learned

- Speech-language pathologists play a key role in assessing skills of auditory processing. However, a formal diagnosis is made by the audiologist.
- Screening for and comprehensive assessment of auditory processing skill weaknesses is a collaborative process using information and data from other professionals, educators, and the child's medical records.
- There is not a single test that can assess the various skills of auditory processing and the speech-language pathologist must be vigilant in making decisions about use of specific standardized and validated instruments.

- Analysis and interpretation of test results should utilize both quantitative and qualitative data.
- Assessment findings should disclose the child's functional abilities of listening, language, communication, and learning.

References

American Speech-Language and Hearing Association. (2004a). Scope of practice in audiology. *ASHA* (Suppl. 24).

Anderson, K., & Matkin, N. H. (1996). *Screening instrument for targeting educational Risk (S.I.F.T.E.R.).* Tampa, FL: Educational Audiology Association.

Anderson, K, & Smaldino, J. J. (1998). *Children's home inventory of listening difficulties (C.H.I.L.D.).* Tampa, FL: Educational Audiology Association.

Anderson, K., & Smaldino, J. J. (2000). *Listening Inventory for Education (L.I.F.E.).* Tampa, FL: Educational Audiology Association.

Barrett, M., Huisingh, R., Bowers, L., Logiudice, C., & Orman, J. (1992). *The Listening Test.* East Moline, IL: LinguiSystems.

Bellis, T. J. (2003). *Assessment and management of central auditory processing disorders in the educational setting: From science to practice* (2nd ed.). Clifton Park, NY: Thomson Learning.

Brownell, R. (2000). *Expressive One-Word Picture Vocabulary Test.* Novato, CA: Academic Therapy Publications.

Brownell, R. (2000). *Receptive One-Word Picture Vocabulary Test.* Novato, CA: Academic Therapy Publications.

California Speech-Language and Hearing Association (2004). *Guidelines for the diagnosis and treatment for auditory processing disorders.* Position paper. Sacramento: California Speech-Language and Hearing Association.

Carrow-Woolfolk, E. (1999). *Comprehensive Assessment of Spoken Language.* Circle Pines, MN: American Guidance Service.

Chermak, G. D. (2001). Auditory processing disorder: An overview for the clinician. *Hearing Journal, 54,* 10–25.

Dunn, L. M., & Dunn, L. M. (1997). *Peabody Picture Vocabulary Test—Third edition.* Circle Pines, MN: American Guidance Service.

Fahey, K. R. (2000). *Language development, differences and disorders.* Austin, TX: ProEd.

Fisher, L. I. (1976). *Fisher's Auditory Problems Checklist.* Bemidji, MN: Life Products.

Geffner, D., & Ross-Swain, D. (2006). *The Listening Inventory.* Novato, CA: Academic Therapy Publications.

German, D. J. (1999). *Test of Word Finding—Second edition.* Austin, TX: ProEd.

Gillet, P. (1993). *Auditory processes.* Novato, CA: Academic Therapy Publications.

Goldman, R., Fristoe, M., & Woodcock, R. W. (2000). *Goldman-Fristoe-Woodcock Test of Auditory Discrimination—Second edition.* Circle Pines, MN: American Guidance Service.

Hammill, D. (1996). *The Detroit Test of Learning Aptitude.* Austin, TX: ProEd

Hammill, D. D., Mather, N., & Roberts, R. (2001). *Illinois Test of Psycholinguistic Abilities—Third edition.* Austin, TX: ProEd.

Huisingh, R., Bowers, L., & Logiudice, C. (2006). *The Listening Comprehension Test-2.* East Moline, IL: LinguiSystems.

Katz, J., & Fletcher, C. H. (1982). *Phonemic Synthesis Picture (PS-P) Test Manual.* Vancouver, WA: Precision Acoustics.

Keith, R. W. (1999). Treatment for central auditory processing disorders: Clinical issues in central auditory processing disorders *Language, Speech and Hearing Services in the Schools, 30*, 339–344.

Lindamood, P. C., & Lindamood, P. (2004). *Lindamood Auditory Conceptualization Test.* Austin, TX: ProEd.

Martin, N., & Brownell, R. (2005). *Test of Auditory Processing Skills—Third edition.* Novato, CA: Academic Therapy Publications.

McGhee, R. L., Ehrler, D. J., & DiSimoni, F. (2007). *The Token Test for Children—Second Edition.* Austin, TX: Pro-Ed.

Moncrieff, D. W., & Musiek, F. E. (2000). Interaural asymmetries revealed by dichotic listening tests in normal and dyslexic children. *Journal of the American Academy of Audiology, 13*, 428–437.

Mueller, G., & Bright, K. (1994). Monolyllabic procedures in central testing. In R. W. Keith (Ed.), *SCAN-C Test For Auditory Processing Disorders in Children—Revised* (p. 3). San Antonio, TX: The Psychological Corporation.

Musiek, F. E., Gollegly, K. M, Lamb, L. E., & Lamb, P. (1990). Selected issues in screening for central auditory processing dysfunction. *Seminars in Hearing, 11*, 372–384.

Newcomer, P. L., & Hammill, D. D. (1997). *The Test of Language Development—Primary—Third edition.* Austin, TX: ProEd.

Porch, B. E. (1981). *The Porch Index of Communicative Ability.* Chicago: Riverside.

Ross-Swain, D., & Long, N. (2004). *Auditory Processing Abilities Test.* Novato, CA: Academic Therapy Publications.

Semel, E., Wiig, E. H., & Secord, W. A. (2003). *Clinical Evaluation of Language Fundamentals—Fourth edition.* San Antonio, TX: The Psychological Corporation.

Sheslow, D., & Adams, W. (2003). *Wide Range Assessment of Memory and Learning—Second edition.* Wilmington, DE: Wide Range.

Smoski, W. J., Brunt, M. A., & Tannahill, J.C. (1998). *Children's Auditory Performance Scale (C.H.A.P.S.).* Tampa, FL: Educational Audiology Association.

Wagner, R. K., Torgesen, J. K., & Rashotte, C. A. (1999). *Comprehensive Test of Phonological Processing.* Austin, TX: ProEd.

Wallace, G., & Hammill, D. D. (2002). *Comprehensive Receptive and Expressive Vocabulary Test—Second edition.* Austin, TX: ProEd.

Wepman, J. M., & Morency, A. (1985). *Wepman Auditory Memory Span Test.* Los Angeles: Western Psychological Services.

Wepman, J. M., & Reynolds, W. M. (1997). *Wepman's Auditory Discrimination Test—Second edition.* Circle Pines, MN: American Guidance Service.

Wiig, E. H., & Secord, W. (1989). *Test of Language Competence—Expanded edition.* San Antonio, TX: The Psychological Corporation.

Williams, K. T. (1997). *The Expressive Vocabulary Test.* Circle Pines, MN: American Guidance Service.

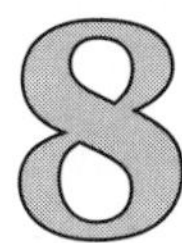

Language Processing Versus Auditory Processing

Gail J. Richard

Overview

Significant confusion currently exists regarding processing disorders. Part of the dilemma is due to confounding terminology used to describe the disorder, for example, auditory processing, central auditory processing, language processing, sensory processing, and speech perception. An additional contributing factor is the complexity inherent within the term "processing" because it encompasses so many different neurological structures and skills. A third aspect is that the area of processing has evolved over the last several decades in response to research, improved technology, and refined diagnostic procedures. As a result, "processing disorder" can have a variety of interpretations, based on who introduced it, when it was introduced, and why it was introduced.

This chapter is designed to assist the professional in delineating aspects of a processing disorder to result in more accurate diagnosis and treatment of individuals who present with the label. An audiologist or speech-language pathologist is the most appropriate professional to differentiate specific symptoms of a communication disorder that need to be addressed. Deficits that can result in a diagnosis of "processing disorder" can range from acoustic to phonemic to linguistic in nature. The professional introducing the label must be able to specifically define the characteristics that comprise the "processing disorder," and be able to differentiate between auditory processing and language processing before recommending treatment options.

Introduction

"Processing disorder" is a generic term frequently used to describe a wide variety of communication disorders. Various professionals introduce the term to describe difficulties a child experiences in an academic setting. Parents could hear "processing disorder" from a psychologist, speech-language pathologist, audiologist, teacher, physician, neurologist, or school administrator. Although all of these professionals are well intentioned, the explanation provided is likely to offer minimal specific information.

An analogy to approach the dilemma would be the Hindu fable by John Godfrey Saxe (1816–1887) about the six blind men exploring an elephant (Figure 8–1, Appendix 8-A). Each man explored a different aspect of the very large animal, resulting in six very different conclusions determined from their isolated perspective.

The blind man exploring the trunk decided the elephant was like a snake. Another blind man who was at the leg and knee decided the elephant was like a tree. A third blind man was at the ear and declared the elephant to be similar to a fan. The blind man exploring the tail declared the elephant to be like a rope. Exploring the tusk determined the elephant to be similar to a spear. A sixth blind man at the side of the elephant resulted in the impression of a wall. In reality, each was correct in regard to one feature of the elephant. However, none of the men were correct in interpreting what the entire entity represented.

The same could be said for "auditory processing." From the perspective of one audiologist, the term could represent transferring the signal through the central auditory nervous system (CANS), or a brainstem function. A second could define the disorder based only on brainstem-evoked potentials. Another audiologist could consider the

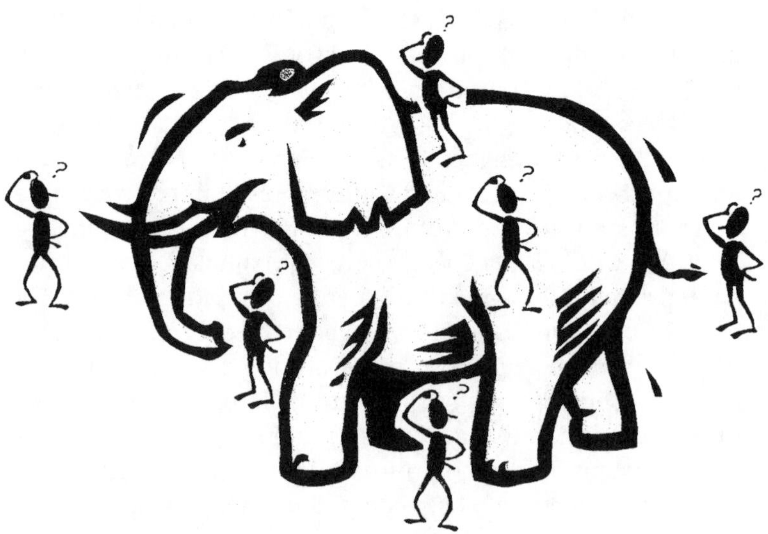

Figure 8–1. The Blind Men and the Elephant.

acoustic characteristics as they are received in the temporal lobe at Heschl's gyrus. Yet a fourth audiologist could functionally interpret the disorder as difficulty with memory and analysis of auditory input. A fifth audiologist could determine the disorder within frequency differences (pitch).

The same confusion can exist within speech-language pathology. One speech-language pathologist might interpret the disorder as phonemic discrimination problems (i.e, hearing acoustic differences), whereas a second might interpret it as a phonic discrimination problem (i.e., representing sounds with grapheme symbols). A third speech-language pathologist might define the disorder as being able to discriminate meaningful versus nonmeaningful acoustic information. A fourth speech-language pathologist could define the differences as being able to understand concrete versus abstract language. Yet another might functionally define the difficulty as understanding and following directions.

As in the Hindu fable, each professional is interpreting one isolated aspect of the disorder and deciding, based on their impression and experience, what a processing disorder is from their own perspective. As in the fable, each professional is correct in identifying one feature or characteristic of the disorder. However, none of them is correctly interpreting the entire entity. Their individual perspective is likely to bias the big picture. Audiologists have approached the definition of "auditory processing" from their perspective, whereas speech-language pathologists have advocated their own viewpoint. The result has further confounded the issue for professionals trying to accurately diagnose and design treatment plans.

Historical Perspective

In 1954, Myklebust introduced the term "auditory processing" to explain difficulty that children were encountering when attempting to comprehend auditory stimuli. At that early stage in the evolution of auditory processing disorders, Myklebust advocated for careful differentiation within auditory problems, explaining that the intervention focus might need to be in language, academic learning, or listening skills (Myklebust, 1954). Careful assessment was essential for the professional to design appropriate treatment, ensuring that a child's potential for learning wasn't compromised. At that point in time, Myklebust's use of the term "auditory processing" was very broad, encompassing all of audiology and speech-language pathology.

Massaro's definition (1975) continued to encompass the entire spectrum of skills by defining processing as the ability to abstract meaning from an acoustic stimulus. He attempted to differentiate processing from auditory perception, which he said occurred at a premeaning, preword stage.

Rees (1973) was among the first to question the premise that auditory perceptual problems were the cause of language disorders. The involvement between auditory perception and language, reading, and learning difficulties was acknowledged, but not within a cause-effect relationship. Dr. Rees discussed the idea of speech versus nonspeech to differentiate between perception of an acoustic utterance and linguistic decoding of an acoustic utterance. She cited several additional researchers who also questioned the importance of speech perception versus phonetic, phonological, lexical, syntactic, and semantic analysis as the basis of language acquisition and academic learning. Rees (1973) concluded that whereas auditory skills appeared to be a critical aspect of language and learning, the auditory processing aspect alone did not account for the difficulties evidenced in language disorders.

As audiology evolved, the term "central auditory processing" was introduced to refer specifically to audiological assessment and function in the central auditory nervous system (CANS) (Keith, 1977). Although this term was more specific than "auditory processing," it further confounded the issue. Keith (1981) cited difficulty in reaching consensus on defining the term. He discussed continuing confusion between auditory processing and language comprehension, acknowledging that in most descriptions of central auditory processing abilities, many language processing and cognitive manipulation abilities were included.

The debate continued, with various aspects of auditory processing being dissected in research studies. A review of the existing literature by Lubert (1981) illustrated the problems with trying to separate auditory processing into distinct and separate clinical entities. She referred to various theories of speech perception that "emphasize different levels of processing of the speech signal" (p. 4). The various theories were divided into "feature detection theories" which focused on early levels of processing (e.g., acoustic and phonetic), whereas "those giving emphasis to semantic and syntactic aspects are called 'analysis-by-synthesis theories'" (p. 4). She concluded that impairment in the ability to detect acoustic features of the auditory signal was the primary difficulty preventing children from performing higher level language tasks.

Language researchers agreed to some extent with the prominence of acoustic and phonetic aspects of processing. The advocates of information processing theories placed emphasis on the adjunct areas of memory capacity and timing components to account for deficits in language comprehension. The ability to perceive and retain auditory input was viewed as critical to facilitate development of higher level language abilities (Stone, Silliman, Ehren, & Apel, 2004). Leonard (1998) emphasized that deficits in phonological skills could negatively impact the development of more advanced language knowledge. In other words, a message had to be acoustically and phonetically received and retained before meaningful interpretation and analysis could occur. At the same time, difficulty with abstract higher levels of language comprehension was attributed to deficits in lower level language skills. The general consensus across information processing theories was that the foundation for abstract higher level language skills was in the acquisition of basic language competency in semantics, phonology, morphology, syntax, and pragmatics.

The initiation of extensive research on literacy skills within the purview of speech-language pathology added to the confusion. Stone et al. (2004) differentiated language as being oral or spoken, while literacy pertained to reading and writing. Phonological awareness seemed to be the bridge between the two, with a focus on teaching graphic symbols to represent sounds. However, the skills involved in auditory analysis of acoustic stimuli, such as sound discrimination, segmentation, and rime, seem to be critical foundation skills for both language and literacy. Anne van Kleeck (2004) discussed this confusion in attempting to define "preliteracy" in regard to the development of phonological awareness and alphabet knowledge. She considers these to be code-related skills that are prerequisite to developing reading and writing, or literacy. The same might be said of auditory processing versus language processing, in that auditory processing, including phonological awareness, is prerequisite to language processing. An acoustic stimulus must first be perceived as having a linguistic component before meaning can be extracted.

Auditory processing gradually came to encompass acoustic, phonologic, and linguistic aspects of analyzing, interpreting, and responding to an auditory signal, depending on the professional discipline and perspective of the individual responsible for diagnosing or treating the disorder. As the professions transitioned to a neuropsychological orientation, observed behaviors were inferred as being mediated by specified neurological structures and sites (Luria, 1970, 1982). This provided a more definitive delineation, but did little to resolve the issue because of the integrated nature of cortical neurological structures involved in processing. Although the central auditory nervous system (CANS) was fairly contained at a brainstem level, when the stimulus entered the temporal lobe of the cortex, it became very difficult to isolate neurological function in a linear fashion. The auditory, phonological, and language aspects all had to work together for accurate processing to occur.

The historical evolution of "auditory processing" illustrates the confusion that exists in trying to define the term. The common theme that emerges among the multiple authors and resources over time is that "auditory processing" encompasses a variety of auditory and language abilities; it is not a simple discrete skill that is easily isolated and defined. Vygotsky (1962) perhaps addressed it best with his discussion of "process" as a continual back and forth movement between thought and word. However, a delineation of the specific aspects of processing into primarily auditory or language areas is necessary for effective treatment.

Can "auditory processing" versus "language processing" be defined? It is difficult to do when relying on behavioral characteristics and described symptoms within tasks. The historical evolution of the term "processing" does little to assist in determining if auditory processing and language processing are the same or different phenomena. The delineation must be determined at a clinical level by observing and isolating specific aspects of speech-language performance to discriminate the salient aspects required for competence.

Continuum of Processing

The major components involved in attaching meaning to an auditory stimulus are acoustic, phonemic, and linguistic. These three types of processing are consistently cited by authors, beginning with Myklebust in 1954 up to the present day. Researchers and clinicians have been in agreement for decades regarding the types of tasks that an individual must be able to competently perform to function adequately in a verbal environment. The challenge becomes how to define and delineate those skills so accurate assessment and treatment can occur.

The starting point for differentiating auditory processing from language processing is to acknowledge the acoustic, phonemic, and linguistic roles, both neurologically and behaviorally. Most professionals would agree that processing an auditory stimulus is initiated by reception of an acoustic signal. Once the acoustic signal has been received, the individual must discriminate the stimulus as being environmental or linguistically encoded within the sound system of a specific language. This necessitates a transition from an acoustic processing task into a phonological processing task. The individual needs to know the phonetic code of the spoken language and be able to discriminate and analyze the signal's component parts. Once the phonemic processing has occurred, then the linguistic code must be applied to interpret or extrapolate the message. The individual must transition into language knowledge to comprehend or understand the intention of the speaker. Figure 8–2 represents this processing continuum.

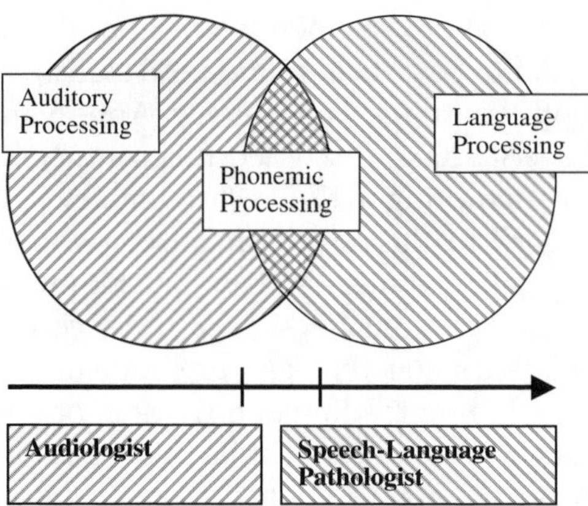

Figure 8–2. The processing continuum: Auditory processing versus language processing.

Although the brain does not work in an isolated linear manner, there are specific structures associated with the primary neurological functions described in the processing continuum (Richard, 2006). The acoustic processing stage involves reception and transference of the acoustic stimulus, which is the responsibility of an audiologist. Neurological structures would include the peripheral auditory system (i.e., outer, middle, and inner ear) as well as the central auditory nervous system, beginning with the eighth auditory nerve and concluding at Heschel's gyrus in the temporal lobe. Assessment tasks to determine if there is a problem would evaluate the integrity of the central auditory nervous system. Typical evaluation involves stressing the auditory system by reducing internal neurologic redundancy through the use of dichotic tasks. Examples of assessment tasks are included in Table 8–1. The goal of auditory processing assessment should be to determine if an individual can accurately receive and transfer an acoustic stimulus through the peripheral and central auditory systems to the upper cortex.

Phonemic processing begins at the level of the temporal lobe. The primary task is to discriminate component parts of the acoustic stimulus received. The ability to analyze the sound components involves a number of phonological skills, such as sound discrimination, blending, and segmentation. This level of processing requires a transition into knowledge of the phonemes of a language. However, the ability to hear and discriminate various sounds doesn't necessarily

Table 8–1. Delineation Within Processing Continuum

	Goal	Professional Responsible	Structures	Sample Assessment Tasks
Acoustic Processing	Receive and transfer signal	Audiologist	Peripheral auditory system	Pure tone thresholds; Tympanometry
			Central auditory system	Electrophysiological; Pitch patterns; Dichotic digits; Figure-ground
Phonemic Processing	Discriminate sound segments in signal	Audiologist; Speech-language pathologist	Heschl's gyrus-temporal lobe	Phoneme discrimination; Sound blending; Auditory segmentation
Linguistic Processing	Attach meaning to signal	Speech-language pathologist	Temporal lobe-Wernicke's area; Angular gyrus; Prefrontal/frontal lobe	Concepts; Antonyms; Idioms, Nonliteral language; Problem solving

require interpretation of linguistic meaning. For example, a person might hear someone speaking a foreign language. They could probably discriminate various phonemes being produced and possibly repeat the phonetic sequences, but they would not be able to comprehend or respond to what was said. The ability to attach meaning to the acoustic signal requires knowledge of the language system, or language processing (Richard, 2001). Examples of assessment tasks to evaluate phonemic processing are included in Table 8–1.

Phonemic processing is part of the preliteracy foundation discussed earlier. The ability to read and write requires development of phonic skills, or grapheme representation of sounds heard. This portion of the processing continuum represents important building blocks for later language and literacy skills. Assessment tasks to evaluate the area of literacy can involve spelling, reading, and writing tasks. The ability to accurately perform these tasks will be based in acoustic, phonologic, and linguistic skills.

Part of the confusion in defining auditory processing versus language processing is that this portion of the processing continuum is encompassed in the scope of practice for both audiologists and speech-language pathologists (see Figure 8–2). Audiologists typically include assessment tasks that evaluate sound discrimination of phonological segments. The stimuli can include both nonsense and meaningful syllables or words. This portion of the continuum is often the highest level of audiological assessment, or central auditory processing evaluations. If an individual encounters difficulty at this level, the audiologist will diagnose a central auditory processing disorder. However, assessment by a speech-language pathologist should begin in this same portion of the continuum. Evaluation of phonemic awareness can include the same types of tasks as those administered by audiologists, utilizing both nonsense and meaningful stimuli. The speech-language pathologist will diagnose a language processing or phonological awareness disorder. Consequently, the exact same deficit can result in three different diagnoses, depending on who first conducts the evaluation.

Linguistic knowledge allows comprehension of a message encoded in an acoustic signal. A phonetic sequence that is heard accurately, transferred to the temporal lobe without being compromised or distorted, and analyzed phonologically, should result in generating images within the cortex of the person who received the signal. If meaning is not attached, then language processing has not occurred.

Language processing is extremely complex. Neurologic structures begin at the level of Heschl's gyrus, but expand to include Wernicke's area, the angular gyrus, and eventually the prefrontal and frontal cortex for planning, organizing. and mediating a response. Language processing begins at a very functional, concrete level in acquisition of basic noun and verb labels. As language develops and matures, the individual progresses from experiential concrete language into abstract conceptual language. The early lower levels of attaching meaning to auditory stimuli continue to refine into higher levels of problem solving and reasoning. Vocabulary knowledge expands with each new venture and exposure. Literal interpretations of language progress into comprehension of figurative language, idiomatic and colloquial expressions, and extrapolating meaning from ambiguous suggestions.

Language processing continues to develop with expectations to interpret nuances encoded in the suprasegmentals of an utterance. The individual must pay attention to inflection, prosody, and tone to determine if a speaker is sincere or teasing. Sarcasm requires that a listener modify the meaning intended, based on how the verbalization is spoken.

The suprasegmental aspects of language processing are mediated in the frontal lobe, but require that the person hear variations in acoustic tone. In other words, the linguistic knowledge is necessary to interpret the words spoken, but the meaning may change based on how the verbalization was spoken. The audiologist evaluates pitch and tone discrimination as part of central auditory processing assessment. The speech-language pathologist evaluates the ability to understand the words spoken. Those isolated segments of processing have to effectively integrate for accurate higher level processing to be successful. A linear delineation is important for understanding how to assess the primary components entailed in processing, but a professional, either audiologist or speech-language pathologist, must acknowledge that there is considerable overlap at a functional level.

Medwetsky (2006) makes a case for use of "spoken language processing" to encompass aspects of auditory, cognitive, and language processing. One of his goals is to advocate an interdisciplinary approach to processing issues, particularly at the assessment level. If professionals share in the responsibility for identifying aspects of a processing problem, then treatment approaches are more likely to be effective and focused.

The concept of "spoken language processing" includes multiple neurological and behavioral aspects of processing (Medwetsky, 2006). Long- and short-term memory are activated for comparison of incoming stimuli. Linguistic information is dealt with in the left hemisphere whereas suprasegmentals are processed in the right hemisphere. Attention to the stimuli, as well as retention and sequencing of the input, occurs as components within the model. The establishment of phonemic representations of sounds is also acknowledged as occurring over time.

It is important for audiologists and speech-language pathologists to work collaboratively on processing disorders. A theoretical framework needs to include consideration of neurological structures and behavioral skills. Assessment should delineate the primary areas of strength or weakness within the processing continuum—acoustic, phonemic, or linguistic processing. Those major components can be divided into a diagnosis of auditory processing or language processing. However, more important than a label of auditory processing or language processing, is a description of deficit skills so effective treatment can be designed to resolve the difficulties.

Conclusions

The term "auditory processing" can be interpreted in a variety of ways, dependent on the personal orientation, experience, or bias. The scope of inclusion can be very broad or very narrow in terms of the specific abilities included in the definition.

Audiologists tend to define "auditory processing" as encompassing the central auditory nervous system (CANS) function. The evaluation is often a "bottom-up" approach, analyzing transference of the acoustic signal through the peripheral auditory system, CANS, and concluding in the upper cortex. Speech-language pathologists tend to use a "top-down" or more holistic approach to auditory processing. The evaluation is often very functional and applied in linguistic interpretation of meaning. Neither approach is complete in addressing the complexity and interdependency of hearing and comprehending auditory stimuli.

Attaching meaning to auditorily presented information is not a simple, linear, isolated neurological task. Consequently, auditory processing cannot be viewed from either a purely audiological or language-based perspective. There is not a distinct separation between auditory processing of information and language processing of the same stimulus. Multiple anatomical and neurological structures overlap and work in cooperation. The tertiary properties of the brain are too efficient for an isolated approach to such a complex, interdependent task.

Processing an acoustic signal is different from processing a linguistic signal in that the response expected is very different. Receiving an auditory signal usually requires a simple repetition of what was heard, with little to no interpretation or extrapolation of meaning. Responding to a linguistic signal requires a much more cortically integrated process of recognizing and decoding sounds to then formulate a response.

In reality, most auditory processing problems are based in difficulty associated with applying meaning within a linguistic code. The acoustic stimulus is not the source of the problem; the challenge lies in trying to decode and interpret the message within the sound-symbol system of language. Most individuals with processing problems do not require acoustic repetition or increased volume; they need contextual cues, prompts, and linguistic assistance as the focus of treatment.

Upon hearing a phrase, ask the following questions:

Did you hear it?	Can you explain what it means?
Can you repeat it?	Will saying it slower help?
Can you identify the first sound?	Will repeating it multiple times help?
Can you identify another sound you heard?	Will making it louder help?
If the answer to these questions is "yes,"	**If the answer to these questions is "no,"**

Then the problem is language processing, not auditory processing.

Summary

Comprehending and responding appropriately to an auditory signal involves a variety of neurological structures and behavioral skills. A mediated response is not a simple linear, isolated procedure; it is a complex, integrated process. Various aspects of the process have been examined and researched since the advent of the professions of speech-language pathology and audiology in the early 1950s. However, consensus has never been reached. In fact, more questions have been raised than answered over the decades.

Processing an auditory stimulus occurs on a continuum that progresses from fairly discrete neurological responses to the acoustic signal, to more complex, abstract interpretations of meaning. A logical division in the past was to refer to the entire continuum as "auditory processing," with a separation between "central auditory processing" (transfer through CANS to cortex) and "language processing" (cortical interpretation) (Richard, 2001). This allowed the professions of audiology and speech-language pathology to clearly identify the types of behaviors under their jurisdiction, with an acknowledgement of overlapping skills in the phonemic area.

However, in 2005, an ASHA task force composed of audiologists generated a technical report and position paper (ASHA, 2005a, 2005b) advocating removal of "central" by moving it to a parenthetic status, and reiterating use of the term "auditory processing" to encompass the responsibilities of audiologists within the disorder. Although removing "central" might help clarify that the audiologist is involved in evaluating auditory skills beyond the central auditory nervous system, it further clouded the differentiation between auditory processing and language processing at a cortical level.

The ASHA task force attempted to promote a more defined description of "auditory processing," which was definitely a positive step for practicing audiologists. In the past, there has not been agreement in what constituted an auditory processing disorder, resulting in a large variety of deficits being categorized as "central auditory processing disorders." This created a significant challenge for parents and speech-language pathologists because diagnostic responsibilities were designated to audiologists, but speech-language pathologists were usually responsible for interpreting the functional problems and designing treatment. A collaborative effort would seem to make more sense, especially in light of the obvious overlap in phonological analysis of the acoustic stimulus.

To ensure quality intervention, accurate diagnosis of processing disorders must be accomplished. The differentiation between auditory processing and language processing can be achieved by determining the primary behavioral task involved—acoustic, phonemic, or linguistic. Auditory processing should be the diagnosis for acoustic challenges in reception and transference of a signal. Language processing should be the diagnosis for problems encountered in interpreting the meaning encoded in the signal. Phonemic problems will be detected in audiological testing, but are usually more representative of difficulty at the early levels of foundation skills for literacy, which is better represented under the diagnosis of language processing.

The key is to determine what the deficit skills are and what treatment strategies will be most effective to resolve the problem. If increased amplitude, signal enhancement, or repetition will facilitate a resolution, then auditory processing methodologies are indicated and auditory processing can be the designated diagnosis. If phoneme/grapheme relationships, phonemic discrimination, or sound segmentation or analysis are indicated, then phonological awareness methodologies under a language processing disorder would be more appropriate.

The issue of auditory processing seems to have come full circle. Myklebust (1954) defined "auditory processing" as encompassing the various listening and language skills involved in successful learning. He advocated careful differentiation of the auditory problems. As in the Hindu fable of *The Blind Men and the Elephant*, professionals must be cautious about narrowing the focus too much, resulting in losing sight of the big picture.

Processing disorders are challenging, intriguing disorders that are becoming more frequently diagnosed to account for the academic deficits occurring in the education setting. Improved differentiation of the primary skills involved will facilitate more accurate diagnosis and intervention. Collaboration between audiology and speech-language pathology is critical to ensure ethical and efficacious delivery of professional services.

Key Points Learned

- Processing occurs on a continuum, progressing from auditory processing to language processing.
- Auditory processing and language processing share overlapping characteristics, but features of each can be differentiated at neurological and behavioral levels.
- Processing an acoustic stimulus should be evaluated using assessment tasks that delineate skills into primarily acoustic, phonemic, and linguistic abilities.
- Processing disorders cannot and should not be diagnosed from one assessment task; a battery of skills must be examined to determine the primary area of deficit.
- A diagnosed processing disorder should be carefully evaluated at a clinical level to determine the functional skills in deficit, regardless of whether the label introduced is auditory processing or language processing.
- Audiologists are responsible for evaluating and diagnosing problems in the reception and/or transference of an acoustic signal in the peripheral auditory system and central auditory nervous system.
- Speech-language pathologists are responsible for evaluating and diagnosing problems in analyzing an acoustic signal in phonological awareness and/or linguistic interpretation.
- Treatment for processing disorders cannot be effective unless the specific skills in deficit are carefully differentiated.

References

American Speech-Language-Hearing Association. (2005a). *Central auditory processing disorders* (Technical report). Rockville, MD: Author.

American Speech-Language-Hearing Association. (2005b). *(Central) auditory processing disorders—The role of the audiologists* [Position statement]. Rockville, MD: Author.

Keith, R. (1977). *Central auditory dysfunction.* New York: Grune & Stratton.

Keith, R. (1981). *Central auditory and language disorders in children.* San Diego, CA: College-Hill Press.

Leonard, L. (1998). *Children with specific language impairment.* Cambridge, MA: MIT Press.

Lubert, N. (1981). Auditory perceptual impairments in children with specific language impairments: A review of the literature. *Journal of Speech and Hearing Disorders, 46*(1), 3–9.

Luria, A. (1970). The functional organization of the brain. *Scientific American, 222,* 66–78.

Luria, A. (1982). *Language and cognition.* New York: John Wiley.

Massaro, D. (1975). *Understanding language: An information-processing analysis of speech perception, reading, and psycholinguistics.* New York: Academic Press.

Medwetsky, L. (2006). Spoken language processing: A convergent approach to conceptualizing (central) auditory processing. *ASHA Leader, 11*(8), 6–7, 30–31, 33.

Myklebust, H. (1954). *Auditory disorders in children.* New York: Grune & Stratton.

Rees, N. (1973). Auditory processing factors in language disorders: The view from Procrustes' bed. *Journal of Speech and Hearing Disorders, 38* (3), 304–315.

Richard, G. (2001). *The source for processing disorders.* East Moline, IL: LinguiSystems.

Richard, G. (2006). Language-based assessment and intervention for APD. In T. K. Parthasarathy (Ed.), *An introduction to auditory processing disorders in children* (pp. 95–108). Mahwah, NJ: Lawrence Erlbaum Associates.

Saxe, J. G. (1816–1887). *The Blind Men and the Elephant.*

Stone, C. A., Silliman, E. R., Ehren, B. J., & Apel, K. (2004). *Handbook of language and literacy: Development and disorders.* New York: The Guilford Press.

van Kleeck, A. (2004). "Fostering preliteracy development via storybook-sharing interactions. In C. A. Stone, E. R. Silliman, B. J. Ehren, & K. Apel (Eds.), *Handbook of language and literacy: Development and disorders* (pp. 175–208). New York: The Guilford Press.

Vygotsky, L. (1962). *Thought and language.* Cambridge, MA: MIT Press.

Appendix 8–A
The Blind Men and the Elephant

A Hindu Fable by John Godfrey Saxe

It was six men of Indostan
To learning much inclined,
Who went to see the Elephant
(Though all of them were blind),
That each by observation
Might satisfy his mind.

The *First* approached the Elephant,
And happening to fall
Against his broad and sturdy side,
At once began to bawl:
"God bless me! but the Elephant
Is very like a wall!"

The *Second*, feeling of the tusk,
Cried, "Ho! what have we here
So very round and smooth and sharp?
To me 'tis mighty clear
This wonder of an Elephant
Is very like a spear!"

The *Third* approached the animal,
And happening to take
The squirming trunk within his hands,
Thus boldly up and spake:
"I see," quoth he, "the Elephant
Is very like a snake."

The *Fourth* reached out his eager hand,
And felt about the knee.
"What most this wondrous beast is like
Is mighty plain," quoth he;
"Tis clear enough the Elephant
Is very like a tree!"

The *Fifth* who chanced to touch the ear,
Said: "E'en the blindest man
Can tell what this resembles most:
Deny the fact who can,
This marvel of an Elephant
Is very like a fan!"

The *Sixth* no sooner had begun
About the beast to grope,
Than, seizing on the swinging tail
That fell within his scope,
"I see," quoth he, "the Elephant
Is very like a rope!"

And so these men of Indostan
Disputed loud and long,
Each in his own opinion
Exceeding stiff and strong,
Though each was partly in the right,
And all were in the wrong!

So, oft in theologic wars,
The disputants, I ween,
Rail on in utter ignorance
Of what each other mean,
And prate about an Elephant
Not one of them has seen!

Note: *The Blind Men and the Elephant* occurs in the Udana, a Canonical Hindu Scripture. http://aries.phys.yorku.ca/~mmdr/elephant_theology.html

9

Auditory Processing Disorders and Literacy

Martha S. Burns

Overview

Although much has been written about the impact of auditory processing disorders in school-age children, only recently has research focused on the specific impact of auditory processing disorders on reading. Certainly, in many clinical practices, first time referrals for assessment and treatment of auditory processing disorders occur after a child begins failing in school. But, commonly the early problems in school center on reading and language arts.

Some young students with a diagnosis of auditory processing disorder (APD) may have a history of speech and language problems. Others may not have experienced significant language, learning, or social difficulties prior to entering school. In fact, occasionally children with APD excel in early academic testing, and even in early reading experiences that depend largely on visual memory of site words and word families (such as those stressed in early reading books like the Dr. Seuss series). Then, suddenly, somewhere around the end of the second or third grade, they exhibit problems decoding longer, less familiar words. Professionals may be at a loss to explain why such a student suddenly starts to experience significant problems with such activities as learning to decode, reading aloud, or in later years, writing essays or taking notes during lectures. (Burns et al., 2005)

This chapter addresses the relationship between APD and literacy. It begins with an overview of literacy and the impact of reading problems on academic success. A discussion of the research linking language problems and reading disorders, specifically dyslexia, follows. The review of the research on the relationship between auditory processing disorders, language disorders, and reading disorders then focuses on the neurological basis of reading, specifically, the underlying cognitive mechanisms required to master reading. A summary of research on the types of neurologically based auditory processing disorders associated with reading disturbances includes an overview of recent neurophysiologic and imaging studies of APD and reading disorders. The chapter concludes with a summary of APD interventions currently being studied for treatment of reading and writing disorders.

Literacy: Impact on School-Age Populations and in Adulthood

Literacy refers to the ability to use a formal written language system to communicate: reading and writing. According to the Alliance for Excellent Education (2004), in the United States, only 34% of 12th graders meet the standard of reading proficiency. Some 70% of older readers require some form of remediation. (Biancarosa & Snow, 2006). The importance of literacy for ability to live a fulfilling and independent life and achieve gainful employment is indisputable. Students in the lowest 25% of achievement are 20 times more likely to drop out of high school than students in the highest 25% (Alliance for Excellent Education, 2004). In fact, adolescents and adults with reduced reading skills are not only more likely to become unemployed; they are more likely to become incarcerated. Project Read conducted a national study that reported that *more than one third* of juvenile offenders at the median age of 15.5 were reading below the fourth-grade level.

For the above reasons the Bush administration, enabled through congressional legislation, initiated "No Child Left Be-hind," a codified initiative to make certain that all American children are reading at grade level by the third grade. Yet, for decades, the goal of a "nation of readers" has eluded educators. Why some children struggle to read, whereas others find learning to read effortless, has puzzled literacy experts for years.

The Language and Literacy Link

Unlike reading, language is a universal cognitive skill that is naturally acquired.

Children with normal intelligence and hearing, acquire language simply through exposure to language in their environment, without being taught (Kuhl, 2004). Reading, on the other hand, must be learned (Snow, Burns, & Griffin, 1998). Not all humans read. In fact even today, there are many nations and cultures where the majority of people are not literate. Yet, despite the differences between the way language and reading are mastered, there is mounting evidence that links early childhood language problems with reading difficulties in school-age children.

As early as 1978, Hall and Tomblin reported a study that demonstrated that children with language and articulation problems were far more likely than controls to exhibit reading problems across all grades. Several years later, Aram, Ekelman, and Nation (1984) performed a 10-year follow-up of 20 children diagnosed with language problems between the ages of 3 and 6 years and found that half of them scored below the 25th percentile in reading and 56% were deficient in spelling skills.

More recent research has led today's reading experts to agree that, in a majority of cases, reading problems stem from underlying language disturbances (Carroll & Snowling, 2004; Flax, et al., 2003; Snow, Burns, & Griffin, 1998). And, although the causes of the underlying language problems remain an area of study, a significant proportion of language, and later, reading problems appear to stem from auditory processing problems (Joanisse et al., 2000; Tallal & Piercy, 1973; Tallal & Stark, 1982; Wible, Nicol, & Kraus, 2002).

Dyslexia

There are two primary reasons that adults may be unable to read: insufficient educational opportunity and dyslexia. Issues of educational opportunity are beyond the scope of this chapter. Most scientific studies of reading and auditory processing have focused on dyslexia.

Dyslexia, as originally defined by Myklebust and Johnson in 1962, is a disturbance in the ability to learn to read among children with normal intelligence, who have no significant emotional disturbance and have had sufficient educational opportunity. Originally termed "word blindness" by Orton in 1937, reading problems were first thought to reflect underlying visual perceptual deficits. Orton discusses a case study of a 13-year-old boy, first described by Hinshelwood at the turn of the century, who could not store visual images but could learn auditorily. However, despite the early focus on visual processing limitations in dyslexia, recent research has pointed to acoustic, memory, and language functions, including phonologic components of language, as core components underlying reading disturbance (Lyon, 1995; Tallal, 2004)

From a neuroscience perspective, learning to read is dependent on language structures of the brain. Linguists and neuroscientists consider reading to be an overlaid cognitive function: that is, dependent on neurocognitive structures that primarily support other cognitive abilities (Hillis & Tuffiash, 2002). Although literacy requires decoding a visual code, the underlying neurocognitive requisite is language, including phonologic systems (Shaywitz et al., 2004), and morphologic systems (Tallal, 2004). As far as the brain is concerned, reading is language (Burns, 1999).

Because language is an auditorily acquired symbol system for all individuals who have adequate hearing, there has been a great deal of research interest on the integrity of the auditory system and the type of perceptual functions necessary to support adequate language acquisition and the overlaid learning of reading. For this reason, some researchers in literacy have begun studying the link between auditory processing disorders and reading problems in school-age children (Galaburda, 1994; Kraus, 2001; Nagarajan et al., 1999; Tallal et al, 1993).

Neurological Foundations: Auditory Processing, Language, and Literacy

In the 1970s, Tallal and Piercy published a remarkable, albeit controversial, paper in which they reported finding that children with developmental language problems had a significant problem with a specific processing task that involved sequencing of two tones of different frequencies. They noted that the children with language problems, when compared to age-matched controls, were equally able to sequence two tones with an interstimulus interval of 350 milliseconds or longer, but when the tones were closer together suddenly the children with language problems showed a marked decrease in their accuracy whereas the controls remained able to accurately sequence the tones down to an interstimulus interval of 20 msec or less. Although the correlation between the two tone sequencing task difficulties and language problems could not be considered causative, based on the design of the study, the finding was provocative.

Controversy surrounding the Tallal and Piercy data stemmed in large part from the prevailing view of causes of language problems in children that centered on emerging psycholinguistic explanations. A widely held view was that the language problems in young children were due to a delay in the normal acquisition of the rules of language. The theory was that all humans have a natural capacity to learn language, a "language acquisition device" (LAD) that is innately wired into the human brain and differentiates humans from other animals (Chomsky, 1965). The LAD set in motion the acquisition of the rules of language simply through exposure to language in the environment (Brown, 1973).

The finding that a nonlinguistic processing deficit could be correlated with language problems posed a theoretical conundrum. If sequencing of nonlinguistic tones was somehow related to language deficits, then language problems in young children might occur independently of the natural capacity for linguistic rule acquisition. Although many language specialists today do not see the two theoretical explanations as mutually exclusive, that is, auditory processing deficits versus natural acquisition of linguistic rules (Leonard, 1998), the controversy over the original research and subsequent corroborative findings has fueled many misconceptions and arguments among language scientists.

Nonetheless, in the decades since early Tallal and Piercy data were reported, many independent neuroscientific studies have corroborated the evidence that rapid auditory processing deficits are a component of reading disturbance and that the differences have observable neurological correlates that correspond to reading deficits (Temple, 2002; Temple et al., 2000). Additional research has demonstrated neurological processing differences between emerging readers and fluent adult readers (Turkeltaub et al., 2003), and that there are marked differences in the regions of the brain used by successful young readers and dyslexic readers during reading and phonologic tasks, (Shaywitz et al., 1998; Temple et al., 2003). To date the research on the neurological basis of reading disorders in young children is strong as is evidence that at least some children who struggle to learn to read have particular problems with the phonological abilities required for decoding and that auditory processing deficits co-occur with phonological problems in young children. Specific neurological research on the links between APD and dyslexia is summarized below.

Neurologic Evidence of the Links Between APD and Dyslexia

Neurological research conducted during the past seven to ten years using neuroanatomical evidence, neurophysiologic measures, and functional imaging has revealed the following about the relationship between APD, language acquisition, and reading:

1. The brains of dyslexic adults studied on autopsy (after death from natural causes) exhibit nonfunctional ectopic (embryonic) cellular collections in the language regions of the left hemisphere; these same ectopic collections when induced in animals cause temporal auditory processing deficits (Galaburda, 1994, Galaburda et al., 1994; Peiffer et al., 2004).
2. Magnetoencephalographic (MEG) studies of adults with poor reading abilities showed electrophysiological evidence of abnormal neural representations of brief and rapidly successive sensory inputs (rapid processing deficits) in auditory cortex (Nagarajan et al., 1999).
3. Electrophysiological studies of children with language and reading problems revealed deficiencies in neural synchrony (timing deficits) in subcortical as well as cortical regions that process speech sounds that were in turn related to speech-sound perception and measures of learning (Kraus, 2001).
4. Functional magnetic resonance (fMRI) studies of dyslexic children and adults revealed that the cortical neurological structures in the left hemisphere that support language learning and working memory also support reading (Temple et al, 2000, 2003).

5. fMRI studies have further indicated that as children learn to read they first rely on temporal/parietal/occipital regions of the left hemisphere that underlie phonological awareness and other aspects of oral language comprehension (Shaywitz et al., 2004).
6. fMRI studies have also shown that as children become more proficient in reading, other regions of the left hemisphere that are active in auditory working memory and language production become part of a reading network (Shaywitz et al., 2004)
7. Electrophysiological studies of young children with a family history of specific language impairment show temporal processing differences in mismatched negativity (MMN) and latency of N_{250} ERP waveforms to 70-msec interstimulus interval (rapid auditory) stimuli as early as 6 months of age. When followed longitudinally, at 48 months and 60 months, poor processors showed significant reductions in language measures when compared to age-matched controls with no rapid auditory processing deficits (Benasich, 2006; Benasich & Tallal, 2002).
8. Four genes that thus far have been linked to developmental dyslexia affect brain development, specifically linked to brain abnormalities linked to auditory and cognitive deficits associated with dyslexia (Galaburda et al., 2006).

In summary, research across many domains is supporting the conclusion that rapid auditory processing impairments are correlated with language and reading disorders in children and adults. The degree to which these disturbances are causative is still debated, but genetic and longitudinal studies are beginning to point to at least a partial causative relationship.

Effect of Auditory Processing Remediation on Reading Achievement

Several research studies using auditory processing interventions in language and reading impaired children have shown improvements in several cognitive domains after treatment directed at increasing auditory processing speed and speech-sound discrimination. In two of the earliest controlled laboratory studies conducted in the 1990s, Paula Tallal, Mike Merzenich, and colleagues conducted clinical trials in which language-impaired children were compared with matched controls. The two groups both received identical direct language intervention except that the experimental group received direct auditory processing training and enhancements as well. The enhancements included an auditory processing exercise as well as speech stimuli that were acoustically modified to increase duration and intensity of rapid acoustic transitions.

These studies revealed that the addition of rapid auditory processing training and use of acoustically modified speech in language intervention, directed at the auditory processing deficit, resulted in significantly increased improvements in rapid auditory processing ability as well as significant improvements in speech discrimination and language comprehension when compared to language intervention without the auditory processing components (Merzenich et al., 1996; Tallal et al., 1996).

Nina Kraus reported results in 2001 in children with auditory processing disorders who were diagnosed with learning and reading problems. She reported preliminary evidence of improvements on measures of perception and learning as well as changes in cortical potentials to stimuli presented both in quiet and in noise after participation in computer-based auditory training programs. She also reported that impaired perception and neurophysiologic encoding of speech sounds in children with learning problems can be improved with training incorporating acoustic cue enhancements (Kraus, 2001).

Improvements in reading skills directly attributable to auditory training and language interventions with acoustically modified speech were studied by Temple and colleagues in two studies conducted at Stanford University using functional magnetic imaging, fMRI. In the most recent study, 20 children with dyslexia and an age-matched control group with normal reading skills were evaluated using a battery of language and reading tests. fMRI recordings were made while performing a phonological awareness task that involved letter rhyming (whether letter pairs rhyme: for example, C and B, or H and F) approximately 8 weeks apart. The dyslexic group completed the Fast ForWord Language training program between assessments. Fast ForWord Language is a computerized intervention with exercises in: rapid auditory processing, speech-sound discrimination, and direct instruction in language structure and working memory exercises. Most of the exercises begin with duration and intensity-enhanced acoustic cues. Then, as the tasks are mastered with enhanced acoustic cues, there is a step-wise decrease into normal acoustic cue ranges until, at the end of training, all exercises are performed with normal acoustic cue duration and intensity.

After only 6 weeks of this combined auditory processing and language training, the group with dyslexia showed significant improvements in measures of language and reading, despite no direct reading intervention. Of particular interest was the finding that reading decoding scores, directly correlated with phonemic awareness skills, increased from one standard deviation below the mean before training to within normal limits after training (Temple et al., 2003).

Summary

There is considerable evidence that auditory processing skills, especially in the domain of rapid auditory processing, underlie language acquisition and reading mastery. Specifically, it appears that rapid auditory processing, at cortical and subcortical levels, represents a core component of phonological awareness. Rapid auditory processing deficits are correlated with problems in phonological decoding of words. Whether these auditory processing disturbances cause phonological awareness problems and, in turn, lead to dyslexia or whether they occur in combination with other neurological processing differences remains an area of intense research interest.

Reading interventions that focus on the phonological component of reading disturbances are effective. And, there is substantial evidence that language and memory intervention in children with dyslexia also substantially improves reading skill. But, perhaps the most exciting aspect of the new neurophysiological and neuroimaging research is that, because auditory processing, language, and reading impairment are so neurologically entwined, the addition of rapid auditory processing training can substantially increase the power and speed of language and phonologically based interventions. The goal of "a nation of readers" may be attainable at last.

Key Points Learned

- Literacy issues impact nearly 70% of adults accounting for issues with high school graduation and eventual employment success. Although literacy requires decoding a visual code, the underlying neurocognitive requisite is language, including phonological systems, and morphologic systems.
- As far as the brain is concerned, reading is language. The causes of the underlying language problems remain an area of study; nonetheless, a significant proportion of language, and later, reading problems appear to stem from auditory processing problems.
- There is substantial research on the specific neurological links between APD and dyslexia. In several research studies using auditory processing interventions with children who have language and reading impairments, subjects have shown improvements in several cognitive domains. Most dramatically, researchers have reported improvements in reading, after treatment directed at increasing auditory processing speed and speech-sound discrimination.

References

Alliance for Education Fact Sheet. (2004) Washington, DC: Author.

Aram, D. A., Ekelman, B. L., & Nation, J. E. (1984). Preschoolers with language disorders: 10 years later. *Journal of Speech and Hearing Research, 27*, 232–234.

Benasich, A. A. (2006). *Predicting childhood language delays: The influence of rapid auditory processing abilities on emerging language.* Seminar on auditory skill development presented at the Royal University Hospital, Saskatoon, Saskatchewan.

Benasich, A, & Tallal, P. (2002). Infant discrimination of rapid auditory cues predicts later language impairment. *Behavioral Brain Research, 136*, 31–49.

Biancarosa, C., & Snow, C. E. (2006). *Reading next—A vision for action and research in middle and high school literacy: A report to Carnegie Corporation of New York* (2nd ed.).Washington, DC: Alliance for Excellent Education.

Brown, R. (1973). *A first language: The early stages.* Cambridge, MA: Harvard University Press.

Burns, M. (1999). *Access to Reading: The Language to literacy link.* San Francisco: Scientific Learning Corporation.

Burns, M., Young, M., Calhoun, B., & Agocs, M. (2005). Treatment of auditory processing disorders in adolescents. *Hearing and Hearing Disorders in Children, 16*(1), 10–18.

Carroll, J. M., & Snowling, M. J. (2004) Language and phonological skills in children at high risk of reading difficulties. *Journal of Child Psychology and Psychology, 45*, 631–640.

Chomsky, N. (1965). *Aspects of the theory of syntax.* Cambridge, MA: MIT Press.

Flax, J. F., Realpe-Bonilla, T., Hirsch, L. S., Brzustowicz, L. M., Bartlett, C. W., & Tallal, P. (2003). Specific Language impairment in families: Evidence for co-occurrence with reading impairments. *Journal of Speech, Language and Hearing Research, 46*, 530–543.

Galaburda, A. (1994). Developmental dyslexia and animal studies: at the interface between cognition and neurology. *Cognition, 50*, 133–149.

Galaburda, A. M., LoTurco, J., Ramus, F., Fitch, R. H., & Rosen, G. D. (2006). From genes to behavior in developmental dyslexia. *Nature Neuroscience, 9*, 1213–1217.

Galaburda, A. M., Menard, M. T., & Rosen, G. (1994). Evidence for aberrant auditory anatomy in developmental dyslexia. *Proceedings of the National Academy of Sciences, 91*, 8010–8013.

Hall, P. K., & Tomblin, J. B. (1978). A follow-up study of children with articulation and language disorders. *Journal of Speech and Hearing Disorders, 43*, 227–241

Hillis, A. E., & Tuffiash, E. (2002). Neuroanatomical aspects of reading. In A. Hillis (Ed.), *The handbook of adult language disorders.* New York: Psychology Press.

Joanisse, M. F., Manis, F. R., Keating, P., & Siedenbery, M. S. (2000). Language deficits in dyslexic children: speech, perception, phonology and morphology. *Journal of Exceptional Child Psychology, 77*, 30–60.

Kraus, N. (2001). Auditory pathway encoding and neural plasticity in children with learning problems. *Audiology and Neuro-Otology, 6*, 221–227.

Kuhl, P. (2004). Early language acquisition: Cracking the speech code. *Nature Reviews Neuroscience, 5*, 831–843.

Leonard, L. (1998). *Children with specific language impairments.* Cambridge, MA: MIT Press.

Lyon, G. R. (1995). Towards a definition of dyslexia. *Annals of Dyslexia, 45*, 3–27.

Merzenich, M., Jenkins, W., Johnston, P., Schreiner, C., Miller, S., & Tallal, P. (1996). Temporal processing deficits of language learning impaired children ameliorated by training. *Science, 271*, 77–81.

Mykelbust, H., & Johnson, D. (1962). Dyslexia in children. *Exceptional Children, 29*(1), 14–25.

Nagarajan, S., Mahncke, H., Salz, T., Tallal, P., Roberts, T., & Merzenich, M. (1999). Cortical auditory signal processing in poor readers. *Proceedings of the National Academy of Sciences, 96*, 6483–6488.

National Center on Education, Disability, and Juvenile Justice. (2002). College Park, MD.

Orton, S. (1937). *Reading, writing and speech problems in children.* New York: W.W. Norton.

Peiffer, A. M., Friedman, J. T., Rosen, G. D., & Fitch, R. H. (2004). Impaired gap detection in microgyric rats. *Developmental Brain Research, 152*, 93–98.

Shaywitz, B. A., Shaywitz, S. E., Blachman, B. B., Pugh, K. R., Fulbright, R. K., Skudlarski, P., et al. (2004). Development of left occipitotemporal systems for skilled reading in children after a phonologically-based intervention. *Biological Psychiatry, 55*, 926–933.

Shaywitz, S. E., Shaywitz, B. A., Pugh, K. R., Fulbright, R. K., Constable, R. T., & Mencl, W. E. (1998). Functional disruption in the organization of the brain for reading in dyslexia. *Proceedings of the National Academy of Science, 82*, 8072–8074.

Skudlarski, P., Meel, K. E., Constable, R. I., Holahan, J. M., Marchione, K. E., Fletcher, J. M., et al. (2004). Development of left occipitotemporal lobe systems for skilled reading in children after a phonologically-based reading intervention. *Biological Psychiatry, 55*, 926–933.

Snow, C. E., Burns, M. S. & Griffin, P. (1998). *Preventing reading difficulties in young children.* Washington, DC: National Academy Press.

Tallal, P. (2004). Improving language and literacy is a matter of time. *Nature Reviews Neuroscience: Perspective, 5*, 721–728.

Tallal, P., Galaburda, A., Von Euler, C., & Linas, R. (Eds.). (1993). *Temporal information processing in the nervous system.* New York: New York Academy of Sciences.

Tallal, P., Miller, S., Bedi, G., Byma, G., Wang, X., Nagarajan, S., et al. (1996). Language comprehension in language learning impaired children improved with acoustically modified speech. *Science, 271*, 81–84.

Tallal, P., & Piercy, M. (1973). Defects of non-verbal auditory perception in children with developmental aphasia. *Nature, 241*, 468–469.

Tallal, P., & Stark, R. E. (1982). Perceptual/motor profiles of reading impaired children with or without concomitant oral language deficits. *Annals of Dyslexia, 32*, 163–176.

Temple, E. (2002). Brain mechanisms in normal and dyslexic readers. *Current Opinion in Neurobiology, 12*, 178–183.

Temple, E., Deutsch, G. K., Poldrack, R. A., Miller, S. L., Tallal, P., Merzenich, M. M., et al. (2003). Neural deficits in children with dyslexia ameliorated by behavioral remediation: evidence from functional fMRI. *Proceedings of the National Academy of Sciences, 100*, 2860–2865.

Temple, E., Poldrack, R. A., Protopapas, A, Nagarajan, S., Salz, T., Tallal, P., et al. (2000). Disruption of the neural response to rapid acoustic stimuli in dyslexia: Evidence from MRI. *Proceedings of the National Academy of Sciences, 97*, 13907–13912.

Turkeltaub, P., Gareau, L., Flowers, D. L., Zeffiro, T. A., & Eden, G. F. (2003). Development of neural mechanisms for reading. *Nature Neuroscence, 6*, 767–773

Wible, B., Nicol, T., & Kraus, N. (2002). Abnormal neural encoding of repeated speech stimuli in noise in children with learning problems. *Clinical Neurophysiology, 113*, 485–494.

II

Management

10

The ABCs of CAP

Practical Strategies for Enhancing Central Auditory Processing Skills

Jeanane M. Ferre

Overview

Central auditory processing disorder (CAPD) is a deficit in the neural processing of auditory information that, although not the result of higher order cognitive or linguistic dysfunction, may lead to secondary difficulties in the understanding and use of language (ASHA, 2005b). In the assessment of CAPD, formal and informal measures are used to diagnose differentially the central auditory deficit from among other deficits having shared symptomatology and to describe specifically the impact of the deficit on the listener's life. In the intervention process, treatment procedures designed to rehabilitate the system are implemented along with management strategies designed to minimize the deficit's adverse effects. The intervention effort is maximized when remediation and management strategies are implemented soon after diagnosis, specific to the needs of the client, and generalized across settings (ASHA, 2005b).

Discussions of specific treatment approaches and management strategies for listeners with CAPD may be found in numerous other chapters in this text. This chapter describes practical, simple, everyday activities, behaviors, and strategies that can influence positively the auditory processing skills not only of the listener with specific CAPD but also of all listeners. These "enhancement tips" include activities designed to rehabilitate central auditory processing skills and strategies designed to minimize the impact of the deficit on communication and related function. By applying the ABCs of CAP, speech and hearing professionals can maximize treatment outcomes, minimize barriers to learning and communication, and achieve effective auditory processing for all listeners.

A. All-Day Processing

Listeners are bombarded daily with an array of sensory stimuli, including auditory, that must be processed quickly and efficiently to ensure effective communication, promote psychosocial wellness, and achieve academic success. Too often, students, especially those with APD, may be led to believe that "processing" is a skill to be practiced only at school or in a therapy session. Similarly, with the rapid increase in commercially available and fairly regimented programs for rehabilitation of specific auditory processing and related skills, parents may be misled to believe that repeated "skill drills" alone will suffice to improve a child's processing. If it is true that processing happens all day, then it is equally true that processing can be enhanced through a variety of activities throughout the day. These activities complement the formal therapy in which the child may be engaged and take the form of simple, often cost-free or low-cost games that can develop specific auditory and related skills.

(Central) auditory processing has been defined broadly as the efficiency and effectiveness with which the central nervous system (CNS) utilizes auditory information (ASHA, 2005b). Basic neuroscientific and clinical research have indicated that these skills include sound localization and lateralization, auditory discrimination, binaural processing, and temporal processing (ASHA, 2005b). A growing body of research indicates that inclusion of direct skills remediation, or bottom-up therapy, can change auditory behavior (ASHA, 2005b; Chermak, 1998; Chermak & Musiek, 1997). In addition, effective auditory processing is associated with other higher order cognitive-communicative skills including, but not limited to, phonological processing, comprehension and interpretation of auditory information, and attention to and memory for auditory information (ASHA, 2005b). Therapy to enhance these skills takes the form of top-down remediation in which metacognitive and metalinguistic strategies are explicitly taught to minimize the impact of the processing deficit on the listener's life (Bellis, 2003; Chermak, 1998; Ferre, 2006). Many formal procedures have been developed to address both top-down and bottom-up processing skills and these are described in detail in Chapter 7 of this text. For many of these programs, informal analogs exist that can be implemented on a daily basis and at little or no cost, at home, in the car, or at school. These "all-day" activities meet the intervention goal of extending rehabilitation beyond the therapy environment to maximize mastery and ensure generalization of skills (ASHA, 2005b) and include games to enhance auditory discrimination, binaural processing, temporal processing, and related visual, linguistic, and cognitive skills.

Auditory Discrimination

In auditory discrimination training, the goal is to improve the listener's ability to discriminate, identify, and recognize fine and/or rapidly changing acoustic cues. Early formal sensory based adaptive auditory training programs include those of Alexander and Frost (1982) and portions of the Central Auditory Abilities (CAA) Teaching Program (Flowers, 1983). More recent efforts include Sloan's phoneme training program (1980, 1995) and those that use computer technology to subtly enhance and/or manipulate the acoustic characteristics of the speech signal, including Fast ForWord (Scientific Learning Corporation, 1997), Earobics (Cognitive Concepts, 1997, 1998) and SoundSmart (Sandford, 2001). Discrimination training for nonspeech targets, including intensity training, frequency training, and duration training (e.g., just noticeable difference training for frequency, intensity of timing cues) is described by a number of authors including Carrell, Bradlow, Nicol, Koch, and Kraus (1999), Chermak and Musiek (1997, 2002) and Bellis (2003). Discrimination skills also can be practiced using low-cost and/or no-cost techniques such as simple rhyming games (e.g., no-cost: Give three rhymes for *cat*; low-cost: A Rhyme in Time, Soundabet), ending sound word-chains (e.g., each player says a word that starts with the *last* sound of the previous word: hiT—ToP—PaTH—THeN—NaMe . . .), and the "telephone game" in which a message is whispered from player to player down a line or around a circle.

Binaural Processing

Training in binaural processing includes activities to enhance binaural integration and separation skills (how the two cerebral hemispheres work together) or binaural interaction skills (how the two ears work together at the brainstem level of the CNS). To improve binaural integration and separation, dichotic listening training is used in which the listener hears two (or more) different targets presented simultaneously, one or more to each ear, and is asked to attend to one (separation) or both (integration) signals. The relative intensities of the targets are varied systematically as is the linguistic complexity of the materials used. Formal dichotic listening training is described by Chermak and Musiek (2002), Bellis (2003), and Musiek (Chapter 15 of this text). Informal binaural separation/integration training can be accomplished by asking the student to repeat one or both targets spoken by individuals standing on either side of the listener. Although not a true dichotic experience, the activity approximates the skill. As with formal dichotic training, relative loudness levels between the two speakers can be varied as can language of the target (e.g., asking the listener to repeat numbers given by two speakers versus repeating sentences or answering questions).

Localization refers to the ability to determine the location of a sound source in space and relies upon intact binaural interaction skills. Localization training can be accomplished in a variety of ways and has been described by a number of authors (Bellis, 2003; Chermak & Musiek, 1997; Kelly, 1995). A simple method for use with young children is "take my keys." In this activity, the child stands with eyes closed and a parent or sibling shakes a set of keys at various locations near the child's head (e.g., above, below, and to the left, etc.) asking the child to try to take the keys. Marco Polo and Blind Man's Bluff are examples of localization games that have been played by children for generations.

Temporal Processing

Temporal processing refers to the listener's ability to use timing aspects of the signal and includes temporal discrimination and temporal patterning. Temporal discrimination can be enhanced using the auditory training activities described previously. Temporal ordering and patterning exercises are designed to improve the ability to recognize and use acoustic patterns such as those that occur in running speech. Formal therapeutic activities of this type include identifying the sweep direction for a short-duration tone burst (Chermak & Musiek, 1997), sequencing a string of words or environmental sounds (Cognitive Concepts, 1997, 1998; Kelly, 1995; Protti et al., 1980), recognizing two- or three-tone patterns (Scientific Learning Corporation, 1997), or imitating rhythmic (e.g., long-short-long) or tonal (e.g., high-low-high) patterns by humming or tapping the response. Phoneme sequencing and sound blending programs such as those described in Chapter 8 enhance both speech-sound discrimination and patterning skills. To extend the benefits of these programs beyond the therapy room, parents may wish to try Mad Gab, Bop It, Bop It Extreme, Simon, Simon^2, or diadochokinetic exercises. In these latter exercises, the listener practices listening to and reproducing nonsense sound chains of up to three targets that vary in sound, rhythm, and/or speed. For example: *puh-tuh-kuh* all spoken with equal stress, *PUH-tuh-kuh* (stress on first target), *bluh-muh-FUH* (stress on last target and first target contains a blend), *spruh, struh, skruh* (equal stress but all targets use three-phoneme blends). Begin with single targets having single phoneme (e.g., *puh)* moving up to "triple-triple" targets (e.g., *spruh, struh, skruh).* Practicing tongue twisters (e.g., Peter Piper picked . . .), reading children's books (e.g., *Hop on Pop, There's a Wocket in My Pocket!*), poems, and nursery rhymes aloud, and singing songs (e.g., *B-I-N-G-O*) are inexpensive activities that enhance right-hemisphere based auditory pattern recognition skills. Enhancement of related visual or motor patterning skills can be accomplished through stringing beads or by playing games such as Simon Says, Scrabble, UpWords, Boggle, dominoes, and Rummikub. Syllable and sound counting, important for phonological awareness, can be initiated with even young children if formatted as a game.

In this whole-body game, the child is asked to "step-out" the sounds or syllables in the target word or phrase. Place number squares (1–4) and a "start/go" square on the floor. A parent, sibling, or caregiver says any one-, two-, three-, or four-syllable word and the child "steps out" the syllable beats, "landing" on the appropriate number square. As recognition skills improve, ask the child to "count the sounds" (e.g., G-O, C-A-T, S-P-EE-CH, etc.). The addition of visual and motor cues enhances the experience for the listener.

Attention to and Vigilance for Auditory Targets

Among the recommendations often given to parents and teachers for enhancing the communication skills of students with auditory processing disorder is to ensure that the speaker has gained the listener's attention before beginning. Activities that can enhance overall attention to auditory information include Simon Says, Battleship, the "telephone game," and Twister. Related to auditory attention is auditory vigilance, or the ability to sustain attention over time and respond to a change in the signal. A teacher or parent may say a string of words, intermittently inserting a "target" word, asking the listener to respond only when the target word is said (e.g., the target word *black* interspersed in a string of other color names). The Earobics program (Cognitive Concepts, 1998) uses pseudoword phonemes and asks the listener to respond only when the target changes. By varying the degree to which the target differs from the common signal (e.g., from /da/ embedded in a string of /bo/ to /dih/ embedded in a string of /deh/), vigilance tasks also train auditory discrimination skills. Other games and activities that require vigilance include musical chairs, cake walks, duck-duck-goose, Bop It, Brain Warp, Simon Says, and Red light-Green light.

Interhemispheric Transfer

Interhemispheric transfer refers to the communication across the corpus callosum and is important for intra- and intersensory integration. Exercises to improve interhemispheric transfer of information involve any task for which cross-hemisphere communication is required. These activities need not be wholly auditory or linguistic in nature. The key criteria are that the activity require a single or double transfer of information across the corpus callosum and include frequent repetitions (Bellis, 2003). Thus, sports, karate, playing a musical instrument, and activities that involve bipedal (e.g., dance) or bimanual coordination (e.g., tossing a ball from one hand to another) can improve communication across the corpus callosum for listeners exhibiting binaural integration and/or interhemispheric deficits. Activities that require intersensory integration such as Simon Says (auditory-motor), Simon (auditory-visual), and the latest generation of interactive video games (e.g., Donkey Kong Jungle Beat, Mario Mix Dance Revolution, Eye-Toy for PlayStation2) that require auditory-visual-motor integration for success can "train" interhemispheric transfer of function in an enjoyable and relatively inexpensive manner. An even less expensive, play anywhere, interhemispheric training game is "Name That Tune" in which the listener recognizes the song title (linguistic labeling—left hemisphere dominated) by recognizing the melodic or tonal pattern (pattern recognition—right hemisphere dominated). For young children, the "feely bag" offers opportunities not only to enhance interhemispheric integration but also auditory-linguistic integration. To play, place several common objects in a bag of box. For *tactile-linguistic* transfer, have the child reach into the bag and name the object without looking at it. For *linguistic-tactile* transfer, have the child "feel around" the bag for an object named by someone else. To enhance linguistic integration, have the child first name the object (noun—labeling) and then give its function (verb—action). Other tasks taxing higher levels of language integration function include asking the child to describe the object verbally, in detail, or name an associated item/object (e.g., if touching a pen the child names "paper").

Visual, Linguistic, and Cognitive Skills

Although not an "auditory" training activity, the inclusion of lip-reading/speech-reading exercises is an important component of the aural rehabilitation program of the listener with auditory processing disorder (Ferre, 1997, 1998). The addition of complementary visual cues enhances the communication experience for most listeners. Using adaptive techniques similar to those described for other types of training, a listener's ability to use lip-reading/speech-reading cues can be quantifiably improved. Ferre's (1997) Processing Power program contains lesson plans for these skills for use with children as young as six years of age. Work on lip-reading also is included, either implicitly or explicitly, in many phoneme training programs (e.g., Sloan, 1995; Lindamood-Bell Learning Processes, 1998). The classic game charades helps children learn the value of gestures and body language in communication. Board games that feature play and practice with lip-reading and other visual cues include Read My Lips, Cranium series, and Pictionary.

Many listeners with auditory processing disorder require the inclusion of top-down therapies designed to improve a listener's ability to use higher level concept driven skills. Metalinguistic strategies refer to the listener's ability to apply higher order linguistic rules when confronted with adverse listening situations. These include auditory closure (i.e., using context to fill in missing pieces), schema induction (i.e., using expectations and experience to fill in the message), use of discourse cohesion devices (e.g., learning to "key-in" to tag words and conjunctions), and prosody training (i.e., learning to use the rhythmic and melodic features of the signal to "get the message"). Metacognitive strategies refer to the listener's ability to think about and plan ways to enhance spoken language comprehension. These include attribution training (i.e., self-identification of the sources of listening difficulties), use of metamemory techniques (e.g., chunking, mnemonics), and self-advocacy (i.e., learning to modify one's own listening environment). Taken together, metalinguistic and metacognitive strategies enable the listener to be an active, rather than passive, participant in a communication event. The listener learns to use all available cues as well as their own knowledge and experience, altering behavior as needed, to enhance communication and improve processing. For a detailed discussion of metacognitive and metalinguistic therapies, the reader is referred to Chermak (1998), Bellis (2003), and Baran's chapter of this text (Chapter 16). Two of the more "auditory" strategies of this type, auditory closure and prosody, are described briefly here.

Auditory Closure

Auditory closure activities are designed to improve the ability to predict a missing target word or sound based upon context. In so doing, the listener learns to listen to the whole message rather than trying to decode each word. Simplest among these is asking the listener to fill in a missing word in a sentence. Tasks usually begin with familiar material such as nursery rhymes (e.g., *Humpty Dumpty sat on a* ____) or predictable everyday sentences (e.g., *When we go to the library, we can get* ____). As skills improve, and/or for older students and adults, use more linguistically challenging materials such as common expressions (e.g., *Don't let the cat out of the* ____) or sentences in which specific parts of speech have been omitted (e.g., omission of the verb: *The pitcher* ____ *the ball to the catcher*). More challenging auditory closure activities include asking the listener to predict targets with a missing syllable (e.g., *wall- __- per)* or missing sound (e.g., *s-p-__ch*). By embedding these activities in a background of noise or playing in an acoustically unfriendly environment (e.g., a car), skills are challenged further. These auditory closure activities require no special equipment or training and can be played virtually anywhere; whereas the children's game of Hangman and its updated counterpart, Wheel of Fortune offer the opportunity to practice auditory (and visual) closure, perhaps during a "family game night."

Prosody

Prosody training, the top-down extension of temporal patterning training, improves the listener's ability to attach meaning to the prosodic or suprasegmental aspects of speech, including melody, rhythm, timing, and emphasis. In prosody training the focus is on the intent of the message rather than the words themselves (i.e., the *way* something is said, not *what* is said). Prosody practice may include recognizing sarcasm or recognizing changes in meaning based upon stress or intonation (e.g., declarative: *Stop.,* interrogative; *Stop?*, exclamatory: *Stop!*). These kinds of recognition tasks will likely include a discussion of the ways in which prosodic cues are coded in print (e.g., commas, exclamation points, question marks) thereby enhancing speech-to-print skills. Crossword puzzles and wordplay books allow students to practice using heteronyms, or words that change meaning depending upon stress pattern (e.g., *OBject* versus *obJECT)*. The *Grammar Rock* video from the Schoolhouse Rock! video series provides an entertaining introduction to a variety of metalinguistic skills, including prosody.

Strengthening higher order linguistic and cognitive skills assists in minimizing the adverse effects of an auditory processing deficit on an individual's listening, communication, and learning (ASHA 2005b). Board games such as Password, Scattergories, Taboo, Rags to Riches, Catch Phrase, Clever Endeavor, and Tribond encourage the development of an array of linguistic and cognitive skills including categorization, labeling, word association, use of idioms, problem-solving, and word retrieval. Word games also can be played without game pieces or equipment almost anywhere. For example, while riding in the car, make up word association chains (e.g., sun-day, daylight, light-time, time-out, out-side . . .) or play "20 questions." Finally, to enhance the listener's linguistic bank, encourage regular use not only of a standard dictionary and thesaurus, but also books for vocabulary building and dictionaries of rhyming words, homonyms, and idioms.

B: BE an Effective Processing Role Model

In addition to engaging children in games and activities throughout the day that promote processing; parents, teachers, and others can enhance auditory processing by serving as good role models of effective communication strategies. For the child with APD these *message modifications* are critical. However, regular use of these simple and practical strategies enhances the acoustic, linguistic, and related aspects of the signal for all listeners. These strategies include using clear speech, adding visual cues, and using clear language.

Clear Speech

In "clear speech" the focus is on enhancing speech recognition by modifying the speech *of the talker*. Schum (1997) noted that in typical conversational speech it is not uncommon for speakers to articulate quickly, fail to project the voice, omit unnecessary or redundant sounds, and to run words and sounds together. These behaviors can adversely affect speech recognition not only for normal hearing listeners (Helfer, 1997), but also for those with hearing loss and auditory-based learning disabilities (Bradlow, Kraus, & Hayes, 2003; Payton, Uchanski, & Braida, 1994; Schum, 1996).

A common complaint among students with (C)APD is mishearing parts or all of a message. In clear speech, the speaker is trained to speak at a slightly reduced rate and to use a slightly increased volume (Picheny, Durlach, & Braida, 1985, 1986). In so doing, spectral boundaries and characteristics are enhanced, signal timing and prosody improves, and relative consonant-to-vowel intensities increase (Bradlow et al., 2003; Ferguson & Kewley-Port, 2002; Krause & Braida, 2004; Picheny et al., 1986).

With a minimal amount of instruction and practice, most talkers can be trained to produce clear speech (Caissie, Campbell, Frenette, Scott, Howell, & Roy, 2005; Schum, 1996). With additional training, clear speech can be achieved without necessarily reducing overall speaking rate (Krause & Braida, 2002, 2004). When a target is "misheard," simple repetition using clear speech often is sufficient to ensure comprehension. By practicing clear speech on a regular basis, parents, teachers, and professionals enhance the listeners' perception and model and encourage the production of clear speech.

Visual Cues

By coupling clear speech with an auditory-visual presentation, speech recognition is enhanced compared to an auditory-only presentation (Helfer, 1997). That is, *looking and listening* should be modeled by parents and teachers if the same behavior is expected from children. However, not all listeners with APD benefit from "looking AND listening" simultaneously. Some listeners are deficient in their ability to integrate auditory and visual information and the addition of visual cues may create further confusion. In these cases, "look *and* listen" should be changed to "look *or* listen" (Bellis, 2003; Ferre, 1997). At times in the home and especially in the classroom, the addition of complementary visual cues or the use of manipulatives, examples, and demonstration (e.g., *show me)* improves understanding, particularly for unfamiliar or abstract information. For some students, these additional cues can be provided with simultaneous auditory input. For others, multisensory cues should be given sequentially, for example, "look *then* listen," to minimize potential overload on integration and/or organization skills (Bellis, 2003; Ferre, 2002). In addition, classroom teachers should be reminded to speak *after* looking down at their notes or writing on a board rather than *while* writing.

Clear Language

As noted above, the use of *clear speech* improves signal perception. By using *clear language*, comprehension is improved. By saying what we *mean* and meaning what we *say* communication between and among speakers and listeners is enhanced regardless of processing skill level. Rephrasing a misunderstood signal provides the listener with a more linguistically familiar and less ambiguous target, thereby fostering improved comprehension. For example, if the word *beverage* is not yet in the child's vocabulary, use *drink* or the specific beverage name (e.g., *water, soda, milk,* etc.). Questions such as "How many times have I told you not to . . . " or "Didn't I tell you last week . . . " may lead to responses considered by adults to be flippant or unresponsive. If clear and precise responses are desired, clear and precise questions should be asked. Similarly, a parent or teacher may say "Stop that!" when the more explicit "Stop tapping your pencil (feet, desk)" would be a more effective use of language, leading to positive results. To gauge the listener's comprehension, the statement "Tell me what you think I said" rather than "Do you understand?" should elicit a paraphrased response rather than a *yes* or *no* answer, allowing the speaker to gauge understanding.

Many speakers are guilty of overusing generic language. Generic labels such as "stuff," "things," and "times" should be replaced by more exact, specific, and communicative terms that apply to the persons, places, and/or events of our lives. Adding or emphasizing "tag" words such as *first, last, before, after, if,* and *then* further enhances the specificity of the communication event leading to positive outcomes. For example, replace "Did you do those *things* I asked you to do?" with "Did you do your homework and *then* pick up your room?" The addition of verbal cues and prompts provides structure to the message, necessary for many students with an auditory processing disorder. Verbal cuing enhances the retrieval of information, especially for the listener experiencing memory difficulties coexisting with or secondary to an auditory processing deficit, rather than asking the listener to pull a response from "thin air." For additional discussion of memory cuing techniques the reader is referred to Richard (2001, and Chapter 8 in this text). In conversation, limiting the overall amount of information given at one time, breaking long messages down into shorter (5–6 word) sequences, adding tag words, and allowing "thinking" or "waiting" time before expecting a response enhances message salience and comprehension as well as the listener's ability to demonstrate understanding.

Familiarity enhances language clarity in a communication event. In general, the more familiar one is with the target, the easier the processing becomes. In the classroom, preteaching or previewing material is designed to enhance familiarity with the target and the task. Books on tape, copies of teachers' notes/texts, CliffNotes, seeing movies, and reading aloud to children can enhance their familiarity with the subject, task demands, main ideas, key elements, and vocabulary. At home and school, knowledge of the rules, structure, and task demands *up front* can minimize overload. For example, before giving the child a list of three tasks to carry out, *tell* the child that there are going to be *three* "things to do" and then itemize each one, numerically or alphabetically. Through a combination of repeated exposure and, as needed, explicit instruction, across a variety of contexts and settings throughout the day, familiarity with and understanding of the "rules" of language are enhanced (Ferre, 2006).

C: CHANGE the Communication Environment

It has been established that by improving room acoustics, the listening and learning skills of all children can be enhanced (ANSI, 2002; Crandell & Smaldino, 2002). A recent report from the American National Standards Institute (ANSI, 2002), estimates that up to 60% of students' classroom activities involve listening to and participating in spoken communication. In addition to this daily "in-school" listening, students participate in a variety of afterschool and "at-home" activities that also require listening and responding to spoken communication. Thus, it is essential that listening environments, especially classrooms, be free of acoustical barriers. When assessing the listening environment, consider both acoustic and nonacoustic variables that can affect speech perception. Acoustic variables include presence, type, and intensity of background noise, room reverberation time, and distance between the speaker and listener (Crandell & Smaldino, 2002). Nonacoustic factors include lighting, presence/absence of visual cues, and presence of visual and/or physical distractions (Ferre, 1997).

Background Noise

Background noise refers to any auditory disturbance in a room that interferes with listening (Crandell & Smaldino, 2002) and can be generated by in-room sources, internal sources (within a building but outside the room), and external sources (outside the building). Background noise adversely affects speech perception by masking the acoustic and linguistic cues in the message and/or by distracting the listener from the communication event (Crandell & Smaldino, 2002). The spectral characteristics of noise can affect the extent to which it will interfere with listening (Nabalek & Nabalek, 1994). Speech spectrum noise, multitalker babble, and "real-life" in-room noise appear to affect more adversely the speech recognition skills of young children, college-age students, and adults with academic difficulties than pink or nonspeech-like noise (Chermak, Vonhof, & Bendel, 1989; Cooper & Cutts, 1971; Jamieson, Kranjc, Yu, & Hodgett, 2004; Papso & Blood, 1989).

Signal-to-noise ratio (SNR) refers to the intensity of the signal relative to the background noise. Holding other factors constant, as the SNR becomes less favorable, speech recognition becomes poorer for all listeners (Cooper & Cutts, 1971). For listeners with normal hearing, speech recognition is not severely reduced until the SNR reaches 0 dB (Crandell & Smaldino, 2002). For very young listeners and those with hearing impairment, speech-language disorders, limited English proficiency, academic disabilities, or (C)APD, SNRs that are at least 2 to 15 dB more favorable than those needed by normal hearing listeners are required (Bradlow, 2003; Bronzaft, 1982; Crandell & Smaldino, 1996, 2002; Evans & Maxwell, 1997; Finitzo-Heiber & Tillman, 1978; Maxwell & Evans, 2000; Plomp & Mimpen, 1979).

Reverberation

Reverberation, or echo, refers to the persistence of a sound in an enclosed space due to the multiple reflections of sound waves off hard surfaces which can adversely affect speech recognition by masking direct sound (Nabalek & Nabalek, 1994). A room's reverberation is expressed in terms of reverberation time (RT), or the amount of time required for the sound pressure level to decrease by 60 dB after the signal has stopped. Although all rooms have some reverberation, large and irregularly-shaped rooms tend to have longer RTs than smaller rooms or those with greater amounts of absorptive material. For normal hearing adults, recognition is not adversely affected until the RT exceeds 1.0 second (Finitzo-Hieber & Tillman, 1978); however, for children with disordered hearing, language, or processing skills, speech perception may be compromised at RTs as low as 0.4 seconds (Crandell, Smaldino, & Flexer, 1995).

Noise Abatement at School and in the Home

Noise abatement programs for classrooms should seek to maintain an SNR of at least +15 with reverberation time of 0.4 seconds or less (ASHA, 1995, 2005a). For normal hearing listeners, large classrooms with reverberation times of up to 0.7 seconds and small to midsize classrooms with RTs of up to 0.6 seconds are acceptable, provided an SNR of +15 or better is maintained (ANSI, 2002). For a complete description of management suggestions, see Chapter 11.

Classroom noise abatement techniques may range from relatively simple to extensive in order to achieve these SNR and RT goals. Extensive, and often expensive, solutions for improving classroom acoustics include: reduction or elimination of open classrooms; relocation of teaching spaces away from playgrounds, gymnasiums, or cafeterias; building changes such as double-paned windows or noise dampening devices on heating, air conditioning, and ventilation systems; changes in lighting fixture location and type (i.e., from fluorescent to incandescent); and lowered ceiling levels. Simpler and less expensive classroom noise abatement can be accomplished by: closing windows; carpeting rooms; using curtains, drapes, and/or acoustic ceiling tiles; placing baffles within the listening space; and damping highly reflective surfaces. Placing bookcases perpendicular to each other or creating a 6 to 8 inch space between side-by-side bookcases can create baffles and minimize noise. Cork bulletin boards and the use of fabric to cover hard surfaces increases sound absorption and dampens reflective surfaces. Felt pads or rubber caps on the bottoms of chair and table legs minimize furniture-to-floor noise.

In the home, parents and caregivers should be reminded about simple ways to reduce noise and minimize acoustic barriers to listening such as closing doors and windows; reducing radio, stereo, and television volume; using carpet and drapes; rearranging furniture and changing lighting; and minimizing the number of speakers talking at the same time. For more detailed information on specific acoustical modifications in the classroom the reader is referred to Crandell and Smaldino (2001, 2004) and Geffner (Chapter 11 of this text).

Distance from Source

Distance between the speaker and listener can affect speech recognition. Generally, sound intensity decreases with increasing distance from the source (Ostergaard, 2000). Sound in a room may be direct or reverberant. Direct sound is the sound reaching the listener without obstruction. Reverberant sound is sound energy composed of reflected waves within the space. As distance from the speaker increases, the amount of reverberant sound tends to increase and dominate the signal. Students seated near the back of a classroom receive a signal composed almost entirely of reverberant sound whereas those near the front receive almost all direct sound (Boothroyd, 2004). For most listeners, a distance of 3 to 6 feet from the sound source creates optimal audibility, with speech recognition decreasing beyond that critical distance (Boothroyd, 2004). For the home, remind parents that this optimal listening distance will likely not be achieved if speaking or shouting to someone from another room or floor in the house.

Nonacoustic Factors

When assessing the physical space, consider also nonacoustic factors such as lighting, presence of visual cues, and presence of visual and physical distractions. Room lighting can affect ability to use visual cues and maintain attention on task. Replacing fluorescent lighting with incandescent lighting not only eliminates the hum often produced by these lights but also improves access to visual cues by reducing harshness and glare. Speakers should avoid being backlit, that is, standing with the light coming from behind the speaker rather than on the speaker's face.

Preferential classroom seating can be used to counteract the adverse effects of distance and poor lighting and enhance the listener's ability to use available relevant visual cues. In preferential seating, an effort is made to maximize both the acoustic and visual aspects of the signal based on the combined benefits of bimodal processing (Erber, 1969; Sanders & Goodrich, 1971). The listener's auditory perception is enhanced when seated nearer the speaker as is the opportunity to use speechreading cues. Speech-reading is optimal at a distance of no more than 5 feet (Schow & Nerbonne, 1996). By placing the listener near and *facing* the speaker at no more than a 45-degree angle and away from distracting noise, both signal audibility and accessibility of speech-reading cues are optimized (Ferre, 1997). Depending upon the type of auditory processing deficit that has been identified, it may be necessary to move students to a different listening, study, or testing environment. Study carrels can be used to minimize visual distractions at school and in the home. Consultation with the occupational therapist (OT) or physical therapist (PT) may lead to changes in desk or chair type or design to minimize physical distractions that can interfere with listening or studying at home and in school.

Summary

Central auditory processing disorders are any one or more of a set of neuroaudiologic deficits that can affect adversely communicative success, academic achievement, and/or psychosocial well-being. Well-designed and controlled diagnostic test procedures exist that can specify the nature of the processing deficit, if present. Having defined as clearly as possible the disorder's nature and impact, one can develop deficit-specific management strategies designed to minimize the adverse effects of the deficit on the listener's life and rehabilitate the system. The management process is incomplete and at risk for being ineffective, however, if not extended beyond the therapeutic environment into all aspects of the listener's daily life. The audiologist and speech-language pathologist are uniquely qualified to provide guidance to listeners, their parents, and caregivers and related professionals regarding the ways in which management goals can be met across a variety of settings. By applying the ABCs of CAP: **A**ll-day processing, **Be** a good processing model, and **C**hange the communication environment; collaborative management is achieved, auditory processing and related skills of the client are improved, and communication is enhanced for all individuals.

Key Points Learned

- Auditory processing occurs all day, every day.
- Deficient auditory processing can adversely affect academics, communication, and social-emotional wellness.
- For listeners with specific auditory processing deficit, intervention involves balancing direct remediation techniques, designed to improve skills, with management strategies, designed to minimize the deficit's effects.
- Effective intervention occurs through collaboration among the client, families, and professionals.
- Although specific therapies have been developed for training a variety of auditory skills; there also exist analogs to these therapies in many inexpensive and simple games.
- Regular game play not only extends the benefits of therapy for listeners with CAPD but also enhances development of healthy processing among all listeners.
- Students' auditory processing skills are enhanced when teachers, parents, caregivers, and other professionals model good communication and processing strategies at home and school.
- By removing acoustic barriers and enhancing complementary multisensory input at home and school, students receive a robust target and efficient processing can be achieved.

References

Alexander, D. W., & Frost, B. P. (1982). Decelerated synthesized speech as a means of shaping speed of auditory processing of children with delayed language. *Perceptual and Motor Skills, 55*, 783–792.

American National Standards Institute. (2002). ANSI S12.60-2002. *Acoustical performance criteria, design requirements and guidelines for schools.* Melville, NY: Author.

American Speech-Language-Hearing Association. (1995). *Guidelines for acoustics in educational settings*. Rockville, MD: Author.

American Speech-Language-Hearing Association. (2005a). *Guidelines for addressing acoustics in educational settings.* Rockville, MD: Author.

American Speech-Language-Hearing Association. (2005b). *(Central) auditory processing disorders* [Technical report]. Rockville, MD: Author.

Bellis, T. (2003). *Assessment and management of central auditory processing disorders in the educational setting* (2nd ed.). Clifton Park, NY: Thomson Delmar Learning.

Boothroyd, A. (2004). Room acoustics and speech perception. *Seminars in Hearing, 25*, 155–166.

Bradlow, A. R. (2003, November). *Sentence perception in noise by children with learning disabilities*. Paper presented at the annual meeting of the American Speech-Language-Hearing Association, Chicago.

Bradlow, A., Kraus, N., & Hayes, E. (2003). Speaking clearly for children with learning disabilities: Sentence perception in noise. *Journal of Speech, Language, Hearing Research, 46*, 80–97.

Bronzaft, A. L. (1982). The effect of a noise abatement program on reading ability. *Journal of Environmental Psychology, 1*, 215–222.

Caissie, R., Campbell, M., Frenette, W., Scott, L., Howell, I., & Roy, A. (2005). Clear speech for adults with a hearing loss: Does intervention with communication partners make a difference? *Journal of the American Academy of Audiology, 15*, 157–171.

Carrell, T. D., Bradlow, A. R., Nicol, T. G., Koch, D. B., & Kraus, N. (1999). Interactive software for evaluating auditory discrimination. *Ear and Hearing, 20*, 175–176.

Chermak, G. D. (1998). Metacognitive approaches to managing central auditory processing disorders. In M. G. Masters, N. A. Stecker, & J. Katz (Eds.), *Central auditory processing disorders: Mostly management* (pp. 49–61). Boston: Allyn & Bacon.

Chermak, G. D., & Musiek, F. E. (1997). *Central auditory processing disorders: New perspectives.* San Diego, CA: Singular Publishing Group.

Chermak, G. D., & Musiek, F. E. (2002). Auditory training principles and approaches for remediating and managing auditory processing disorders. *Seminars in Hearing, 23*, 297–308.

Chermak, G. D., Vonhoff, M. R., & Bendel, R. B. (1989). Word identification performance in the presence of competing speech and noise in learning disabled adults. *Ear and Hearing, 10*, 90–93.

Cognitive Concepts, Inc. (1997). *Earobics® auditory development and phonics program* [Computer software]. Evanston, IL. Author.

Cognitive Concepts, Inc. (1998). *Earobics®, step two auditory development and phonics program* [Computer software]. Evanston, IL. Author.

Cooper, J., & Cutts, B. (1971). Speech discrimination in noise. *Journal of Speech and Hearing Research, 14*, 332–337.

Crandell, C., & Smaldino, J. (1996). Speech perception in noise by children for whom English is a second language. *American Journal of Audiology, 5*, 47–51.

Crandell, C., & Smaldino, J. (2001). Acoustical modifications for the classroom. In C. Crandell & J. Smaldino (Eds), Classroom acoustics: Understanding barriers to learning. *The Volta Review, 101*(5), 33–46.

Crandell, C., & Smaldino J. (2002). Room acoustics and auditory rehabilitation technology. In J. Katz (Ed.), *Handbook of clinical audiology* (5th ed., pp. 607–630). Philadelphia: Lippincott Williams & Wilkins.

Crandell, C., & Smaldino, J. (Eds.). (2004). Classroom acoustics. *Seminars in Hearing, 25*(2).

Crandell, C., Smaldino, J., & Flexer, C. (1995). *Soundfield FM amplification: Theory and practical applications.* San Diego, CA: Singular Publishing Group.

Erber, N. (1969). An interaction of audition and vision in recognition of oral speech stimuli. *Journal of Speech and Hearing Research, 12*, 423–425.

Evans, G. W., & Maxwell, L. (1997). Chronic noise exposure and reading deficits: The mediating effects of language acquisition. *Environment and Behavior, 29*, 638–656.

Ferguson, S., & Kewley-Port, D. (2002). Vowel intelligibility in clear and conversational speech for normal-hearing and hearing-impaired listeners. *Journal of the Acoustical Society of America, 112*, 259–271.

Ferre, J. (1997). *Processing power: A guide to CAPD assessment and management.* San Antonio, TX: The Psychological Corporation.

Ferre, J. M. (1998). The M3 model for treating central auditory processing disorders. In M. G. Masters, N. A. Stecker, & J. Katz (Eds.), *Central auditory processing: Mostly management* (pp. 103–116). Boston: Allyn & Bacon.

Ferre, J. M. (2002). Managing children's central auditory processing deficits in the real world: What teachers and parents want to know. *Seminars in Hearing, 23,* 319–326.

Ferre, J. (2006). Management strategies for APD. In T. K. Parthasarathy (Ed.), *An introduction to auditory processing disorders in children*. Mahwah, NJ: Lawrence Erlbaum Associates.

Finitzo-Heiber, T., & Tillman, T. (1978). Room acoustical effects on monosyllabic word discrimination ability for normal and hearing impaired children. *Journal of Speech and Hearing Research, 21,* 440–448.

Flowers, A. (1983). *Auditory perception, speech, language, and learning*. Dearborn, MI: Perceptual Learning Systems.

Helfer, K.(1997). Auditory and auditory-visual perception of clear and conversational speech. *Journal of Speech Language and Hearing Research, 40,* 432–443.

Jamieson, D. G., Kranjc, G.,Yu, K., & Hodgett, W. E. (2004). Speech intelligibility of young school-aged children in the presence of real-life classroom noise. *Journal of the American Academy of Audiology, 15,* 508–517.

Kelly, D. A. (1995). *Central auditory processing disorders: Strategies for use with children and adolescents*. San Antonio, TX: Communication Skill Builders/The Psychological Corporation.

Krause, J., & Braida, L. (2002). Investigating alternative forms of clear speech: The effects of speaking rate and speaking mode on intelligibility. *Journal of the Acoustical Society of America, 112,* 2165–2172.

Krause, J., & Braida, L. (2004). Acoustic properties of naturally produced clear speech at normal speaking rates. *Journal of the Acoustical Society of America, 115,* 362–378.

Lindamood-Bell Learning Processes, Inc. (1998). *LiPS: Lindamood Phoneme Sequencing Program*. San Luis Obispo, CA: Author.

Maxwell, L.,& Evans, G.(2000).The effects of noise on pre-school children's pre-reading skills. *Environmental Psychology, 20,* 91–98.

Nabalek, A., & Nabalek, I. (1994). Room acoustics and speech perception. In J. Katz (Ed.), *Handbook of clinical audiology* (4th ed., pp. 624–637). Baltimore: Williams & Wilkins.

Ostergaard. P. (2000). Physics of sound and vibration. In E. Berger, L. Royster, J. Royster, D. Driscoll, & M. Layne (Eds.), *The noise manual* (pp. 19–39). Fairfax, VA: American Industrial Hygiene Association.

Papso, C. F., & Blood, I. M. (1989). Word recognition skills of children and adults in background noise. *Ear and Hearing, 10,* 235–236.

Payton, K., Uchanski, R., & Braida, L. (1994). Intelligibility of conversational and clear speech in noise and reverberation for listeners with normal and impaired hearing. *Journal of the Acoustical Society of America, 95,* 1581–1592.

Picheny, M., Durlach, N., & Braida, L. (1985). Speaking clearly for the hard of hearing I: Intelligibility differences between clear and conversational speech. *Journal of Speech and Hearing Research, 28,* 96–103.

Picheny, M., Durlach, N., & Braida, L. (1986). Speaking clearly for the hard of hearing. II: Acoustic characteristics of clear and conversational speech. *Journal of Speech and Hearing Research, 29,* 434–446.

Plomp, R., & Mimpen, A. (1979). Speech-reception threshold for sentences as a function of age and noise level. *Journal of the Acoustical Society of America, 66,* 1333–1342.

Protti, E., Young, M., & Bryne, P. (1980). The evaluation of a child with auditory perceptual deficiencies: an interdisciplinary approach. *Seminars in Speech, Language, and Hearing, 1,* 167–180.

Richard, G. J. (2001). *The source for processing disorders*. Rock Island, IL: LinguiSystems, Inc.

Sanders, D., & Goodrich, S. (1971). Relative contribution of visual and auditory components of speech intelligibility as a function of three conditions of frequency distortion. *Journal of Speech and Hearing Research, 14,* 154–159.

Sandford, J. (2001). *BrainTrain* [Computer software and manual]. Richmond, VA: SoundSmart™.

Schow, R., & Nerbonne, M. (1996). *Introduction to audiologic rehabilitation* (3rd ed.). Boston: Allyn & Bacon.

Schum, D. (1996). Intelligibility of clear and conversational speech of young and elderly talkers. *Journal of the American Academy of Audiology*, *7*, 212–218.

Schum, D. (1997). Beyond hearing aids: clear speech training as an intervention strategy. *Hearing Journal*, *50*, 36–39.

Scientific Learning Corporation. (1997). *Fast ForWord training program for children. Procedure manual for professionals.* Berkeley, CA. Author.

Sloan, C. (1980). Auditory processing disorders in children: Diagnosis and treatment. In P. J. Levinson & C. Sloan (Eds.), *Auditory processing and language: Clinical and research perspectives* (pp. 117–133). New York: Grune & Stratton.

Sloan, C. (1995). *Treating auditory processing difficulties in children*. San Diego, CA: Singular Publishing Group.

Registered Trademarks

A Rhyme in Time is a registered trademark of Poet and Didn't Know It.

Battleship and *Twister* are registered trademarks of Milton Bradley, Inc.

Boggle, Scattergories, Simon, Simon², *Scrabble, Bopit, Bopit Extreme, Catch Phrase, Brainwarp, Taboo,* and *UpWords* are registered trademarks of Hasbro, Inc.

Clever Endeavor is a registered trademark of Mind Games, Inc.

Cliffs Notes is a registered trademark of Hungry Minds, Inc.

Cranium is a registered trademark of Cranium, Inc.

Donkey Kong Jungle Beat is a registered trademark of Nintendo.

Earobics is a registered trademark of Cognitive Concepts, Inc.

Eye-Toy and *Playstation2* are registered trademarks of Sony Computer Entertainment, Inc.

Fast ForWord is a registered trademark of Scientific Learning Corporation.

Hop on Pop and *There's a Wocket in My Pocket!* are registered copyrights of Dr. Seuss and A. S. Geisel through Random House.

Mad Gab is a registered trademark of Patch Products.

Mario Mix Dance Revolution is a registered trademark of Nintendo.

Password is a registered trademark of Mark Goodson Productions, LLC.

Pictionary is a registered trademark of Pictionary, Inc. and Parker Brothers.

Rags to Riches is a registered trademark of Super Duper Publications.

Read My Lips and *Rummikub* are registered trademarks of Pressman Toy Corporation.

Schoolhouse Rock! is a registered trademark of Walt Disney Video.

Soundabet is a registered copyright of The Psychological Corporation, a division of Harcourt Assessment, Inc.

SoundSmart is a registered trademark of BrainTrain.

Tribond is a registered trademark of Big Fun A Go Go, Inc.

Wheel of Fortune is a registered trademark of Merv Griffin Enterprises, LLC.

Appendix 10–A
Summary of Games/Toys and Related Processing Skills Described in This Chapter

Game	Auditory Processing or Related Skill(s)
A Rhyme in Time	speech sound discrimination, auditory closure
Battleship	active listening, visual patterning, integration
Blind Man's Bluff	localization, binaural interaction
Boggle	pattern recognition, integration
Bop It, Bop It Extreme	integration, vigilance
Brain Warp	vigilance, integration, problem-solving
Catch Phrase	integration, vocabulary development, output/organization
Charades	use of visual cues, metalinguistic strategies
Clever Endeavor	metalinguistic strategies, critical listening
Cranium	bottom-up and top-down strategies
Diadochokinetics	patterning, output skills, discrimination
Feely Bag	interhemispheric communication
HangMan	auditory closure
Interactive video games	interhemispheric communication
Mad Gab	temporal patterning, metalinguistic skills
Marco Polo	localization, binaural interaction
Musical Chairs/Cake Walks	auditory vigilance
Name That Tune	interhemispheric transfer of function
Password	vocabulary building, metalinguistic skills
Pictionary	using visual cues, metalinguistic strategies
Rags to Riches	metalinguistic skills (idioms)
Read My Lips	lip-reading/speech-reading
Red Light-Green Light	auditory vigilance, active listening
Rummikub	patterning, problem-solving, integration
Scattergories	vocabulary building, metalinguistic strategies
Scrabble	integration, linguistic skills, visual patterning

Game	Auditory Processing or Related Skill(s)
Simon, Simon[2]	auditory-visual patterning
Simon Says	auditory vigilance, active listening
Soundabet	discrimination, integration, organization
Sound Chains	auditory discrimination, active listening
Taboo	vocabulary building, metalinguistic strategies
Telephone game	attention, active listening, discrimination
Tribond	metalinguistic, metamemory strategies
Twister	integration, critical listening
UpWords	integration, visual patterning
Wheel of Fortune	auditory closure

11

Management Strategies

Donna Geffner

Overview

Any discussion of management of (C)APD has to take into account three approaches: compensatory strategies, environmental modification, and direct treatment. The latter area is covered in subsequent chapters. This chapter addresses environmental modifications/engineering including suggestions for the home, classroom, school, and work environment, compensatory strategies, sound enhancement, FM and other sound enhancement systems and their efficacies for use by individuals with (C)APD.

Management goals should be determined on the basis of the diagnostic outcomes and the specific test measures that identified particular problems in processing the auditory message. Often the intake history and parent/client report provides a sufficient indication of areas that are compromised and need adjusting or intervention. A good listening environment is essential as children spend at least 45% of their school day in listening activities (Berg, 1987). Hearing accurately is essential in the classroom with the maximum desirable noise level for children having normal hearing at 35 dB. However, classrooms can have noise levels reach as high as 44 dB, in an empty classroom. With traffic from the street, and a class of 25 students and a teacher, the noise level can reach 60 dB, twice the level appropriate for most children to hear adequately. Thus, making a classroom conducive to hearing accurately is a critical step in environmental engineering so that the child with (C)APD can function in the classroom. This chapter addresses environmental modification engineering and assistive technologies to ameliorate the noise, increase the signal, and make the listening environment conducive to accurate listening as well as provide suggestions for individuals and their families as to what can be done to compensate for their auditory processing deficits.

Compensatory Strategies

Compensatory strategies are often quite effective in getting the adult client or child to adjust his environment without any alterations, but by simply moving his chair, putting himself far from a window or distracting noises, or moving away from a talkative friend. This type of behavior is called "self-advocacy," the ability to advocate for oneself. In some communication situations, it is essential. By teaching one assertiveness, to indicate to his listener or communicative partner that he didn't hear it, it was too noisy, or the speaker was talking too quickly, can accomplish a solution with little outlay of costs. Often "assertiveness training" is what is needed to get a youngster to defend himself and "speak up" about his difficulties. Motivating the child or adult client may be necessary. To accomplish this goal, it is helpful to practice and rehearse in mock settings. Encouragement to use these strategies may be necessary with continued and consistent use throughout the day. Other strategies include support from the school to provide notes for classes in which there is a lot of language spoken, and preteaching support so that vocabulary used in the class is known ahead of the class to improve the predictability. Getting notes from a "buddy" will help the youngster stay on top of his class. Using a tape recorder in class can help capture information that the listener is unable to get initially. The tape recorder with a reduced speed playback could be useful when the youngster goes to replay the lecture, as rapid speech is often too difficult for the person with (C)APD to grasp initially. Having the person take notes can be an unmanageable task, as listening and taking notes are too difficult tasks to accomplish together, thus the need for notes ahead of class or the use of a buddy's notes. Using lip reading to enhance the signal reception can assist with understanding the entire message. Often, when one looks on the lips of the speaker, the information becomes clearer and the visualizing helps to fill in the missing sounds of the word that was "misheard." Use of visuals is helpful so that teachers should be encouraged to use visuals (pictures, graphs, clippings, photos, computer images) in the classroom. Youngsters should be taught through a visualizing technique to take it all in. Such youngsters will do better on tests most of the time, when the test is not oral. Alternative methods of testing should be employed. Use of metacognitive skills may prove useful in interpreting the spoken message. Teaching one to utilize these skills in understanding the nonliteral and inferential meaning in language can help the person participate fully in the classroom. Multisensory learning is often the most effective for this population. However, strategies alone are not sufficient to solve the problem. Other methods that include environmental modifications should be employed.

Environmental Modifications

Environmental modifications include altering the environment in which the person functions, enhancing the signal to which the person is exposed, and improving access to information needed in the classroom, work, or other communicative environments.

Suggestions for the Classroom

Environmental accommodations to make the listening conditions better, with less noise in the background, include placing the child's seat in a favorable position, up front, next to the teacher, with his stronger ear proximal to the teacher (if a stronger ear exists). The use of visual aids, having the teacher provide notes ahead of the class, and study notes in advance of the week are helpful so the child knows what to expect and does not have to rely on his auditory system to process it all. Placing the children in a classroom situated away from noise, with insulation where needed, and limiting distractions are necessary.

The American Speech-Language-Hearing Association (ASHA) recommends an appropriate acoustical environment for all students in educational settings. ASHA endorses the ANSI S12.60-2002 *Acoustical Performance Criteria Design Requirements and Guidelines for Schools* (ANSI S12.60-2002) as the national standard for classroom acoustics. Acoustic conditions in the classroom or other environments in which learning takes place are critical in the academic, psychological, and psychosocial development for all children, not just for those with hearing loss, or auditory processing disorders. Inappropriate noise levels, reverberation, and poor insulation conditions can affect learning, speech perception, reading, spelling, classroom behavior, attention, concentration, and achievement in school. Teacher performance in the classroom is also compromised resulting in more absenteeism and voice conditions (ASHA, 2005b). When referring to acoustical factors in the classroom, one usually means reducing the level of background noise, known as "ambient" noise in the room, and using an improved "signal-to-noise level," (a better level of the speech signal in comparison to the nonspeech/informational signal or noise), and eliminating the reverberation.

Reverberation is the sound that persists in a room once the sound source has ceased. It is the time in seconds that a sound dies down by 60 decibels or to 1/1,000,000 of its level at the moment the sound source ceases. Reverberation is the prolongation of sound by multiple reflections (Stach, 2003). Reverberation time is the rate of sound decay that occurs as a sound decays in time units to a specified level following cessation of the sound source. In a large hard-surfaced area, the reverberation can be heard quite distinctly as an echo or persistent sound for several seconds once the original sound has stopped. Reverberation is still present in classrooms, to a lesser extent, which can interfere with speech intelligibility through what is called a "smearing effect" (Nixon, 2002). That occurs when the reflected sounds are still present and interfere with the newly uttered sounds, resulting in an overlap that "smears" the speech signal. In the ANSI Acoustic Standards, the reverberation time allowed in an average classroom (up to 10,000 cubic feet) should not exceed 0.6 seconds at frequencies of 500 Hz, 1000 Hz, and 2000 Hz. Reverberation can be controlled by acoustical absorption in the room. Such absorption is determined by the size of the room and the absorptive properties of the room. To measure reverberation one calculates the reverberation time in seconds equal to 0.05 times the product of room volume over total absorption of the room surfaces (Stach, 2003). Often correcting reverberation is simple as it involves additional acoustical treatment such as acoustic tiles and damping materials added to walls and furniture to comply with the standards.

Classroom Acoustics Recommendation

The following recommendations were made by ASHA's Working Group on Classroom Acoustics (2005a):

1. Unoccupied classroom noise level must not exceed 35 dBA.
2. The signal-to-noise ratio (SNR) should be at least +15 dB at the child's ears.
3. Unoccupied classroom reverberation times must not surpass 0.6 seconds in smaller classroom (<10,000 cu. ft.) or 0.7 seconds in larger rooms (>10,000 to 20,000 cu. ft.).

These criteria are identical to the approved ANSI Standards (ANSI S12.60) on classroom acoustics.

There is a need for all new school building construction to adhere to these acoustical criteria. Now it is only voluntary. In order to effect such a change in the construction of new classrooms, an architect, acoustical engineer and an audiologist should participate together in its design and construct.

What Is the Impact of Poor Acoustics?

What can happen if there are bad acoustics in the classroom? Results of studies indicate that children have a reduced speech perception, resulting in mishearing and spelling errors. There is reduced academic achievement and a decrease in attention. Reading ability declines and on-task behavior is compromised. Unfavorable psychosocial behaviors arise (Crandell & Smaldino, 2000). Of concern is the current state of classrooms with reported conditions registering signal-to-noise ratios in classrooms at −7 to +5 dB. Given the fact that children spend nearly half (45%) of their days focusing on listening and that children's ability to hear in noise does not reach adult-like levels until adolescence, then it follows that young children can be placed at risk for auditory misperceptions because of unfavorable listening environments (Berg, 1987).

What Can Be Done to Improve Classroom Acoustics?

To begin with, it is important to determine where the child sits. Since not all children can sit in the first row, facing the teacher, it is preferable to arrange seating so that the compromised child can see the teacher's lips and face. Enabling the child to take advantage of visual information is essential. Today, many early childhood classes have children sit in a semicircle. That would work, providing that the child can see the teacher's lips. Teaching a child to look and listen, and read the lips and face is a good strategy that can be adopted quickly.

Another approach is to reduce the overall noise levels in the school and classroom. To accomplish this, it is suggested that if the classrooms have movable chairs, the legs be furnished with tennis balls at the end to ward off the screeching sounds when the chairs are moved. "Hushh-Ups" (http://www.hushh-ups.com) is a company, (Sound Listening Environments, Inc.) that produces tennis balls already prepared to be fitted to the edge of the chair leg. Any rubber tip can absorb noise vibrations.

A rather simple, yet helpful, suggestion is to close the door. This is important as is the use of acoustic tiles on the ceilings and walls to help insulate the room. Even suggesting to the parents that they insulate the child's room or study area by using acoustic tile, draperies, carpeting, or study carrels will help reduce noise and distractions. Using permanent walls in place of wall partitions is far more preferable. Any moving partition, or classroom walls that are not permanent creates the wrong environment for a child with (C)APD.

Noise reduction headsets are helpful. Have the child use them during study time to complete his or her assignment. Even during a class study time, such a headset should prove valuable. The classroom itself should have a quiet study area, free from auditory and visual distractions. Use of study carrels or partitions for individual students is recommended.

Furthermore, teachers can play an important part in improving the classroom acoustics. First, teachers need to practice slowing down and speaking more slowly, using pauses. A slow speaking rate will improve speech perception, as will taking pauses to give a child time to catch up and digest what was said. Use of visuals for models, plans, and curriculum is most helpful. The teacher can alert the child when he or she wants his or her attention, by touching/tapping him or her sensibly to gain the student's attention or by saying his or her name or speaking softly to him or her. The use of a sign like a tap on the shoulder, or a finger cue can help remind the child to pay attention. Other suggestions for the classroom teacher include using pauses for extra processing and informing the child about any changes in topic, or transitions that will be coming up. Giving the child a preview of what's coming up, like telling him there are more interesting slides and how many there are of them are useful techniques. The teacher should allow the child to tape-record the teacher or lecturer, so the student can play it back later when there is less distraction.

Although the child's comprehension may appear to be good, the teacher should be responsible for confirming whether the child has heard appropriately. Ask the child to repeat back the story read aloud to him, or repeat the directions given. Ask the child to paraphrase information given to him, in his own words to check for understanding.

The *ASHA Guidelines for Addressing Acoustics in Educational Settings* (2005a) make it clear that the audiologist has the responsibility to advocate for good acoustics in the classroom by being available to measure the physical environment and assess behavioral performance and effects on achievement and speech recognition. The audiologist along with an acoustical engineer may design noise attenuating devices to meet the 35 dBA background noise requirement. Such mechanical devices might include an insulation box around a noisy piece of equipment, or a closet around a heating unit, a sealant on walls and doors, and the use of duck liners to minimize sound escaping into the classroom. When investigating and ameliorating the noise level of the school building, it would be helpful to have the maintenance crew plant shrubbery around the building to serve as an absorbent.

When attempts fail to attenuate the noise level sufficiently, or when there are children in the classroom that have compromised hearing either because of a hearing loss or a central auditory processing disorder, the next best approach is to bring assistive technology into the classroom.

Suggestions for the Home and Work Environment

It is generally agreed that reducing the noise level in the home and insulating the home are important. Lack of insulation and poor noise attenuation lead to poor study habits and distractions in learning, which result in poor grades.

There is a need to provide carpeting, remove the telephone or cell phone from study areas, and remove siblings or other distractions. Parents would be wise to provide "coaching" to help their child meet the deadlines and work expectations. Use of ear plugs and noise canceling headphones are an alternative, if the home environment cannot be altered.

In the work environment, it is better to work in a quiet area, where possible, away from doors and windows and other distractions, which include talkative colleagues. Placing oneself away from the distractions, insulating the desk by closing doors and windows, and setting up a "study carrel" around the work space is often helpful to heed off noise and interferences. Noise reduction ear plugs should also be considered. When these easy, economic methods are not sufficient, there are assistive listening devices to improve the listening conditions.

Assistive Technology

FM Systems

What is an FM system? It is a wireless communication technology in common use with telephones, two-way radios, alarms, and wireless headset. This frequency modulated system consists of a transmitter, which picks up the voice at the speaker's mouth and transmits it through radio waves to the FM receiver, which is in the form of a headset, ear bud, hearing aid, or speaker.

To describe it in laymen's terms to parents: It is an assistive device that can improve the student's ability to hear in background noise. For youngsters with APD, listening in background noise is often very difficult. The effectiveness of an FM unit is that it provides an increase in the signal (teacher's voice) from the noise (N) in a favorable signal-to-noise ratio (SNR). The signal is what we want to hear; the noise is what we don't. Noise can be defined as other students speaking, sneezing and whispering, fluorescent lights, heating, and air conditioner units. The best SNR is typically +15 dB or better in a classroom. Thus, the teacher's voice should be 15 dB louder than the background noise. Unfortunately, not all classrooms have maintained this ratio. Some have undesirable ratios like +5 or as poor as –7 dB (Crandell & Smaldino, 2000). The best way to compensate for that and improve the SNR is to use an FM unit.

Why Is an FM System Needed?

The alteration of a classroom or room design to make it less noisy is not enough to ensure good quality listening. Improvement of room acoustics is helpful; however, children with learning disabilities and auditory processing problems need a greater signal-to-noise level to ensure accurate hearing and acoustic design changes may not be sufficient to meet those needs. Furthermore, what may be needed in a classroom may not be financially feasible to a school district. Typically FM units have been individualized so that each child has his or her own unit, connected to the teacher's transmitter and microphone.

How Do You Know if a Child Needs an FM Unit ?

There are a few factors to consider when preselecting a child for a sound enhancement personal unit which include (ASHA, 1999):

1. The child's poor speech-in-noise discrimination (he or she asks what?; often mishears words spoken) and needs repetition.
2. The child's ability to wear and adjust to the unit. Many AD/HD children will fidget too much with the unit to make it useful.
3. The support available in the classroom or district to be sure that the unit is functioning properly and fitted appropriately.
4. The youngster's willingness to accept and wear it without feeling stigmatized.
5. The classroom teacher's willingness to wear the microphone and transmitter and knowledge about how to wear it and troubleshoot it, to be sure it is functioning. (The selection of appropriate settings should be decided upon by the audiologist as it doesn't have to be worn all the time. A time schedule can be devised for its use in the school day.)
6. The unit's compatibility with other aids or FM units in the classroom. Often the frequency has to be changed to match the frequency being transmitted by the teacher's microphone in the class.
7. Interferences from other external sources such as radio stations, computers, and pagers.

8. The cost of the unit should be taken into account. Often families may opt to purchase their own unit so that it can be used on weekends and during summer months while the child receives other support therapies.
9. The mandate from the school. As this is a technology device, it can be mandated by law to be put on the child's IEP or on a 504 and be covered by the school district.

Who Should Be Responsible for the FM Unit?

The audiologist by virtue of the scope of practice (ASHA, 2004, ASHA Preferred Practice Patterns for the Profession of Audiology, 1997; ASHA Guidelines, 1999) and by education, training, and experience is the appropriate person to be responsible for the fitting and maintenance of the unit(s). If the audiologist cannot provide daily monitoring, then another person should be designated. It is necessary that the audiologist provide monitoring, preferably daily, but other professionals can be trained to do checks.

Furthermore, the audiologist should make the selection based on appropriate speech recognition data, according to the child's developmental age and language skills; make sure that all controls on the FM are set for use and that it is working. The audiologist should instruct the teachers on its use and placement of the microphone, as proximity to the speaker's voice is critical to its efficacy. The audiologist should physically place the unit on the child and instruct the family and teacher on its use, and teach them how to check the battery and change or charge the unit. The FM microphone should be 6 to 8 inches from the talker's mouth leaving an overall level of speech at approximately 80 to 85 dB SPL. This would intensify the signal by 15 to 20 dB more than a traditional hearing aid.

Should the Audiologist Fit One Ear or Both Ears?

It is usually recommended that both ears be fitted with an FM so that there is adequate amplification of the signal, better speech discrimination in noise, and better sound localization. It also simulates normal hearing. Binaural stimulation has been proven to be important for optimum auditory development and recommended for learning disabled children (http://www.phonak.com). FM systems can also be an additional add-on unit in the form of a "boot" to a hearing aid. For those children with hearing loss, an FM may prove more helpful because of the favorable signal-to-noise level. Such devices are available from most hearing aid manufacturers and enhance the capability of the personal hearing aid.

The complexity of FM systems can be divided into its component parts, namely, its microphone and receiver, each with its own variation. For microphones, the input to the system, there are the lapel, lavaliere, boom, and conference types for the transmitter and ear-level or body-worn microphones. The microphone may be omnidirectional or directional. There may be more than one volume control wheel, depending on whether there are two microphones. The gain and frequency response should be based on the distance of 3 to 6 feet from the local microphone, over a wide frequency range.

The saturation sound pressure level should be high enough to provide an adequate dynamic range above the threshold of audibility but low enough to avoid discomfort from loud sounds. The input/output characteristics should be sufficient so that the talker distance variation of a few inches can be accommodated without loss of intelligibility and an increase in talker distance beyond 6 feet should be accommodated without further loss of intelligibility. There should be low acoustic feedback to permit gains without whistling.

For the receiver, there are individual headphones, behind-the-ear hearing units, speakers, and toteables.

Types of Personal Units

The personal FM unit contains a teacher-worn transmitter with three microphone options, and a student-worn receiver with four listening options. The personal unit is intended for one-to-one use from teacher to student to several individual students. The teacher clips or places the microphone 6 inches from her mouth and speaks normally. This will carry the teacher's voice to the child's ear directly without any wires. Thus, they are not connected, as one would be with a "hard wired system. See Figures 11–1, 11–2, and 11–3.

Phonak-Edu-Link (http://www.phonak.com)

Designed specifically for listeners with normal hearing acuity, this device is a miniaturized FM receiver that can be utilized with all Phonak transmitters. The child wears a small receiver which can be fit quickly by the audiologist. No mold or custom fitting is needed. The transmitter is small and portable so it can be used by the classroom teacher and travel with the child to other classes. It can be used in many settings such as art, music, and school assemblies, and does not have to be used in a formal class setting. The receiver is an open fitting—nonocclusive to the canal which allows the child to take

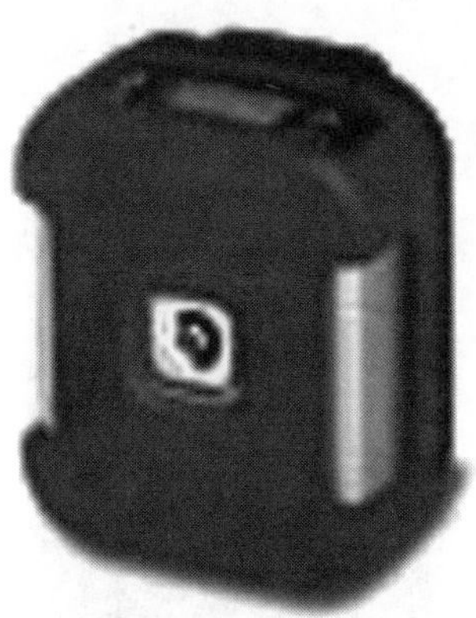

Figure 11–1. EduLink transmitter.

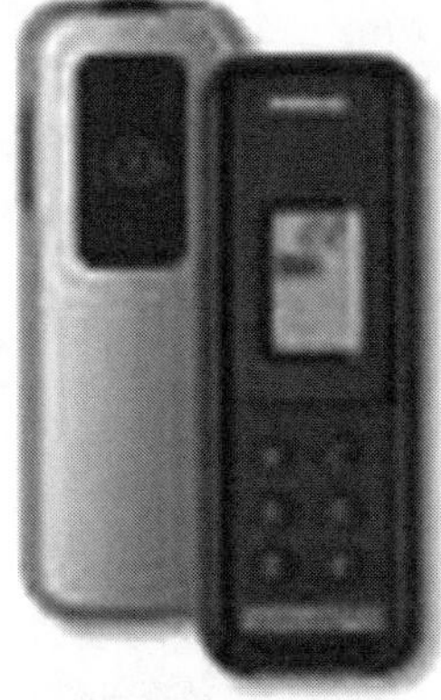

Figure 11–2. EduLink transmitter.

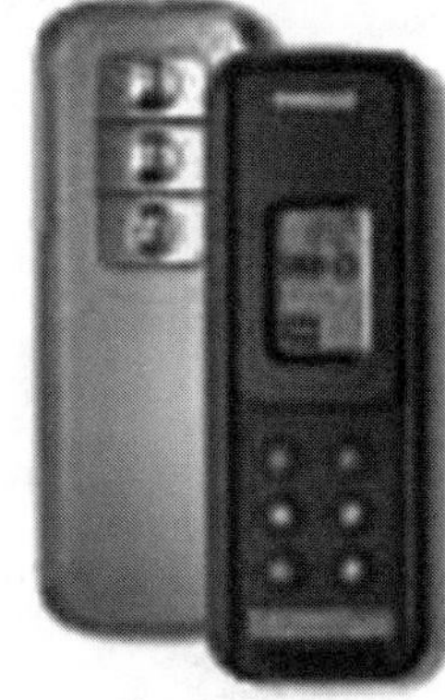

Figure 11–3. Edulink transmitter.

(Photos courtesy of Phonak Hearing Systems)

in the natural ambient sounds and feel part of the natural environment. It provides a favorable signal. A careful fitting process is necessary to determine its effectiveness and training in its use and care are important. A pre- and postassessment is useful to determine its efficacy. Some recommend using a Listening questionnaire to determine the child's or individual's personal benefits. "Although it is not a panacea for APD," claims the company, its use allows the student greater control over his or her listening environment and improves access to auditory information, an important component to learning (http://www.phonak.com). It provides students with a good signal-to-noise level, and speech clarity with little stigma attached. The unit is hardly visible and preferred by older students (Figure 11–4).

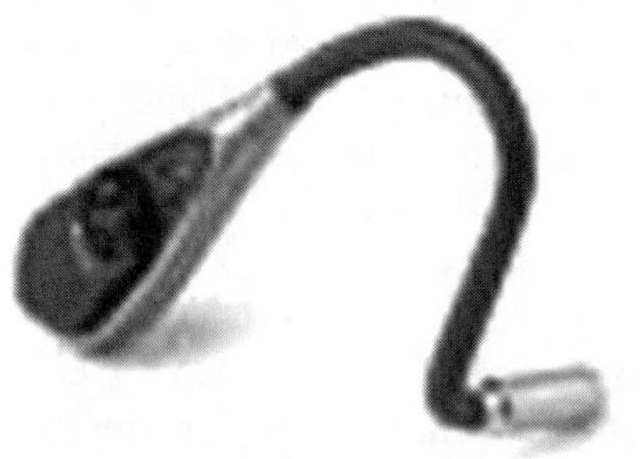

Figure 11–4. Receiver. (Courtesy of Phonak Hearing Systems)

For children with hearing loss who are aided, a "boot" can be attached to their hearing aid to serve as an FM receiver with direct audio input from the teacher's transmitter (Figures 11–5, 11–6, and 11–7).

Phonic Ear-Oticon EASY LISTENER (http://www.oticon.com)

The personal receivers provide amplification for mild hearing losses in the 10- to 40-dB range. The receiver may be used by a person with normal hearing, with an appropriate accessory. With on/off switch and a volume control, the instrument is easy to use and customized. A single-channel receiver has a large number of channels available that must be set at the manufacturer. Some units have switches in the back and can be changed by the user. For the Easy Listener, the receiver needs to be

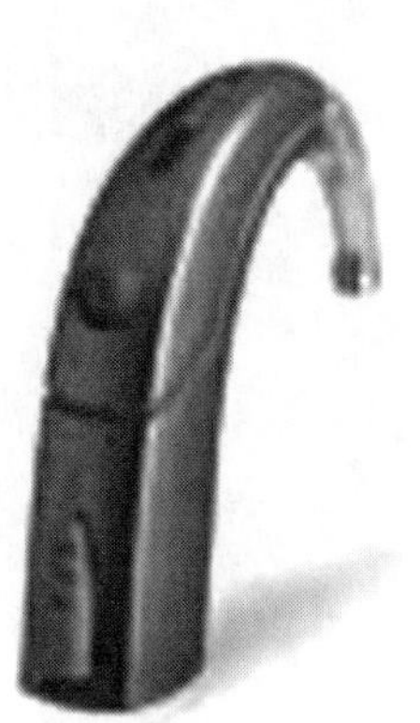

Figure 11–5. Receiver HA with boot.

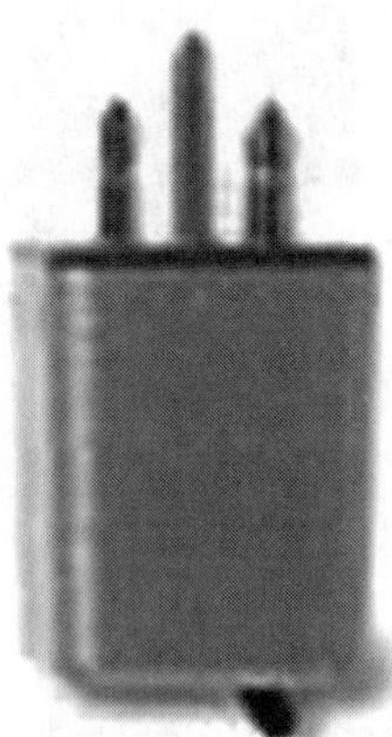

Figure 11–6. Boot attached to HA receiver.

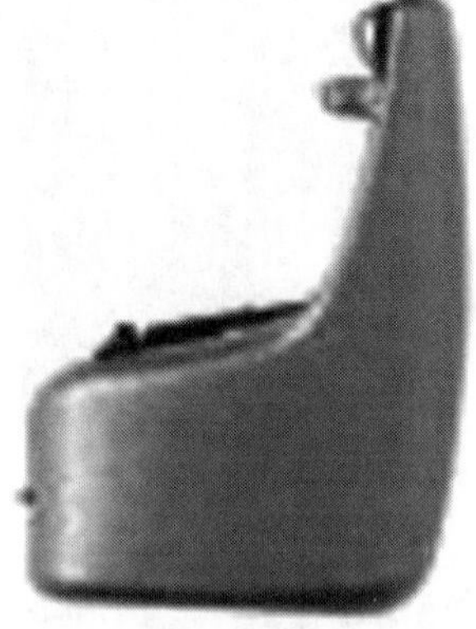

Figure 11–7. Boot.

(Photos courtesy of Phonak Hearing Systems)

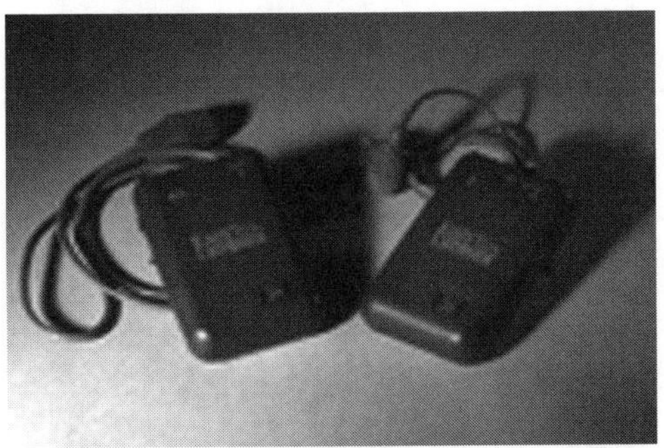

A.

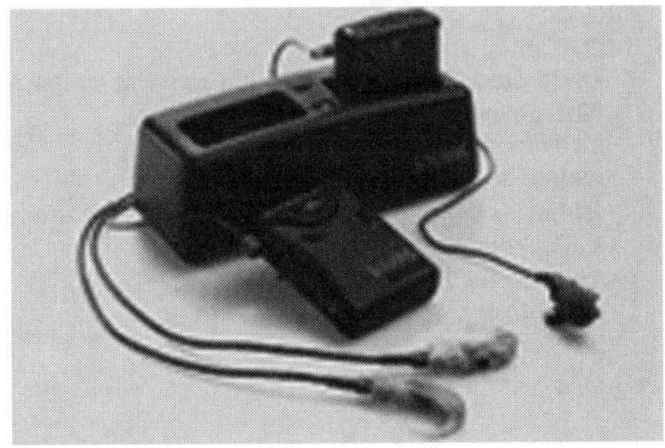

B.

Figure 11–8. **A.** Easy Listener Personal FM system. **B.** Solaris Personal FM System. (Photos courtesy of Phonic Ear, http://www.phonic ear.com)

set to the channel that matches the transmitter appropriately (Figure 11–8A).

Solaris (http://www.phonicear.com/ http://www.oticon.com)

The Solaris is a personal FM system that works with a hearing aid to enhance speech clarity and overcomes the effects of noise, distance, and echo. The FM transmitter and receiver which interface with hearing aids suppress background sounds whenever the teacher speaks. Different channels from class to class can be used to tune away from another person's frequency. It can supplement the performance of cochlear implants and hearing aids, or it can be used alone with headsets or earbuds (see Figure 11–8B).

Desktop Model—Toteable System (http://www.phonicear.com/ http://www.oticon.com)

There is the desktop model that presents the teacher's voice to the child through a speaker in a desktop lunchbox-like model that sits on the child's desk. The teacher wears a transmitter in the form of a lapel, lavaliere, or boom microphone. The child does not wear anything on his ears. The "lunchbox" can be placed on the teacher's desk, with the child seated proximal to it, if the child fidgets with the device (Figure 11–9).

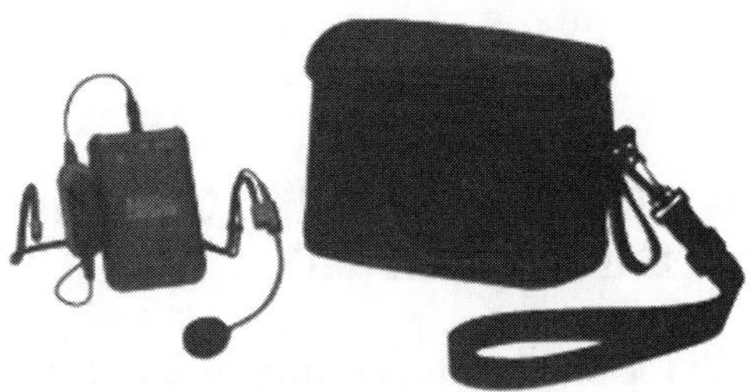

Figure 11–9. Toteable sound field system. (Photo courtesy of Phonic Ear, http://www.phonicear.com)

Light Speed Desktop Unit (http://www.lightspeed-tek.com)

This is used for children with (C)APD, ADD, mild hearing loss, cochlear implants, and English language learners to help students understand phonemes and soft consonants that the teacher pronounces. The LES 391 Sound Pak System has a dedicated frequency band, and reduces FM interference with a noise canceling microphone which eliminates feedback (Figure 11–10).

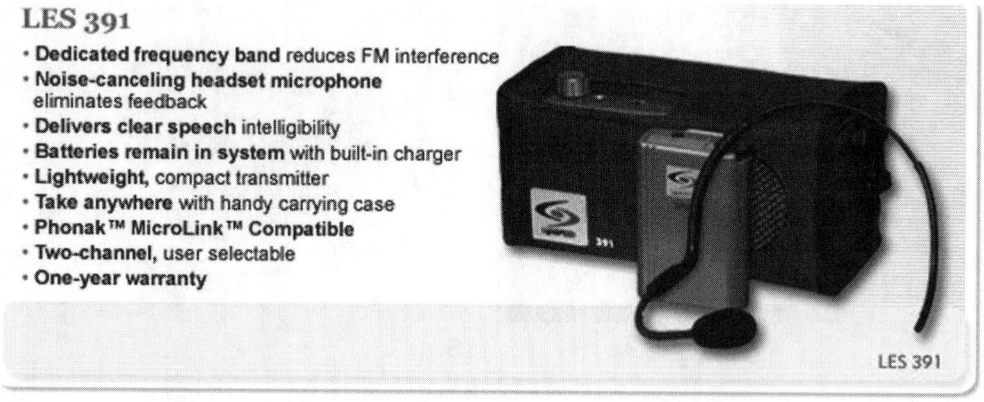

LES 391

- **Dedicated frequency band** reduces FM interference
- **Noise-canceling headset microphone** eliminates feedback
- **Delivers clear speech** intelligibility
- **Batteries remain in system** with built-in charger
- **Lightweight,** compact transmitter
- **Take anywhere** with handy carrying case
- **Phonak™ MicroLink™ Compatible**
- **Two-channel,** user selectable
- **One-year warranty**

LES 391

Figure 11–10. Desktop SoundPak (Photo courtesy of Lightspeed Technologies, http://www.lighspeed-tek.com).

Is a Desktop Model as Good as an Ear Level Model?

When an ear-level model is used, youngsters get a better speech perception performance, with an improvement in speech discrimination up to approximately 20% (Picard & LeFrancois, 1986). An improvement of 25% can be seen in word discrimination in nonreverberant classrooms. In addition, these devices help to foster increased attention and reduced dependency on note-taking (Anderson et al., 2003; Toe, 1999). There are other technology aids available to foster better listening and improve note-taking, such as the Kurzweil reading program (http://www.kurzweiledu.com).

Researchers have found that performance is better with devices that improve the signal-to-noise ratio within the critical listening distance than for sound field or infrared devices presenting the teacher's voice throughout the classroom (Nabelek & Donahue, 1986; Noe et al., 1997).

Efficacy of Personal FM Units

Children who wear the binaural BTE FM or body-worn FM systems are better at speech recognition (Crandell et al., 2005).

A study by Frederichs and Frederichs (2005) examined whether electrophysiologic and psychoacoustic auditory measures would reflect changes following use of a personal ear-level FM system in children with (C)APD. Ten children between the ages of 7 and 14 were provided with a personal ear-level FM system that was mainly used during school time for 1 year. The children underwent a comprehensive audiologic evaluation (pure-tone air and bone conduction threshold, tympanometry, and acoustic reflex, otoacoustic emissions) prior to the study and at 6 months and 1 year following the study. The data indicate that these children exhibited improved performance on tests of auditory function. The electrophysiologic late event–related potentials revealed significant changes in the functioning of the children using the FM system, suggesting an accelerated neuromaturational process when using the FM system. Parents and teachers reported a significant improvement in speech understanding and in overall school performance and conduct (Frederichs & Frederichs, 2005).

In a recent study of FM technology for individuals with multiple sclerosis, (Lewis et al., 2006) found that the use of FM systems had merit, given the prevalence of hearing difficulty in a population of MS patients (approximately 50% complains of hearing difficulty).

The subjects with MS had significantly more subjective complaints about their hearing than their matched-control subjects did. These complaints were correlated with reduced performance on the speech-perception in noise task. As it has been shown that frequency modulation (FM) systems can improve speech perception in noise for individuals with normal and sensorineural hearing loss in adverse conditions (Crandell & Smaldino, 1995), the utilization of the FM SNL system by children with (C)APD can result in an improvement in SNR (signal-to-noise ratio). It can achieve a 50% word recognition score with an increase by as much as 26.6 dB over the unaided listening condition (Phonak Hearing Systems, 2004). The population of MS patients was studied to determine if they would benefit. Lewis et al. (2006) attempted to evaluate whether the FM technology would have the same effect on speech perception in noise for adults with and without multiple sclerosis. All 10 subjects utilized the Phonic Ear Easy Listener FM system, designed for individuals with normal hearing to moderate degrees of hearing loss. Results indicated that at different signal-to-noise ratios there was a significant difference in speech perception in noise for the MS subjects between the unaided and aided condition with the FM system. On average, subjects obtained a 38% improvement in the number of key words correct at difficult signal-to-noise ratios. An average improvement of 3.5 SNR was obtained in speech perception. This finding is consistent with other previous studies indicating that FM systems can improve the SNR needed for 50% word recognition (Lewis et al., 2004). As the results obtained for both the MS subjects and those without MS were positive, it was postulated that the improvements may be the result of having the remote microphone located near the speaker's mouth, where the effects of reverberation, distance, and noise are minimal.

Sound Field Amplification

With the use of a microphone at the teacher's voice and the use of a receiver in the classroom in the form of a speaker, the person's voice can be projected over the drone of noise. Sound-field amplification improves the signal-to-noise ratio in the classroom. Where the speaker is placed in the classroom can make the difference.

The benefits of sound field amplification are not new to the literature. The first study to show its benefits was the MARRS Project, Mainstream Amplification Resource Room Project in 1978, (ASHA, 2005a). This was a 15-year project to describe the benefits of sound-field amplification for children with normal hearing and mild hearing loss. Greater academic achievement was seen at a faster rate for all children at a tenth of the cost of instruction in the amplified classroom than in the unamplified classroom. Other researchers found improvement in word recognition, and sentence recognition (Crandell & Bess, 1986). Students benefiting included those with developmental disabilities, non-native English speaking students, and those with hearing loss (Crandell & Smaldino, 1996). Furthermore, sound-field amplification can improve the problems of speaker distance in the classroom and speech degradation. What it cannot improve are the effects of sound reverberation beyond the 0.6 seconds limit. For that there are acoustic engineers, and materials such as acoustic tiles that can be installed with double-faced tape or hook and loop fasteners. These new, more flexible tiles are manufactured from recycled cotton and comply with building code standards for fire safety and carry an ASTM E-84 Class A certification. A suspended ceiling is not assurance enough that it will be acoustically effective. If there are hard walls, or tile floors, the reverberation time may be a problem. Carpeting may help, although not in a significant way, it provides protection against floor generated noise by students in the occupied room. Placing acoustical treatment on walls and furniture may be sufficient (Nixon, 2002).

Types of Sound Field Listening Enhancement Systems

Phonic Ear Front Row to Go for Active Learning (http://www.phonicear.com/ http://www.oticon.com)

Formally known as The Radium, this system's dispersion pattern is elliptical thereby reducing reverberation from the ceiling and floor. The teacher wears a transmitter, either a lavaliere or handheld microphone and the speaker/receiver is placed at the front of the room. The entire room is amplified (see Figure 11–11).

Light Speed Listening Enhancement Systems (http://www.lightspeed-tek.com)

This is used for children with APD, ADD, mild hearing loss, cochlear implants, and English language learners to help students understand phonemes and soft consonants that the teacher pronounces. The Redcat is an all in one system with integrated amplifier, speaker, receiver, and infrared sensors (see Figure 11–12).

Infrared System (http://www.phonicear.com/ http://www.oticon.com)

This newer system provides clearer signals, reduces interference, and covers from 4,000 to 12,000 sq. ft. The trans-

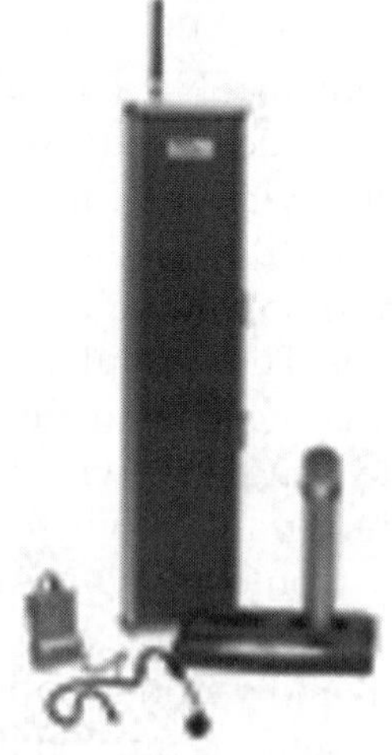

Figure 11–11. Front Row to Go. (Photo courtesy of Phonic Ear, http://www.phonicear.com)

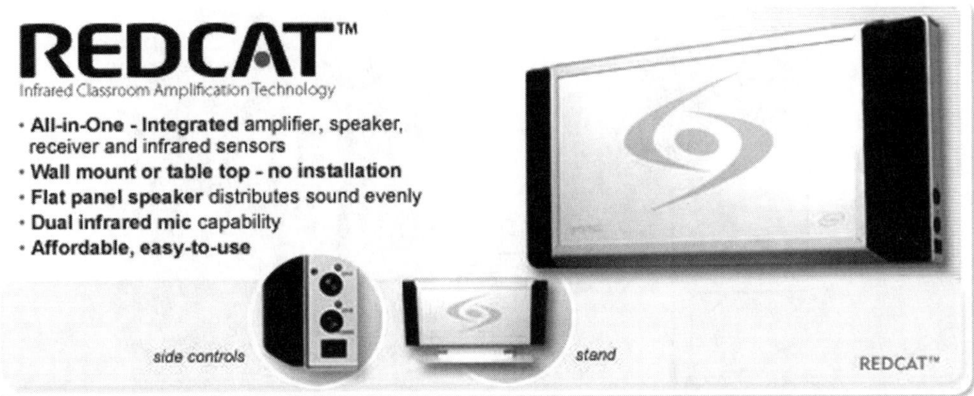

Figure 11–12. Infrared Classroom Amplification Technology. (Courtesy of Lightspeed, http://www. lightspeed-tek.com)

mitter is a light signal (infrared light) which transposes sound into a light energy and transmits it to a receiver that receives the light signal and converts it into sound energy. It is used in theaters, multiplex facilities, and in dark places. If there is any interference with the light beam, the signal will not be received. If one rubs one's hand over the light beam it will obviate the signal. It does not penetrate through walls. It can be a body-worn system, and offers a selection of receiving options, such as: stetoclip, monaural earbuds, binaural earbuds, standard headset, and teleloop. The Star Sound 400 Infrared Enhancement System is seen in Figure 11–13.

Infrared System, Califone (http://www.califone.com)

This system is used in a classroom and provides sound-field amplification without interference between classrooms. Using two ceiling mounted infrared receivers with mini-internal sensors for improved reception and increased coverage in larger classrooms, and a powerful belt-pack transmitter with lapel microphone, enables transmission in a 40-foot range. Sound is evenly distributed at the front and rear of the room (Figure 11–14).

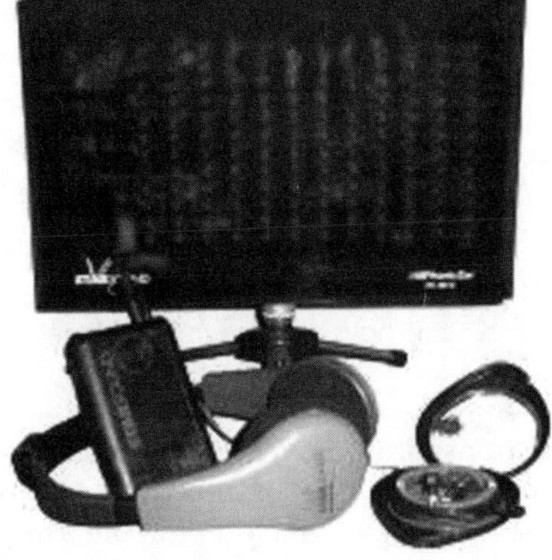

Figure 11–13. StarSound 400 Infrared Hearing Enhancement System. (Photo courtesy of Phonic Ear, http://www.phonicear.com)

AudiSee-AudiSoft (http://www.audisoft.net)

This is a wireless system that transmits the image of the teacher to a small screen on the student's desk. The audio

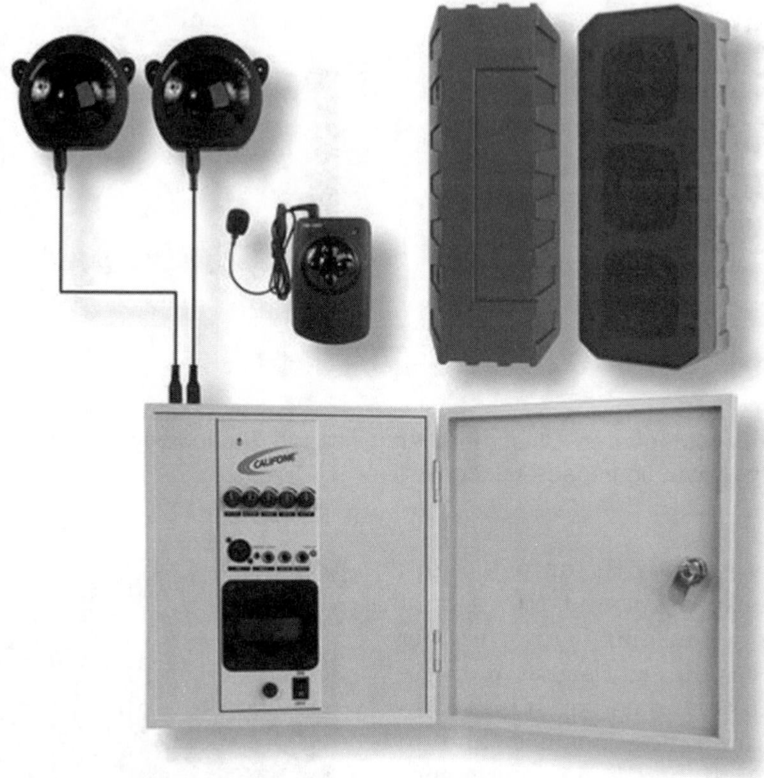

Figure 11–14. Classroom Infrared System, Model P`20-IRSSYS. (Photo courtesy of Califone, http://www.califone.com)

is transmitted either to the student's current FM system or directly to a hearing aid. It is meant for hearing-impaired children to take advantage of both auditory and visual cues of the speaker. It is an assistive listening device that provides students with a hearing loss the opportunity to access the entire message, by combining hearing capabilities with visual cues (Gagne, 2001) (Figures 11–15A and 11–15B).

HearIt-3 Step Phonologic Amplification Tool (http://www.hearitllc.com)

This system was developed for students with language/learning disabilities, articulation difficulties, AD/HD, autism, CAPD, CP, Down syndrome, language fluency, otitis media, and hearing loss. This durable acoustic device was engineered to minimize acoustic distortion and feedback on higher volume settings. It has amplified speech-range frequencies to "pluck-out" speech from noise and sustain attention. Hearit SE with enhanced speech "banana frequencies" and built-in directional microphone and noise cancellation system, is specifically designed for the distractible student. It can help improve attention and content mastery.

The clinician can work with one to four students each wearing a receiver headset. The amplified speech frequencies help students identify speech cues for improved phonological awareness.

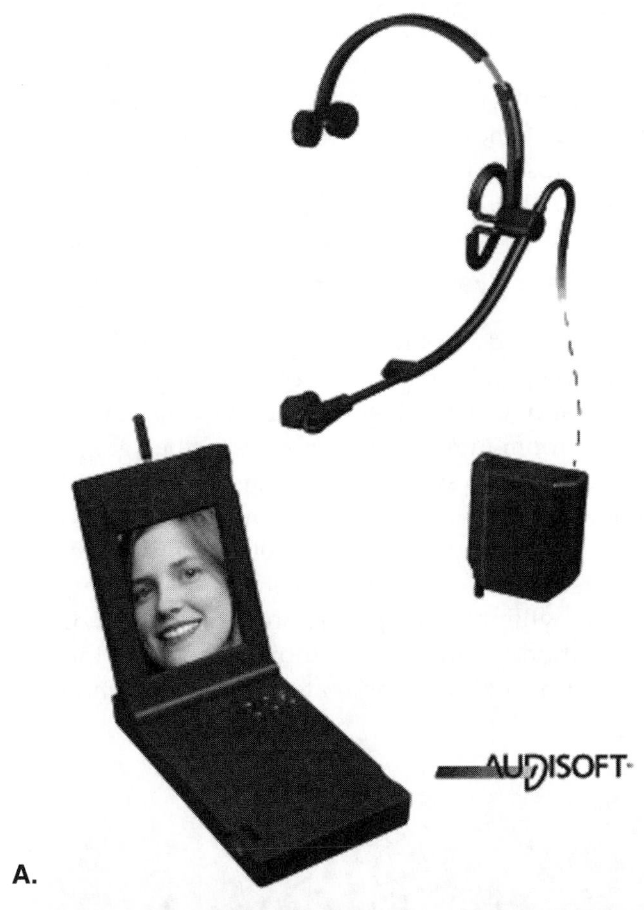

A.

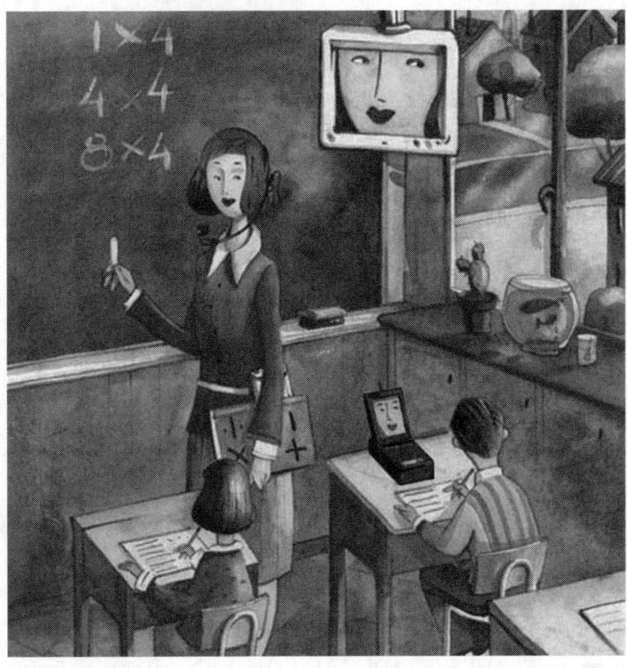

B.

Figure 11–15. The Audisee by AudiSoft Technologies. **A.** Details. (Courtesy of AudiSoft Technologies. http://www.audisoft.net) **B.** Use in the classroom.

Its automatic gain control protects listeners from damage due to noise. It can be used in small groups and a classroom as well (Figure 11–16).

Efficacy of Sound-Field Systems

The advantage to sound-field amplification is that students accept it better. As they learn about it and use it, they report improved classroom interaction and participation. Sound-field systems can be used to enhance other instructional equipment, such as televisions, cassette tape recorders, and compact disk players. Parents willingly accept sound field amplification (Crandell et al., 2005). Crandell et al. (2005) upon studying its efficacy found that the sample of subjects tested had improved eye contact, attending skills, reduced figure-ground listening difficulties, reduced listener fatigue, and reduced teacher's stress and vocal strain.

Allen and Patton, (1990) reported decreased distractibility and increased on-task behaviors (17%) with sound-field systems in first and second-graders. Other gains reported include improved eye contact, attending skills, improved speech perception, and reduction of listener fatigue. Preschoolers with severe language impairment showed an increase in attending behaviors and improvements in the use of appropriate comments (Benafield, 1990).

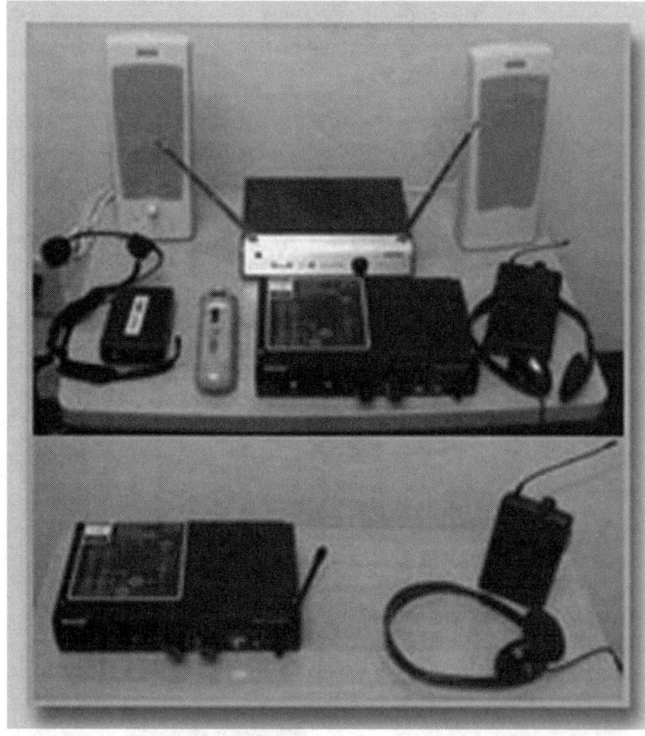

Figure 11–16. Personal Listening System by Hearit (Model 551PLS/551PLSA). (Photo Courtesy of Hearit, http://www.hearitlc.com)

Higher SIFTER scores were computed for at-risk and no-risk students in amplified classes, and lower scores were reported for at-risk students in unamplified classes (Flexer, Richards, & Buie, 1993).

Higher scores were obtained by students in amplified classes for listening, academic/preacademic behaviors, and academic/preacademic skills (Rosenberg et al., 1999). Improvements were noted in speech intelligibility scores for students with hearing loss and students with normal hearing with sound-field amplification (Eriks-Brophy & Ayukawa, 2000). Attention to task improved and clients demonstrated greater gains in achieving therapy outcomes during therapy sessions (ASHA, 2005a).

Overall, findings support the use of sound-enhancement systems for children with normal hearing, children with hearing loss or listening problems, as well as for children who are non-native English speakers. Even in classrooms that meet the acoustical standards, these systems provide advantages.

In support of these findings, there are school systems that are adding sound-field amplification systems in preconstruction plans in the building of the school. Others are putting them into already constructed classrooms. Amplification systems are moving into the mainstream and are no longer reserved for special education classrooms. There are approximately 160,000 classrooms in the United States that have sound-field systems and that number grows by 20% each year, according to manufacturer's estimates (Boswell, 2006).

Given the knowledge that children's auditory systems are not mature until they reach 13 to 15 years of age, and younger children need a quieter setting for learning the sounds of the language, particularly as it relates to reading skills, there is no question as to the benefit such a classroom enhancement can provide. Results of performance on national tests indicated improved scores. Reports show that scores for children in the first grade on a reading test began at or above grade level in September (59%), for a school district in West Orange, New Jersey. By May of that year, 89% were at or above grade level. Most of the children improved in their reading scores. In reality the cost to the school was only 3% more to install a sound-enhancement system than to fit one child with an amplification system. Thus, in an urban community with noise surrounding the building and many children crowded into one classroom, it serves the school well to have a sound enhancement system. Informal data gathered for a lead article for the *ASHA Leader* (Boswell, 2006) revealed benefits also to teachers including less vocal fatigue, throat infections, and overall stress. One hundred percent of the teachers wanted to keep the device.

Public Law

The Public Law, originally known as PL94-142 and now called IDEA, is responsible for state funding that reaches the district. In the law, all children are entitled to an assessment and an education in a free and appropriate public school setting. The education is to take place in the least restrictive setting. Placing the child with disabilities with other children who are not disabled has become known as a mainstream environment. Children who have been designated as having a disability, or who are in need of accommodations, supplementary aids, and services in their educational plan, can be entitled to technology and assistive devices. Such devices can be put on the child's IEP—Individualized Educational Plan. Children with hearing loss are protected by the law for counseling, identification, habilitative services, and need for amplification. Children with all degrees of hearing impairment, permanent or fluctuating, are entitled to audiology rehabilitative services to support their educational performance, if their performance has been negatively affected by their impairment.

The Technology-Related Assistance Act of 1994 for IDEA Amendments provides access to assistive technology services and devices for individuals with disabilities of all ages. Assistive technology and services may be needed to assist that child to obtain a free and appropriate education in the least restrictive setting. Sound field units can be seen as improving the environment for the youngsters with auditory disabilities. With the later law— No Child Left Behind (2001) (NCLB), provision was made to provide access to, or inclusion in, the instruction of the general classroom. General education classrooms need to be equipped with sound-field amplification. Thus, sound-field technology has a place in the law and provides the necessary materials to help the child succeed in the classroom.

504 Accommodations

This is a federal civil rights act that prohibits recipients of federal funds (agencies) from discrimination against qualified individuals with disabilities in the United States. A recipient of federal funds that operates a public elementary or secondary education program shall provide a free appropriate public education (FAPE) to each qualified person with a disability who is in that jurisdiction regardless of the nature and severity of the person's disability (Flexer, 2005). Section 504 can outline access support with accommodations for the individual in need. It may be necessary to apply for a Section 504 accommodation when the child is classifiable to obtain the assistive listening device needed. However, some districts do not yet recognize the use of FM for non-hearing-impaired children.

Summary

This chapter addressed the various approaches to managing a (central) auditory processing disorder. For one, compensatory strategies can be taught to allow the individual to obtain the clarity by requesting repetition, reclarification and positioning oneself in the best place to take advantage of the signal. Furthermore, there are changes one can make to improve the listening environment by reducing noise and distractions and by using sound-absorbent materials. Environmental modifications were discussed for the classroom, home, and workplace. Such changes can allow the person with (C)APD to understand and process the auditory message. Furthermore, even in the face of modified environments, there are assistive listening devices that make the listening environment more favorable for individuals with (C)APD. A particular challenge is listening in a background of noise which can be ameliorated by the use of FM systems. The value of individual personal versus classroom amplification was discussed with support for personal units as they provide improved speech recognition. Their advantages and disadvantages, with recommendations for fitting different types of FM units including classroom, toteable, and ear-level models were discussed. A description of different FM units along with efficacy data support their use in both personal, classroom, and social situations. There is evidence to suspect that as one becomes a better listener through the use of assistive listening devices, there are concomitant measurable neuromaturational changes that occur to support their use. The federal educational laws and regulations protecting disabled individuals make the implementation of assistive devices more viable and accessible.

Key Points Learned

- Children spend at least 45% of their school day listening.
- All children need favorable listening conditions in the classroom with a favorable signal-to-noise ratio of +15 dB.
- To manage the child with (C)APD, environmental alternations are needed to reduce noise, limit distractions, and provide acoustic insulation.
- There are advantages to an ear level unit in that it is more direct. The FM microphone should be 6 to 8 inches from the talker's mouth leaving an overall level of speech at approximately 80 to 85 dB SPL.
- There are allowable noise levels established by ANSI (S12.60-2002) for the unoccupied classroom (35 dBA) with a recommended signal-to-noise ratio of +15 and a reverberation limit of 0.06 in a typical classroom.
- Personal FM units can increase the speech signal by as much as 12 to 15 dB, making the message easier to process. It serves to improve speech recognition, attention, and ability to receive the spoken message.
- Sound-enhancement systems provide enhanced signal-to-noise ratios in a classroom via speakers or infrared receivers, reducing the level of background noise for all children in the room.
- Research supports the efficacy of using sound-enhancement devices to improve sound/speech reception
- Federal Education law protects individuals with disabilities by providing them with access to a free and appropriate education in the least restrictive environment (FAPE), thus making the use of assistive devices a viable alternative for those with hearing and auditory processing disorders.

References

Allen, L., & Patton, D. (1990). *Effects of sound-field amplification on students' on-task behavior.* Paper presented at the American Speech, Language and Hearing Convention, Seattle, WA.

American National Standards Institute. (2002). *Acoustical performance criteria design requirements and guidelines for schools.* ANSI S12.60. New York: ANSI.

American Speech-Language Hearing Association. (1997, March). *Preferred practice patterns for the profession of audiology.* Rockville, MD: Author.

American Speech-Language Hearing Association. (1999). *Guidelines for fitting and monitoring FM systems.* Rockville, MD: Author.

American Speech-Language Hearing Association. (2004). Scope of practice in audiology. *ASHA, 38*(Suppl. 16), 12–15.

American Speech-Language Hearing Association. (2005a). *Guidelines for addressing acoustics in educational setting.* Rockville: MD: Author.

American Speech-Language Hearing Association. (2005b). *Acoustics in educational settings: Position statement.* Rockville, MD: Author.

Anderson, K. A., Colodzin, H, G., Iglehart, F., & Goldstein, H. (2003). *Benefit of personal FM, desktop FM, and infrared sound field devices to speech perception of children with hearing aids or cochlear implants.* Unpublished manuscript.

Benafield, N. (1990). *The effects of sound field amplification on the attending behaviors of speech and language-delayed preschool children.* Unpublished master's thesis. University of Arkansas at Little Rock.

Berg, F. S. (1987). *Facilitating classroom listening: Handbook for teacher of normal hearing students.* Boston: College-Hill Press/Little, Brown.

Boswell, S. (2006). Sound field systems on the rise in school: Improved test scores cited as benefit. *ASHA Leader, 11*(7), 1, 32–33.

Crandell, C., & Bess, F. (1986, November). Speech recognition of children in a "typical" classroom setting. *ASHA, 29,* 87.

Crandell, C., Flexer, C., & Smaldino, J. J. (2005). *Sound field amplification: Applications to speech perception and classroom acoustics* (2nd ed.). Clifton Park, NY: Thomson Delmar Learning.

Crandell, C., & Smaldino, J. (1995). An update of classroom acoustics for children with hearing impairment. *Volta Reviews, 1,* 4-12.

Crandell, C., & Smaldino, J. (1996). Speech perception in noise by children for whom English is a second language. *American Journal of Audiology, 5*(3), 47–51.

Crandell, C., & Smaldino, J. (2000). Room acoustics for listeners with normal-hearing and hearing impairments. In M. Valente, H. Hosford-Dunn, & R. Roeser (Eds.) *Auditory treatment* (pp. 601–623). New York: Thieme Medical Publishers.

Eriks-Brophy, A. & Ayukawa, H. (2000). The benefits of sound field amplification in classroom of Inuit students of Nunavik: A pilot project. *Language, Speech, and Hearing Services in Schools,* 3(4), 324–335.

Flexer, C. (2005). Laws and regulations that govern the utilization of sound field amplification. In C. C. Crandell, J. J. Smaldino, & C. Flexer, *Sound field amplification: Applications to speech perception and classroom acoustics* (2nd ed.). Clifton Park, NY: Thomson Delmar Learning.

Flexer, C., Richards, C., & Buie, C. (1993, April). *Sound field amplification for regular kindergarten and first grade classrooms: A longitudinal study of fluctuating hearing loss and pupil performance.* Paper presented at the American Academy of Audiology Convention, Phoenix, AZ.

Frederichs, E., & Frederichs, P. (2005). Electrophysiologic and psycho-acoustic findings following one ear application of a personal ear lever FM device in children with attention deficit and suspected central auditory processing disorder. *Journal of Educational Audiology*, *12*, 19–34.

Gagne, J. P. (2001). Audiovisual-FM system is found more beneficial in classroom than auditory only. *The Hearing Journal*, *54*(1), 48–51.

Lewis, M. S., Crandell, C., Valente, M., & Horn, J. (2004). Speech perception in noise: Directional microphones versus frequency modulation (FM) systems. *Journal of the American Academy of Audiology*, *15*(6), 424–437.

Lewis, M. S., Hutter, M., Lilly, D. J., Bourdette, D., Saunders, J., & Fausti, S. (2006). Frequency-modulation (FM) technology as a method for improving speech perception in noise for individuals with multiple sclerosis. *Journal of the American Academy of Audiology*, *17*(8), 605–616.

Nabalek, A. K., & Donahue, A. M. (1986). Comparison of amplification systems in an auditorium. *Journal of the Acoustical Society of America*, *79*, 2078–2082.

Nixon, M. (2002, May/June). Assessing the acoustics in your child's classroom: A guide for parents. *Hearing Loss: The Journal of Self-Help for Hearing Impaired People*, 15–19. Available from: http://www.hdhearing.com/Learning/

No Child Left Behind Act. (2001). Education. Intergovernmental Relations. 20 USC 6301 *et seq.* note.

Noe, C. M., Davidson, S. A., & Mishler, P. J. (1997). The use of large group assistive listening devices with and without hearing aids in an adult classroom setting. *American Journal of Audiology*, *6*, 48–64.

Picard, M., & LaFrancois, J. (1986). Speech perception through FM auditory trainer in noise and reverberation. *Journal of Rehabilitation Research and Development*, *23*(1), 53–62.

Rosenberg, G. G., Blake-Rahter, P., Heavner, J., Allen, I., Redmond, B. M., Phillips, J., & Stigers, K. (1999). Improving classroom acoustics (ICA): A three year FM sound field classroom amplification study. *Journal of Educational Audiology*, *7*, 8–28.

Stach. B. A. (2003). *Comprehensive dictionary of audiology: Illustrated*. Clifton Park, NY: Thomson Delmar Learning.

Toe, D. (1999). Impact of FM aid use on the classroom behavior of profoundly deaf secondary students. *Seminars in Hearing*, *20*(3), 223–235.

Resources

AudiSoft Technologies—http://audisoft.net

Califone—Classroom Infrared System—http://www.califone.com

Hearit—3 Step Phonologic Amplification Tool—http://www.hearitllc.com

Kurzweil—www.kurzweiledu.com

Light Speed Listening Enhancement Systems—http://www.lightspeed-tek.com

Oticon People First—http://www.oticon.com

Phonak Hearing Systems—http://www.phonak.com

Phonic Ear, Inc.—http://www.phonicear.com

12

Parenting the Child with Auditory Processing Disorders

A Dynamic and Challenging Role

Dorothy A. Kelly

Overview

This chapter emphasizes the perspective of the parent, addressing both emotional and practical concerns specific to raising a child with auditory processing disorder. It recognizes that an involved, informed, and respected parent becomes a more effective member of the educational and clinical intervention management team.

The information that follows helps prepare parents for their role as team members, communication facilitators, organization strategists, and managers of their children's socioemotional growth. It provides strategies for functional outcomes in the home, while recognizing the enormity of a challenging task.

The chapter is divided into six major sections. These address: Parents as team members: understanding the basics and understanding the legal terrain; parents as managers: communication facilitators and organization strategists; parents as facilitators of socioemotional growth; parents and children having fun; looking ahead: children with APD become adults; and resources.

Introduction

Harvard Medical School recently implemented a program designed to encourage empathy for patients in their medical students. Following the lead of an earlier program at the University of Pennsylvania (1997), administrators realized that empathy is a valuable clinical tool, resulting in mutual respect and partnership between patient and physician (Thornburgh, 2006). Treating the whole individual, rather than a series of symptoms, adds humanity to an often difficult process.

Speech-language pathologists and audiologists have long recognized the importance of such notions. However, even the most well-intentioned, involved clinician may need a reminder occasionally. Living with a disorder (as patient or caretaker) is always more difficult than treating it. Furthermore, parenting a child with a disorder carries its own set of unique concerns and challenges.

Among other challenges, parents must come to terms with the realities of their child's diagnosis. This troubling information is often received after an exhaustive and frustrating search. Even when the diagnosis of auditory processing disorder (APD) has been made, a sense of relief is usually accompanied by feelings of loss, grief, and guilt (Bellis, 2002). Anger, denial, and depression may follow. Left unaddressed, such feelings can be destructive to both parent and child.

Parents as Team Members

From the clinician's perspective, auditory processing disorder (APD) describes the functional impairment of the auditory nervous system, negatively impacting skills such as auditory discrimination, sound localization, and auditory integration (Ferre, 2002a). In addition, APD frequently affects language and language-dependent behaviors such as reading, spelling, and writing. This description is abstract and impersonal, failing to capture the impact of a complex disorder on the lives of children and their families.

From the parent's perspective, auditory processing disorder makes home and school life challenging. The child with APD experiences a myriad of social, emotional, academic, language, and communication deficits, affecting virtually every aspect of his or her life.

The following list of possible symptoms offers situational context from a parent's perspective:

> The child may not follow directions *. . . homework is misunderstood, buses are missed;*
>
> The child demonstrates impulse and behavioral problems . . . *an increase in risk-taking behaviors requiring greater parent vigilance, a greater number sibling arguments;*
>
> The child daydreams excessively *. . . chores aren't completed, homework becomes laborious;*
>
> The child has academic and/or speech-language problems . . . *child hates to go to school, comprehension of conversations may be difficult, self-esteem is low;*
>
> The child has poor long-and short-term memory difficulties . . . *child may not learn from past mistakes, studying for tests is difficult, ability to follow directions is uneven;* (Richard, 2001);

The child has poor peer relations . . . *the child is socially rejected, lonely;*

The child is easily distracted . . . *the typical home environment is fraught with distractions (e.g., competing conversations, phones ringing, video games, etc.), attention has to be continually redirected; tasks take much longer to complete;*

The child has difficulty with background noise . . . *households are filled with challenging ambient noises (aperiodic, low predictability), excursions to family restaurants and playgrounds can be problematic;*

The child gives slow or delayed responses . . . *it may be difficult to wait for a response during high activity times (e.g., getting ready for school), other children may interpret auditory latency as a sign of low intelligence;*

The child has problems interpreting other's emotions . . . *the child may appear not to care about the feelings of others, others may identify him or her as "weird," the child appears confused in social situations* (Keller, 1998);

The child has problems remembering names and places heard, gives inappropriate responses to age-appropriate questions . . . *others may interpret this as evidence of low intelligence, poor effort, or inattention* (Gillet, 1993);

The child often has a history of ear infections . . . .*some of these infections may involve temporary hearing loss which complicates auditory responses even more, child may be absent from school making it more difficult to keep up academically, child-care issues for working parents may become more challenging* (Fisher, 1976);

The child demonstrates unusual expressions or body postures while listening . . . *other children may consider the child odd; child becomes self-conscious and avoids social interactions;*

The child tends to use the same words or phrases over and over instead of responding appropriately to changing verbal information . . . *the child can't maintain conversations or respond to teacher's questions in class resulting in withdrawn behavior and poor self-esteem, child may becomes frustrated and act out;*

The child seems confused about where sounds are coming from and has trouble locating them quickly . . . *the parent can never relax when the child is playing outside, simple activities such as crossing the street with the child become stressful, child may feel smothered or overprotected* (http://www.firn.edu/doe/commhome/pdf/y2001-9.pdf)

It is apparent that auditory processing/language processing deficits can negatively impact home activities, resulting in stress and frustration for the child and family members. In addition, the child with APD often commands more of the parent's attention, perhaps leaving siblings feeling neglected or resentful.

Parenting a child with a disorder is different today than in the past. Contemporary parents enjoy unprecedented access to information about their child's mental, emotional, social, and learning needs. Answers to troubling concerns (*Is my child like other children his or her age? If there is a problem, what can be done?*) can be obtained through media and electronic options unavailable to earlier generations.

Because of the Internet and other electronic innovations, parents interact with one another in a highly effective manner. For example, listservs (hosted by computer programs of the same name) are often dedicated to a specific disorder (such as APD). One such dedicated listserv is http://AuditoryProcessing@yahoogroups.com. These interactive chats allow parents to vent frustrations or share cutting-edge information (Kuster, 2006). Blogs (electronic opinion venting) offer another communication option for parents with concerns about education, therapy, or other child-related issues.

Podcasting (a type of radio on demand) is an evolving electronic communication option for parents and professionals. Subscribers can access a podcast on the Web at their convenience with free software (e.g., iTunes and Juice) or through use of any MP3 player, such as the iPod from Apple Computers (Banotai, 2006b). Podcasts about language, attention deficit hyperactivity disorder, disability concerns, health politics, and clinical neurology are currently available, with new additions appearing regularly.

Professional organizations such as The American Speech-Language-Hearing Association (ASHA), The American Audiological Association, and The American Academy of Audiology (AAA) offer parent-friendly/consumer information on their Web sites. Here parents can directly access information, as well as follow links to related internet sites. A list of parent-friendly sites may be found in Resources near the end of the chapter.

In some cases, media and electronic innovations have altered the dynamic between school and home. The school is no longer the exclusive source of educational and clinical information. Now, it is sometimes the informed parent who drives the search for more appropriate assessment and programming for a child's complicated learning profile. Children and Adults with Attention-Deficit/Hyperactivity Disorder (CHADD/http://www.chadd.org) is an organization founded by parents seeking information about the educational needs of children with ADHD. Founders realized that organized, prepared parents could share information and positively impact school programming. The National Coalition on Auditory Processing Disorders (http://www.ncapd.org) is an example of a parent-driven Web site designed to increase awareness about APD.

Some information available on the Internet can be misleading. Without educational or clinical context, it is possible for a parent (or professional) to misinterpret information. With only a piece of the diagnostic puzzle, it is easy to miss the big picture. For example, although a child with a comorbid diagnosis (e.g. APD, learning disabilities, and attention deficit hyperactivity disorder) demonstrates auditory processing disorder, it may not be *the* diagnosis (i.e., *the answer*). That is, this child may not respond to educational or therapeutic programs designed for only one specific diagnosis (e.g., programs for APD or learning disabilities). As children with APD often present symptoms on a secondary diagnostic level, this is of particular interest. For example, a significant proportion of individuals with learning disabilities

(LDs) (approximately one-third) demonstrate auditory processing deficits, as well (Medwetsky, 2006).

In addition, not all Internet sources provide legitimate (objectively researched and reviewed) information. For example, a well-meaning parent may discover an advertised therapy program for children with auditory processing disorder. This parent may not realize that no single program suits *all* children with APD. In fact, it may be argued that misapplication of programs can be counterproductive. In general, time spent on misguided programs is time lost. Although it is not appropriate here to comment on particular programs, the parent is well advised to discuss all clinical or educational programs with team members.

Parents are important to the programming and intervention process in the school. As their child's principal advocate, they know what motivates positive behaviors (what works and what does not). Sometimes a parent can advocate for a small change in setting or learning style that can significantly improve their child's behavior in school. For example, allowing an inattentive child to get out of his or her seat (occasionally) without punishment may increase attention markedly (Honos-Webb, 2006).

To become the most effective advocate, Pierangelo and Jacoby (1996) make recommendations for parents when dealing with the school team:

View yourself as an equal member of the intervention team;

Know your rights and activate them when needed;

Keep copies of all records;

Resolve problems as early as possible and be willing to file a complaint if needed;

Ask professionals why particular services are recommended; and

Be involved in every step of program planning and implementation (adapted for present purposes).

Knowledgeable parents realize that auditory processing disorder must often be *managed*, rather than *remediated*. Effective intervention necessitates a comprehensive, cooperative approach including direct intervention, environmental modifications, and compensatory strategies (Ferre, 2002b). As the child with APD spends the vast majority of his or her life outside the therapy setting, parents become the principal home management strategists.

Although parents may need to apply strategies at home that complement therapy programs (Ferre, 2002b), their principal role is parent, not teacher or therapist. Children with APD need escape from the demands of school life. It may be possible to weave constructive auditory and language learning experiences into everyday life without the necessity of structured practice. The section on Parents and Children Having Fun gives suggestions for informal, naturalistic learning activities.

Understanding the Basics

The informed parent understands basic concepts about auditory processing and auditory processing disorder. Specifically, parents know that auditory processing involves the recognition and interpretation of auditory stimuli—the ability to hold, sequence, and process accurately what is heard (Rowe, Rowe, & Pollard, 2004). APD suggests that something adversely affects the processing or interpretation of the information. Succinctly, APD is a problem with processing of information somewhere in the auditory system (Jerger & Musiek, 2004). Informed parents know that the development of auditory processing skills parallel language abilities in many children (Nicolosi, Harryman, & Kresheck, 1996).

The knowledgeable parent also understands the importance of accurate and thorough assessment of auditory processing disorder. Even if the child is too young for a formal auditory processing evaluation (typically under the age of 7 or 8), a parent with questions should not adopt a *wait and see* attitude. Concerns should be discussed with a pediatrician who may then make a referral to an audiologist and speech-language pathologist (Krauss, 2002).

County health departments and local school districts often offer screening services for children 3 years of age and younger. If the child demonstrates speech-language delays (or other identifiable difficulties), he or she may qualify for early intervention services through state programs. For children over age 3, local school districts can complete a screening or assessment of the child's speech-language/processing abilities.

Unfortunately, a diagnosis of auditory processing disorder may not qualify a child for special education services. School districts, however, may provide special learning accommodations in the classroom under a Section 504 plan (Krauss, 2002). Additional information about this option is discussed next in The Legal Terrain.

Just as a parent should not adopt a *wait and see* attitude when observing their child's questionable behaviors, they should also be aware of critical windows of opportunity. In general, the earlier the intervention, the better the prognosis for positive outcomes. While a formal diagnosis of APD may not be possible until age 7 (or thereabouts), children who demonstrate at-risk behaviors for language processing or auditory processing disorders (e.g., academic underachievement, auditory distractibility, and phonological/phonemic difficulties) may benefit from targeted auditory activities designed to increase neural connections and improve auditory functions (Kelly, 2001).

Some of these activities can be implemented by parents under the guidance of a speech-language pathologist or audiologist. Activities that involve auditory attention are particularly helpful. For example, parent and child may play a sound game (*I'm thinking of an animal that says . . .*). Other suggestions include using phrases and words that encourage and reinforce listening, such as *I heard you, You heard that,* or *You know Daddy was speaking,* and asking the child to watch the speaker's face when listening (Minnesota Department of Children, Families and Learning, 2003). Activities involving sound-symbol associations (verbal and nonverbal), simple instruments, voice cues, identification/imitation, and rhythms are also recommended (Kelly, 2001).

The Legal Terrain

Special education law is a category associated with laws and regulations pertaining to the education of students with special needs. These needs include: learning disabilities; physical disabilities; behavioral disorders; talents; or academic aptitude difficulties that cannot be addressed in regular classrooms (http://www.lawyers.com/lawyers/A~1016043`OVT/Special+Education+Law.html)

The Individuals with Disabilities in Education Act (IDEA/formerly PL94-142) guarantees a free public education to children demonstrating speech, hearing, or visual impairments, brain injury, mental impairment, severe emotional or health issues, autism, or identifiable learning disability.

The Amendments of 1997 known as Public Law 105-17, reauthorized the IDEA and identified increased, meaningful parental involvement in evaluations, including parental access to reports, test results, and other materials containing personal identifiable information (Roseberry-McKibbon & Hegde, 2000). Auditory processing disorder is not a category identified under the IDEA. However, children with APD may receive considerations under a civil rights law known as Section 504 of The Rehabilitation Act of 1973.

Section 504 prohibits discrimination against individuals with disabilities. It makes certain that children and adults have equal access to appropriate education including necessary accommodations and modifications. In contrast to IDEA, Section 504 does not involve an Individual Education Plan designed to meet the child's unique and specific educational needs. It uses a broad identification format, not a limited list of specific disabilities (http://www.wrightslaw.com/info/section.index.htm) Examples of modifications on a Section 504 plan include seating the child near the teacher or next to a helpful peer, allowing use of a calculator, or using a computer for writing projects.

In some cases it is helpful for parents to engage the services of an education lawyer, a specialist in education advocacy from a parent's perspective. Although it is hoped that parents and school professionals can agree upon services and procedures, occasionally the process stagnates. Education lawyers may help mediate and resolve complicated education issues. Some lawyers maintain Web sites offering message boards, chats, and special education articles, among other helpful services for parents.

The process of diagnosis and intervention for children with auditory processing disorder is fraught with hazards and pitfalls. Parents must be prepared to navigate a complicated legal and educational maze. Common mistakes include:

1. Not making requests in writing;
2. Requesting a related service instead of an assessment that supports the need for a related service;
3. Accepting assessment results that do not recommend the services you think your child needs;
4. Accepting goals and objectives that are not measurable;
5. Allowing placement decisions to be made before IEP goals and objectives are written;
6. Not asking questions (Foley & Hyatt-Foley, 2001).

Other mistakes include:

1. Requesting programs that may not be appropriate to the child's particular profile and challenges;
2. Accepting assessment results that are incomplete;

3. Accepting assessment results that are not timely;
4. Accepting assessment results that do not make sense;
5. Accepting assessment results from professionals who may lack expertise;
6. Accepting programs that do not reflect assessment results specifically;
7. Not understanding the educational implications of placement options (i.e., push in; pull-out; etc.);
8. Accepting the services of a parent advocate who lacks adequate background information;
9. Failing to request evidence of functional outcomes for goals, services, and programs.

Beyond these mistakes, miscommunication between team members can occur. Although participants are well intended, each comes from a different background, experience, and perspective. Team members (e.g., parent, speech-language pathologist, classroom teacher, and psychologist) understand auditory processing disorders from different educational and experiential perspectives. Whereas this may work quite well in some settings, in others it results in miscommunication (often unknown to team members). There may be an appearance of communication; however, in realty, there may be little. Although the information shared by a team member may be accurate, it is limited to the perspective of a single discipline.

What can be done to reduce such communication hazards? First, in all team meeting environments, there should be a common set of understood terms. Terms such as *progress, listening, paying attention, effort, processing, cooperation, motivation,* and others can be the most problematic. For example, a team member may describe a child's efforts to pay attention as *inadequate* exclusively from their perspective (e.g., as a teacher or parent) and miss the more subtle factors (such as the role of listening environment or the negative impact of poor memory skills on attention). Even more troubling, a team member may consider the child uncooperative (suggesting a choice) or unmotivated. In reality, very few children *choose* the social repercussions of inadequate attention (i.e., public humiliation and irritation of others).

Team members (including parents) should understand and agree upon concepts such as:

- What is AP?
- What is APD?
- What are the differences between APD, LD, and ADHD (or others as needed)?
- How do these disorders present on a comorbid basis?
- How does each impact language, learning, listening, and behavior?
- What are different kinds of auditory memory, attention, and listening?
- How do emotions and environment impact on the child's behavior and performance?

Parents may have questions for the team specific to their child's individual profile of APD:

- What is my child's unique profile of APD?
- What are your educational goals for my child and how will you achieve them? Why are these goals important?

- How do each of these goals relate to classroom functions?
- How will you document/assess progress?
- How will the classroom teacher modify his or her teaching style to accommodate my child?
- Where do you see my child in 5 months . . . 1 year . . . 2 years?
- What are my child's responsibilities in the *process* of intervention?
- What technology (if any) will be used in therapy and/or the classroom? Why is it necessary? How long will it be used?
- How will team members share information?
- What other supportive technologies or other means of assistance would be helpful to my child ?
- How can we improve (if necessary) my child's self-esteem?
- What support services (e.g., reading lab) will be available?
- Where will therapy take place? Why is that the best location?
- Will my child be grouped with other children? How do you determine groups?
- How will skills gained in therapy carry over into the classroom and at home? (Kelly, 1995).
- How much time out of the classroom is too much time?

Other simple strategies may reduce miscommunications at team meetings. Parents should bring a tape recorder to meetings (if permitted), ask for clarifications of ambiguous information, and request a follow-up meeting, if desired. The IEP or Section 504 plan should not be signed unless the parent is satisfied that it reflects their child's best interests (http://ww.angelfire.com/ny/Debsimms/education.html).

Parents as Managers

In terms of functional family outcomes, parents are responsible for making certain everything that should be done is done at the end of each day. To achieve that end, parents must expeditiously structure schedules and activities for all family members. In typical families, this is a daunting task considering two or more work schedules, as well as school and social activities. In families dealing with auditory processing disorder, the challenges are even more difficult. This section examines two broad areas of family activities that can improve practical outcomes (i.e., make certain everything runs more smoothly). To this end, Parents as Managers can act as Communication Facilitators and as Organization Strategists. Children with APD often demonstrate both communication and organization deficits.

Communication Facilitators

Although communication strategies may be targeted to particular profiles of auditory processing disorder, some general recommendations for many children are possible. Parents (and other family members) should remember two important guidelines: *Keep it short and simple* (KISS) and *Don't say it, show it* (Ferre, 2002). Repetition of a message may be helpful, but an enhanced, repeated message is better. Adding emphasis, timing, and other linguistic cues facilitates recall. Some children process information slowly (auditory latency); premature repetition of information is counterproductive. Many children with auditory latency will eventually respond to the original message; when it is repeated, the child may have to begin again (this time with greater emotional stress). However, the difficulty may involve an auditory memory, executive function, or language comprehension component (among other possibilities) if, even with extended time, the child does not respond to the message or direction.

When a message is ambiguous or unclear, repetition will do little to improve communication. A simple direction, such as *Find something to do* or *Straighten your room,* can be confusing to some children with language processing/comprehension/executive function difficulties. Examples of specific directions are: *You seem bored. Would you like to read or play video games?* or *Go to your room. Pick up your toys. Then make your bed. Then vacuum.* Tone of voice is important, as well. A perception of irritation or impatience may negatively affect auditory processing. Children are often keenly aware of the emotional climate of communication.

The environment in which communication takes place greatly affects both transmission and reception of information. Parents should speak to their child in a quiet (distraction-free) environment, at a slightly elevated volume, and with increased intonation and expressive, natural gestures. Simple memory strategies such as tying a piece of string on the wrist, placing daily chore and homework charts on the refrigerator, and sounds cues (e.g., grocery list/M . . . milk, A . . . apples, P . . . potatoes/MAP) can facilitate recall of directions and tasks. Mnemonic strategies and verbal rehearsal may also prove helpful.

Everyday conversations can be opportunities to enhance the child's vocabulary. Parents can use new words in exchanges while informally encouraging context cue awareness and offering synonyms. Discussions about school and social experiences can be opportunities to increase language and listening skills, as well as to deepen socioemotional awareness as discussed in the next section.

Some children with APD have difficulty processing auditory and visual information (and perhaps other sensory input) simultaneously. For these children, information should be presented consecutively. For example, in the classroom, some children should not be asked to copy notes from the board as the teacher is speaking. In fact, taking a spelling test in the usual manner may be too challenging. It is more effective when the teacher asks the child to: *First, look at me while I present the word (e.g., spell geography or measure). Then, look down at your paper and write the word. I won't present the next word until you are finished.* Although this strategy of *look* or *listen* is recommended for teachers (Bellis, 1996), if helpful, parents may adopt a similar strategy at home. For example, *First, look at me. Now listen to what I want you to do. Take the laundry up to your room. Here's the laundry.*

Bellis (2002) advocates *active listening* in children with APD. This behavior is helpful during difficult listening tasks. It involves sitting or standing alertly, maintaining eye contact with the speaker, eliminating unnecessary movements, and forcing the mind back to attention when drifting occurs. It is important for many children with APD to actively listen in school. However, parents may wish to gently remind their child of key features when helpful at home (e.g., *Keep your eyes on whomever is talking* and *Don't do anything else while you are listening*). This type of mindful listening may become automatic over time, especially with parent modeling.

Other practical communication strategies for parents include:

- Don't try to carry on a conversation across large rooms, while media is playing, or if the child is in another room.
- Be aware that places such as classrooms or churches have large, flat surfaces that reverberate. Children often have difficulty processing information in such reflective environments.
- Help the child to be responsible. Encourage the child to check that he or she has "heard" all of the instructions. Numbers, dates, addresses, and names can often be written down in a small notepad (http:d3.k12.id.us/~sservice/CAPDhandout.html)

It is important for parents to realize that many listening skills are developmental and are related in part to time and the quality of auditory experiences. Structures within the auditory nervous system do not reach maturity until age 9 in typically developing children (Martin, 1994). The ability to screen out secondary signal sources (i.e., background noises) and to attend to primary signal sources (e.g., a parent's or teacher's voice) may not develop until 6 to 8 years of age (Greenberg, Bray, & Beasley, 1970). The ability to recognize speech in reverberant environments (e.g., classrooms) may not develop until the teen years (Johnson, 2000). In children with APD, some milestones may be achieved late, if ever. Although apparently approximately 60% children with APD eventually grow out of it, for the remaining 40%, symptoms linger indefinitely (Burleigh, Skinner, & Norris, 1982).

In general, parents should remember that the desire to communicate is as strong in their children as in more typically developing children. The difference lies less in the intent than in the technical ability to receive and transfer information.

Organization Strategists

Parent managers may find simple organization strategies make daily routines and activities run smoother. In general, the more structured and predicable the environment, the less stressful it is for a child with processing limitations. However, although many children with APD perform better within structured environments (e.g., daily chores, regular times for dinner, bedtime, and homework), children also need to relax at home. The home environment shouldn't be so structured that it does not feel like a place to escape at the end of the day (Bellis, 2002). Children cannot be expected to maintain the same degree and type of focus at home as is needed in school.

Despite the need for acceptance in the home, it is important for the child with APD to make an effort. Chores, instructions, and other communications are better understood when strategies acquired at school are implemented (more informally) at home. For example, just as the classroom teacher may write daily schedules (e.g., music class/9:15; art class/12:30) on the blackboard, the parent can place similar lists on the refrigerator or a corkboard (e.g., soccer practice/5:30; homework/7:30). Morning instructions recorded on a WalkMan, MP3 Player, or Discman provide the child with repeated reminders until tasks are completed (Vinson, 1999). Cell phones offer another recording option.

Behavioral or attentional problems can occur at home and negatively impact routines and schedules. When such problems arise, Bellis (2002) advises, *Blame the disorder, not the child.* Although it is understandable to become frustrated, parents should objectively analyze major incidents. *What can be attributed to behavior or inattention and what was due to the processing disorder?* When parents realize that their child wants to comply, but lacks the necessary tools for success, patience comes more easily. Often poor behavior is the result of frustration, inadequate language or social skills, or poor self-esteem, rather than misguided intent.

Homework can be a significant organization management problem for parents and children with APD. Because school is often exhausting, the child may have little patience for schoolwork at home. In addition, the child with APD may receive extra tutoring which further depletes his or her energy and motivation to learn.

Teachers may wish to consider shorter, more directed homework assignments, rather than prolonged tasks. In this case, more is not necessarily better. A child who is drained from a difficult day at school is not likely to benefit from lengthy homework tasks. Parents are advised to start with short work periods that gradually increase with better tolerance. Stop at the point of success rather than at the point of frustration and failure (Colorado Department of Education, 1997). Praise successes rather than emphasize failures. The overall efficacy of homework in general (for all children) may be a long overdue discussion for all parents, teachers, clinicians, and administrators.

Studying for spelling tests can also pose a management problem. A child can apparently *know* the spelling list the night before a test only to fail the next day. Here again, more studying is not the answer. In fact, more ineffective studying may increase frustration and decrease productivity. Studying more efficiently (in a different way) is often helpful.

This strategy may produce better results:

The child should use his or her own voice to make a tape recording of the spelling list.

Read the list aloud, as if the student were the teacher administering the test (e.g., *Spell . . .* , *Spell . . .* , and so on). Leave a little time in between words.

Practice each word by looking at it, *while* spelling it aloud. Repeat this procedure, as needed.

Then play the tape recording of the child's voice reading the spelling list (as if the teacher). Take the test by spelling the words aloud (only looking at the list when necessary).

Do this as many times as needed, until the child is able to spell all (or almost all) of the words.

Lastly, listen to the tape recording of the list again. This time, take the test as if in class—without looking at the list. Repeat this procedure, as needed (Kelly, 1995).

Some children consistently receive high grades on spelling tests, yet do not apply spelling skills to their writing. Words spelled correctly on a test one day can be misspelled in a paragraph the next day. Such a child does not demonstrate competent spelling skills; rather, he or she has simply memorized symbol sequences for the short-term purpose of passing a test. This pattern should be viewed as a possible symptom of memory and/or phonologic/phonemic difficulties.

Parents as Facilitators of Socioemotional Growth

In recent years, researchers have explored the relationship between language ability and social/emotional skills (Fujiki, Brinton, Isaacson, & Summers, 2001; Fujiki, Brinton, Morgan, & Hart, 1999; Fujiki, Brinton, & Todd, 1996; Hart, Fujiki, Brinton, & Hart, 2004). In general, it has been found that children with language deficits appear to desire the same social interactions as typically developing children, but may lack the linguistic tools to initiate and maintain social interactions.

Without language tools to think about emotions and understand them, it is difficult to associate them with behavior and consequences. Children with weak language resources may resort to inappropriate nonverbal expressions (e.g., anger/hitting, frustration/throwing objects) in the absence of adequate verbal abilities to express emotions. Other effects may include poor self-esteem, depression, and withdrawn behavior.

Language impairment not only affects the ability to regulate one's own emotions, but it may also affect one's ability to identify emotions in others. For example, kindergarteners with language impairment have been found unable to read a conversation partner's emotional reactions through facial expressions (Ford & Milosky, 2003). The potential impact on social interactions is apparent. A child, even as young as kindergarten-age, may be perceived by peers as inadequate conversation partners.

Rice (1993) offers additional insights in socioemotional communication skills in children with language impairment. A *negative social spiral* describes the relationship between language development and social experiences in children with language limitations. Specifically, because of language deficits language-impaired children are often rejected in social settings resulting in fewer opportunities to refine social/conversation skills. Fewer social interactions may result in deficient language development. In this way, language impairment and social limitations may negatively impact one another (i.e., *The sum becomes greater than the parts.)*

Not *all* children with language impairment demonstrate deficits in socioemotional communication skills, although many do. However, many children with *various* diagnoses involving language impairment experience social problems (Anita & Kreimeyer, 1992, Guralnick, 1992). Furthermore, children with language impairment display difficulties in a *variety* of social settings in which language plays a role (Windsor, 1995).

Similarly, not all children with auditory processing disorder demonstrate language impairment or socioemotional communication deficits. However, many children with APD display limitations in both areas (Bellis, 1996; Keith, 2000; Keller, 1998; Kelly, 1995, 1998, 2005). For example, children with APD may seek playmates who are younger than themselves because of repeated failures with age-peers (Willeford, 1985). Parents often describe their children with APD as loners. For these compelling reasons, it is useful for parents to understand the impact of language deficits on their child's social and emotional behaviors. With valuable insights, parents may help their children identify and resolve frustrating and upsetting social situations.

Parents may use everyday experiences (e.g., going to the supermarket, talking about school, etc.) to improve their child's socioemotional/language skills. As opportunities arise, a parent may help their child with social problem-solving. For example, if an unfortunate incident happens on the school bus, parents may discuss behavior options, intentions, and effective ways to say things. Facial expressions and body language can be identified as social cues.

Children with APD sometimes do not understand the finer aspects of conversations. Parents may discuss appropriate topics of conversation, timing aspects, and telephone protocols, among other pragmatic skills. Role-playing may help encourage empathy and listener perspectives. Discussions may also involve the child's feelings about social rejection and qualities that make strong friendships.

A parent's model of competent socioemotional skills is invaluable. Under challenging social circumstances, the parent who maintains composure and chooses effective language and behavior strategies provides a strong learning opportunity to their child.

Parents and Children Having Fun

Time set aside during the day for just parent and child is time well spent (Colorado Department of Education, 1997). Sometimes, parents and children can just *be* together, without schedules, chores, or obligations. All interactions do not have to be viewed as opportunities for learning. However, familiar games can improve language and auditory processing skills (without the atmosphere of drills or therapy). Activities and games (e.g., rhyming games, telephone game, I Spy, Red Light-Green Light, Scrabble, Name That Tune, Password, Simon Says, chess, checkers, and card games) that involve active listening, memory, judgment, discrimination, soundmakers, or analysis are particularly helpful (Ferre, 2002b).

Other helpful activities include imitating sounds; memorizing jingles, songs, and rhymes; play-acting using different voices; developing a sense of rhythm and tonality; developing a concept of time, direction, space, rate, and size; relating happenings in sequence; and engaging in activities that involve the giving and receiving of directions (adapted from Gillet, 1974). Singing, dancing, dramatic arts, karate, gymnastics, and listening to music are also beneficial.

Research suggests that music activities may afford an added bonus; lessons may boost IQ as well as grades in some children (Munsey, 2006). However, all such activities should be discontinued if not pleasurable to the child. Parents should be careful about overscheduling of activities. Too many activities (no matter how beneficial) can be counterproductive. Children with APD are especially in need of adequate quiet time.

In order for families with challenges to function, parents need to care for themselves first. Parent who see to their own physical and emotional needs are acting responsibly (i.e., to be a healthy caretaker). To truly be present, parents need to resolve any emotional issues that may impact their effectiveness as a parent and advocate. Although difficult, parents should acknowledge feelings of denial, guilt, anger, or depression about their child's disorder. Parents must realize that such emotional debris is understandable under very stressful parenting conditions. Key to emotional resolution is a simple reality—no parent intended, nor caused their child to have a disorder. In fact, the vast majority of parents of children with disabilities make extraordinary efforts under difficult conditions.

The dreams a parent may have for their child may not be realistic (considering the severity of the disorder). Unfortunately, for some children with APD, it is not a matter of time until *they grow out of it.* Sadly, not all children will be able to attend college, become lawyers, doctors, or teachers. Many parents face such disappointments (not just parents of children with learning or language issues). Sometimes it is helpful to ask, *Am I disappointed for myself or for my child? Can my child find other avenues for success*? The answer to the latter question is a resounding *Yes*. It is a matter of changing perspective a little and redefining success. All success does not have to be measured by academic achievements. Talents come in many forms. Here again, counseling and support from other parents may prove helpful.

Looking Ahead: Children with APD Become Adults

As children with auditory processing disorder become adults with auditory processing disorder, emotional, social, and academic transitions are necessary. In general, adults with disabilities must become their own advocates. Whereas the IDEA identifies responsibilities of the parent and school district for a child's disability, the Americans with Disabilities Act (ADA), transfers responsibilities to students or employees. Section 504 plans transition from high school to college, university, or work settings. It is the adult's responsibility to declare and document their disability in the postsecondary education or work setting to receive services and accommodations. Students with disabilities may receive academic support services from the college or university *only* if such services are available to all students.

Under Section 504, colleges and universities must make "appropriate academic adjustments" and "reasonable modifications" that provide students with disabilities access to the educational programs and activities available to other students. These modifications may include extended test times, quiet work environments, access to large print or audio books, or parking permits (Banotai, 2006a).

Baran (1998) maintains that counseling is helpful to a smoother transition from school-age to career-age for the student with APD. The emerging adult who has enjoyed a strong educational and therapy support system throughout school years may feel at a loss when required to independently transition to the work world.

Successful transition from school-age to career-age responsibilities necessitates an understanding of how auditory processing limitations may affect job performance. The young adult may be asked to realistically consider careers that are suited to their particular skills and challenges. Poor job performance in an ill-suited position may result in a downward spiral involving a loss of self-esteem and motivation. Positive, challenging goals rooted in reality are most constructive.

Resources for Parents

Support and information for parents of children with APD is available through Internet Web sites:

http://www.home.earthlink.net/~mcoleman/cpdadd.html

http://www.schoolmatch.com

http://www.cthome.net/cbristol/capd-1dx.html

http://www.cshassoc.org/capdpres.html

http://www.members.aol.com/HERDEWE/page2html

http://www.braingym.org/faas.html

http://www.mcs.brandonu.ca/~education/myranbj/resource.htm

http://www.home.ptd.net/~blnelson/SIDWEBPAGE2.htm

http://www.ldaca.org/gram/thompson

http://www.allkindsofminds.org

http://www.exploratorium.edu/exhibits/ladle/index.html

http://www.apduk.org

http://www.help4adhd.org

http://members.tripod.com/dolfrog/iep_page.htm

http://specialed.about.com/education/specialed/msubcapd.htm

http://www.angelfire.com/home/capddownunder/

http://www.cde.state.co.us/cdesped/download/pdf/CI-APD-Gu.pdf

http://arkedu.state.ar.us/

http://cfl.state.mn.us/stellent/groups/public/documents/translatedcontent/pub_010368.pdf

http://www.firn.edu/doe/commhome/pdf/y2001-9.pdf

http://www.access-board.gov/publications/acoustic-factsheet.htm

http://www.tsbvi.edu/Outreach/seehear/spring00/centralauditory.htm

http://kidshealth.org/parent/medical/ears/central_auditory.html

http://www.ldonline.org/ld_indepth/process_deficit/capd_paton.html

http://capdlinks.homestead.com/AA_index_ZZ.html

http://www.nidcd.nih.gov/health/spanish/audidsrdr_span.asp

http://www.nidcd.nih.gov/health/voice/auditory.asp#5

http://www.nidcd.nih.gov/health/pubs_vsl/auditory.htm

http://capdlinks.homestead.com/useful_CAPD_links.html

http://www.ncapd.org/

http://www.dolfrog.com/

http://www.angelfirecom/f/4/ncapd

http://www. hearingreview.com

http://www.theshopnet/campbell/central.html

http://www.kidspeech.com/tips.html

http://www.audiologyinfo.com/email/capd.htm

http://www.maelstrom.stjohns.edu/archives/capd.html/

Summary

Parents of children with auditory processing disorder are advised to be their child's strongest and most effective advocate. For the most functional management outcomes, parents should be informed, proactive team members, appropriately aware of technology, therapy, placement options, legal rights, and the Individual Education Plan process. Parent should avail themselves of the many information resources available today, including electronic media and parent support organizations. Contact with clinicians and teachers are critical to their child's education progress.

At home, parents should be parents first. Children with APD need a place to escape and relax from the stresses of school. While providing a balance between work and play, parents can manage listening conditions within the home environment, and stimulate listening, processing, and language skills within natural contexts. With knowledge, support, and purpose, parents realize that life can progress normally and efficiently, perhaps just with more management and organization.

The messages of this chapter can be further summarized succinctly. Perhaps the best advice for parents of children with auditory processing disorder is to: find out, feel, get real, seek others, find perspective, find balance, and get going. The child's best parent is one that is healthy, compassionate, loving, resilient, and strong.

Key Points Learned

- Parents should identify themselves as critical team members in their child's educational and therapy programming.
- Parents should come to terms with the realities of their child's diagnosis, including having reasonable expectations for academic performance and future goals.
- If applicable, parents should identify and manage their own feelings of loss, grief, and guilt.
- Parents should wisely make use of the Internet and other electronic innovations (e.g., support groups, chat groups, listservs, and podcasts) to access important information

about their child's challenges (e.g., legal rights and therapy innovations), as well as to find support for themselves.

- Simple organizational (e.g., homework, chore, and bedtime schedules) and communication (e.g., one person speaks at a time; *keep it short and simple*) strategies at home can make daily routines flow more efficiently and less stressfully.
- Parents can use everyday experiences such as an unfortunate incident on the school bus or playground to talk about behavior options, language choices, and social problem-solving.
- Parents should be cognizant of their responsibility to prepare their child for adulthood and independence (to whatever extent possible). The legal terrain for children is different from that for adults.
- Parents need balance in their personal and family lives. It is possible to be a responsible, involved parent of a child with challenges and still make time for relaxation and fun.

References

Anita, S. D., & Kreimeyer, K. H. (1992). Social competence intervention for young children with hearing impairment. In S. L. Odom, S. R. McConnell, & M. A. McEvoy (Eds.), *Social competence of young children with disabilities: Issues and strategies for intervention* (pp. 135–164) Baltimore: Paul H. Brooks.

Auditory processing disorders. [Technical Assistance Paper/10967]. Florida Department of Education (http://www.firn.edu/doe/commhome/pdf/y2001-9.pdf)

Banotai, A. (2006a). Post-secondary transition: Strategies for students with special needs. *Advance for Speech-Language Pathologists and Audiologists*, *16*(3), 6–8.

Banotai, A. (2006b). The power of portable information: Potential podcasting in future of continuing education, *Advance for Speech-Language Pathologists and Audiologists*, *16*(23), 6–8.

Baran, J. A. (1998). Management of adolescents and adults with central auditory processing disorders. In M. G. Masters, N. A. Stecker, & J. Katz (Eds.), *Central auditory processing disorders: Mostly management* (pp. 195–214). Boston: Allyn & Bacon.

Bellis, T. (1996). *Assessment and management of central auditory processing disorders in the educational settings.* San Diego, CA: Singular Publishing Group.

Bellis, T. J. (2002). *When the brain can't hear.* New York: Pocket Books.

Burleigh, A., Skinner, B., & Norris, R. (1982, November). *Central auditory processing disorders in children: A five-year study.* A paper presented at the American Speech-Language-Hearing Association Convention. Toronto, Ontario.

CAPD Handout for Parents and Teachers. Available at: http://d93.k12.id.us/sservice/CAPDhandout.html

Colorado Department of Education. (1997). *Auditory processing disorders: A team approach to screening, assessment and inter-*

vention practice. Denver, CO: Task Force on APDs.

Ferre, J. (2002a). Behavioral therapeutic approaches for central auditory problems. (pp. 525–531). In J. Katz (Ed), *Handbook of clinical audiology* (5th ed.). Baltimore: Lippincott Williams & Wilkins.

Ferre, J. (2002b). Managing children's central auditory processing deficits in the real world: What teachers and parents want to know. *Seminars in Hearing, 23,* 319–326.

Fisher, L. I. (1976). *Fisher's Auditory Problem Checklist.* Cedar Rapids, IA: Grant Woods Area Educational Agency.

Foley, M., & Hyatt-Foley, D. (2001, Winter). Ten common mistakes parents make during the individual education plan meeting, *SEE/Hear Quarterly Newsletter, 6*(1), 4–7.

Ford, J., & Milosky, L. (2003. Inferring emotional reactions in social situations: Differences in children with language impairment. *Journal of Speech-Language, and Hearing Research, 46*(1), 21–30.

Fujiki, M, Brinton, B., & Clarke, D. (2002). Emotion regulation in children with specific language impairment. *Language, Language, Speech, and Hearing Services in Schools, 33,* 102–111.

Fujiki, M., Brinton B., Isaacson, T., & Summers, C. (2001). Social behaviors of children with language impairment on the playground: A pilot study. *Language, Speech, and Hearing Services in Schools, 32,* 101–113.

Fujiki, M., Brinton, B., Morgan, M., & Hart, C. H. (1999). Withdrawn and sociable behavior of children with language impairment. *Language, Speech, and Hearing Services in Schools, 30*(2), 183–195.

Fujiki, M., Brinton, B., Morgan, M., & Todd, C. M. (1996). Social skills of children with specific language impairment. *Language, Speech, and Hearing Services in Schools, 27*(3), 195–202.

Gillet, P. (1974). *Auditory processes.* Novato CA: Academic Therapy Publications.

Gillet, P. (1993). *Auditory processes.* Novato CA: Academic Therapy Publications.

Greenberg, G. Z., Bray, N. W., & Beasley, D. S. (1970). Children's frequency-selective detection of signals in noise. *Perception and Psychophysics, 8,* 173–175.

Guralnick, M. J. (1992). A hierarchical model for understanding children's peer-related social competence. In S. L. Odom, S. R. McConnell, & M. A. McEvoy (Eds.), *Social competence of young children with disabilities: Issues and strategies for intervention* (pp. 37–64). Baltimore: Paul H. Brookes.

Hart, K. I., Fujiki, M., Brinton, B., & Hart, C. H. (2004). The relationship between social behavior and severity of language impairment. *Journal of Speech-Language-Hearing Research, 47,* 647–662.

Honos-Webb, L. (April, 2006). Ways to help your ADHD child pay attention. *New Living Magazine, 16*(2). Available at http://newlivingmagazine.com/issues_apr2006/articles/adhd/htm/

Jerger, J., & Musiek, F. E. (2004). Report of consensus conference on the diagnosis of auditory processing disorders in school-aged children. *Journal of the American Academy of Audiology, 11,* 467–474.

Johnson, C. E. (2000). Children's phoneme identification in reverberation and noise. *Journal of Speech, Language, and Hearing Research, 43,* 144–157.

Keith, R. W. (2000). *SCAN-C: Test of Auditory Processing Abilities in Children* (rev. ed.). San Antonio, TX: The Psychological Corporation.

Keller,W. D. (1998). The relationship between attention deficit disorder, central auditory processing disorders, and specific learning disorders. In M. G. Masters, N. A. Stecker, & J. Katz, J. (Eds.), *Central auditory processing disorders: Mostly management* (pp. 33–47). Boston: MA: Allyn & Bacon.

Kelly, D. (1995). *Central auditory processing disorder: Strategies for use with children and adolescents*. Tucson, AZ: Communication Skill Builders.

Kelly, D. (1998). *Understanding central auditory processing disorder: TheraGuide*. San Antonio, TX: Communication Skill Builders.

Kelly, D. (2001). *Screening for central auditory processing difficulties*. Oceanside: CA: Academic Communication Associates.

Kelly, D. (2005). Suggestions for patents, teachers, speech-language pathologists, and students: Enhancing functional outcomes in children with APD. In T. K. Parthasarathy (Ed.), *An introduction to auditory processing disorders in children* (pp. 229–245). Mahwah, NJ: Lawrence Erlbaum Associates.

Krauss, K. (2002.) Auditory processing: "What we do with what we hear." *Community Times* (Geneva, IL Community Therapy Services). Available from: http://www.commtx.com/communitytimes/winter03

Kuster, J. (2006). Hidden treasures from mailing lists. *The Asha Leader*, *11*(6), 36.

Martin, F. N. (1994). *Introduction to audiology* (5th ed.). Englewood Cliff, NJ: Prentice-Hall.

Medwetsky, L. (2006). Spoken language processing: A convergent approach to conceptualizing (central) auditory processing, *The ASHA Leader*, *112*(8), 6,7, 30, 31, 33.

Minnesota Department of Children, Families and Learning. (2003). *Introduction to auditory processing disorders: Ideas for developing listening behaviors for the preschool child at home and school APD work team*. Roseville, MN: Author. Available at: http://www.nesc.K12mn.us/special_ed/mauals/documents/APD.pdf

Munsey, C. (2006). Music lessons may boost IQ and grades. *Monitor on Psychology*, *37*(6), 13.

Nicolosi, L, E., Harryman, E., & Kresheck, J. (1996). *Terminology of communication disorders: Speech-language-hearing* (4th ed.) Baltimore: Lippincott Williams & Wilkins.

Pierangelo, R., & Jacoby, R. (1996). *Parents' complete special education guide: Tips, techniques and materials for helping your child succeed in school and life*. West Nyack, NY: The Center for Applied Research and Education.

Resources on special education, IEPS, IDEA, inclusion, and Section 504. Updated April 13, 2005; retrieved January 23, 2006 from: http://www.angelfire.com/ny/Debsimms/education.html

Rice, M. L. (1993). Don't talk to him; he's weird: A social consequences account of language and social interactions. In A. P. Kaiser & D. B. Gray (Eds.), *Communication and language intervention series, Vol. 2, Enhancing children's communication: Research foundations for intervention* (pp. 139–158). Baltimore: Paul H. Brookes.

Richard, G. (2001). *The source for processing disorders*. East Moline: IL: LinguiSystems.

Roseberry-McKibbon, C., & Hegde, M. N. (2000). *An advanced review of speech-language pathology*. Austin,TX: Pro-Ed.

Rowe, K., Rowe K., & Pollard J. (2004). *Literacy, behaviour and auditory processing: Building "fences" at the top of the "cliff" in preference to "ambulance services" at the bottom*. Paper presented at the Literacy, Behaviour and Auditory Processing Research Conference, Adelaide, Australia.

Section 504. Wrightslaw. Available from: http://www.wrightslaw.com/info/sec504.index.htm

Special Education Law. Available from: http://www.lawyers.com/lawyers/A~1016043`OVT/Special+Education+Law.html.

Thornburgh, N. (2006, May 29). Teaching doctors to care. *Time*, *167*(22), 58–59.

Vinson, B. P. (1999). *Language disorders across the lifespan*. San Diego, CA: Singular Publishing Group

Willeford, J. A. (1985). Assessment of central auditory disorders in children. In M. L. Pinheiro & F. E. Musiek (Eds.), *Assessment of central auditory dysfunction: Foun-*

dation and clinical correlates (pp. 239–255). Baltimore: Williams & Wilkins.

Windsor, J. (1995). Language impairment and social competence. In M. E. Fey, J. Windsor, & F. Warren (Eds.), *Language intervention: Preschool through the elementary years* (Vol. 5, pp. 213–238). Baltimore: Paul H. Brookes.

III

Treatment and Intervention

13

Phonemic Training and Phonemic Synthesis Programs

Jack Katz

Overview

When parents learn that their child has an auditory processing disorder (APD) their next concern is what can be done to help the child improve. Decoding disorders are very common in those who have auditory processing (AP) problems. This chapter discusses two straightforward approaches to improve Decoding. These procedures have been used most successfully for many years and require relatively little time in therapy (Katz & Burge, 1971). There are three basic principles: Simplify the task to encourage correct responses; Repeat because repetition is needed to train the brain; and increase the difficulty level gradually to facilitate learning and minimize frustration.

Introduction and Theoretical Framework

The decoding category of the Buffalo model is defined as the ability to quickly and accurately digest speech (Katz, 1992). It is a skill that is closely associated with the auditory cortex of the temporal lobe (Luria, 1966, 1970). The specific auditory skills that are listed by Luria for this part of the brain are the ability to discriminate phonemes, remember phonemes, and to analyze-synthesize phonemes. When these basic functions of the auditory system are compromised as a result of early otitis media, genetic factors, or other etiologies, the child may be slow in learning to speak, have poor articulation, misunderstand what is said, as well as have problems in phonics and reading-word accuracy (see Holm & Kunze, 1969; Duane, 1977; Katz, 1992).

Although the effect of a Decoding problem can have major academic and communicative consequences, remediation of the problem may not be too difficult. However, it does take knowledge, planning, and time to do an effective job in remediating this disorder. This chapter reviews two therapy programs designed to improve Decoding skills. These therapies complement one another and provide basic skills that facilitate speech and reading therapies as well as improve accuracy in oral comprehension.

Decoding problems are conceptualized as faulty engrams in the brain, that is, for whatever reason, the brain has encoded vague or incorrect information regarding the specific sounds of speech. It is perhaps most easily visualized as a result of early otitis media when speech sounds are reduced in intensity and distorted by the fluid in the middle ear. The fluctuating fluid levels produce inconsistent acoustic stimulation of the brain which has its most potent effect during the critical periods of development. This likely causes the brain to have vague or inaccurate concepts for many phonemes and makes the listener more willing to accept a broader range of utterances for specific speech sounds.

Phonemic Training Program (PTP)

The PTP is a basic approach for improving a person's phonemic knowledge. Because the purpose of this therapy is to improve the brain's auditory concepts (i.e., engrams) it is presented auditory-only, except in certain situations. The only equipment needed is a cross-stitch hoop covered by loudspeaker material (to conceal the therapist's lower face from view while permitting the sounds to be transmitted relatively unimpeded to the listener) and a deck of cards with letters representing the sounds to be taught. The latter can be made inexpensively by using half-sized index cards with the letters printed on them (including markings to show, e.g., long and short vowels).

For PTP, and most APD training programs, we start with minimal challenges and increase the difficulty of the material as the patient demonstrates improved skills. Many of the concepts and procedures are based on the work of Winitz (1973). Generally, four new phonemes are introduced in each lesson. The four sounds are chosen to be easily discriminated from one another. We generally begin with three or all four of those sounds that were among the most challenging for the individual (based on pretest information or on sounds that are generally difficult, e.g., liquids and short vowels). A reasonable plan would be to introduce the following sounds: *d*, short-*e*, *l*, and *m*. Although these are difficult sounds for most children with Decoding problems; importantly, each of them is easy to distinguish from the other three. The advantage of starting with difficult sounds is that they are reviewed each succeeding session and, therefore, by the time the child is faced with discriminating among many sounds, the most difficult ones are much improved and the child can tolerate the challenge. Figure 13–1 shows the basic steps for PTP.

Session One

The program for the first two sessions differs from the subsequent ones. On the first visit one starts with the introduction of the new sounds. This is called "Introduction Without Bias" because the individual is not told what sound will be heard. This is an important step in training because it helps the individual to realize, perhaps, that he or she has a faulty concept of the sound. If the person is told that they will be hearing for example, the /l/ sound, they will not be surprised when they hear it. But if they are not told what sound it will be, especially in older children and adults, often there is a surprised look when they are finally told what the sound is.

Introduction Without Bias: the individual is instructed to listen carefully to the sound that will be presented a number of times but *not* to repeat the sound. The cross-stitch hoop conceals the therapist's lips and facial movements and in a clear voice the therapist says the sound, aperiodically about three times. For example, /d/. . . /d/ . . . . /d/. At this point the card with the letter "D" is shown and the individual is told (without the face obscured), "That was the /d/ sound that we hear in words like dog, daddy and good." The card is placed in front of the individual and he or she is asked to point to the card each time the /d/ sound is heard. The sound is presented a few times in a clear fashion (behind the hoop) and the individual is expected to point each time. To keep the individual "honest" indicate that occasionally you will say a different sound than the card(s) on the table. In that case the person should point to a spot over to the side. This is not meant as a discrimination task but only to keep the person alert and not to go on "automatic pilot" when the person anticipates the sound before it is said.

Now the first sound card is removed and a second sound is introduced without bias. In this case the short-*e* is said a few times aperiodically, then, as before, the therapist's face and the card are shown and the person is told that it was the /ɛ/ sound that we hear in words like end and ten. After the person responds correctly a few times; the two cards are placed in front of the person and each one is given once or twice in a random order. When a person anticipates a sound by preparing to point to a card it is preferable to give the other sound or some third sound to help ensure that the person is tuned-in to the sounds presented.

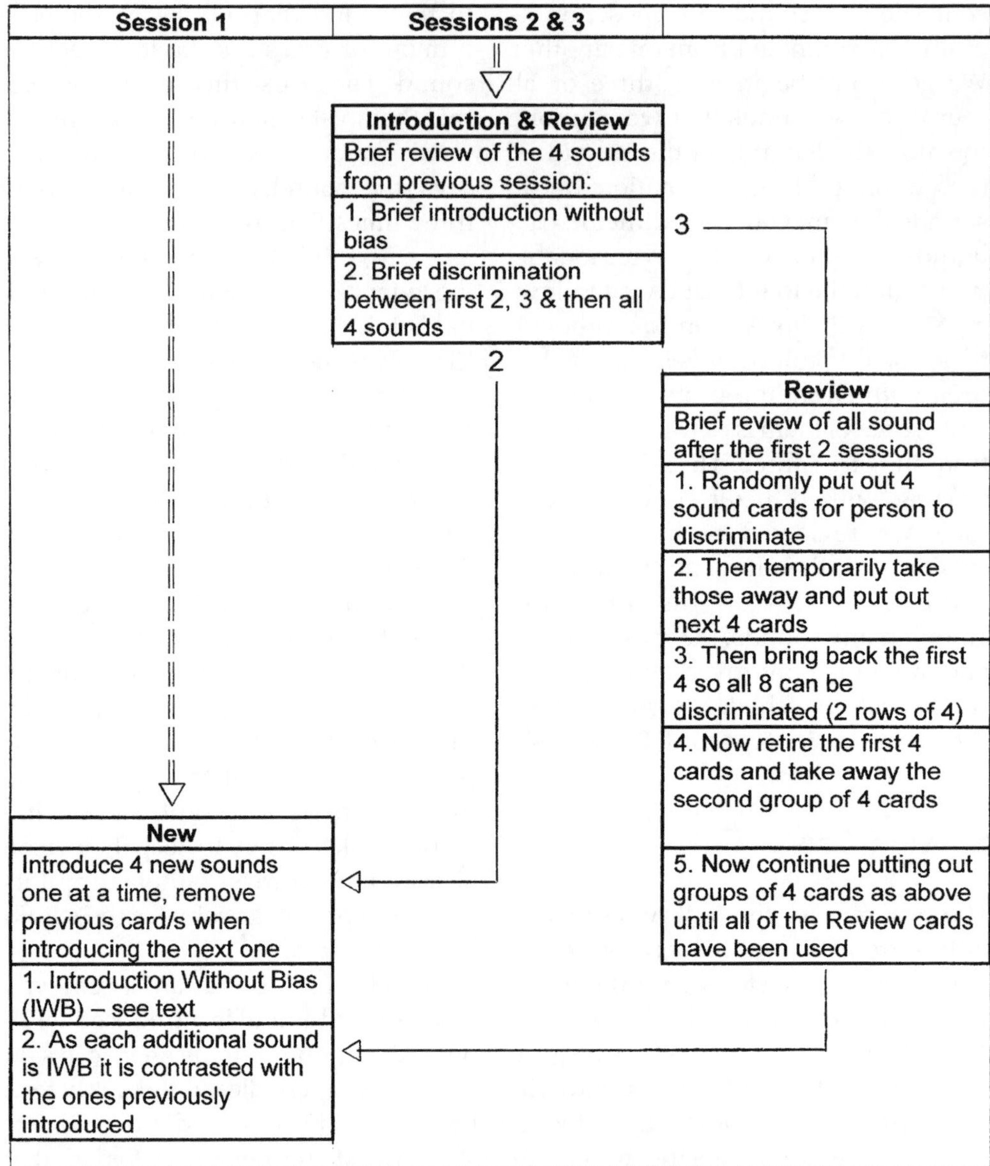

Figure 13–1. PTP flow chart showing the increasing number of steps for the first three therapy sessions. The succeeding sessions basically follow the procedures diagrammed for the third session.

Now, the third sound is presented without bias and then test discrimination with the two previous sounds proceeds. Finally the fourth sound is introduced in the same way and all four sounds are tested. Although this is not difficult for the listener it gives the person more and more opportunities to hear the clear sounds spoken in isolation and to associate them with the letters on the cards.

Session Two

Based on the work of Winitz (1973), first review the previous material and later introduce the new material. To reinforce the material that was presented in the previous session do a modified Introduction Without Bias that is called "Introduction and Review (IR)." Each of the sounds that were introduced in the previous session is introduced again more briefly. After one or two presentations indicate, "That was the /d/ sound that we talked about last time." After Introduction and Review (IR) each sound is contrasted with the other three sounds as in session one.

After IR four new sounds are introduced without bias and discriminated as above. Circle sounds on the lesson plan that need further reinforcement if the person had confusions or it took longer to figure out what the sound was (even with these easy contrasts).

Session Three

The third session contains each of the three major steps of PTP. Again start with IR, but this time a "Review" step is introduced next and new sounds come last. While the clinician usually sticks to a specific order of presentation of sounds for new and IR sounds, by the third presentation the person should be ready to handle all four cards that are put out at once in any order. This review is rather brief, going over the sounds once or perhaps twice if needed.

For the Following Sessions

The standard procedure for most of the remaining sessions follows the three steps as in session three. However, at each of the succeeding visits there are likely four new sounds to be introduced; the four new ones from the previous week are given in Introduction and Review and the previous IR sounds go into the Review step. The first two steps employ four sounds each time but each week four more are added to the Review. The Review sounds are all mixed together in a more or less randomized order and presented four at a time. After reviewing the first four; they are moved away from the person and four new ones put in front of the individual. After the second four are reviewed then all eight are given at the same time (in two rows of four). When completed the first four are "retired" and the second group of cards is pushed back and a new set of four is put down and so forth.

Repair Strategies

When an individual has difficulty easily recognizing a sound, remembering a sound, or distinguishing one from another it is appropriate to use a repair strategy. Leave repair of the confusion until the next session when the person's brain is clear of the error.

Key-Word Cards

These cards have words on them that represent the various speech sounds. They are used to reinforce sounds that may be difficult for the child by providing an association and coarticulation. The clinician introduces one card at a time without bias. Using the hoop the clinician can say, "The first sound is

/m/ and the key word is "mud." Show the card and say, "When I say /m/ you tell me 'mud' and point to the card." Put the card in front of the person and behind the hoop say the sound once or twice, hopefully, getting the appropriate answer each time. Then introduce the next one, train it, and then use both words and so forth.

Focus Cards

This is a powerful tool that helps one to narrow the phoneme boundaries (so it does not overlap with similar sounds). The most frequent use of focusing is for short-*e* versus short-a, /v/ versus /ð/, and especially /f/ versus /ʃ/. After showing the two cards say, "I'm going to say the /f/ three times and then I'll say the /ʃ/. Please point to the card I say each time." After this, if successful, indicate that you will always start with the /f/ but this time you will not tell how many times you will say it; however, the client is to point to whichever card is said. Then say /f/ one to four times followed by the /ʃ/. Do it again a few times varying the number of /f/ sounds. Repeat this procedure the next session or two. That is generally all that is needed for most sounds. At first accentuate the differences between the sounds but reduce the clues as you go along.

The PTP is so simple and so effective that it can be used with the most severe cases and those with very limited cognitive abilities as well as the brightest people. To the latter explain that each time they attend and hear the sounds and point, it improves the system until the sounds are quickly and accurately processed. This procedure has been used most effectively with mentally challenged individuals, those with cochlear implants (Katz, 1998), those who are learning English as a second language, and aphasics. These groups are among those with the most severe Decoding problems.

Phonemic Synthesis (PS)

The author has used Phonemic Synthesis (PS) therapy most effectively for the past 50 years. It is available commercially[1] (CD or cassette). This provides consistency as well as a carefully arranged progression of challenges from very easy to quite difficult. It works very well with PTP. In particular it aids the person in associating the sounds with words. It is at this point that we often hear spontaneously improved articulation without specific attention or training.

PS is a form of sound blending, phonemic build-up, and other labels used for this sound-by-sound presentation of words (real or pseudo) (Orton, 1937; Stovall et al., 1977; Van Riper, 1954). The individual is to say the word, point to the word, or point to a picture of the word. For those who use the recorded program the sounds are presented slowly and clearly. The words are organized to provide a great deal of success even as the difficulty level is increased. For those who will be presenting the therapy by live voice the sounds are presented in 1.0 to 1.5-second intervals. This provides an easily digested

[1]Phonemic Synthesis Kit from Precision Acoustics, 505 NE 87th Avenue, Suite 150, Vancouver, WA 98664. Or phone (360) 892-9367.

sound along with a pause to enable the person to figure out what was heard without other sounds confounding the experience. The sounds are presented individually and without coarticulation. For example, the individual sound /b/ is said but not the two sounds /bə/ and the sounds should not show the influence of the abutting sounds of the target word.

In the recorded program the first three lessons have picture multiple-choice support. For older children and those who have demonstrated reasonably good performance on the Phonemic Synthesis test, these three lessons can be skipped but the words that are on these earlier lessons should be given by live voice before starting the more difficult lessons. In lesson number 1 the children are told that they will be hearing words that are said in a funny way and asked to point to the picture of the word. Two practice items are given so that children can be instructed if they cannot figure out the word that was said. For example, the first practice item shows a picture of "cow" and "chair" and the child is given /k au/. The word contrasts are so easy that chances are children with even meager phonemic knowledge will choose the correct one. After the practice items the regular items are begun. The child sees a picture of a girl eating and a pencil and hears the sounds /i t/ and should point to the child eating. The item is repeated and for each administration the response is recorded by the therapist. Four more words are presented in the same way and then the same five words are presented again with the same pictures and yet a third time. The score correct for the 15 items is entered on the score form. Only 13 correct responses are needed to complete the lesson. Completion means that this lesson does not have to be repeated. Lesson number 2 (presumably in the next session or after a break or work on a nonphonemic activity) repeats the same five words, first with the same two picture choices and then with three choices. In lesson number 3 the words are given with three picture choices and then again with no picture choices. For the first time the children must generate their own answers. This should not be too difficult because they have already heard and responded to these words several times each. The third go-round in the lesson is with three picture choices again.

Because most of the children have had considerable academic challenges they are greatly encouraged by their initial successes in PS. Although it is fine to acknowledge some correct responses with encouragement (e.g., "Good listening") it is not good form to point out when one was in error (especially in the first go-round) because generally the program teaches it by the next administration. However, at the end of the lesson the clinician tells the child how many correct responses he or she had and has him or her enter this on the summary sheet. After a not-so-good performance the first time, children are likely to show improvement so you can point out that they are going up the steps of the chart (getting better and better). When the program was first designed we waited for a few sessions before using repair strategies, but now we speed up the process by "branching." Branching refers to going off the program (usually prior to redoing a lesson) to give some needed training. We usually use Word Charts (see below) but avoid training the specific error words, so when the child gets it right we know that it was not because we gave away the answer. If the child reaches the completion level but does not get all of the items correct, it is a good idea to give those error words by live voice. If necessary the clinician can tell the word and present it once again.

If the clinician is not using the PS program the general order of difficulty is vowel-consonant (v-c), c-v, c-v-c, consonant blend-vowel (bl-v), v-bl, bl-v-c, bl-v-bl. Longer sounds are generally easier for poor Decoders than short ones but there are notable exceptions (e.g., /l/ and /n/). Familiar words are generally easier than less familiar. Consonant blends may be quite difficult so at first it is a good idea before starting with a word like "bride" to first present "ride" sound by sound and then say, "Now this one is longer" and give "bride." If it is not successful do "ride" again and say, "Now let's put a /b/ sound in front of it."

Word Charts: Generally for PS repairs word charts are the most effective. A word chart (or a picture chart for someone who can't read) is a method to teach the skills that the individual has not yet gotten from the program. If the person made an error on a lesson in which the word "steel" was repeated as "seal" then it suggests that the person is having difficulty with the "st" blend. On another word there might have been a short-*e*/short-*a* confusion. A blank sheet of paper is usually folded into eight boxes. Avoid using the actual error words (unless all else fails), but use similar ones. In the top two spaces the words "store" and "sore" are entered. The next set is the words "bet" and "bat." In the third pair "sake" and "stake" are entered and in the last 2 boxes are "sad" and "said." They are presented first (sound-by-sound) for each pair and then all eight are shown and they are presented randomly. If there are errors try it again and exaggerate the difference (in desperation indicate the word and repeat it once again). Usually this is sufficient to remediate the problem. Later on in the program the same words or similar words are given in other contexts so the therapist is able to verify that the issue is resolved.

Evidence-Based Results of Phonemic Training

Our first controlled study, Katz and Medol (1972), compared two matched groups of children with *functional* articulation problems; one received Phonemic Synthesis (PS) training for one semester and the other received their regular speech therapy. Following the therapy the experimental group performed significantly better than the controls on the PS test. The more important finding, however, was that the improvement for the experimental group on the Goldman-Fristoe Articulation test was at the 0.01 level, whereas the control group did not improve significantly.

Katz and Harmon (1981) conducted a field study in four states (by four SLPs, one audiologist, and one reading specialist) including 54 children who received PS therapy and 31 controls who received their standard therapies. In this study the PS trained group (mean = 11 therapy sessions) was significantly improved on the three independent variables over the control group: Lindamood Auditory Conceptualization Test (p = 0.01), Arizona Articulation Proficiency Scale (p = 0.001), and the Phonemic Synthesis Test (p = 0.001) (Katz, 1983, p. 287). It appears that the PS therapy had a positive effect that generalized to other AP skills and speech articulation.

Kahler (1983) carried out a study with 60 children entering first grade all of whom were given the Phonemic Synthesis test and California Achievement Test (CAT) for reading. The top half on the PS test was considered "not-at-risk" for reading deficiency. The other 30 children were considered "at-risk" for reading. They were randomly divided into two groups: an experimental PS-trained group and a control group that received their normal programming. At the end of the semester the re-evaluation indicated that both the PS-trained and the not-at-risk groups were within normal limits on the CAT and PS tests and significantly better than the not treated at-risk group, which remained below normal on both tests. There was no significant difference between the two top groups.

These three studies indicate that Phonemic Synthesis training is a very effective therapeutic approach. They have shown impressive improvements in speech articulation and reading as well as stronger Decoding skills in other auditory processing tasks. In addition, as expected, the children showed much improved PS test performance.

In our current work we have been even more successful than in our previous therapy likely because of the addition of PTP to the PS training (Table 13–1). The average number of hours for 35 children who received Decoding training was 6.5 hours over an average of 13 sessions. The PS Quantitative Score is the number of words correct out of 25 on the Phonemic Synthesis test. The Qualitative Score is the Quantitative Score minus delayed and quick responses and quiet rehearsals on items that were otherwise correct. The Qualitative Score is considered the more informative score for those who

Table 13–1. Data for three measures (see text) to assess phonemic decoding improvement are shown. This initial PS and PTP therapy program consisted of an average of 13 therapy sessions for a mean of 6.5 hours devoted to Decoding. The subjects were 35 children (5 to 16 years of age) who were seen for Phonemic Decoding therapies and Speech-in-Noise training.

Test	Mean *(SD)* Pre	Mean *(SD)* Post	Mean *(SD)* Diff	t-Test *P*-value
PS Quantitative (# correct)	13.8 *(6.6)*	20.6 *(4.1)*	6.9 *(4.7)*	<0.001
PS Qualitative (# correct)	9.3 *(4.1)*	19.7 *(4.6)*	10.4 *(3.5)*	<0.001
Phonemic Error Analysis (# error)	51.9 *(20.1)*	30.5 *(12.8)*	21.4 *(14.5)*	<0.001

have had prior speech therapy, auditory training. or phonological awareness training. The average child had one such prior therapy. The third measure, the Phonemic Error Analysis is a tally of the phonemic confusions, omissions, and additions on the speech in quiet, speech in noise, SSW, and PS tests based on a total of 926 phonemes.

A Final Comment About Phonemic Decoding

An audiologist questioned whether working with phonemes was outside the scope of audiology and if phonemes should be considered part of auditory processing. The answers appeared obvious to this author, but apparently not to everyone. The audiologist was asked whether pure tones, noise, words, nonsense words, and sentences were processed auditorily and to each the answer was "yes." So the final question was, so why not phonemes? There was no response.

In regard to the scope of audiology all manner of sounds are part of audiology, why not phonemes? But more should be said regarding the importance of phonemes in audiology. From the beginning of central testing the temporal lobe and most specifically the middle-posterior superior portion was the audiologist's main interest and concern (Bocca et al., 1954; Katz, 1968). Importantly, recall that the three functions uniquely associated with the auditory cortex are phonemic discrimination, phonemic memory, and phonemic synthesis-analysis (Luria, 1966, 1970). These are the very same functions evaluated by the Phonemic Synthesis test (Katz, 1983) and remediated by the Phonemic Synthesis therapy (Katz & Harmon, 1981). Thus, there is no reason to exclude phonemic testing or therapy from the scope of audiology and there are many good reasons to include them. No central function is more basic to audiology and auditory processing than the phoneme.

Case Study

In therapy, generally children improve more than adults and those with developmental problems improve more than those with organic disorders. This case study looks at the therapeutic results for an adult with an organic disorder, mitochondrial myopathy (MM) (Pavlakis et al., 1988). MM is a progressive condition in which the mitochondria within certain cells of the body lose their potency to provide sufficient energy. When a large number of cells are affected it can lead to organ failure (e.g., lungs, parts of the brain). There is no known cure for MM and no effective treatment. "Sue" was in her early 20s when she began having symptoms of MM but it was not diagnosed until 20 years later. Sue had been a very good student and an excellent athlete, but MM caused major reading and spelling problems, cognitive decline, aphasic-type communication, and considerable physical limitations. She was 47 years old when first seen for central testing.

Unlike other patients seen for this therapy, initially Sue did not absorb or retain enough skill in the typical 14-week therapy program, so it was extended by five sessions followed by retest. The therapy consisted of the Phonemic Training Program followed by a Speech-in-Noise desensitization program and finally a

Phonemic Synthesis lesson. The total time spent on Decoding was about 9.5 hours. Table 13–2 shows the initial test findings and the post therapy results.

These results are most impressive. To gauge the level of her success on the three Decoding tasks, Sue's results in Table 13–2 can be compared to the means for the 35 children shown in Table 13–1.

Summary

This chapter provides a rationale for phonemic therapies to remediate phonemic Decoding problems as well as detailed information for two powerful approaches that have been used successfully for years to remediate Decoding problems were presented.

Table 13–2. Test results for the Phonemic Synthesis test, Phonemic Error Analysis, SSW, and the Speech-in Noise Difference (Quiet minus Noise) scores for the right and left ears for an adult patient with Mitochondrial Myopathy. For PS higher numbers are better, but for the other four measures lower numbers are better.

Test	Norm	Pretest	Posttest	Difference
PS Quantitative (# correct)	23	8	17*	+9
PS Qualitative (# correct)	22	3	15*	+12
Phonemic Error Analysis (# errors)	not normed	58	42**	+16
SSW (# errors)	6	38	19*	+19
Speech-in-Noise Diff (% error) Right	17	20	16	+4
Speech-in-Noise Diff (% error) Left	17	20	12	+8

*still significant on retest; ** apparently still significant; + = improved.

Key Points Learned

- The decoding category is often noted in those with APD.
- Phonemic Synthesis and Phonemic Training Program are two procedures that specifically target decoding difficulties.
- These approaches have been used most successfully for many years.
- Several studies have shown the effectiveness of PS therapy and current findings suggest further progress using both PS and PTP.
- Details for successful implementation of these approaches are discussed.

References

Bocca, E., Calearo, C., & Cassinari, V. (1954). A new method for testing hearing in temporal lobe tumors. *Acta Otolaryngogica, 44,* 219–221.

Duane, D. D. (1977). A neurological perspective of central auditory dysfunction. In R. W. Keith (Ed.), *Central auditory dysfunction* (pp. 1–42). New York Grune & Stratton.

Holm, V. A., & Kunze, L. H... (1969). Effect of chronic otitis media on language and speech development. *Pediatrics, 43,* 833–839.

Kahler, L. B. (1983, November). *Phonemic synthesis: A prediction of early reading success.* Paper presented at American Speech-Language-Hearing convention, Cincinnati, OH.

Katz, J. (1968). The SSW test: An interim report. *Journal of Speech and Hearing Disorders, 33,* 132–146.

Katz, J. (1983). Phonemic synthesis and other auditory skills. In E. Lasky & J. Katz (Eds.), *Central auditory processing disorders: Problems of speech, language and learning* (pp. 269–296). Baltimore: University Park Press.

Katz, J. (1992). Classification of auditory processing disorders In J. Katz, N. Stecker, & D. Henderson (Eds.), *Central auditory processing: A transdisciplinary-view* (pp. 81–92). Chicago: Mosby Yearbook.

Katz, J. (1998). Central auditory processing and cochlear implant therapy. In M. G. Masters, N. Stecker, & J. Katz (Eds.), *Central auditory processing disorders: Mostly management* (pp. 215–232). Boston: Allyn & Bacon.

Katz, J., & Burge, C. (1971). Auditory perception training for children with learning disabilities. *Menorah Medical Journal, 2,* 18–29.

Katz, J., & Harmon, C. (1981). Phonemic Synthesis: Diagnostic and training program. In R. Keith (Ed.), *Central auditory and language disorders in children* (pp. 145–147). San Diego, CA: College-Hill Press.

Katz, J., & Medol, E. (1972). The use of Phonemic Synthesis in speech therapy, *Menorah Medical Journal, 3,* 10–13.

Luria, A. R. (1966). *Higher cortical functions in man* (pp. 106–107). New York: Basic Books.

Luria, A. R. (1970). *Traumatic aphasias: Its syndrome, psychology and treatment* (pp. 118–119, 122). The Hague: Mouton.

Orton, S. T. (1937). *Reading, writing and speech problems in children* (pp. 158–159). New York: W. W. Norton.

Pavlakis, S., Rowland, L., DeVivo, D., Bonilla, E., & DiMauro, S. (1988). *Mitochondrial myopathies and encephalomyopathies. Advances in contemporary neurology* (pp. 95–133). Philadelphia: F.A. Davis.

Stovall, J. V., Manning, W. H., & Shaw, C. K. (1977). Auditory assembly of children with mild and severe articulations. *Folia Phoniatrica, 29,* 162–172.

Van Riper, C. (1954). *Speech correction: Principles and methods* (3rd ed., pp. 122–123). Englewood Cliffs, NJ: Prentice-Hall.

Winitz, H. (1973). Problem solving and the delaying of speech as strategies in the teaching of language. *Asha, 15,* 583–586.

14

Metacognitive Therapy Approaches

Patricia McAleer Hamaguchi

Overview

In this chapter, metacognition, and the important role it plays in the top-down piece of an intervention plan is discussed. A metacognitive therapy approach for APD emphasizes increasing our awareness of the listening process itself, then appropriately adjusting our listening "set" and actions accordingly. In this chapter, the history of the study of metacognition, its application in other fields, and the features of a successful metacognitive program that helps to enhance the processing of spoken language are examined.

What Is Metacognition?

Imagine you are on your way to an airport. Time is running short, and somewhere you made a wrong turn. As your heart starts to race a bit, you pull over to a gas station to ask someone how to find the airport. The conversation goes something like this:

> *You:* "Excuse me, I'm looking for the airport. Do you know how I can get there?"
>
> *Helpful Man:* "Oh, yes, sure! You just go back out to the road and go r . . . (Loud truck zooms by, so you move closer and follow his lips even more closely), then when you get to the light, turn right at the McDonald's." His arm is waving and he is pointing in that direction, so you quickly transfer your gaze to his body language. "You'll probably go down—oh, I don't know—maybe 2 miles, then you—"
>
> *You:* "Would you mind if I grabbed a pen and started jotting this down? (You grab a piece of paper and pen and begin writing) So— when I pull out of this parking lot I turn right? (On the paper, you simply put R)
>
> *Helpful Man:* "Yes, turn right, and when you get to the light, you'll make a right at McDonald's."
>
> *You:* "Do you know the name of that street?"
>
> *Helpful Man:* "Uh . . . Cooper Avenue. Turn right there, and go about 2 miles and then you'll see the airport on your left."

On your paper, you just write the key words and letters that will help jog your memory:

1. R
2. LT: McD-R (Cooper)
3. 2 mi. on L

When you get back into the car, your friend who is driving asks you where to go. She turns down the talk radio station she has been listening to, but doesn't turn her head, keeping her eyes on the road. You use your handy info that has been scrawled onto the back of an old envelope to give her the directions. As she is driving, she doesn't have the luxury of reading it, instead she repeats them back to you, which she has boiled down this way, "Ok, so we go right—right on Cooper—2 miles, got it." As she restates it, she is sketching the pathway in the air with her right index finger. For a moment she is looking in one spot and visualizing the path, committing it to memory.

You arrive at the airport, in time.

How did you do it? Without even realizing it, you both utilized a number of metacognitive strategies that were helpful in getting the information in, processing it, and remembering it. Some of these include:

1. Taking action to improve the signal-to-noise ratio (when you moved closer to the man giving directions to compensate for the ambient truck noise).
2. Lip-reading (to aid in the poor acoustic environment).
3. Utilizing body language and gestures to aid in comprehension (when you transferred your gaze from the man's mouth to his gestures).
4. Taking action to aid in remembering the information (getting the paper and pen).

5. Pulling out the salient, key words to aid in recall (writing down just key words and abbreviations).
6. Checking back with the speaker to reconfirm comprehension, including giving some acoustic highlighting to the information in question (I take a right?)
7. Chunking important information together (McDonald's—Right)
8. Establishing a good listening set (When the driver anticipated the need to attend to the directions, she first turned down the radio).
9. Supplementing verbal directions with gestures to help commit them to memory (when the driver used her hand to indicate the path she needed to take).
10. Visualizing (when the driver pictured turning right at the McDonald's in her room).
11. Verbal rehearsal, also known as subvocalizing and reauditorization (repeating the information to commit to memory).

Most of us use these strategies without even thinking about it. They are automatic, and an integrated part of our communication process. For many people with auditory processing disorders, as well as language processing disorders, these steps require careful teaching and practice to become habituated. When we bring this thinking process to the conscious level, we are tapping into metacognition: "thinking about the thinking process." A metacognitive approach requires that we analyze the demands of the listening task and make behavioral changes in the way we carry out the task. Metacognitive strategies are an important tool in facilitating a more successful communication exchange, and for maximizing the auditory processing function.

There are some misconceptions about metacognitive strategies. Metacognition is not just about "repair strategies," which are helpful during a communication breakdown. They are not merely "compensatory strategies" which are designed to make up for the auditory weakness, such as note-taking skills. Metacognitive strategies require anticipating the listening/attending demands of the task and regulating one's thinking process in response to those demands, to *reduce* the need for repair strategies. They are a "top-down" piece to the intervention of auditory processing disorders. In this section, more information about how to integrate metacognitive approaches into your therapy plan is presented.

History/Theoretical Background on the Topic of Metacognition

In the 1960s, J. H. Flavell, a psychologist, first began writing about metacognition. His early works and research focused on the application of metacognition during the learning process, including how infants learn. He sought to find out and define the thinking process itself, and how it relates not only to cognition, but also processing and memory tasks, and how direct intervention in these areas can impact the learning process. His later works (*Cognitive Development*, 2002) have looked at social cognition and language learning, and what we know about these now, given current research and understanding. Flavell acknowledged the difficulty in defining metacognition. It is typically described, rather than defined, but Flavell (1979) said it is "knowledge and cognition about cognitive phenomena" (p. 906).

Metacognition involves a higher order thinking ability and is linked to intelligence (Borkowski, Carr, & Pressley, 1990). Inner knowledge of our thinking process requires a level of self-regulation and executive control. Developmentally, younger children (first grade) tend to be less insightful as to whether or not their responses are correct or not (Bisanz, Vesonder, & Voss, 1978). An analysis by Kail (1991) of 72 studies suggests processing speed is also affected by developmental maturity. Flavell (2002) suggests that "the faster the processing, the greater the amount of information that can be kept "alive" or "on stage" at once in active, working memory." The development of executive function, insight, and working memory are all factors which aid in the ability of children to perform language processing tasks, particularly through the auditory modality.

This might lead one to ask, "What are the cognitive requirements of a metacognitive intervention program?" Research in early literacy has shown that even young children (first grade) are able to utilize and report metacognitive strategies they employed during reading and writing activities (Brenna, 1995; Cox 1994). Piaget's model of cognitive development tells us that from about the age of 7, a child begins to acquire perspective-taking and higher order cognitive skills that would lend themselves well to metacognitive approaches. However, Flavell (2002) challenges the assumption that a child moves neatly from one phase to the next, and that a host of influences, including biology, environment, and so forth interact within the child to mold his or her cognitive process. Therefore, one is cautioned to individualize any intervention program, based on the child's needs and developmental readiness for any given approach.

Researchers in other fields have examined how metacognition is useful in tasks such as memory, music, learning match concepts, addressing emotional and psychological problems, and attention. The application of metacognitive learning principles can also extend to literacy learning. In *Metacognition in Literacy Learning* (Israel et al., 2005), the authors lay a groundwork in which a reader is taught how to apply metacognitive strategies to the reading process. This is accomplished through self-questioning, self-regulation, application of specified rubrics, and the use of strategies, which are carefully selected by the reader before, during, and after the reading task.

Metacognition and the Field of Auditory Processing Disorders

In the field of auditory processing disorders, experts have long advocated utilizing metacognitive therapy approaches (Bellis, 2003; Chermak, 2003; Geffner & Wynne, 2001; Hamaguchi, 2002a) to supplement the intensive auditory training that often is required for those with APD. Metacognitive intervention is not meant to supplant the need for auditory skills training and should not be considered the complete, or comprehensive, program for someone with APD. It is always a piece—albeit an important one—in the intervention plan.

Chermak and Musiek (1997) describe a metacognitive approach which they refer to as *attribution training*, as well as cognitive behavior training. The components of these approaches, as well as the one discussed later in this section, have several common features. Most importantly, the participants must take an active and willing role in the therapeutic process, as well as possess the cognitive ability to make analytical judgments about their role in the auditory processing task.

Metacognitive intervention strategies for APD are the application of a psychological principle against the backdrop of a disordered auditory system. The resulting APD symptoms (missing part of the message, "mishearing" what was said, auditory fatigue or inattention, etc.) often overlap other disorders, which are discussed in other chapters. To that end, applying these principles within the context of an intervention plan that addresses these coexisting conditions, such as language processing weakness or attention deficits, can be appropriate as well, with individual modifications as needed.

Within the larger category of metacognition, there are two related subcategories: metalinguistics (conscious knowledge of the structure and use of language) and metamemory (awareness and use of memory strategies). Certain skills, such as "phonemic awareness" can be considered metalinguistic in nature when the child is taught to recognize sound or syllable patterns, as well as define word and sound boundaries. The role of auditory memory for language continues to be a somewhat controversial topic among those who work in the field of APD. Audiologists tend to view auditory memory as a function of the language system and not necessarily a component of APD. SLPs tend to regard auditory memory as a function of both the language and auditory system and therefore assess it and treat it in the context of an auditory processing disorder. Strategies designed to enhance one's working memory, such as subvocalizing, chunking, and mnemonics can also accurately be called "metamemory" strategies. In this chapter, they are included as part of a comprehensive metacognitive intervention program.

Visualization occurs when one hears a word (e.g., "cat") and is able mentally to conjure a picture or representation of the word in the mind. It is usually done automatically by the listener, at a rate that can keep up with the input of language, whether it is a verbal stimulus or a written one. It requires quick modification ("a huge, white hairy cat") of the initial image, as more information becomes known. The ability to visualize—rapidly and accurately—is essential in order to translate the auditory input into something meaningful to the listener. Although getting the auditory input into the listener's ear accurately is the function of auditory training, visualization can be considered the "end stage" of this process. For some, it requires careful teaching, practice, and conscious implementation. When it is utilized as a tool to aid in the successful processing of auditory language, I consider it an additional component in the metacognitive "bag of tricks" which may need direct intervention, and thus, it is included in this discussion on metacognitive intervention strategies.

Developing a Metacognitive Intervention Plan

"Thinking about thinking" can be a useful strategy; however, because mental "multi-tasking" (listening to the content + simultaneously analyzing one's environment and thought process) can be distracting unto itself, it is important not to overdo it. Communication is best done in a spontaneous and interactive way. A metacognitive intervention program should be utilized as a way to help habituate behaviors which in most people are already instinctive. By integrating them into one's daily life, the need for conscious and deliberate application should diminish, or at the very most, provide tools to employ during higher- demand listening tasks.

At this time, there are no commercially-available standardized tests to assess one's metacognitive skills, although their successful application should be observable in higher scores on certain tests, such as auditory comprehension of language or auditory memory. The power in using metacognitive strategies is that the listener not only improves his ability to perform discrete tasks in a clinical setting, but that all these pieces are then put together in a functional listening environment, where the listener can then thoughtfully choose where and when to employ these tools in a more naturalistic context.

To decide which metacognitive skills to target, the clinician needs to analyze listening behaviors during assessment tasks, as well as informal conversational interchanges, and to take careful notes. The school-based clinician is in a particularly advantageous position in that these behaviors can also be clinically observed during directed teaching lessons and group discussions. Do the responses indicate the client forgot part of the message? Misheard it? Did he apply any strategies when the tasks became too difficult? Is he attending to the message? Where is the breakdown? How is the client responding to it? What could have been done to avoid the breakdown? Does he say anything when his communicative partner is talking way too fast or mumbling? Does the client have insight into his listening behaviors? Does he possess the lexicon to express it? By paying careful attention to these issues, the clinician can assist in developing behaviors and skills that will increase the likelihood for more success during the auditory processing task.

The steps below are part of a comprehensive metacognitive system I call "**ARCA**," and are a handy way to help the client remember to implement the strategies taught in daily life. The client is told:

1. **A**nticipate and adjust your listening set
2. **R**egulate your thought process and behavior accordingly
3. **C**ommunicate and/or
4. **A**ct to solve listening challenges.

Table 14–1 provides further suggestions for ways in which the SLP can survey the client's metacognitive skills during the assessment process.

Table 14–1. Metacognitive Behaviors Observed During the Auditory and Language Assessment Process Using the ARCA Process

1. Anticipating and adjusting the child's listening set:

- ☐ Does the child straighten up and stop moving when told he will have to listen carefully (such as during a rote word memory task)?
- ☐ Does he interrupt during the instructions or when listening to the testing prompts?

2. Regulating his thought process and behavior

- ☐ Does he appear to use subvocalizing (reauditorization) when attempting to hold and recall a series of numbers or words? (Look for moving lips or an actual repetition of the prompts under his breath)
- ☐ During rote auditory memory tasks, when the number of words to recall becomes longer, does he "blank out" and have difficulty remembering anything? (Indication there is a need for teaching strategies)
- ☐ When making errors on rote auditory memory tasks, does he substitute words with no relationship in meaning, but similar in phonemic content ("bell" for "ball")? (Indication there is memory for the phonemic shape of the words, but no visualization)
- ☐ When making errors on rote auditory memory tasks, does he substitute words with similar meanings ("kitten" for "cat")? Indicates he did visualize the prompt, but did not note the phonemic shape.
- ☐ When given inordinately long or complex oral directions that are too difficult, does the child seem to know that he "doesn't know it" or does he seem unaware of his errors?
- ☐ Does the child shift visual focus to the testing pictures (such as during the CELF "Following Directions" subtest) or look around the room/pick at his fingers until he is required to respond?

3. Communicate to Solve Listening Challenges

- ☐ When you set up foils (such as purposely mumbling or coughing during a conversation and then asking a question) does the child indicate he couldn't hear you?
- ☐ Does the child articulate the nature of the listening challenge or simply say, "I don't know"?

4. Act to Solve Listening Challenges

- ☐ Does the child attend to your lips during listening tasks when you purposely have set up loud music or talking in the background? (It helps to speak real softly to elicit this)
- ☐ Does the parent or teacher report that the child takes action (turning down the TV, moving closer to the speaker) when it is difficult to hear?

A metacognitive approach requires the listener to transition from one who is a passive listener, to an *active listener*. Although educational modifications and visual supports are excellent compensatory strategies, they require action on the part of the professionals working with the child with the disorder. They require very little of the child. As we know that APD is in large part a long-term challenge, it is critical that children with APD become keen observers of their environment and the requirements of each listening demand. It is the clinician's job to provide them with a "bag of tricks" from which they can pull strategies at a time when they need them. Teaching them which strategy to utilize and when, is part of the intervention plan. Often taught initially in a controlled therapy setting, carryover to a naturalistic context is the key to a successful transference of these skills. Our goal is to transition a child from being a passive or inattentive listener to an active one who attends, processes, and initiates action to increase the likelihood of an accurate response.

Application of Metacognitive Strategies with the ARCA Model

In working with children who have spoken language processing weaknesses, including APD, the following activities are particularly helpful in facilitating a change in the approach to the listening process. When introducing these concepts in the context of a metacognitive therapy intervention, clinicians should guide the child, rather than directly provide the answer. The process works best when the participant finds the information for himself, rather than by having it spoon-fed. Remember that "thinking about thinking" will most likely take place when the child makes the discoveries by himself. When information is presented—and the child is merely told what to do and how to do it—it ceases to be a metacognitive intervention. Self-discovery helps lead to self-regulation.

Although there is no specified order in which these are to be introduced, it helps to address attention and "listening-set" issues first, if there are weaknesses in these areas. The rest of the activities should be selected according to the child's individual needs. The use of the ARCA model can help implement metacognitive strategies as follows:

1. Anticipate and Adjust your Listening Set

- *Survey the listening environment.* What level of attention is needed?

Together, you can develop a grading system to gauge the level of attention one would anticipate, given the listening task. Children who like numbers may prefer a numeric-based system, whereas others may prefer to have something visual that they can color or draw.

Remember to use situations that are most likely to come up in the child's everyday life. Take note that for one child, a particular situation may require a different level of focus than another. For example, when one child is given a verbal list of items to retrieve from upstairs, it may or may *not* be the highest demand auditory task for him, depending on his auditory memory strength. For some, listening with background noise or distortion, such as in a reverberant gymnasium, is the ultimate listening challenge, but for others it may not be. Remember that there are different strengths and weaknesses within the category of "APD" and so it is important that the client's individuality be appropriately considered.

Here are some samples of grading systems:

Numeric:

1 to 10 (10 being most difficult listening environment)

Mnemonic device:

A—Alert for specific information, but perhaps multitasking (e.g. name being called)

B—Be a polite listener (e.g. during classmates' presentations, routine social conversations)

C—Clearly time to be in CHARGE (e.g. oral directions, new information)

Visual display: Thermometers with different levels of red

- *Make adjustments in the level of attention needed.*

This requires the child take action, once the listening environment has been defined, if needed. Varying the level of attention for one with APD is particularly important. Experience has shown that sometimes children with APD underattend ("tune-out") because they are not assigning enough significance to the task, or are "overattending," resulting in auditory fatigue and missing the main idea or salient details. Modulating one's listening set could be compared to approaching reading with a specific purpose, and therefore selecting the reading rate accordingly (Slow and careful? Just skim?). For example, with a high-demand listening task, the child will need to know how to ready his body and mind to receive auditory input. There are programs (*It's Time to Listen,* 2002, Hamaguchi) that provide instruction on how to lead a child to developing a listening set, usually involving a stable body position and eye contact.

It is important to note here that in some subtypes of APD (Bellis, 2006) it is in fact better for the child to avoid a focused listening task while maintaining eye-contact at the same time, due to the poor integration of the left/right hemispheres. Likewise, for children with AD/HD or certain balance weaknesses, it may be preferable for the child to be allowed to move in a quiet way, such as squeezing a squishy ball. It is thought that this extraneous motion can sometimes give the extra energy somewhere to go so that the child does not have to expend mental energy on the task of staying still.

- *Reduce interrupting behaviors to maintain listening set.*

When the child attempts to respond or act before the auditory input has been completed, he misses part of the incoming message. It jolts his attentive "listening set." Likewise, it also means the child is busy formulating his own plan of action and reducing his attention on the listening task itself. Work directly on having the child practice waiting until the auditory input has been completed before responding.

2. Regulate Your Thought Process and Behavior Accordingly

- *Shift your visual focus during the listening task according to the demands of the situation.*

While we often stress maintaining eye contact with the speaker, there are times when the listener is required to look at something else, such as what is written on the board, or a page in a book, while still listening to auditory input. Knowing when to transfer the visual focus back to the speaker, or even to another target (such as a classmate who is asking a question), is a practical skill that sometimes needs direct practice. The "back and forth" reference points we need to follow during a conversation assist us in comprehension. For some, particularly those with interhemispheric transfer weakness, combining these two tasks is a challenge, as it stimulates the left and right hemispheres simultaneously. Likewise, noting body language, facial expression, and gestures and comparing the information against the actual words/tone presented requires executive function and integrative skills that are often weak in those with APD. In a metacognitive intervention program, it is important to help the listener become alert to these kinds of challenges and make a plan so that auditory focus can be maintained while still visually scanning something else.

- *Attend to and select the most salient part of the message.*

"Ok, class. Please take out your pencils and your open up your math book to page 82. Jim, hurry up and get your drink, and then get back to your seat. Okay, I'd like all of you to work on the first three rows, then we'll go over it together. Any questions?"

Let's pretend your client is now really good at recognizing when he needs to get focused and utilize his very best "listening set." How, then, does he know which part of this message he needs to listen to? Which part to remember? Before he can apply memory techniques and note-taking strategies, he needs to know what is important. Whereas it is usually quite obvious to us, it is often not so obvious to someone who has struggled to assign the proper degree of attention to the right parts of the message. To improve this skill, consider the following in Table 14–2.

- *Remember the salient parts of the spoken message.*

There are a number of metamemory devices that are helpful in keeping

Table 14–2. What's Important?

• Pick out key words from directions
• Listen for voice emphasis and watch body language in conversations
• Attend to information that answers "who, what, where, when, how and why" questions
• Focus on temporal concepts (before, after, during)
• Names, names, names! Use strategies to commit names and related details to memory

auditory input in our mental "holding tank" long enough for us to attach meaning to it, as well as remember it for short and long periods of time. These include: subvocalizing (reauditorizing), chunking, self-gesturing (particularly for spatial concepts and adjectives) mnemonics, and setting words to music or using a sing-song pattern.

Once a client is able to identify the salient parts of a direction, story, lecture, and conversation, the clinician can work on integrating the metamemory strategies with note-taking skills, particularly in upper–grade elementary and older children. For example, if the teacher gives an assignment (e.g., "For tonight's homework, I'd like you to do the first two rows on the top of page 34") what part of this direction should be held in one's working memory? What is the best way to keep it there until you can grab a pencil and write it down? What should you write down? Lots of role-playing in typical school and home situations will help the child learn how to do this.

- *Visualize what is heard.*

There are two primary methods that are used to help facilitate the increased visualization of language. The Lindamood-Bell Visualizing and Verbalizing™ program (Bell, 1991) utilizes a systematic self-questioning technique to help the client visualize and verbally describe the image in greater detail, facilitated by core words (e.g., size?). It was developed as a tool for aiding reading comprehension, but has some application for auditory processing disorders, particularly those with a well-developed vocabulary and auditory memory.

Another method described by Dr. Musiek (2003), as well as this author (2002), is designed to guide the visualization process by tapping into the right hemisphere, (e.g., drawing/sketching) which is particularly helpful for those with less developed verbal strengths, poor auditory memory, and who need to work on interhemispheric transfer activities. Because quick sketching requires the ability to hear and pick out the salient aspects of a sentence or story, it is particularly helpful for those who need work in this area. It is this author's experience that this method is most effective for those who need assistance in visualizing language at its most basic level (e.g., "his socks" would need to depict a male figure and at least two socks) and for those who struggle with word retrieval. The client then uses his sketch to stimulate the verbal description of what he heard. In time, the steps are compressed so that the process is more mental than actually drawn out. For some children, working at this level first and then moving on to a higher level program, such as the Visualizing and Verbalizaing™ can be quite effective.

3. Communicate to Solve Listening Challenges

- *Verbal repair strategies.*

Once a client has learned to recognize communication breakdowns due to a listening "challenge," it becomes imperative to work on the specific language one would need to use to troubleshoot listening dilemmas. Asking the other communicative partner to say or do something specific is a key element in this process. Through role-playing and simulated situations, one can begin to teach and reinforce the use of these language structures. It is also helpful to work with adults in the child's academic and home environment. Some examples:

a. "I'm sorry. I couldn't hear what you said. Could you repeat that a little louder, please?"
b. "I'm sorry. Could just tell me one direction at a time? It's hard for me to remember all that."
c. "I don't know what the word, "explicit" means. Could you explain that to me?"
d. "I'm sorry. Could you say that again a little more slowly?"
e. "Can we turn down the TV so I can hear you better?"
f. "Mom, it's hard for me to have this conversation from the back seat. Can you speak up a little?"

4. Act to Solve Listening Challenges

- *Take steps to improve your listening environment.*

When analyzing our listening environment, we need to determine if, in fact, the speech signal is reaching us with sufficient clarity and volume, so that we can then process the information accurately. Is the fan humming too loudly? Is the teacher too far away? The clinician should lead the child toward a fairly comprehensive list of situations that might be encountered, and encourage the use of a daily "listening challenges" journal. This can be reviewed to help bring this awareness to a more conscious level.

Being alert to a compromised signal is the first step, but taking action to change it requires initiation. For some, this aspect is the greater challenge. By using puppets or role-playing, we can help the child learn to develop a mental "tool kit" to use when the speech signal cannot be heard well. Some examples are given in Table 14-3.

Work on transferring these concepts into functional settings. Reward and praise the child for taking action and responsibility for his own listening, regardless of whether the ultimate outcome (e.g., responding to a verbal question) is correct. Improving the child's listening behavior is a critical part of the process. The accuracy of the auditory processing is the long-term goal, but taking action to improve the clarity of the input, is a short-term goal that will lead there, and should be encouraged and practiced as well.

Table 14–3. Mental Tool Kit

a. Move closer to the person talking
b. Close the window or door
c. Attend to the person's lips when acoustics are poor
d. Ask the person to stand closer to you
e. Turn off/down the noise-producing object
f. Use an assistive listening device
g. Move the conversation to another location

Summary

Metacognition is a cognitive-based teaching strategy that is utilized in a variety of learning contexts. It is advocated by many experts in the field of auditory processing disorders as a helpful, "top-down" component to a comprehensive intervention plan, including the introduction of metamemory and metalinguistic strategies. The underlying principles of metacognitive intervention require a deeper awareness of one's individual thought process, and the desire and ability to regulate it in response to the cognitive demands of each situation. By providing our clients with a variety of strategies (e.g. establishing a listening "set," chunking, subvocalizing, visualizing, self-questioning, etc.) they can pick and choose when and where to employ the most appropriate tools to process what they hear with greater accuracy.

Key Points Learned

- Metacognition involves increasing our awareness of our own internal thought and learning process.
- Metacognitive approaches can be utilized in the teaching of other subjects.
- Metacognitive strategies are referred to as "top-down" interventions.
- Metacognitive strategies are only one piece in a comprehensive intervention plan for those with APD.
- A successful metacognitive program requires motivation and action on the part of the participant.
- A suggested model by this author is called ARCA:
  1. **A**nticipate and adjust your listening set
  2. **R**egulate your thought process and behavior accordingly
  3. **C**ommunicate to solve listening challenges
  4. **A**ct to solve listening challenges

References

American Speech-Language-Hearing Association. (2004). *(Central) auditory processing disorders: Working Group on Auditory Processing Disorders* [Technical report]. Rockville, MD: Author.

Bell, N. (1991). *Visualizing and verbalizing.* Paso Robles, CA: Academy of Reading Publications.

Bellis, T. (2003). *Assessment and management of central auditory processing disorders in the education setting* (2nd ed.). Clifton Park, NY: Thomson Delmar Learning.

Bellis, T. (2006) *Definition, diagnosis and treatment of auditory processing disorders: Current perspectives.* Presentation; Roseville, CA.

Bisanz, G. L., Vesonder, G. T., & Voss, J. (1978). Knowledge of one's own responding and the relation of such knowledge to learning: A developmental study. *Journal of Experimental Child Psychology*, 25, 116–128.

Borkowski, J. G., Carr, M., Rellinger, E., & Pressley, M. (1990) Self-regulated cognition: Interdependence of metacognition, attributions, and self-esteem. In B. F. Jones & L. Idol (Eds.), *Dimensions of thinking and cognitive instruction* (pp. 53–92). Hillsdale, NJ: Lawrence Erlbaum.

Brenna, B. A. (1995). The metacognitive reading strategies of five early readers. *Journal of Research in Reading, 18*(1), 53–62.

Chermak, G. D. (2003, November). *Auditory processing disorders: Identification, intervention, and management with school-age children.* Presentation at ASHA Conference, Scottsdale, AZ.

Chermak, G. D., & Musiek, F. E. (1997). *Central auditory processing disorders: New perspectives.* San Diego, CA: Singular Publishing Group.

Cox, B. E. (1994). Young children's regulatory talk: Evidence of emergent metacognitive control over literary products and processes. In R. Ruddell, M. Rudell, & H. Singer (Eds.), *Theoretical models and processes of reading* (4th ed., pp. 733–756). Neward, DE: International Reading Association.

Flavell, J. H. (1979). Metacognition and cognitive monitoring: A new area of cognitive-developmental inquiry. *American Psychologist, 34,* 906–911.

Flavell, J. H., Miller, P. H, Miller, S. A. 2002. *Cognitive development* (4th ed.). Upper Saddle River, NJ: Prentice-Hall.

Geffner, D., & Wynne, M. (2001). *Identification and remediation of central auditory processing disorders.* Paper presented at the California Speech-Language-Hearing Association, San Diego, CA.

Hamaguchi, P. M. (2002a). *A metacognitive program for treating auditory processing disorders.* San Antonio, TX: Pro-Ed.

Hamaguchi, P. M. (2002b). *It's time to listen: metacognitive activities for improving auditory processing in the classroom.* San Antonio, TX: Pro-Ed.

Israel, S., Block, C. C., Bauserman, K., & Kinnucan-Welsch, K. (2005). *Metacognition in literacy learning.* Mawah, NJ: Lawrence Erlbaum.

Kail, R. V. (1991). Development of processing speed in childhood and adolescence. In H. W. Reese (Ed.), *Advances in child development and behavior* (Vol. 23). San Diego, CA: Academic Press.

Musiek, F. (2003, November). *Auditory processing disorders: Identification, intervention, and management with school-age children.* Presentation at ASHA Conference. Scottsdale, AZ.

15

Dichotic Interaural Intensity Difference (DIID) Training

Principles and Procedures

Jeffrey A. Weihing
Frank E. Musiek

Overview

Dichotic Interaural Intensity Difference training was designed to address deficits in dichotic processing. In dichotic processing tasks, a different stimulus is presented simultaneously to each ear and the patient is asked to repeat back one or both stimuli. Individuals who have lesions of the corpus callosum generally show left ear deficits when asked to complete a dichotic processing task. This training protocol attempts to strengthen these weaker left ear pathways by manipulating interaural intensity differences. The flexibility of administration makes this a technique that can be utilized formally in most clinical settings. Additionally, case studies and group data have shown this protocol to be efficacious.

Introduction

Dichotic Interaural Intensity Difference (DIID) training is an auditory rehabilitation procedure that has its roots in "split brain" case studies conducted in the late 1970s. It was then that Musiek et al. (1979) showed that auditory deficits in these patients, caused by a processing disorder of the central nervous system, could be alleviated when the interaural intensity difference between the ears was manipulated. That is, if sound was made softer in one ear, performance in the other ear tended to improve.

It is only within the past decade or so, however, that these observations have made their way into a formal auditory training procedure that can be used clinically. Interestingly, this procedure is most commonly applied, not in cases of "split brain" patients, but in children with learning disabilities in which an auditory system deficit plays some role. Although there are obvious differences between these two clinical groups, a similar physiological mechanism may contribute to both (Milner et al, 1968; Musiek et al., 1979; Musiek et al., 1982; Musiek et al., 1984; Sparks & Geschwind, 1968).

The following chapter discusses the conceptual and physiological foundations of the DIID, in addition to detailing how the procedure can be conducted in the clinic. Although research is still ongoing, initial studies suggest the DIID is an efficacious auditory training procedure.

Dichotic Processing

Background

The DIID is a form of auditory training that addresses central auditory deficits in dichotic processing (Baran et al., 2006; Musiek et al., 2002; Musiek & Schochat, 1998). It utilizes plasticity in an attempt to establish beneficial, long-term changes in the central auditory system (Musiek et al., 2002). Because the DIID specifically targets dichotic processing, it is necessary to consider the nature and measurement of this process before providing a detailed discussion of the training. Although the DIID may generalize to other types of auditory deficits, it was designed to address this specific mechanism.

The term dichotic refers to the fact that a different stimulus is presented to each ear simultaneously, and is distinguished from diotic tasks, in which the same stimulus is presented to both ears at the same time, and monotic tasks, in which a stimulus is being presented to only one ear. In a clinical dichotic paradigm, a patient is asked to recall one or both the auditory stimuli being presented. If both left and right ear stimuli are asked to be recalled, then the task is one of binaural integration. If the stimulus from only one ear is to be recalled, and the other ignored, then the task is one of binaural separation (Musiek, 1999; Musiek et al., 2002; Musiek & Pinheiro, 1985). For example, in a binaural integration paradigm, if the word "hot dog" was presented to the left ear and "pancake" was presented to the right ear, the expected response would be "hot dog, pancake." In a binaural separation paradigm, the patient might be asked to repeat the right ear stimulus only and would say "pancake." Although both binaural integration and separation tasks are similar in execution, the physiological mechanism underlying these two tasks varies somewhat.

A variety of tests can be used to diagnose dichotic processing deficits in the clinic. Most of these tests utilize single words or utterances, although several tests have been developed that make use of sentence material. Table 15–1 summarizes some of the dichotic tests more commonly used in clinical practice. For reasons that are discussed below, left ear performance is commonly below normal limits in cases of dichotic processing deficits (Musiek et al., 2002; Musiek & Schochat, 1998). Therefore, a patient with this deficit might score 50% in the left ear and 90% in the right ear on the dichotic digits.

Table 15–1. Dichotic Tests

Test	Stimulus Example	Citation
Dichotic Digits	Left Ear—1, 2 Right Ear—5, 8	Musiek, F. E. (1983). Assessment of central auditory dysfunction: The dichotic digit test revisited. *Ear and Hearing*, *4*, 79–83.
Dichotic Rhyme	Left Ear—pill Right Ear—bill	Wexler, B., & Halwes, T. (1983). Increasing the power of dichotic methods: The fused rhymed words test. *Neuropsychologia*, *21*, 59–66.
Dichotic CVs	Left Ear—ta Right Ear—da	Berlin, C. I., Lowe-Bell, S. S., Jannetta, P. J., & Kline, D. G. (1972). Central auditory deficits after temporal lobectomy. *Archives of Otolaryngology*, *96*, 4–10.
Staggered Spondaic Words (SSW)	Left Ear—wash**tub** Right Ear—**black**board (bold portions are simultaneous)	Katz, J. (1962). The use of staggered spondaic words for assessing the integrity of the central auditory system. *Journal of Auditory Research*, *2*, 327–337.
Competing Sentences Test	Left Ear—I'm expecting a phone call. Right Ear—Please answer the doorbell.	Willeford, J. (1978). Sentence tests of central auditory function. In J. Katz (Ed.), *Handbook of Clinical Audiology*. Baltimore: Williams & Wilkins.
SSI	Left Ear—A small boat with a picture has become. Right Ear—[a competing passage about Davy Crockett]	Jerger, J. F., & Jerger, S. W. (1974). Auditory findings in brainstem disorders. *Archives of Otolaryngology*, *99*, 342–349.

These scores would indicate that, while the right is performing normally, the left ear performance is beyond normal limits. Ultimately, the goal of the DIID is to bring the performance of the left ear up into the normal range while retaining the good right ear performance. Although similar gains might be expected in cases of right ear deficits, this pattern is much less common.

Clinicians are encouraged to establish their own normative values for each of the dichotic tests in the population that they treat. Because unpredictable variations in performance may occur with certain populations, clinic-specific norms are very important. However, normative values have been published for most of the dichotic tests shown in Table 15–1, and these norms can be used as a guideline for testing in the absence of other norms. Special consideration should be given to the patient with hearing loss, as this will undoubtedly affect test performance. For instance, dichotic digits normative values of 90% for both the left and right ears have been suggested for normal hearing individuals, but 80% is a more reasonable norm for individuals with hearing loss (Musiek, 1999).

There is a neuromaturational time course to dichotic processing that must also be taken into consideration when interpreting test results (Musiek & Gollegly, 1988). This time course applies more to left than right ear performance, as right ear performance is usually quite good even at an early age. For left ear performance, the age of maturation can be as late as 10 years of age, especially for more linguistically loaded dichotic tasks (e.g., sentence material) (Musiek & Gollegly, 1988). Therefore, consideration of age-related variations in normative values is important for the pediatric patient.

Regardless of the age of the patient, it should be noted that lesions which contribute to dichotic processing deficits can also lead to abnormal performance on other types of auditory processing tests. For instance, scores on some temporal processing tests, like the frequency and duration patterns, will often be below normal limits in cases of dichotic processing deficits (Musiek et al., 1980). These tests can be used in conjunction with dichotic tests to aid in diagnosis.

Physiological Mechanisms

The current application of the DIID is built upon what is known of the physiological mechanisms underlying dichotic processing. In the central auditory nervous system, two main pathways extend from the periphery to the auditory cortex. The stronger of these two pathways consists of the contralateral connections, which connect the left periphery to the right hemisphere and the right periphery to the left hemisphere. However, there also exist weaker ipsilateral connections which connect, for instance, the left periphery to the left hemisphere (Pickles, 1982). As animal models have shown, the ipsilateral connections may be weaker, in part, because there are more contralateral connections in the central nervous system (Rosenzweig, 1951; Tunturi, 1946).

Utilization of these two pathways depends on the mode of stimulation. When a stimulus is presented monotically, both the contralateral and ipsilateral pathways are used to bring the neural signal to the cerebrum. For instance, if "hot dog" is presented to the right ear, the ipsilateral connections will bring the signal to the right hemisphere, whereas the contralateral connections will bring the signal to the left hemisphere. The situation changes, however, when stimuli are presented dichotically at equal sensation levels. The contralateral connections will still carry the signal, but the ipsilateral connections will now be suppressed to some degree (Hall & Goldstein, 1968; Rosenzweig, 1951). This means that, under dichotic conditions, the pathways contributing to auditory processing are mainly the stronger contralateral connections. Presumably, this suppression of the ipsilateral connections occurs because of overlap between the two pathways at some point along the ascending route (Kimura, 1961). Competition by the two pathways for critical neural substrate may also contribute to suppression of the ipsilateral connections.

The conditions described above assume passive stimulation without requiring the patient to make a response. How does the situation change when the patient is asked to repeat back what is heard in a dichotic task? Figure 15–1 depicts this scenario. Both signals, again presented at equal sensation levels, need to reach the language areas in the left hemisphere in order to be produced as speech. The right ear stimulus can reach this area directly along the contralateral pathway. However, the left ear cannot directly reach the left hemisphere because the ipsilateral pathway is being suppressed. Instead, the left ear signal must first go to the right hemisphere via the contralateral connections, and then travel to the left hemisphere via the interhemispheric connections (i.e., corpus callosum).

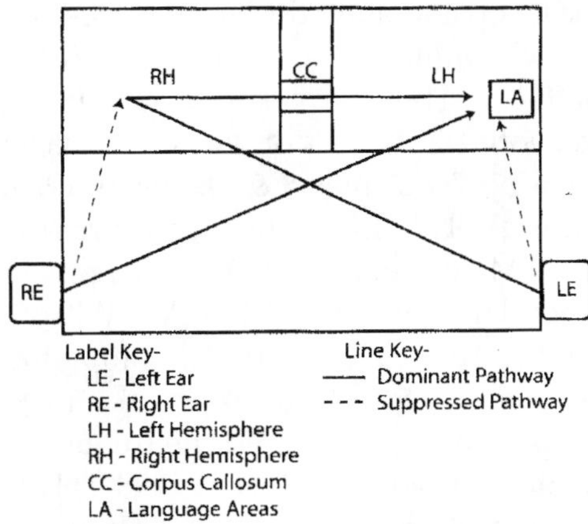

Figure 15–1. Dominance of the contralateral pathways and suppression of the ipsilateral pathways during verbal labeling of dichotically presented stimuli.

The ability to respond to stimuli in a dichotic task, therefore, requires different neurologic precursors depending on which ear is being considered. For the right ear, the contralateral pathway and language areas in the left hemisphere need to be uncompromised. For the left ear, the contralateral pathway, the right hemisphere, the corpus callosum, and the language areas in the left hemisphere need to be uncompromised. In a healthy auditory system, both of these routes are able to function appropriately and dichotic stimuli can be repeated verbally.

Function will change, however, when compromise of either pathway occurs. Of interest is the effect of a callosotomy, which is sometimes used to treat intractable epilepsy. When the auditory (posterior) region of the corpus callosum is sectioned, the result is an often drastic decrease in performance on tests that require interhemispheric interaction (Milner et al., 1968; Sparks & Geschwind, 1968;). Specifically, the patient has considerable difficulty repeating back stimuli that are presented to the left ear. This has been shown using dichotic digits and/or words (Damasio et al., 1976; Damasio & Damasio, 1979; Musiek et al., 1979), the dichotic rhyme test (Musiek et al., 1989), the staggered spondaic words test (Musiek & Wilson, 1979; Musiek et al., 1981), competing sentences tests (Musiek et al., 1979; Musiek et al., 1981), and the frequency patterns test (Musiek et al., 1980). This pattern of performance for cases of callosal involvement is often referred to as the auditory disconnection model (Musiek et al., 1984). When a lesion is created in the corpus callosum, the neural signal can no longer travel between hemispheres because of the damaged fibers. Hence, the right and left auditory cortices have become disconnected.

Consider again the dichotic scenario presented above in which the patient must repeat back all stimuli that are heard. If the corpus callosum is damaged, the right ear pathway will likely be unaffected. The signal will travel from the right ear, along the contralateral connections, to the language areas in the left hemisphere. The left ear pathway, however, will no longer behave normally. The signal will travel to the right hemisphere via the contralateral connections. However, upon reaching the right hemisphere, the signal can no longer be transmitted to the left hemisphere language areas. This is because the route of transmission, the corpus callosum, is no longer functioning properly. Therefore, the callosotomy patient will be able to say the right ear stimulus but not the left ear stimulus when the stimuli are presented dichotically. This is why callosal lesions typically yield a left ear deficit.

Thus far, it has only been considered how the auditory system would behave when dichotic stimuli are presented at equal sensation levels. An important change in the auditory system occurs when stimuli are presented at *unequal* sensation levels. Specifically, when the intensity level in the better ear (e.g., usually right ear) is decreased while the level in the poorer ear (e.g., usually left ear) is kept constant, the patient can respond more easily to poorer ear stimuli. This was observed by Musiek et al. (1979), who reported that patients with callosal lesions could correctly identify more left ear stimuli when the right ear presentation level was decreased (i.e., creating an interaural difference of about 25–30 dB). Figure 15–2 demonstrates this principle. It is not entirely clear what the mechanism is behind this change. However, it is thought that decreasing the better ear presentation level releases some of the other path-

Right Ear ("Better Ear")
Left Ear ("Poorer Ear")
Hot Dog at 50 dB SL
Pancake at 50 dB SL
Response: "Hot Dog and ?"
Hot Dog at 35 dB SL
Pancake at 50 dB SL
Response: "Hot Dog and ?"
Hot Dog at 25 dB SL
Pancake at 50 dB SL
Response: "Hot Dog and Pan Cake"

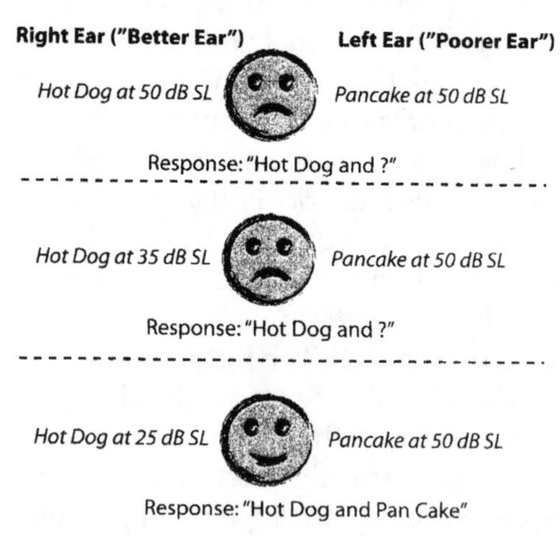

Figure 15–2. Correct repetition of left ear stimuli by decreasing the intensity of the stimulus in the right ear. Notable increases in left ear performance usually begin to appear at IIDs between 25 and 30 dB.

ways, including the left ear ipsilateral pathway, from suppression. This occurs because the greater the intensity of a stimulus, the greater the amount of neural substrate that is activated. As a result, utilization of this ipsilateral pathway allows the left ear signal to reach the left hemisphere language areas with greater ease. As discussed in the sections that follow, it is this interaural intensity difference phenomenon upon which the DIID is based.

Learning Disabilities and the Corpus Callosum

Due to the relatively high prevalence of learning disabilities (Boyle et al., 1994; Brown et al, 2001) and the increasing awareness of auditory involvement in this disorder (Musiek et al., 1984), the DIID has considerable potential as a treatment for this population. As suggested previously, there are auditory system similarities between patients with callosal lesions and those with learning disabilities. From where do these similarities arise? The common finding in both groups is a reduction in the ability of the corpus callosum to transfer the neural signal between hemispheres. In patients with neurologically based callosal lesions, this reduction arises from damage to the corpus callosum. In some children with learning disabilities, it has been theorized that a similar reduction may arise from a maturational delay in myelin development (Musiek et al., 1984).

Myelin is a fatty substance that surrounds axons. Axons transmit the neural signal between neuron groups. The greater the amount of myelin surrounding an axon, the faster the signal can travel within the cerebrum and the more efficient auditory processing may become. Relative to other parts of the central nervous system, the corpus callosum is especially highly myelinated and requires this myelin in order to perform optimally (Bear et al., 2007; Musiek et al., 1984). Unlike some other components of the central nervous system, myelin is not completely developed at birth and takes some time to fully mature. For instance, it may take some auditory regions of the cerebrum up to 10 to 12 years of age or more to become fully myelinated (Salamy, 1978; Yakovlev & LeCours, 1967). Interestingly, left ear performance on dichotic processing tests shares a similar maturational time course (Musiek & Gollegly, 1988).

It should be noted that the 10- to 12-year maturational milestone for myelin development is not, however, a time course that applies to all children. There is considerable variability in myelin development across individuals. Salamy (1978) reports that the age at which adult levels of myelin are reached can vary between 10 and 20 years of age. Therefore, there is potential for considerable delays in myelin maturation. It is for those children who exhibit these delays that a reduction in callosal efficiency becomes noteworthy (Musiek et al., 1984).

The fact that myelin maturation varies across individuals is central to the similarities witnessed between patients with callosal lesions and those with learning disabilities. Incomplete myelin production in learning-disabled children may lead to a temporary lesion which is not that much different from the neurologically induced lesion of "split-brain" patients. In both cases, there is an inability to transfer the neural signal efficiently from the right to the left hemisphere, and left ear deficits would be expected as a result.

The connection between myelin delays and learning disabilities has thus far been one of inference. Indirect evidence includes the fact that similar dichotic deficits are also witnessed in cases of neurological callosal lesions (Milner et al, 1968; Musiek et al., 1979; Musiek et al., 1982; Musiek et al., 1984; Sparks & Geschwind, 1968) and that a similar neuromaturational time course is observed for both left ear performance on dichotic processing tasks and myelin development. However, does any direct evidence link corpus callosum abnormalities to children with learning disabilities? Although the research is somewhat inconsistent on these grounds, there does appear to be some tendency for the corpus callosum to appear different in children with learning disabilities. Hynd et al. (1991) and Semrud-Clikeman et al. (1994) used magnetic resonance imaging (MRI) to compare the structure of the corpus callosum in children with learning disabilities and/or attention deficit disorder (ADD) to normal controls. In both cases, it was found that the auditory (posterior) region of the corpus callosum was significantly smaller in the experimental group than in the control group. The researchers suggested that the smaller posterior region may negatively affect modulation of cerebral activity in the experimental group (Hynd et al., 1991). Additionally, the number of fibers in the posterior region may be smaller in the experimental group (Semrud-Clikeman et al., 1994).

Basic research with nonhuman animals has also provided some additional evidence for callosal involvement in cases of learning disabilities. Specifically, it has been suggested that lesions created in the corpus callosum can produce behaviors not dissimilar to those exhibited by children with learning disabilities and/or ADD. Sechzer et al. (1977) completely sectioned the corpus callosum and psalterium in a group of neonatal cats and compared their behavioral development to normal controls. It was found that the experimental group tended to be more hyperactive than the control group. For instance, whereas control cats huddled around the parent and slept, the experimental group continually roamed around the cage and over the parent's body. The experimental group also had difficulties with a memory task. When having to learn which of two patterns signified food, it took the experimental group almost twice the number of trials compared to controls to reach a 90% correct criterion. Both of these behaviors, hyperactivity and difficulties with memory, are often exhibited by children with learning disabilities and suggest a possible link between structure and behavior.

Dichotic Interaural Intensity Difference Training

Procedure

The DIID makes use of the physiological principles delineated thus far to train the neural connections involved in dichotic processing. Specifically, patients involved in DIID training participate in a variety of dichotic tasks, not unlike the clinical dichotic tasks that are used diagnostically. However, unlike diagnostic dichotic tests, which are presented at equal sensation levels bilaterally, the DIID stimuli are presented at various interaural intensity differences (IID). The purpose of the procedure is to, first, reduce the amount that the weaker connections are suppressed by the stronger connections and, second, to strengthen the weaker connections under progressively more challenging listening conditions. To reduce the amount of suppression, the presentation level in the better ear is decreased until the left ear performs normally. To then strengthen the weaker connections under challenging conditions, the presentation level in the better ear is gradually increased over time. The ultimate goal of DIID training is to have the poorer ear perform normally when the IID is near zero.[1] Conceptually, DIID training is similar to the research conducted by Wiesel and Hubel (1965) and Hubel and Wiesel (1970), who examined the effects of visual deprivation and subsequent rehabilitation in the cat.

The first step in conducting the DIID is to establish that a dichotic processing deficit is present. Considerations for this have already been discussed in previous sections. Again, the left ear will typically be the poorer ear on these tasks. Following diagnosis, the cross-over point should be established. The crossover point is the IID at which performance in the poorer ear exceeds performance in the better ear. If performance never crosses over, the patient will likely not benefit from the DIID. Stimuli are presented to both ears at equal sensation levels re: speech recognition threshold, generally at 50 dB SL. The presentation level in the better ear is then systematically decreased in 7-dB steps before beginning each dichotically presented list of stimuli. When the poorer ear performance exceeds the better ear performance, crossover has been reached. This is typically accomplished at 20 to 30 dB IID.

When establishing crossover, it is important to take two criteria into consideration. The first criterion is that performance in the poorer ear should be close to normal limits when stimuli are presented at the crossover levels. For instance, consider the case where a patient scores 20% in the better ear and 30% in the poorer ear at crossover. This patient may have achieved crossover, but the performance in the poorer ear is still considerably below normal limits. If patients are unable to achieve near normal levels in the poorer ear when stimuli are presented at crossover levels, they may not be good candidates for the DIID procedure. The second criterion is that the stimulus presented to the better ear should never be presented below the level of audibility. Although performance in the better ear will become poorer as the presentation level in that ear is decreased, performance should never extinguish completely. In order for this to remain a dichotic task, both stimuli need to be audible.

Once the crossover point has been properly established, training can begin.

[1]It has also been suggested that making the onset of the two stimuli progressively less synchronous can also accomplish the same end (Musiek et al., 2002). This method, however, will not be discussed in the present chapter.

The initial session should begin at an IID that is slightly larger than that needed for crossover. Typically, the initial IID used is 3 to 5 dB greater than the crossover amount. In other words, if crossover is obtained when the sensation level is 30 dB in the better ear and 50 dB in the poorer ear, then the presentation level for the better ear during the initial session should be approximately 25 dB SL. At this IID, the patient should be administered a variety of dichotic tasks. The tasks should be conducted using both binaural integration and binaural separation paradigms, and different types of stimuli should be presented (e.g., words, digits, CVs, sentences). It is thought that the more varied the tasks and stimuli, the more likely it will be that learning is generalized. It is essential to maintain a log of what types of tasks were conducted, which stimuli were used, what the presentation level was in each ear, and how the patient performed. This log will be used to document progress obtained by the patient over the course of training.

A typical formal training schedule is to have the patient complete the DIID in the clinic for 15 to 30 minutes, three to four times a week. Informal training can be used to supplement formal training, and will be discussed in more detail below. Following the initial week of training, an attempt should be made to make the task more challenging by decreasing the IID. In the first attempt, the IID should be decreased by 5 dB. From our example above, if the presentation level is 25-dB SL in the better ear, it should be raised to 30-dB SL at the beginning of the second week. If performance in the poorer ear is 80% or greater at this smaller IID, then training should continue for the next week at this presentation level. If not, then a second attempt should made in which the IID is decreased in 1-dB increments. If the patient performance is 80% or greater in the poorer ear with even a 1-dB decrease in the IID, this new presentation level should be used. If the patient is unable to tolerate even a 1-dB change in the IID, then training for the week should continue with the IID unchanged. However, another attempt should be made to modify the IID at the beginning of the following week. It is important to realize that it can take several weeks for a patient to tolerate any change in the initial IID, and sometimes improvement in auditory processing happens in an incremental, and not a continuous, fashion.

Subsequent weeks should continue in the manner described, with each week beginning with an attempt to decrease the IID. If the patient begins to show a rapid increase in improvement, decrements in the IID can be attempted at the beginning of each session. For the patient who benefits from the DIID, the log should demonstrate a decrease in the IID over the course of the training period. As previously stated, the ultimate goal of the training protocol is to have the patient perform dichotic processing tasks within normal limits bilaterally when stimuli are presented at or near equal sensation levels. However, it has been our experience that if this goal has not been achieved by approximately 3 months time, then it is unlikely the patient will receive any further benefit from the procedure.

As part of our current DIID protocol, we generally retest patients approximately 1 year after they have completed training. This is done to determine how well the effects of training have been maintained. Although not essential, a reevaluation has the obvious benefit of long-term monitoring of the patient's condition and can speak to the efficacy of the DIID training. It is not usually the case that performance decreases in the absence of training. This is likely due, in part, to the fact that almost any natural listening situation is a dichotic situation. Therefore, rather than being completely removed from dichotic tasks, the patient is exposed to them throughout most of the day.

Special Considerations

Hardware

When conducting formal DIID training, no additional hardware is needed beyond a calibrated two-channel device. In the clinic, the most common of these devices would be a two-channel audiometer, which can receive an external input from a compact disc player or a tape deck and is calibrated to ANSI standards. However, if such equipment is unavailable, a good substitute is a laptop which is able to present a stereo signal and can be calibrated. The bottom line is that it is not necessary to have a high-tech clinic to conduct the DIID. In fact, perhaps one of the greatest advantages of this procedure is that it can be administered using equipment and materials that most audiologists already own.

It is often also beneficial to have the patient conduct informal training at home to supplement the formal clinical training. Such informal training can be accomplished in a variety of ways. For instance, if the patient owns a portable audio device that has a balance between left and right stereo channels, this balance can be adjusted to create an IID. If the left ear is the poorer ear, then the balance can be turned toward the left channel so that the signal emitted from that channel is stronger. Alternatively, a laptop could be used in the same manner. Most computer operating systems allow the user to adjust the output balance. Again, the signal will become stronger on the channel toward which the balance is shifted. Of course, it is difficult to determine precisely at what IID the stimuli are being presented using this equipment. The patient should simply be instructed to modify the balance until the stimulus becomes just easy enough to understand in the poorer ear without removing the better ear stimulus entirely.

Many other informal training procedures can be conducted in addition to those described above. Almost anything which can create an IID is acceptable. Recently, a patient seen in our lab has been completing a binaural separation task by listening to words through a portable compact disc player with one ear and exposing himself to a competing signal through a television speaker with his other ear. He uses a television channel that broadcasts mostly talk programming, like a news station. He then adjusts the presentation level of the compact disc player until his performance repeating back the CD words is around 70 to 80%, and trains at this level for around 20 minutes.

The DIID has been conducted both over headphones and through speakers in the sound field. Although the headphones create a more controlled environment, presenting stimuli in the sound field may create a more challenging listening situation because the two stimuli are mixed at the ear level (Musiek & Schochat, 1998). In other words, the left ear will still receive the majority of the left stimulus, but the right stimulus will reach the left ear as well, albeit to a lesser degree. Certainly training in the sound field can provide an ecologically valid alternative to headphones, and may benefit the patient if done in moderation or if it is the only transducer available. However, the majority of training should be conducted over headphones as it is important to maintain a specific IID.

Stimuli

As mentioned previously, it is important to use a variety of stimuli when conducting the DIID formally. For formal training, any material that can be calibrated and has a different stimulus on each channel can be used. The onsets of the stimuli should be relatively aligned, but precise alignment is not essential. Any combination of stimulus types can be used. For instance, patients could also be asked to repeat back words from the poorer ear while sentences in the better ear are ignored, or they can be asked to repeat back a CV from one ear and a digit in the other ear. The most important thing is that dichotic tasks are completed and that they are done so with a variety of stimulus types. In our lab, we have found the following materials to be useful: Qualitone (Q/MASS)—Speech Audiometry Volume 1; Department of Veterans Affairs —Speech Recognition and Identification Materials; Department of Veterans Affairs—Tonal and Speech Materials; and Audiology Illustrated—Extended Dichotic Digits. We also use audio recording software (e.g., Cool Edit, Praat) to record our own stimuli for use in training. Without a doubt, many additional stimulus materials can be used in DIID training and, if administered correctly, are probably adequate.

When training the patient, it is important to limit the use of diagnostic tests as training materials. Tests that will be used as pre- and post-training measures should mostly be reserved for the evaluation sessions only. Obviously, if these tests are overused during the training, the patient may become familiar with the stimuli. The list then becomes a closed set and demands placed on the auditory system are decreased. Additionally, as a post-training measure, the test may become invalid. Although it may not always be possible to limit use of these tests entirely during training, special attention should be given to nondiagnostic stimulus sets during the training proper.

Behavioral Tasks

The majority of DIID training requires the patient to complete binaural integration and binaural separation type tasks. There are, however, other types of tasks the patient can be asked to complete. It is thought that the more varied the tasks, the greater the area of the central nervous that will be trained. Cognitive-based approaches, for instance, can also tap auditory processes and may increase the generalization of training. These approaches to DIID training involve having patients make some sort of decision with the stimuli that are presented. For instance, four numbers could be presented to each ear and patients could be asked to repeat back only the first and third numbers in each ear. They might also be asked to label each word that is heard as person, place, or thing.

Other types of tasks the patient can be asked to complete include quality judgments of the acoustic signal. Is the stimulus in one ear louder or clearer than the stimulus in the other ear? They could be asked where the intracranial acoustic image is located; that is, to where in their head do the stimuli appear to lateralize? Some patients with dichotic processing deficits will never lateralize to the poorer ear even if the IID is greater than 8 to 10 dB. Asking patients to complete these types of tasks may make it easier for them to make these decisions in the future.

Efficacy

Although the collection of efficacy data for the DIID is ongoing, several studies and preliminary data have shown the DIID to provide a benefit. Behaviorally, improvements are witnessed on dichotic processing tasks. In a sample of children with auditory processing disorder, Musiek (unpublished data) recorded left (poorer) ear improvement on the dichotic digits ($N = 11$) and the competing sentences ($N = 10$) tests and compared this improvement to a control group ($N = 7$). Following DIID training, the left ear improvement observed in the experimental groups was between 10 and 15% on the two tests, whereas the control group only improved approximately 6%. Wertz and Moncrieff (unpublished data) conducted a similar study, comparing the improvement on the dichotic digits in a pediatric auditory processing disorder group pre- and post-training ($N = 8$). Left ear improvement was again approximately 15% following training.

Case studies that incorporate behavioral measures have also shown some evidence of DIID benefits. Musiek and Schochat (1998) administered the DIID as part of an auditory training battery to a 15-year-old boy with learning disabilities. Pretraining, the patient showed a bilateral deficit on the dichotic digits with worse performance in the left ear. Following 6 weeks of training, performance on this measure returned to normal limits in both ears. Benefits were also observed on speech-language measures and in academic performance; however it is unclear whether these secondary benefits can be attributed to the DIID (Musiek & Schochat, 1998). Musiek et al. (2004) also administered the DIID as part of an informal auditory training protocol for an adult who had suffered a closed head injury. Prior to beginning the training protocol, the patient showed a left ear deficit on the dichotic digits and the competing sentences tests. At the end of training, the left ear performance on the dichotic digits was within normal limits and on the competing sentences it was borderline normal. This patient also reported that she was now able to engage in activities she previously had not been able to do (e.g., listen on the phone with her left ear), although her ability to complete these activities still had not returned to their initial state.

Effects of the DIID have also been investigated electrophysiologically. Schochat et al. (submitted) administered an auditory training protocol, in which the DIID was a component, to 30 children with auditory processing disorder and a control group. Results showed that, not only did children demonstrate benefits behaviorally, but that their evoked potentials improved as well. Specifically, the middle latency response Na-Pa amplitude at the C3 electrode (i.e., electrode over the left hemisphere) was greater in the auditory processing group following training, but not in a control group. These results demonstrate that changes induced by an auditory training protocol that includes the DIID may be measured electrophysiologically as well as behaviorally.

Finally, there is some evidence to indicate that DIID training may translate into benefits in natural listening situations. Lau (unpublished data) asked parents and teachers to rate children's improvement across several dimensions of a Communication-Education questionnaire following a training battery that included the DIID. Dimensions included areas like: ability to follow directions, communication ability, academic performance, attention, ability to hear in noise, and others. Each area was rated from 0 to 5, with 0 indicating no improvement and 5 indicating a 100% improvement. Results showed that all dimensions were scored at least a 3 on average, with some, like academic performance, scoring around 4 on average. This suggests that improvements caused by batteries that include the DIID may generalize to other modalities, although these results cannot show with certainty if these gains are auditorily based.

Illustrative Case (from Weihing et al., 2006)

The patient was a 58-year old male who experienced a cerebrovascular accident in June 2002. A CT scan revealed a large subcortical bleed in the left parietotemporal region, very near the motor strip. A diagnosis of arteriovenous malformation (AVM) was made and a left vertebral angiography conducted postoperatively revealed an occlusion of the left posterior parietal and angular branches of the middle cerebral artery. Prior to the CVA, the patient did not notice any difficulties hearing. Currently, he has difficulty comprehending rapid speech, particularly in group situations and when listening on the telephone with his right ear. In such cases, he generally "tunes out." He reports that, when in the presence of background noise, his ability to understand speech is severely affected. There is a significant history of noise exposure (i.e., right-handed shooter). He is right-handed.

The patient had a significant speech and language history. Following the CVA, he presented with global aphasia, which had resolved to a mild-to-moderate anomia for both nouns and verbs by October 2004. Aphasia was accompanied by mild apraxia of speech. Comprehension of orally presented materials continued to be mildly to moderately impaired, with severity depending on the complexity of the material. He easily comprehended short sentences with simple syntax, but had more difficulty with longer, more syntactically complex productions.

Due to the reported auditory symptoms, the patient completed peripheral hearing and central auditory processing evaluations. These pretraining results are presented in Figures 15–3A and 15–3B. Most notable was that the patient had much poorer "central" hearing in the right ear and much poorer peripheral hearing in the left ear. Although his anomia likely played

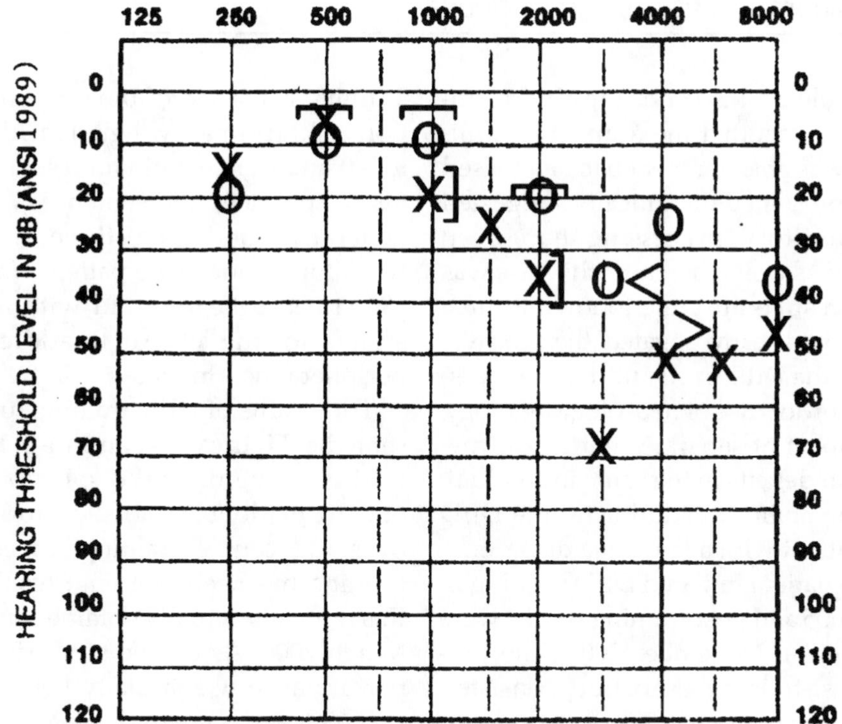

A.

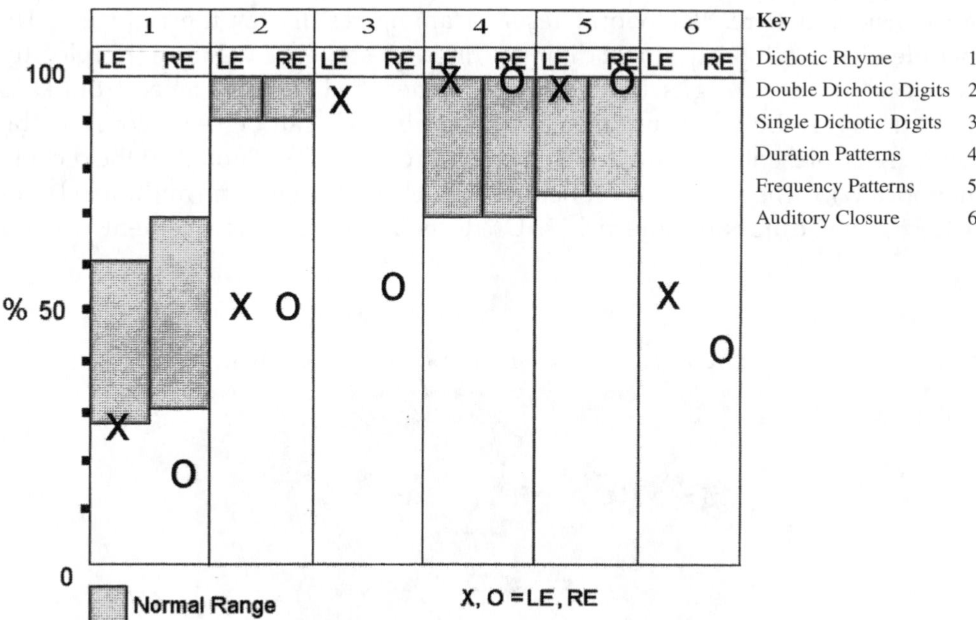

B.

Figure 15–3. A. Pretraining pure tone audiogram for subject in the case study. **B.** Case study showing results of pretraining central auditory test battery

some role on his central test performance, the fact that the number of stimuli he was able to repeat back increased when presented monotically suggested that auditory processing had been affected as well. Therefore, this case was of interest because the following three goals could be investigated: the effectiveness of the DIID in an auditory processing disorder case of neurologic etiology, the impact of separate central and peripheral deficits in the same individual, and the ability to administer the DIID to a patient with a language disorder.

The patient initiated DIID training in May 2005 and post-training results were obtained in November 2005. The pre- and post-training test battery consisted of six behavioral auditory processing tests and several electrophysiological tests, although only the behavioral data are considered here. Behavioral tests include dichotic digits (a single digit to each ear), dichotic digits (two digits to each ear), auditory closure measure (two digits presented simultaneously, monotically), dichotic rhyme, frequency patterns, and duration patterns. DIID Training consisted of binaural integration tasks (primarily digits) in addition to left and right ear binaural separation tasks (spondees and sentences). It was generally conducted three times a week for an hour. The patient was also prescribed a hearing aid with an FM system for the left ear to address his peripheral hearing loss.

The results of DIID training are presented in Figures 15–4 and 15–5. Figure 15–4 is a longitudinal display of dichotic digits (double digits) performance over the course training. Since this training has been ongoing, results for this test were actually obtained up until March 2006. As can be seen, right ear performance was initially between 50 and 65% and increased to around 85% at the last formal session. Figure 15–5 shows the post-training minus pre-training results for the right ear. The more positive the value on this plot, the greater the benefit received from DIID training. As can be seen, considerable improvement was noted on the dichotic digits-single digits and auditory closure tests. Although improvement was not

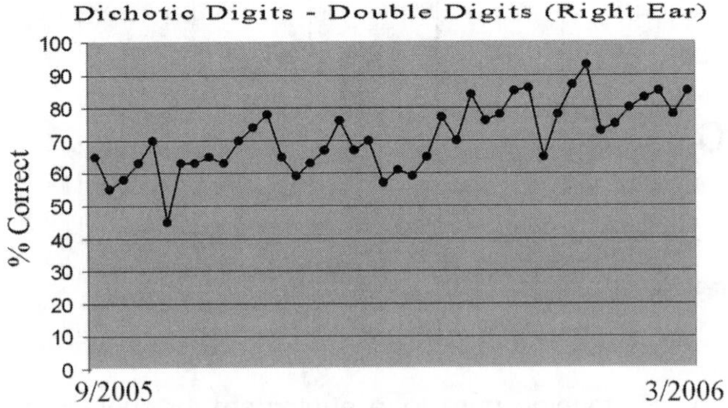

Figure 15–4. Case study showing performance on the dichotic digits (two digits to each ear) over the course of DIID training.

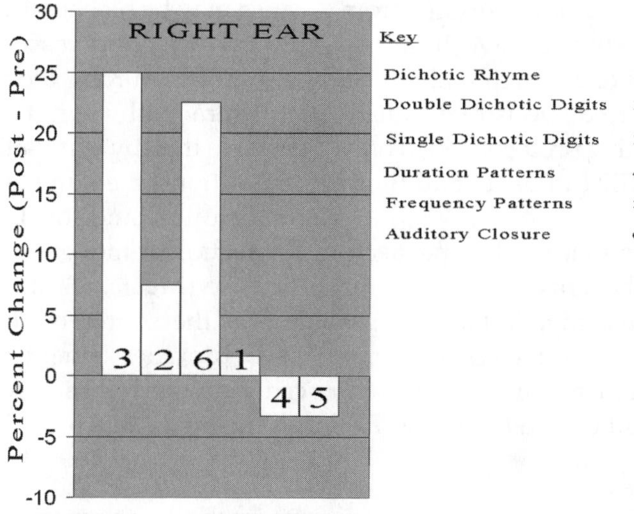

Figure 15–5. Case study showing post-training minus pretraining test performance expressed as a percentage change.

apparent on the double dichotic digits, Figure 15–4 shows that gains were eventually obtained on this measure.

This case showed the DIID can provide benefits in cases of neurologically based auditory processing disorders. Although the corpus callosum may have been affected indirectly by the lesion, the primary influence on test performance is likely damage to auditory regions of the cerebrum. Additionally, the case also demonstrated the difficulties of conducting the DIID in cases of hearing loss. Because increasing the presentation level in the left ear to a sensation level that would overcome the hearing loss was inconsistent with the goals of the DIID (i.e., in this case, decreased left ear intensity), it was not possible to have much high frequency information above threshold in the left ear. However, despite this limitation, right ear benefits were still obtained. Finally, this is the first instance of administration of the DIID to a patient with a language deficit and, as such, is very revealing. The patient's anomia proved a challenge in repeating back some stimuli. However, although semantic errors were encountered, improvements were still noted over time for digit, spondee, and sentence stimuli. This indicates that, in some cases, the DIID may be used effectively even when a language disorder of mild severity is present and there is compromise of the auditory cortex.

Summary

This chapter detailed the nature of dichotic processing deficits and how the DIID can be used to treat this condition. Conceptual and procedural foundations for the DIID have been described, with an emphasis on logistical consideration. Although results from initial efficacy studies have been encouraging, further research with group data is needed to demonstrate statistically that a training protocol which only contains the DIID can benefit auditory processing.

It is not entirely clear what the mechanisms behind benefits gained from the DIID are. Because myelin takes longer than 3 months to develop, it seems unlikely that more myelin is being generated as a result of DIID training. The cause may be biochemical, or may simply involve an increase in the number of usable neurons along the weaker ipsilateral pathways. It is certainly conceivable that, by stimulating the weaker connections, the number of viable neuron groups and/or the number of connections among such groups will increase (Musiek et al., 2002). Regardless of the source of change, that the DIID provides benefit is the ultimate criterion and initial research seems promising in this regard.

Key Points Learned

- Dichotic processing deficits typically manifest as poor left ear performance and may be attributed to pathology of the corpus callosum.
- Reducing intensity in the right (better) ear can increase left (poorer) ear performance on dichotic tasks.
- Conducting dichotic processing tasks using interaural intensity differences which favor the poorer ear can yield long-term changes in dichotic processing over time.
- The DIID is characterized by flexibility, and can be administered both formally in the clinic and informally at home.
- Initial research has shown that patients with dichotic processing deficits tend to improve over time when enrolled in auditory training programs which include the DIID alone or as part of a larger battery.

References

Baran, J., Shinn, J., & Musiek, F. (2006). New developments in the assessment and management of auditory processing disorders. *Audiological Medicine*, *4*, 35–45.

Bear, M., Connors, B., & Paradiso, M. (2007). *Neuroscience—Exploring the brain* (3rd ed.). New York: Lippincott, Williams, & Wilkins.

Boyle, C., Decoufle, P., & Yeargin-Allsopp, M. (1994). Prevalence and health impact of developmental disabilities in U.S. children. *Pediatrics*, *93*, 399–403.

Brown, R., Freeman, W., Perrin, J., Stein, M., Amler, R., Feldman, H., et al. (2001). Prevalence and assessment of attention deficit/hyperactivity disorder in primary care settings. *Pediatrics*, *107*, 43–53.

Damasio, H., & Damasio, A. (1979). Paradoxic ear extinction in dichotic listening:

Possible anatomical significance. *Neurology, 29*, 644–653.

Damasio, H., Damasio, A., Castro-Caldas, A., & Ferro, J. (1976). Dichotic listening pattern in relation to inerhemispheric disconnection. *Neuropsychologia, 14*, 247–250.

Hall, J., & Goldstein, M. (1968). Representations of binaural stimuli by single units in primary auditory cortex of unanesthetized cats. *Journal of the Acoustical Society of America, 43*, 456–561.

Hubel, D., & Wiesel, T. (1970). The period of susceptibility to the physiological effects of unilateral eye closure in kittens. *Journal of Physiology, 206*, 419–436.

Hynd, G., Semrud-Clikeman, M., Lorys, A., Novey, E., Eliopulos, D., & Lyytinen, H. (1991). Corpus callosum morphology in attention deficit-hyperactivity disorder: Morphometric analysis of MRI. *Journal of Learning Disabilities, 24*, 141–146.

Kimura, D. (1961). Some effects of temporal-lobe damage on auditory perception. *Canadian Journal of Psychology, 15*, 156–165.

Lau, C. (unpublished data). Dichotic interaural intensity difference training.

Milner, B., Taylor, S., & Sperry, R. (1968). Lateralized suppression of dichotically presented digits after commissural section in man. *Science, 161*, 184–185.

Musiek, F. (1999). Central auditory tests. *Scandinavian Audiology, 28*(Suppl. 51), 33–46.

Musiek, F. (unpublished data). Dichotic interaural intensity difference training.

Musiek, F., Baran, J., & Shinn, J. (2004). Assessment and remediation of an auditory processing disorder associated with head trauma. *Journal of the American Academy of Audiology, 15*, 117–132.

Musiek, F., Geurkink, N., & Kietel, S. (1982). Test battery assessment of auditory perceptual dysfunction in children. *Laryngoscope, 92*, 251–257.

Musiek, F., & Gollegly, K. (1988). Maturational considerations in the neuroauditory evaluation of children. In F. H. Bess (Ed.), *Hearing impairment in children.* Baltimore: York Press.

Musiek, F., Gollegly, K., & Baran, J. (1984). Myelination of the corpus callosum and auditory processing problems in children: Theoretical and clinical correlates. *Seminars in Hearing, 5*, 231–241.

Musiek, F., Kurdziel-Schwan, S., Kibbe, K., Gollegly, K., Baran, J., & Rintelmann, W. (1989). The dichotic rhyme test: results in split brain patients. *Ear and Hearing, 10*, 33–39.

Musiek, F., & Pinheiro, M. (1985). Dichotic speech tests in the detection of central auditory dysfunction. In M. Pinheiro & F. Musiek (Eds.), *Assessment of central auditory dysfunction: Foundations and clinical correlates.* Baltimore: Williams & Wilkins.

Musiek, F., Pinheiro, M., & Wilson, D. (1980). Auditory pattern perception in "split brain" patients. *Archives of Otolaryngology, 106*, 610–612.

Musiek, F., & Schochat, E. (1998). Auditory training and central auditory processing disorders—a case study. *Seminars in Hearing, 19*, 357–366.

Musiek, F., Shinn,. J., & Hare, C. (2002). Plasticity, auditory training, and auditory processing disorders. *Seminars in Hearing, 23*, 263–275.

Musiek, F., & Wilson, D. (1979). SSW and dichotic digit results pre- and post-commissurotomy: A case report. *Journal of Speech, Language, and Hearing Disorders, 44*, 528–533.

Musiek, F., Wilson, D., & Pinheiro, M. (1979). Audiological manifestations in "split brain" patients. *Journal of the American Auditory Society, 5*, 25–29.

Musiek, F., Wilson, D., & Reeves, G. (1981). Staged commissurotomy and central auditory function. *Archives of Otolaryngology, 107*, 233–236.

Pickles, J. O. (1982). *An introduction to the physiology of hearing.* London, Academic Press.

Rosenzweig, M. (1951). Representations of two ears at the auditory cortex. *American Journal of Physiology, 167*, 147–158.

Salamy, A. (1978). Commissural transmission: Maturational changes in humans. *Science, 200,* 1409–1410.

Sechzer. J., Folstein, S., Geiger, E., & Mervis, D. (1977). Effects of neonatal hemispheric disconnection in kittens. In S. Harnard, R. Doty, L. Goldstein, J. Jaynes, & G. Krauthamer (Eds.), *Lateralization in the nervous system.* New York: Academic Press.

Semrud-Clikeman, M., Filipek, P., Biederman, J., Steingard, R., Kennedy, D., Renshaw, P., & Bekken, K. (1994). Attention-deficit hyperactivity disorder: Magnetic resonance imaging morphometric analysis of the corpus callosum. *Journal of the American Academy of Child and Adolescent Psychiatry, 33,* 875–881.

Sparks, R., & Geschwind, N. (1968). Dichotic listening in man after section of neocortical commissures. *Cortex, 4,* 3–16.

Tunturi, A. (1946). A study of the pathway from the medial geniculate body to the acoustic cortex in the dog. *American Journal of Physiology, 147,* 311–319.

Weihing, J., Munroe, S., Swainson, S., Cho, Y., & Musiek, F. (2006, March). *Dichotic interaural intensity difference (DIID) training in a case of left hemisphere stroke.* Poster presentation at the convention for the American Academy of Audiology, Minneapolis, MN.

Wertz, D., & Moncrieff, D. (unpublished data). Dichotic interaural intensity difference training.

Wiesel, T., & Hubel, D. (1965). Extent of recovery from the effects of visual deprivation in kittens. *Journal of Neurophysiology, 28,* 1060–1072.

Yakovlev, P. & LeCours, A. (1967). Myelogenetic cycles of regional maturation of the brain. In A. Minkowski (Ed.), *Regional development of the brain in early life.* Philadelphia: F.A. Davis.

16

Metalinguistic Approaches

Jane A. Baran

Overview

Individuals with (central) auditory processing disorders ([C]APD) face many challenges in processing spoken language and these challenges can vary considerably with both extrinsic factors (e.g., tasks demands, situational contexts, etc.), as well as with a number of intrinsic variables (e.g., listener fatigue, alertness, motivation level). Although the use and application of the signal enhancement technologies and the environmental modifications that are discussed in Chapters 11 and 20 of this text and the auditory training procedures that are presented in Chapters 10 and 15 can often help to remediate, or at least moderate, the auditory difficulties that many individuals with (C)APD experience in some linguistic contexts and listening environments, it is unlikely that such interventions will completely eliminate the auditory deficits being experienced by the individual with (C)APD in all contexts and in every listening situation/environment. This situation is especially true when working with the older individual with a (C)APD as brain plasticity is less robust in the more mature brain than in the younger (and more "plastic") brain—a situation that limits the potential extent of the neurobiologic changes that can be realized with auditory training in the central auditory nervous system of the older individual with (C)APD (Baran, 2002; Musiek, Shinn, & Hare, 2002). For many individuals with (C)APD, the use of alternative knowledge bases and cognitive skills can be used to effectively "fill in" or supplement what is being "missed" during the perceptual processing of an auditory stimulus. Utilization of central resources (i.e., the alternative knowledge bases and cognitive skills) if appropriately and effectively deployed when conversing or attempting to process a speech message (e.g., as in a lecture setting) can help to minimize both the extent and the impact of the functional consequences of the (C)APD that the individual experiences (ASHA, 2005; Baran, 1998, 2002, 2007; Bellis, 2003; Chermak, 1998, 2007; Chermak & Musiek, 1992, 1997, 2002; Ferre, 2002; Musiek, 1999; Musiek, Baran, & Schochat, 1999; Musiek & Schochat, 1998).

A number of chapters in this text have focused on the cognitive, language, and metacognitive approaches that can be used to help manage or remediate (C)APD (see Chapters 13, 14, 17, and 19). This chapter discusses the intervention approaches that focus specifically on metalinguistic skill development and the application of metalinguistic strategies to help the individual with (C)APD comprehend spoken language when auditory language processing challenges and/or deficits are encountered. It is important to note at the outset that the procedures highlighted in this chapter should not be used in isolation when working with individuals with (C)APD, but rather they should be incorporated into a comprehensive intervention program, which may include auditory training approaches, other types of central resources training (i.e., language, cognitive, and metacognitive approaches), and the provision and application of environmental modifications and sound enhancement technologies, as would be appropriate to the individual's age, his or her unique listening needs, and his or her auditory, cognitive, and language abilities (ASHA, 2005, Baran, 1998, 2002, 2007; Bellis, 2003; Chermak, 1998, 2007; Chermak & Musiek, 1992, 1997, 2002; Ferre, 2002; Masters, Stecker, & Katz, 1998; Musiek, 1999; Musiek et al., 1999; Musiek & Schochat, 1998).

Introduction

Defining the Term

Metalinguistic skill, or language awareness refers to the ability to reflect consciously on the nature and properties of language (van Kleeck, 1994, p. 53). There is, in fact, not a single metalinguistic skill, but a rather a number of metalinguistic skills that collectively form the basis of "language awareness." These skills include the cognitive-linguistic processes that allow a person to think about language and to analyze language in a critical manner. They enable the individual not only to make judgments about the accuracy of the linguistic code and the appropriate (or inappropriate) use of language both in terms of form and function, but they also provide the listener with the ability to talk about language in meaningful ways (Bernstein, 1997; van Kleeck, 1984a, 1994).

With the emergence and development of metalinguistic abilities comes the realization that language is more than a tool that enables communication, but that it is a complex system that is governed by linguistic rules and conventions (van Kleeck, 1984a, 1984b, 1994). As the child acquires new metalinguistic skills, he or she becomes increasingly adept at manipulating the various components of language (phonology, morphology, syntax, semantics). Such skills and abilities are essential to the understanding of humor, idioms, multiple word meanings, inferences, and figurative language (Hakes, 1982; Kamhi, 1987; Vinson, 2007; Westby, 1998). They also subserve the ability of the individual to provide definitions of words and to use phonemic awareness skills, such as the blending of speech sounds and sound segmentation processes, to produce words and to facilitate speech-to-print skills—skills that will be important for the subsequent literacy development and academic success of the individual (Hempenstall, 1997; Roth & Worthington, 2001; van Kleeck, 1984a, 1984b, 1994; Westby, 1998).

Normal Development

In the normally developing child, metalinguistic skills begin to emerge early in life and then continue to develop well into the adolescent years. The most marked period of development typically occurs between 4 and 8 years of age (Bernstein, 1997), during which time many of the basic metalinguistic skills develop. With the development of metalinguistic skills and abilities, children begin to actively think about language and to make judgments about the accuracy and the appropriate use of language, both in terms of its form and function. At the same time that metalinguistic skills are developing, the normally developing child also is in a period of rapid and pronounced cognitive development (Saywitz & Wilkinson, 1982; Siegler & Shipley, 1995; van Kleeck, 1984b, 1994). With the development of these cognitive skills, the child is able to consider alternative ways to solve a problem—he or she is able to analyze the tasks involved in the solving of the problem, to form hypotheses about the problem and its potential solution(s), and then to make informed decisions based upon these analyses (Larson & McKinley, 1987). Although these abilities are important for the processing of information in many cognitive domains, in the linguistic domain they function to help facilitate the developing child's ability to critically analyze language, to recognize incongruous or anomalous information in the language being processed, and to articulate and explain the incongruities or anomalies being noted.

As discussed above, language awareness does not include a single metalinguistic skill but rather a number of component skill areas. These component skills include (1) the ability to repair communication breakdowns, (2) the ability to adjust one's language to the level of the conversational partner, (3) the ability to make judgments about the accuracy and appropriateness of language content and form, (4) the ability to analyze and dissect language into smaller linguistic units, (5) the ability to understand and appreciate rhymes, riddles, puns, and humor, and (6) the ability to comprehend and use figurative language (i.e., similes, proverbs, metaphors, and idioms) (Hakes, 1982; Kamhi, 1987; Westby, 1998). The first among these component skills/abilities to emerge are the ability to utilize conversational repair strategies when communication breakdowns occur and the ability to adjust the content and structure of one's language to the perceived level of the listener (Shatz & Gelman, 1973). These skills tend to emerge during the preschool years, whereas other metalinguistic skills, such as the ability to make judgments about linguistic form and content do not typically begin to emerge before the age of 4 years, and often not until the ages of 7 to 8 years of age or later (Hakes, 1980, 1982; Smith & Tager-Flusberg, 1982; Westby, 1998). More advanced and higher order metalinguistic skills (e.g., the ability to recognize and appreciate multiple word meanings, which is an aspect of both semantic and metalinguistic development; the ability to recognize and process linguistic ambiguity, which is necessary if the individual is to understand puns, riddles, and humor; and the ability to produce and comprehend figurative language) begin to emerge at the age of 6 years or older in normally developing children and have a much longer course of development, often not achieving full development until the adolescent years (Douglas & Peel, 1979; Hakes, 1982; Nippold, 1988; Saywitz & Wilkinson, 1982; Shultz & Horibe, 1974; Westby, 1998; Wiig, 1989). The reader interested in more detailed information on this topic is referred to Hakes (1982), Saywitz and Wilkinson (1982), and Westby (1998).

Although most adults may not have a sophisticated understanding of the components of language, they tend to have at least a basic understanding of the components of language (phonology, morphology, syntax, and semantics) and are cognizant of the rules that govern these various dimensions of language. It is the individual's metalinguistic ability that allows him or her to make judgments about the grammaticality of a sentence, its semantic appropriateness, and so forth. When speaking or conversing, individuals do so automatically with little conscious attention to the rules that are being applied. However, if called upon to make a judgment about a language form, then one consciously attends to the form and applies internalized knowledge about the rules to determine if it is correct. As Hulit and Howard (2002) have indicated, "the production of language is a linguistic function, while the evaluation of language is a metalinguistic function" (p. 258).

A review of the literature reveals a large number of resources that discuss the normal and/or the abnormal development of metalinguistic skills and devices in young children and adolescents. For the most part, however, these informational texts and research papers have focused on the link between the development of normal metalinguistic skills and the subsequent development of literacy skills. Although there is no doubt that the appropriate development of metalinguistic skills is central to the development of reading and writing skills, the development and subsequent deployment of metalinguistic skills and strategies can also be an important supplement to auditory language processing. Take for example, the listener who is listening to a conversation in a noisy environment. If the speaker states, *"I have two cats"* when sharing information about his or her pets, the listener who may not accurately perceive the plural marker (-*s*) in this spoken sentence due to its relatively weak acoustic energy, its brief duration, and its partial or complete masking by noise in the environment is not likely to misunderstand this message since plurality in this sentence is marked by more than just the plural marker. The use of the adjective, *two*, also signals plurality in this statement and thus a certain level of redundancy is built into the language used in this sentence—this intrinsic redundancy is a common feature of the English language. If the listener in this situation were asked to transcribe the sentence perceived, it is highly unlikely that he or she would actually write down the statement as it was actually perceived through the auditory sensory modality (i.e., *I have two cat*), rather the individual is much more likely to transcribe what he or she perceived auditorily supplemented by his or her linguistic/metalinguistic knowledge and experience. That is, he or she is more likely to add the appropriate morphological marker (-*s*) to the object of this sentence, thus appropriately denoting the number (i.e., the plurality) of the cats intended by the speaker and signaled by the plural adjective, *two*, by transcribing the following sentence, *"I have two cats."*

Metalinguistic Skills and Strategies

As indicated above, much of the information in the literature that addresses metalinguistic skill development and the application of these skills has appeared in the context of literacy development. Although the development of these skills is critical to the subsequent development of literacy skills and academic success, each of these individual metalinguistic skills is not reviewed here. Rather the following discussion centers on only those metalinguistic skills that are important for the individual to be able to effectively process language in the auditory modality; that is, when listening to and processing spoken speech messages.

In earlier sections of this chapter, the discussion has focused largely on the development of *"metalinguistic skills."* Although these constitute important foundational skills that must be developed in order that the individual can use these skills in the processing of written language, it is also equally important that the individual be able to deploy or evoke *"metalinguistic strategies"* when auditory comprehension or processing difficulties occur (or when they are expected to occur). Hence the effective listener must not only possess the requisite language competence and metalinguistic skills that are needed to understand the language that the speaker is using, but also be capable of shifting from a passive listening stance to being a more "active" listener when the need arises. To do so, the individual must be able to deploy or utilize *"meta-" strategies*[1] that will help to move the individual from being a more passive participant in a conversational situation or other listening context (e.g., an attendee at a religious service, a movie viewer, a student in a lecture, etc.) to being a more active participant in the specific listening activity. These *"meta-" strategies* include both metacognitive as well as metalinguistic strategies. As the metacognitive strategies have been discussed in detail in Chapter 14 of this text, they are not reviewed here. However, it should be noted that these strategies can help to facilitate the efficient reception and/or processing of auditory information— and in some cases may well be the strategy or strategies of choice. Therefore, when implementing central resources training with the individual with a (C)APD, it will be important to consider all potential "central resources" approaches that can be used (and that may be needed) to facilitate specific skill development (i.e., linguistic, cognitive, metacognitive, and metalinguistic skills), if delayed or disordered, and to encourage the use of those specific "meta-" strategies (metacognitive and metalinguistic) that will meet the individual's personal abilities and needs.

In the context of the following discussion the term, metalinguistic strategy, is used to refer to the listener's ability to consciously apply higher order linguistic rules when attempting to process language in adverse or challenging situations (Chermak, 1998). The specific metalinguistic devices, skills, and strategies discussed include phonemic segmentation and sound blending, auditory closure, vocabulary building and derivation, prosody training, discourse cohesion devices, and schema induction.

Segmentation (Analysis and Synthesis)

Segmentation skills (both phonemic analysis and synthesis) form the basis of phonological awareness, which is a metalinguistic skill that tends to emerge relatively early in the course of the normal child's development. Phonological awareness and phonemic awareness are terms that are often used interchangeably by some authors when referring to the ability to recognize and manipulate the sounds of language (see Hempenstall, 2003), whereas other authors (e.g., Goswami & Bryant, 1990) differentiate between these two terms, reserving the term, *phonemic awareness,* to imply an awareness of and the ability to manipulate individual phonemes and the term, *phonological awareness,* to refer to a more global skill that encompasses the earlier stages of segmentation abilities, such as rhyme and syllable segmentation (Hempenstall, 1997). Regardless of

[1]*"Meta-"* is a prefix that is used to indicate *"after; mounted or built upon"* (Singh & Kent, 2000, pg. 185). "Meta-" skills (i.e., metalinguistic, metacognitive, metamemory, etc.) are skills or abilities that are built upon an individual's cognitive and language knowledge bases that allow the individual to think and talk about cognition, memory, attention, language, and so forth. In the context of auditory language processing, meta-strategies represent conscious and deliberate actions to effectively use such skills to assist in processing of a linguistic message.

the term or terms used to define these metalinguistic skills, what is apparent is that normally developing children quickly learn that sentences, phrases, words, and syllables can be segmented or divided into smaller units, as young children (as young as preschoolers) are often observed playing with words in creative ways that demonstrate their emerging metalinguistic abilities.

The typical course of the development of segmentation skills tends to progress from the larger units to the smaller units. Children first segment or divide sentences into phrases or words, then they segment words into syllables, and finally they segment syllables into individual speech sounds. Westby (1998) outlined the following sequence of phonological awareness (and phonemic awareness skills) as they tend to emerge in the normally developing child. The typical sequence is as follows: (1) syllable segmentation (e.g., fire/truck; ba/na/na), (2) rhyme recognition (e.g., Do *cat* and *hat* rhyme? What rhymes with *ball*—*call* or *bait*?), (3) blending of sounds (e.g., What is /c/ /ae/ /t/?), (4) sound segmentation (e.g., What is the first sound in *cat*? What is the last sound in *boat*?), and (5) sound manipulation (e.g., Say *soak* without the /s/.). The first two of these skills develop during the preschool years, the second two during kindergarten and first grade, and the final skill during the second grade (Westby, 1998, p. 328). Slight variations in the sequence of steps or stages through which a normally developing child progresses as he or she moves from a more global phonological awareness to a deep phonemic awareness have been suggested by some authors (see Hempenstall, 1997 for a review of these alternatives). However, common to all of the sequences is the development of the ability to recognize and manipulate smaller and smaller units of sounds.

Unlike normally developing children, many children with (C)APD do not have well-developed phonological awareness skills and as a result face challenges when it comes to the accurate identification and manipulation of the sounds of the language. In some cases, these deficits or difficulties are secondary to a primary auditory processing deficit, but in others, they may be related to some other comorbid condition, such as a specific language impairment. In either case, efforts should be directed at improving the child's phonological and phonemic awareness skills. Specific skill areas that can be targeted for remediation include auditory discrimination, sound segmentation, sound blending, sound deletion, recognition of the position of a phoneme in a word, and rime and rhyming. The ultimate goal of such activities is to develop accurate phonemic representations and improve speech-to-print skills, but in doing so temporal auditory processing skills can be improved (Chermak, 2007).

When working on any of these skills, it is advisable to work on them in the appropriate developmental order, working from larger to smaller units (Chermak, 2007; Westby, 1998). For example, if a child has segmentation difficulties, then it is advisable to start with activities focusing initially on the segmenting of sentences into words and then to progress in the following order: segmenting compound words into component words, multisyllabic words into syllables, words to onset/rimes (i.e., onset—initial consonant or cluster before the vowel and rime—vowel and consonant following the onset), and finally words to sounds. If deletion is a problem area for the individual then therapy can start by having the individual delete one morpheme from a compound word, which is a relatively easy task (e.g., delete *hot* in *hotdog*). Then training activities can train deletion skills in the following sequence: delete syllables from single words, delete initial phonemes from single words, and delete final phonemes from single words. In each case, work would begin with at the level where difficulties are first encountered. For example, in the latter example, if the child is able to delete one syllable from a multisyllabic word, then work can begin deleting initial phonemes from single words and then progress through the more difficult deletion task levels.

There are a number of formal programs that have been developed to train phonological awareness/phonemic awareness skills. These programs in-clude the Lindamood *Phoneme Sequencing Program (LiPS)* (1999), *Earobics* (1996), and *Fast ForWord* (1999). The latter two are computer-based programs, which have received much interest in the past decade or so (see Chapters 17, and 19 of this text). In addition, there are a number of other resources that are available to assist in the development of these skills. These include, but are not limited to, *Treating Auditory Processing Difficulties*, a program developed by Sloan (1986) and the *Phonemic Synthesis Program* developed by Katz and Harmon (1982) (see Chapter 13 in this text). Additional information on these programs can be found in Chapters 17, 18, 19, and 20 of this text as well as in a number of other resources (Chermak, 2007; Richard, 2007; Thibodeau, 2007). In addition to these formalized programs, there are a number of educational companies that offer a variety of workbooks and programmed training activities that can be used to facilitate the development of phonological/phonemic awareness skills. Finally, comprehensive reviews of the normal development of phonological awareness skills in children and suggestions for intervention protocols when delayed or disordered phonological awareness and segmentation skills are noted can be found in Catts (1991), Gillam and van Kleeck (1998), van Kleeck (1994), and Westby (1998).

Auditory Closure

Auditory closure refers to the ability to reorganize or process a message in spite of the fact that part of the message may be missing or not perceived. It is a conscious attempt to make whole an incomplete message. Listeners achieve auditory closure by filling in gaps in the acoustic signal through a process in which they invoke language, contextual, or world knowledge. Auditory closure can operate at a number of levels including the acoustic-phonetic level wherein the listener utilizes the inherent redundancy that is built into speech due to features such as coarticulation effects. Grammatical closure functions at a different level and is achieved by listener's invoking his or her knowledge of the syntax and/or morphology of the language (as demonstrated in the example provided above), and auditory-verbal closure is a function that allows the listener to use semantic information to achieve closure (discussed in greater detail below).

Individuals with (C)APD often demonstrate deficits in word knowledge, limited receptive and expressive vocabularies, difficulties in recognizing and interpreting multiple word meanings, and difficulties in interpreting figurative language (Keith & Novak, 1984; Matkin & Hook, 1983; Willeford & Burleigh, 1985). Given the importance of an individual's receptive vocabulary or lexicon to the comprehension of the spoken message, a viable approach to intervention with the individual with deficits in any of these areas would be to incorporate vocabulary building activities into the individual's intervention program, with a particular focus on establishing semantic relationships between and among words in an effort to foster semantic networks. The ultimate goal would be the construction of meaning (Chermak, 2007; Chermak & Musiek, 1997).

Approaches that can be used to increase both the depth and breadth of an individual's vocabulary and semantic networks include context-derived vocabulary building, word derivation training, training in the identification and appreciation of multiple word meanings, and inferencing activities (Chermak, 2007). Specific intervention activities can focus on activities that help the individual examine the relationships between root words and their derivatives (e.g., know/knowledge, declare/declaration, able/ability, etc.). They can also include activities which help to foster the individual's ability to recognize and comprehend the multiple and varied meanings that a single lexical item can share.

Multiple Word Meanings

A single word or lexical item can be used to refer to different concrete objects and/or actions, and it may additionally have a figurative meaning (Westby, 1998) as depicted in this example:

(1) Lexical item: bank

Alternative meanings:

1a. *The young could sit on the river bank.* (concrete object)

1b. *I am going to withdraw some money from the bank.* (concrete object)

1c. *It is important to bank your car when making a sharp turn.* (concrete action)

1d. *You can bank on it.* (figurative)

Other lexical items can have both concrete/physical and psychological referents (as shown in the second example) (Westby, 1998; Wiig, 1989).

(2) Lexical item: crooked

Alternative meanings:

2a. *John walked down the crooked path to the cabin in the woods.* (physical attribute)

2b. *The crooked accountant overcharged his clients.* (psychological attribute)

Work on helping the individual recognize and become facile with the multiple meanings of words such as those shown in the examples above should help bolster the individual's ability to correctly and efficiently comprehend the intended message of a speaker. The individual will need to be prepared to use this knowledge to quickly select the correct "meaning" of the word by using his or her knowledge of all of the potential word meanings, especially when this knowledge is coupled with information contained in the linguistic or situational context.

Homophones

Work can also focus on development of an appreciation and comprehension of homophones (see example below). If the individual is aware that a word with the same phonological representation can have different referents, he or she will be better able to correctly comprehend the meaning of the particular homophone when it is encountered in conversational exchanges or in other listening situations (e.g., movies, lectures, etc.).

(3) Homophonous pair: medal/meddle

3a. *John won a silver medal in the art competition.*

3b. *You do not want to meddle in your neighbor's business.*

Training in these areas will encourage facility and flexibility in the comprehension of both written and auditory language (Gerber, 1993), while at the same time providing the client with opportunities to expand semantic networks and increase the individual's expressive and receptive vocabularies (Chermak & Musiek, 1997).

Context-Derived Vocabulary

Linguistic contexts can be used to derive word meaning and enhance message comprehension when an individual encounters a novel or an unfamiliar lexical item embedded within the message (Miller & Gildea, 1987). Unfortunately many individuals with (C)APD are not adept at using information that is either contained in the message itself or in the situational context within which the message is occurring to assist in the derivation of the meaning. Often they inefficiently attempt to identify the word by using bottom-up processing procedures wherein they focus on acoustic processing of the sequence of individual speech sounds within the word to achieve word recognition, rather than using the context of the message to assist in comprehension (a top-down or central resources process). By using the linguistic information contained in an utterance to derive meaning, the efficient listener can achieve closure in spite of the fact that they have no knowledge or experience with one or more of the lexical items contained in the message. Take for example, the following sentence, *"The CEO pilfered $800,000 from his company's assets before his illegal activities were uncovered."* The meaning of the word, *pilfered*, which may be unfamiliar to the listener, can be deduced from the semantic information contained in this message, thus allowing the listener the ability to comprehend the meaning of the sentence. As individuals with (C)APD are often not efficient at the use of such strategies (i.e., context-derived meaning), intervention efforts focused on building such skills can and should be incorporated into the intervention plan for the individual with (C)APD. Thus teaching a new vocabulary word should incorporate a technique that employs the use of that word within a sentence that conveys its meaning (Chermak, 2007; Chermak & Musiek, 1997; Musiek et al., 1999).

Inferencing

Efficient comprehension of auditory information also can require that the individual be capable of inferring or predicting meaning from the context—a skill that has often been figuratively referred to as "reading between the lines" (Westby, 1998). Inferring meaning and predicting meaning are rooted in the ability to bring one's world and/or linguistic knowledge to the auditory listening event. Inferences can either be pragmatic or logical in nature. Pragmatic inferences are not based on information contained within the message itself, but rather on information that the listener possesses (Westby, 1998). If a listener heard the following statement, *"In the afternoon, John retuned home to find his back door kicked in and the contents of his house in disarray,"* then he might infer that John's house had been broken into over the course of the day and that a robbery had occurred. These inferences were not based in the text itself (i.e., there is nothing explicit in the statement that specifies that a robbery occurred), but rather on the listener's world knowledge (i.e., that it is common to find that a burglary or robbery has taken place if a door is kicked in and the contents of the home are in disarray). In contrast, logical inferences are based on information that is contained within the text itself (Westby, 1998). Take for example the following statements. *"Marsupials are warm-blooded mammals who carry their newborns in pouches on their stomachs for several months following their birth. A bandicoot is a marsupial."* Although the individual to whom these statements may be made may not know what a bandicoot is (as this is a mammal that few individuals have had the opportunity to see), the individual can deduce or infer a considerable amount of information about what a bandicoot actually is (i.e., it is a warm-blooded mammal, it carries its newborns in a pouch).

Grammatical Closure

Although most of the discussion included in this section of this chapter has focused on auditory-verbal closure activities, similar procedures and strategies can be used to achieve grammatical closure (Chermak, 2007; Chermak & Musiek, 1997; Musiek et al., 1999). For example, if an individual is not accurately perceiving weak morphological endings or other brief and unstressed morphemes within a message, then encouraging the individual to use internalized linguistic knowledge to fill in the missing information can achieve closure and result in accurate comprehension during conversation (as shown in the example provided on page 305) or during academic activities that rely heavily on accurate auditory perception (e.g., spelling tests—where the teacher might say "Spell *adolescents* as in 'The adolescents *were* ready to become adults.").

Prosody

Prosody refers to the suprasegmental aspects of spoken language and is critical for the processing of speech and language at a number of levels. Efficient and accurate language processing of a speaker's message and intent involves the ability to recognize and interpret the use of rhythm, stress and intonation, and timing in the spoken message. Subtle differences in stress, inflections, timing, and pauses within the spoken message are used by the speaker to differentiate verbs from nouns, to convey humor, and to distinguish potentially ambiguous information. Also conveyed in the suprasegmental information contained in the spoken message is information about the emotional status of the speaker and the nature of a spoken statement. Take for example, the sentence, *"It is hot in here."* If this sentence is interpreted solely on the basis of the sentence structure it would appear to be a simple declarative sentence. However, when spoken in the right context with a certain suprasegmental pattern it may be interpreted as an indirect request to open the window or even a stronger imperative/directive to open a window.

Prosody is used to link phonetic segments, to direct attention to the important part of the message, and to provide clues about the lexical, semantic, and syntactic content of the utterance. The use of intonation and stress within an utterance gives clues to word meanings and can be used to resolve ambiguity. Take for example the following two sentences, the stress patterns (shown by the capitalization of the word) clearly differentiate the meanings of these two sentences.

1. FLYING planes can be dangerous.
2. Flying PLANES can be dangerous.

Stress is also used by the speaker to differentiate heteronyms (i.e., words that share the same spelling, but differ in pronunciation and meaning) by differentially placing the stress on the first syllable of the word (if it is a noun) and on the second syllable of the word (if it is a verb) as in the examples shown below. Accurate "perception" of such differential stress patterns can aid in the accurate and "efficient" recognition of the semantic meanings of the heteronyms, CONvict and conVICT, in sentences (1) and (2) and the heteronyms, REcord and reCORD, in sentences (3) and (4).

1. The CONvict was released early.
2. The decision was to conVICT the defendant.
3. John went to the music store to purchase a new REcord.
4. The new parents went to the town hall to reCORD their child's birth.

Stress and prosody are also used by the speaker to disambiguate temporally cued differences in words or phrase as in the following samples.

1. You'll love them all.
2. You'll love the mall.
3. It's parked.
4. It sparked.

Training activities to facilitate the use of prosody to aid in the processing of auditory language can involve such activities as key word extraction, where the individual is taught to listen for specific words, phrases, or sentences within spoken texts, reading and/or listening to poetry, reading aloud with animated intonation, and presentation of series of temporally cued sentence pairs that contrast one versus two word segmentation of words (e.g., *fair grounds* versus *fairgrounds*) as well as the types of temporally cued information depicted above (e.g., *it's parked* versus *it sparked*) (Chermak, 2007; Chemak & Musiek, 1997).

Discourse Cohesion Devices

Discourse cohesion devices are linguistic terms or forms that either imply or clearly establish relationships among parts of messages or ideas (Halliday & Hasan, 1976). They function to connect ideas or propositions into efficient and complex messages and in doing so they typically reduce the overall number of words in a message. For a child or an adult with an auditory processing disorder, the reduction in the number of words that must be processed is a desirable outcome. However, this reduction in the auditory processing load does come with a cost. Although cohesive ties or devices serve to increase transmission efficiency by reducing the number of words needed to convey a message, they generally increase the memory and language processing demands that are placed upon the listener (Musiek et al., 1999). To be used effectively listeners must be able to recognize the relationships signaled by these cohesive devices. If and when individuals can identify and understand these terms they will be better able to separate the message into smaller, more manageable units for linguistic processing.

Cohesive devices are special classes of words that are used by speakers to signal relationships between propositions and/or to build cohesive trains of thought through the use of linguistic forms that either make explicit the referent as in the case of the use of pronouns or that must be inferred by the listener as in the case of ellipsis (Chermak, 2007; Musiek et al., 1999).

Conjunctions are one category of discourse cohesion devices. These can signal additive, adversative, or disjunctive relationships or they may signal causal or temporal relationships between elements within and across propositions as shown in the examples below. These devices do not require the listener to make any assumptions or presumptions about the information that either precedes or follows the device (Chermak, 2007; Chermak & Musiek, 1997).

Additive: The freshmen *and* sophomores planned a holiday party for the upperclassmen.

Adversative: *Although* Mary wanted to go the beach with her classmates, no one invited her.

Disjunctive: Mary chose to bake a pie *instead* of a cake for the party even though baking a cake would have been easier for her.

Causal: The student cheated on the final exam; *therefore*, the professor gave her a failing grade for the course.

Temporal: It is important to fasten your seat beat *before* turning on your car.

Referents such as pronouns, proverbs, and comparatives constitute another group of cohesive device mechanisms (Chermak, 2007; Chermak & Musiek, 1997). In these cases, the referent refers back to an individual, action, or situation that is specified in an earlier statement or phrase (see examples below).

Pronoun: John completed his term paper. *He* then turned it in to his professor

Pro-verb: The darkness of the night enveloped the town. When it *did* all of the street lights came on.

Comparative: The members of the U.S. diving team completed their dives with agility and excellent form. *Similarly*, the members of the gymnastic team executed their balance beam programs with grace and impeccable technical form.

Finally, there is a class of cohesion devices that (1) delete part of a message that can be inferred from the information available (ellipsis), (2) use different terminology to refer to the same or a similar referent or activity (substitution), or (3) activate known versus new information (definitiveness) (Chermak, 2007; Chermak & Musiek, 1997).

Ellipsis: Mary enjoys her anatomy class. John does too. [John enjoys anatomy class too.]

Substitution: The university's *football team* won the NCAA championship. The spectators were amazed at the performance of *the players*.

Definitiveness: The automobile's fuel injection system failed to work. The mechanic at the repair shop was unable to fix *the* problem.

Intervention activities in this area should focus on having the individual identify the presence of these lexical items in spoken statements and then describe the relationships being signaled by the lexical items. The reader interested in additional discussion of this metalinguistic skill and its application in the processing of spoken language is referred to Chermak (2007), Chermak and Musiek (1997), and Musiek et al. (1999).

Schema Induction

Schema theory tries to explain how knowledge and experience are mapped in the mind and how those underlying representations or maps facilitate comprehension and learning (Kintsch, 1980, 1988). A schema is a conceptual framework connecting related ideas that can be used by an individual to predict and infer unmentioned or illusive aspects of a situation (Kintsch, 1980, 1988). It consists of "a structured cluster of concepts, a set of expectations, an abstract and generic knowledge structure stored in memory that preserves the relations among constituent concepts and generalized knowledge about a text, event, situation, or object (Mandler, 1984; Miller, 1988; Rumelhart, 1980, 1984)" (cited in Chermak & Musiek, 1997, p. 194). The schema does not specify meaning but rather it helps create a set of expectations that serves to narrow the range of possibilities and gives direction to the construction of meaning by connecting interrelated ideas. As explained by Rumelhart (1980), "schemata are employed "in the process of interpreting sensory data (linguistic and nonlinguistic), in retrieving information from memory, in organizing actions, in determining of goals and subgoals, in allocating resources, and generally in guiding the flow of processing in the system" (pp. 33–34). When confronting a novel situation the use of schemata can assist the individual in identifying the "best fit" between the data and the structure. Schemata if used effectively can help increase the likelihood that a message or a behavior will be understand by an individual through the deployment of the top-down processes mentioned above.

Formal schemata include a collection of linguistic markers that function to organize, integrate, and predict relationships across ideas and propositions (Dillon, 1987). The discourse cohesion devices discussed above represent format schemata as they can be used to organize, integrate, and predict relationships about propositions. Other linguistic conventions that also can be used to organize, integrate, and predict relationships include those linguistic markers that signal parallelism or correlative state (e.g., *not only . . . but also*, *neither . . . nor*), causation or speculation (e.g., *if . . . then*), temporal relationships (e.g., *first, secondly, finally*), and so forth. Use of these types of linguistic conventions serves to help reduce the linguistic-cognitive demands involved in the processing of complex utterances, but they require a knowledge of discourse conventions that give form and structure to the message.

Content or contextual schemata provide a generalized interpretation of the content of experience (Dillon, 1981). Content or contextual can also be thought of as "scripts." They function to organize facts in a framework that allows the listener to impose structure on events and situations to facilitate interpretation and comprehension (Rumelhart, 1980). Listeners utilize the sequential steps or actions involved in common events to anticipate the way in which a message will unfold. Having accessed a particular script, the listener anticipates the major actions or behaviors of characters in a story or assumes an ongoing event will progress in a logical order with an "ending" coming at the end of the script (Chermak & Musiek, 1997).

There is evidence that children with language disorders have difficulty with the formulation of these types of schemata (Liles, 1985, 1987). It is anticipated that individuals with (C)APD will also have similar difficulties. For these individuals efforts should be directed at developing the ability to recognize the presence of cohesive ties and formal schemata within utterances so that the individual will be able to use this information to discern the unique relationships between the propositions and events that are signaled by these discourse elements. In addition, intervention activities can focus on the application and use of "scripts" to aid in establishing expectations about the nature of the event that is being described. These types of intervention will assist the individual with a (C)APD in the processing of complex spoken messages, as deployment of these skills and abilities during listening activities should (1) evoke certain expectations about the message, (2) narrow the possible alternatives for explanation, and (3) provide the individual with direction in processing the information (Chermak & Musiek, 1997; Musiek et al., 1999).

Strategy Instruction

For many individuals the metalinguistic skills and strategies discussed in this chapter are automatic and require little conscious effort to be used effectively (Flavell, 1985; Siegler, & Sharger, 1984). However, for some individuals this is not the case. In these individuals a much more conscious and effortful approach to applying these skills or strategies is necessary. Such an approach typically involves (1) a deliberate assessment of the cognitive demands associated with the context or behavior that is causing (or may ultimately cause) inefficiencies in processing, (2) a determination of one's personal goal (or goals) with respect to the context or behavior, and (3) the identification of the mental processes needed to meet both the demands and the goals associated with the context or behavior (Siegler & Shipley, 1995). The latter situation is often the case with individuals with (C)APD. For these individuals, the simple identification of a strategy (or strategies) that could result in the improved reception and decoding of an auditory message may not be sufficient to encourage use of the strategy (or strategies) to aid in comprehension. Moreover, it should be realized that if the individual is not already using one or more of these strategies, then the use of such strategies is not automatic or effortless for the individual and more formalized strategy instruction may be needed (Baran, 2002, 2007; Bellis, 2003, Chermak, 2007; Chermak & Musiek, 1997).

There have been a number of different instructional approaches that have been developed in an effort to provide effective instruction in the use of strategies (e.g., Deschler, Alley, Warner, & Schumaker, 1981; Deschler, Shumaker, Lenz, & Ellis, 1984; Harris, Graham, & Pressley, 1991). Common to these procedures are a number of essential activities or steps. These include: (1) some type of preassessment of current strategy use and a commitment to the use of newly acquired strategies, (2) the identification and description of the strategies, (3) the modeling of the strategies, (4) verbal rehearsal of the strategies, (5) controlled practice and feedback on the application of the strategies, and (6) generalization of the strategies to new contexts (Baran, 2007, p. 251). An exhaustive review of these various approaches to strategy instruction is beyond the scope of this chapter. The reader interested in detailed information on the application of strategy instruction procedures is referred to the following sources (Baran, 1998, 2002, 2007; Bender, 2004; Chermak, 2007; Chermak & Musiek, 1997; Deschler, Alley, Warner, & Schumaker, 1981; Deschler, Shumaker, Lenz, & Ellis, 1984; Hallahan, Lloyd, Kauffman, Weiss, & Martinez, 2005; Harris, Graham, & Pressley, 1991; Wynn-Dancy & Gillam, 1997, 1998).

Although the application and use of the strategies that have been detailed in these publications may appear to be obvious to most mature language users, they may not be as readily apparent to some individuals with auditory processing deficits (Baran, 2002, 2007). If they were, then it is likely that the individual would have adopted the use of the strategy (or strategies) without the need for any type of specific instruction. Moreover, even if an individual with (C)APD "self" identifies a strategy that works well in a particular situation or context, it is possible that he or she will continue to experience processing deficits and communication breakdowns in other settings if that individual has not learned how to generalize the adopted strategy to new situations or contexts. For these reasons, it is recommended that formalized, strategy instruction (beyond just the simple identification of strategies) be considered as a potential component of a comprehensive management plan that is being developed for the individual with (C)APD (Baran, 2007, p. 251).

Target Populations

Efforts directed at either the development of new metalinguistic skills or the individual's ability to use existing and internalized metalinguistic skills can be used with both children and adults with (C)APD. The use of specific metalinguistic strategies, however, should be developmentally appropriate. With young children, intervention may focus more on actual skill development (e.g., phonological awareness training) than on strategy development. In older children and adults it is much more likely that the metalinguistic skills discussed in this chapter will already have been developed—especially if one is working with individuals with acquired (C)APDs. In these cases, it is unlikely that efforts will be directed at metalinguistic skill development, but rather on the identification of metalinguistic skills and strategies that can be used by the individual when he or she encounters a communication breakdown or a problem processing auditory information. As part of this intervention, it will be important to help the individual identify when and where difficulties are likely to arise. As mentioned above, the impact of a (C)APD on one's ability to process language is likely to change with a number of variables. These can include the language context, the characteristics of the conversational partner, teacher, or other speaker, the room acoustics, the individual's state (e.g., level of alertness, motivation level, and attention) and so forth. Therefore, it is possible and, in fact, likely that the individual with (C)APD may not experience listening and comprehension difficulties in every listening situation or context, but that certain listening environments and situations will provide listening challenges for him or her. Moreover, even within a given situation or context the deficits that an individual may experience may be variable. Being able to predict when and where auditory processing difficulties are likely to be encountered will enable the individual to be both flexible and efficient in his or her strategy selection and application procedures.

Although many of the metalinguistic strategies discussed in this chapter may provide some assistance, it is important to explore the metacognitive strategies that may also be helpful. An integrated approach to dealing with difficult listening situations is essential if the individual is to be successful. As has been suggested by several authors, the successful individual needs not only to learn metacognitive and/or metalinguistic strategies, he or she needs to learn how to become "strategic" (Baran, 2002, 2007; Chermak, 2007; Wynn-Dancy & Gilliam, 1997, 1998). A strategy that works well in one context may prove to be of little assistance in another context. Reliance on a single strategy or even a small group of strategies is not likely to serve an individual well if he or she is not able to critically evaluate the listening demands, analyze where the difficulties are likely to occur, consider the strategies that may be useful in the given context, and be able to switch strategies if the chosen strategy fails to provide the support that is needed.

Summary

Metalinguistic strategies as discussed within the context of this chapter are one subset of a larger number of central resources that an individual can use to help facilitate the accurate and efficient processing of auditorily presented information. Metalinguistic skills allow the individual to think about and use language in meaningful contexts. For many listeners, metalinguistic skills are deployed automatically and require little conscious effort. Unfortunately this is not typically the case for many individuals with (C)APD. For these individuals, it may be necessary for the audiologist and/or speech-language pathologist to provide direct instruction in the ways in which these skills can be used to help ensure correct and efficient processing of auditory information; that is, assuming that the individual has mastered the appropriate metalinguistic skills. If delays in the development of the metalinguistic skills are noted, then the initial remedial efforts should be directed toward the development of normal and age-appropriate metalinguistic skills and abilities.

As with any "meta-strategy" to be used, it will be important not only to identity the strategy or strategies that can provide assistance in the processing of spoken language, but also to provide formalized instruction in the application and use of the strategy or strategies. This typically involves a number of important steps during which the individual learns how to analyze the listening situation, predict the listening problems that are likely to be encountered in the listening situation, generate potential solutions for these problems, and identify and implement the most effective solution(s). Other important components of the instructional program will include the provision of opportunities for the application, reinforcement, and generalization of these learned strategies.

As some strategies may work well in some situations and contexts, but not be effective in other situations and contexts, it is important that intervention efforts focus on helping the individual become "strategic." With each new listening context, it is important that the individual be prepared to analyze the new listening context or environment, to identify potential processing challenges, and to select and deploy the strategy (strategies) that is (are) the best fit for the given context. Interventions that combine metalinguistic strategies instruction with self-regulation and other metacognitive approaches are likely to be more successful than use of either approach in isolation.

Key Points Learned

- Metalinguistic skills are cognitive-linguistic skills that allow an individual to "think" about language in a critical manner, to "make informed judgments" about the accurate and appropriate use of language, and to "talk" about language in meaningful ways.
- Metalinguistic strategies are purposeful actions that are used to accomplish specific language processing goals. In regard to the processing of auditory language, these strategies allow the individual to become more of an active as opposed to a passive listener when processing spoken language.
- For most individuals, the use of metalinguistic knowledge to aid in comprehension occurs automatically at a subconscious level; however, for many individuals, such as many individuals with (C)APD, specific strategy instruction is needed.
- Metalinguistic approaches to the management of auditory processing deficits can include basic skill development, as in the case of phonological awareness training, as well as strategy instruction, as in the identification and application of the metalinguistic strategies discussed in this chapter that can be used when processing challenges are encountered.
- Metalinguistic approaches should not be used in isolation but rather should be included in a comprehensive intervention plan/program used for the remediation and/or management of a (C)APD. Such a plan/program is likely to include other approaches, such as auditory training, signal enhancement strategies and environmental modification interventions, and additional central resource training, including cognitive, metacognitive, and language training.
- The relative reliance on the various approaches to intervention will be determined by a number of factors, including but not limited to, the patient's age and cognitive abilities, the specific auditory deficits that are uncovered during a diagnostic workup, a consideration of the individual's listening demands and contexts, and the presence of other comorbid conditions.
- Unlike auditory training intervention, metalinguistic approaches are not targeted at directly remediating the auditory deficits, but rather are designed to help the individual with (C)APD identify, internalize, and use a variety of cognitive-linguistic strategies that can be used to help "fill in"

information that is either not perceived or not perceived accurately through the auditory modality.

- Finally, the successful approach to management of an individual's auditory processing disorders through the use of "meta-strategies" cannot end with the identification and application of the strategies in a given context or contexts (which are often artificially created in the clinical setting). Rather the approach must include opportunities for the individual to (1) generalize the newly acquired and/or deployed strategies in novel contexts; (2) evaluate new contexts to determine if auditory processing difficulties are likely to be encountered, and if so, which strategy or strategies would work best in the new listening situation; (3) quickly re-evaluate the context, listening demands, and so forth when a selected strategy fails to provide the assistance anticipated; and (4) effectively and efficiently deploy an alternative strategy or strategies when the need arises. In other words, the ultimate goal of "meta-training" would be to train the individual with (C)APD to be "strategic" in his or her selection, use, and application of the various "meta-strategies" available to him or her.

References

American Speech-Language-Hearing Association. (2005). *(Central) auditory processing disorders.* Available at http://www.asha.org/members/deskref-journals/deskref/default.

Baran, J. A. (1998). Management of adolescents and adults with central auditory processing disorders. In G. A. Masters, N. A. Stecker, & J. Katz (Eds.), *Central auditory processing disorders: Mostly management* (pp. 195–214). Boston: Allyn & Bacon.

Baran, J. A. (2002). Managing auditory processing disorders in adolescents and adults. *Seminars in Hearing, 23,* 327–335.

Baran, J. A. (2007). Managing (central) auditory processing disorders in adolescents and adults. In G. D. Chermak & F. E. Musiek (Eds.), *Handbook of (central) auditory processing disorder: Comprehensive intervention* (Vol. 2, pp. 243–272). San Diego, CA: Plural Publishing.

Bellis, T. J. (2003). *Assessment and management of central auditory processing disorders in the educational setting: From science to practice* (2nd ed.). Clifton Park, NY: Thomson Learning.

Bender, W. A. (2004). *Learning disabilities: Characteristics, identification, and teaching strategies* (5th ed.). Boston: Allyn & Bacon.

Bernstein, D. K. (1997). Language development. The school age years. In D. K. Bernstein & E. Tiegerman-Faber (Eds.), *Language and communication disorders in children* (4th ed., pp. 127–151). Boston: Allyn & Bacon.

Catts, H. W. (1991). Facilitating phonological awareness: Role of speech-language pathologists. *Language, Speech and Hearing Services in Schools, 22,* 11–28.

Chermak, G. D. (1998). Metacognitive approaches to managing central auditory processing disorders. In G. A. Masters, N. A. Stecker, & J. Katz (Eds.), *Central auditory processing disorders: Mostly management* (pp. 49–62). Boston: Allyn & Bacon.

Chermak, G. D. (2007). Central resources training: Metacognitive and metalinguistic skills and strategies. In G. D. Chermak & F. E. Musiek (Eds.), *Handbook of (central) auditory processing disorder: Comprehensive intervention* (Vol. 2, pp. 107–166). San Diego, CA: Plural Publishing.

Chermak, G. D., & Musiek, F. E. (1992). Managing central auditory processing disorders in children and youth. *American Journal of Audiology, 1*, 62–65.

Chermak, G. D., & Musiek, F. E. (1997). *Central auditory processing disorders: New perspectives*. San Diego, CA: Singular Publishing Group.

Chermak, G. D., & Musiek, F. E. (2002). Auditory training: Principles and approaches for remediating and managing auditory processing disorders. *Seminars in Hearing, 23*, 297–308.

Deschler, D. D., Alley, G. R., Warner, M. M., & Schumaker, J. B. (1981). Instructional practices for promoting skill acquisition and generalization in severely learning disabled adolescents. *Learning Disability Quarterly, 4*, 415–421.

Deschler, D. D., Schumaker, J. B., Lenz, B. K., & Ellis, E. S. (1984). Academic and cognitive interactions for LD adolescents. Part II. *Journal of Learning Disabilities, 17*, 170–187.

Dillon, G. L. (1981). *Connecting texts*. Bloomington: Indiana University Press.

Douglas, J. D., & Peel, B. (1979). The development of metaphor and proverb translation in children grades one through seven. *Journal of Educational Research, 73*, 116–119.

Earobics. (1996). Evanston, IL: Cognitive Concepts.

Fast ForWord. (1999). Berkeley, CA: Scientific Learning Corporation.

Ferre, J. (2002). Management strategies for APD. In T. K. Partasarsarathy (Ed.), *An introduction to auditory processing disorders in children* (pp. 161–183). Mahwah, NJ: Lawrence Erlbaum Associates.

Flavell, J. H. (1985). *Cognitive development*. (2nd ed.). Englewood Cliffs, NJ: Prentice-Hall.

Gerber, A. (1993). Intervention: Preventing or reversing the failure cycle. In A. Gerber (Ed.), *Language-related learning disabilities: Their nature and treatment* (pp. 323–393). Baltimore: Paul H. Brookes.

Gillam, R. B. & van Kleeck, A. (1998). Phonological awareness training and short-term working memory: Clinical implications. In R. B. Gillam (Ed.), *Memory and language impairment in children and adults: New perspectives* (pp. 83–96). Gaithersburg, MD: Aspen Publishers.

Goswami, U., & Bryant, P. E. (1990). *Phonological skills and learning to read*. Hillsdale, NJ: Lawrence Erlbaum Associates.

Hakes, D. (1980). *The development of metalinguistic abilities*. New York: Springer-Verlag.

Hakes, D. (1982). The development of metalinguistic abilities: What develops. In S. Kuczaj, II (Ed.), *Language development: Language, thought and culture* (Vol. 2, pp. 163–210). Hillsdale, NJ: Lawrence Erlbaum Associates.

Hallahan, D. P., Lloyd, J. W., Kauffman, J. M., Weiss, M. P., & Martinez, E. A. (2005). *Learning disabilities: Foundations, characteristics, and effective teaching* (3rd ed.). Boston: Allyn & Bacon.

Halliday, M. A. K., & Hasan, R. (1996). *Cohesion in English*. London: Longman.

Harris, K. R., Graham, S., & Pressley, M. (1991). Cognitive-behavioral approaches in reading and written language: Developing self-regulated learners. In N. N. Singh & L. L. Beale (Eds.), *Learning disabilities: Nature, theory, and treatment* (pp. 415–541). New York: Springer-Verlag.

Hempenstall, K. (1997). The role of phonemic awareness in beginning reading: A review. *Behaviour Change, 14*(4), 201–214.

Hempenstall, K. (2003). Phonemic awareness: What does it mean? *Education Oasis.* Retrieved 2/8/07 from: http://www.educationoasis.com/resources/Articles/phomenic_awareness.htm.

Hulit, L. M., & Howard, M. R. (2002). *Born to talk: An introduction to speech and language development*. Boston: Allyn & Bacon.

Kamhi, A. G. (1987). Metalinguistic abilities in language-impaired children. *Topics in Language Disorders*, *7*(2), 1–12.

Katz, J., & Harmon, C. (1982). *Phonemic synthesis*. Allen, TX: Developmental Learning Materials.

Keith, R. W., & Novak, K. K. (1984). Relationships between tests of central auditory function and receptive language. *Seminars in Hearing*, *5*(3), 243–250.

Kintsch, W. (1988). The role of knowledge in discourse comprehension: A construction-integration model. *Psychological Review*, *95*, 163–182.

Larson, V. I., & McKinley, N. (1987). *Communication assessment and intervention strategies for adolescents*. Eau Claire, WI: Thinking Publications.

Liles, B. Z. (1985). Cohesion in narratives of normal and language disordered children. *Journal of Speech and Hearing Research*, *28*, 123–133.

Liles, B. Z. (1987). Episode organization and cohesive conjunctions in narratives of children with and without language disorders. *Journal of Speech and Hearing Research*, *30*, 165–196.

Lindamood Phoneme Sequencing Program-LiPS. (1999). San Luis Obispo, CA: Lindamood-Bell Learning Center.

Mandler, J. M. (1984). *Stories, scripts, and scenes: Aspects of schema theory.* Hillsdale, NJ: Lawrence Erlbaum Associates.

Masters, G. A., Stecker, N. A., & J. Katz (Eds.). (1998). *Central auditory processing disorders: Mostly management*. Boston: Allyn & Bacon.

Matkin, N., & Hook, P. (1983). A multidisciplinary approach to central auditory evaluations. In E. Lasky & J. Katz (Eds.), *Central auditory processing disorders* (pp. 133–148). Cambridge, MA: MIT Press.

Miller, G. A. (1988). The challenge of universal literacy. *Science*, *241*, 1293–1299.

Miller, G. A., & Gildea, P. M. (1987). How children learn words. *Scientific American*, *257*, 94–99.

Musiek, F. E. (1999). Habilitation and management of auditory processing disorders: Overview of selected procedures. *Journal of the American Academy of Audiology*, *10*, 329–342.

Musiek, F. E., Baran, J. A., & Schochat, E. (1999). Selected management approaches to central auditory processing disorders. *Scandinavian Audiology*, *28*(Suppl. 51), 63–76.

Musiek, F. E., & Schochat, E. (1998). Auditory training and central auditory processing disorders. *Seminars in Hearing*, *19*, 357–365.

Musiek, F. E., Shinn, J., & Hare, C. (2002). Plasticity, auditory training and auditory processing disorders. *Seminars in Hearing*, *23*, 263–276.

Nippold, M. A. (1988). *Later language development: Age nine through nineteen.* Austin, TX: Pro-Ed.

Richard, G. J. (2007). Intervention for cognitive-communicative and language factors associated with (C)APD. In G. D. Chermak & F. E. Musiek (Eds.), *Handbook of (central) auditory processing disorder: Comprehensive intervention* (Vol. 2, pp. 291–308). San Diego, CA: Plural Publishing.

Roth, R. P., & Worthington, C. K. (2001). *Treatment resource manual for speech-language pathology* (2nd ed.). Albany, NY: Delmar Publishers.

Rumelhart, D. E. (1980). Schemata: The basic building blocks of cognition. In R. Shapiro, B. Bruce, & W. Brewer (Eds.), *Theoretical issues in reading comprehension* (pp. 1–20). Newark, DE: International Reading Association.

Rumelhart, D. E. (1984). Understanding understanding. In J. Flood (Ed.), *Understanding reading comprehension* (pp. 1–20).

Newark, DE: International Reading Association.

Saywitz, K., & Wilkinson, L. (1982). Age-related differences in metalinguistic awareness. In S. Kuczaj, II (Ed.), *Language development: Language, thought and culture* (Vol. 2, pp. 229–250). Hillsdale, NJ: Lawrence Erlbaum Associates.

Shatz, M., & Gelman, R. (1973). The development of communication skills: Modification of speech of young children. *Monograph Society for Research in Child Development*, *38*, 1–37.

Shultz, T. R., & Horibe, R. (1974). Development of the appreciation of verbal jokes. *Developmental Psychology*, *10*, 13–20.

Siegler, R., & Sharger, J. (1984). Strategy choices in addition and subtraction: How do children know what to do? In C. Sophian (Ed.), *Origins of cognitive skills* (pp. 229–293). Hillsdale, NJ: Lawrence Erlbaum Associates.

Siegler, R., & Shipley, C. (1995). Variation, selection, and cognitive change. In T. E. Simon (Ed.), *Developing cognitive competence* (pp. 31–76). Hillsdale, NJ: Lawrence Erlbaum Associates.

Singh, S., & Kent, R. D. (2000). *Singular's pocket dictionary of speech-language pathology*. San Diego, CA: Singular Publishing Group.

Sloan, C. (1986). *Treating auditory processing difficulties in children*. San Diego, CA: College-Hill Press.

Smith, C., & Tager-Flusberg, H. (1982). Metalinguistic awareness and language development. *Journal of Exceptional Child Psychology*, *34*, 449–468.

Thibodeau, L. M. (2007). Computer-based auditory training for (central) auditory processing disorder. In G. D. Chermak & F. E. Musiek (Eds.), *Handbook of (central) auditory processing disorder: Comprehensive intervention* (Vol. 2, pp. 167–206). San Diego, CA: Plural Publishing.

van Kleeck, A. (1984a). Assessment and intervention. Does "meta" matter? In G. Wallach & K. Butler (Eds.), *Language learning disabilities in school age children* (pp. 179–198). Baltimore: Williams & Wilkins.

van Kleeck, A. (1984b). Metalinguistic skills: Cutting across spoken and written language and problem-solving abilities. In G. Wallach & K. Butler (Eds.), *Language learning disabilities in school age children* (pp. 128–153). Baltimore: Williams & Wilkins.

van Kleeck, A. (1994). Metalinguistic development. In G. P. Wallach & K. G. Butler (Eds.), *Language learning disabilities in school-age children and adolescents: Some principles and applications* (pp. 53–98). New York: Macmillan College Publishing Company.

Vinson, B. (2007). *Language disorders across the lifespan* (2nd ed.). Clifton Park, NY: Thomson Delmar Learning.

Westby, C. E. (1998). Communicative refinement in school age and adolescence. In W. O. Haynes & B. B. Shulman (Eds.), *Communication development: Foundations, processes, and clinical applications* (pp. 311–350). Baltimore: Williams & Wilkins.

Wiig, E. (1989). *Steps to language competence*. San Antonio, TX: The Psychological Corporation.

Willeford, J. A., & Burleigh, J. M. (1985). *Handbook of auditory processing disorders in children*. Orlando, FL: Grune & Stratton.

Wynn-Dancy, M. L., & Gillam, R. B. (1997). Accessing long-term memory: Metacognitive struggles and strategic actions in adolescents. *Topics in Language Disorders*, 18, 32–44.

Wynn-Dancy, M. L., & Gilliam, R. B. (1998). Accessing long-term memory: Metacognitive strategies and strategic action in adolescents. In R. B. Gillam (Ed.), *Memory and language impairment in children and adults: New perspectives* (pp. 156–172). Gaithersburg, MD: Aspen Publishers.

17

Lindamood-Bell Instruction

Dual Coding with Imagery and Verbal Processing for Language and Literacy Skills

Nanci Bell

Overview

This chapter discusses the importance of Dual Coding Theory for language and literacy skills. First, this theory of cognition is explained and its history elucidated. Then its direct effect on the discrete skills of decoding/encoding and comprehension/critical thinking is revealed. There are three Lindamood-Bell® programs that develop dual coding by bringing sensory information to consciousness, each program having its own primary sensory focus. Both the *Seeing Stars*® program and the *LiPS*® program develop phonemic awareness for reading and spelling. The *Seeing Stars*® program focuses on the sensory development of symbol imagery whereas the *LiPS* program focuses on the sensory development of articulatory feedback. The *Visualizing and Verbalizing*® program develops concept imagery for comprehension and critical thinking. Each Lindamood-Bell® program is described in detail, with its steps listed and explained. Finally, evidence from an independent longitudinal study is presented, demonstrating the effectiveness of Lindamood-Bell instruction. In this study, reviewers from Texas A&M University examined the large-scale implementation of Lindamood-Bell instruction in an urban multicultural public school district.

Dual Coding: Cognition for Language and Literacy Skills

The human brain receives information through the senses, and the efficient integration of that sensory information is a critical base for acquisition of and competency in language and literacy skills. Lindamood-Bell instruction brings sensory processing to a conscious level to facilitate dual coding—the interplay between verbal and nonverbal information.

Allan Paivio, a cognitive psychologist, researcher, and originator of Dual Coding Theory (DCT), wrote extensively about the role of imagery as the nonverbal code in cognition. He believed all performance is mediated by the joint activity of verbal and nonverbal systems (Paivio, 1969). He suggested that linguistic competence and performance are based on a substrate of imagery, and that imagery includes not only static representations but also dynamic representations of action sequences and relationships between objects and events. He further suggested that individuals differ in the extent, manner, and efficiency of employment of each of the systems according to their verbal and nonverbal habits and skills.

According to DCT, cognition is always an interplay between the verbal and the nonverbal systems. Mark Sadoski (personal communication, March 21, 2006) expanded on a definition of DCT: "Dual Coding Theory is a theory of mind in which all cognition consists of the independent activity of, or interplay between, two great mental codes: a verbal code specialized for language and a nonverbal code specialized for knowledge of the world in the form of mental images."

Lindamood-Bell instruction focuses not on just multisensory integration, but on *imaginistic* multisensory integration. The goal is to bring the nonverbal code of imagery to consciousness so it can be integrated with the verbal code for oral and written language processing.

Imagery and Cognition: A Long History

The importance of imagery's role as a nonverbal source of sensory information cannot be overstated, and it is crucial to understanding Lindamood-Bell's sensory-cognitive programs. Imagery has been presented as a cornerstone of cognition as far back as 348 BC when Aristotle, in his contemplations on the ability to reason, theorized that man cannot think without mental imagery. His summation of memory concludes that memory or remembering is a state induced by mental images related as a likeness to that of which it is an image (Sorabji,

1972). References to imagery abound through the years. Even before Aristotle, Simonides (556–468 BC) taught imagery as a system to improve memory. The Greek and Roman orators used imagery as a memory system enabling them to speak for hours without written notes. Imagery as a sensory function for memory and thinking prevailed for thousands of years, fell out of favor, and was then revived in the eleventh and twelfth centuries. Thomas Aquinas was among those responsible for renewing interest in imagery as a cognitive tool when he argued that the mind could not comprehend ideas without imagery for them.

More recently, Jean Piaget (1971) wrote that knowledge, structures, or schemata are acquired when an infant actively manipulates, touches, and interacts with his environment. Piaget believed that as objects are manipulated, sensory-motor schemata are developed and changed to accommodate new information becoming internalized in the form of imaged thought (Bleasdale, 1983). Given the individual differences in the ability to access mental imagery, individuals with weakness in the sensory function of creating mental representations may have difficulty taking the last step of *internalizing the schemata in the form of imaged thought.* Piaget believed that imaginal representations are not formed with the same facility in each case, that there is a hierarchy of image levels, which may correspond to stages of development. He saw the evolution of images as a kind of intermediate between that of the perceptions and that of intelligence.

In 1969, Rudolf Arnheim wrote that thinking is concerned with the objects and events of our world and when the objects are not physically present, they are represented in the shape of memory images. He states that experiences create the images.

Paivio has written extensively on the role of imagery in cognition, stating that imagery was widely regarded as the mental representative of meaning, especially concrete meaning. He cited William James (1890) who suggested that the static meaning of concrete words consists of sensory images awakened (Paivio, 1969).

The cognitive psychologist Karl Pribram hypothesized that all thinking has, in addition to sign and symbol manipulation, a holographic component (Pribram, 1971). Stephen Kosslyn (1976) conducted a developmental study on the effects and role of imagery in retrieving information from long-term memory and determined that *imagery provided more opportunity for retrieval.* In 1983, Kosslyn further noted that a number of great thinkers, most notably Albert Einstein, professed to rely heavily on imagery in their problem solving. Einstein indicated that thoughts are images, which can be voluntarily reproduced as an essential feature of productive thought before there is any connection with the logical construction of words.

Einstein's achievements are milestones in the history of science, altering and expanding the understanding of our universe. His esteemed contributions were the result of his ability to make his thinking concrete by accessing the sensory function of mental imagery. He stated that if he couldn't picture it, he couldn't understand it. This illuminates his genius and also embodies a truth about the role imagery plays on the language processing spectrum as we dual code for cognition.

Two Types of Processing: Parts and Wholes

There are two primary language-processing deficits that are causal in preventing individuals from performing to their potential: weak decoding and weak comprehension. These two processes each use imagery in a specific and unique manner, distinct but related, like two sides of a coin. The two types of imagery are symbol imagery for processing parts, and concept imagery for processing wholes.

Symbol imagery is the ability to create mental representations *for sounds and letters* within words, the parts of the whole. Individuals with good symbol imagery have good phoneme awareness, good word attack skills, good word recognition skills, good contextual reading skills, and good spelling skills. A measure of symbol imagery confirms not only a correlation between the above skills, but also a stronger causal relationship than phoneme awareness.

Concept imagery is the ability to create a mental representation *for the whole*—an imaged gestalt. Individuals with good concept imagery have good language comprehension. They get the big picture—the whole concept—from which they can think critically and logically. They are apt at higher order thinking skills such as understanding the main idea, drawing a conclusion, making an inference, predicting, and extending. They easily follow directions and connect to oral language.

Although the ability to rapidly create mental representations for and from language is an important base for processing language, there are individual differences in the ability to access symbol and concept imagery. Some individuals have weakness in symbol imagery but strength in concept imagery, subsequently they have difficulty reading and spelling words, but they have good comprehension. On the other side of the coin, some individuals have strength in symbol imagery but weakness in concept imagery. They easily read and spell words, but experience moderate to significant difficulty in comprehension. Words appear to go in one ear and out the other.

Lindamood-Bell's Programs Bring Sensory Information to Consciousness

We can visualize language processing as a spectrum ranging from processing words (reading and spelling words) to processing concepts (comprehending and expressing language). When there is weakness on the left side of the spectrum, it may be labeled "dyslexia," and when there is weakness on the right side of the spectrum, it may be labeled "hyperlexia" and/or "autism" (Figure 17–1).

As a core sensory deficit is identified, instruction needs to be specific to that deficit to bring the appropriate sensory processing to a conscious level. For example, on the left side of the language-processing spectrum—the processing of single words—research shows that we need to auditorily perceive and create mental representations for sounds and letters within syllables, sensory-cognitive functions referred to as phoneme awareness and symbol imagery. The *Seeing Stars: Symbol Imagery for Phonemic Awareness, Sight Words and Spelling*

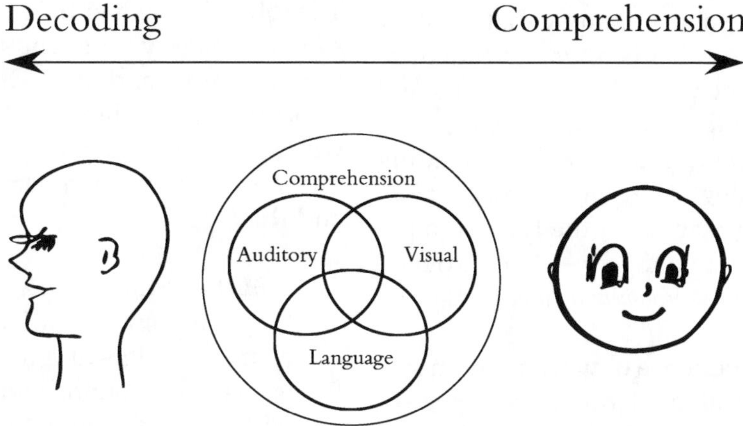

Figure 17–1. Language processing is a spectrum ranging from processing words (reading and spelling words) to processing concepts (comprehending and expressing language).

and the *Lindamood Phoneme Sequencing*® (*LiPS*) programs both develop phonological and orthographic awareness for reading and spelling words.

However, on the right side of the language-processing spectrum—the processing of concepts—research shows that we need to create mental representations for an imaged whole, a sensory-cognitive function referred to as concept imagery. Concept imagery is developed by the *Visualizing and Verbalizing for Language Comprehension and Thinking*® (V/V) program.

Seeing Stars: Symbol Imagery for Phonemic Awareness, Sight Words, and Spelling

The primary sensory focus of the *Seeing Stars* program is the development and application of symbol imagery to reading and spelling. As noted earlier, symbol imagery is causal to a range of reading skills and is also highly correlated to phonemic awareness. However, this knowledge was not known years ago. Prior to the development of the *Seeing Stars* program, we noted that students often made significant gains in word attack skills, but only modest gains in word recognition and contextual reading. Although the students could phonetically process words, too often their processing was slow, and they had difficulty establishing a strong sight word base. This attention to phonological processing—often at the expense of orthographic processing—contributed to substantial difficulty reading in context. Without a strong sight word base for orthographic processing, students often had to use phonological processing for too many words, which slowed their contextual reading. Their slow contextual reading contributed to their excessive guessing at words in an attempt to improve their fluency—and this interfered with their comprehension.

It was soon apparent that another sensory mechanism was needed to establish memory for sight words and attention to both phonological and orthographic processing for reading and spelling. The sensory mechanism was imagery but not the type of imagery—concept imagery—that we developed with the *Visualizing and Verbalizing* program.

The experience of working with students illuminated this new aspect of imagery for us. To our surprise, we found that individuals with good concept imagery, who could describe dynamic, colorful mental representations from connected text, could often not visualize even a few letters in a simple word. For example, a college student with difficulty reading and spelling words (but exceptional reading comprehension) described making "movies" when he read, and although he could give elaborate descriptions of contextual scenes and concepts, he couldn't visualize letters in words. When asked what letters he saw for the word *enough*, he looked puzzled and said he didn't see anything. When then asked what letters he saw for the word *cat*, he said he still didn't see anything. It was dark. Then he said, excitedly, "But I can see a cat. I can make it a black cat. I can make it a white cat. I can put it in the kitchen, sitting on a red chair near a table . . . but I can't see any letters."

As we worked with numerous students, specific steps to develop symbol imagery were created and applied to phonological and orthographic awareness for reading, and spelling words.

The Steps of the Seeing Stars Program

The following sequential steps develop symbol imagery for sounds and letters within words, and apply that sensory information to phonemic awareness, word attack, word recognition, spelling, and paragraph reading accuracy and fluency.

1. *Climate*—Students learn what they are doing and why. They come to understand that learning to visualize sounds and letters within words will help them read and spell words better.
2. *Imaging Letters*—Students are shown consonant and vowel letter cards to develop their ability to image, say, and write single letters by name and sound. The Sounds and Symbols Chart presents ten levels of consonants and vowels based on ease and frequency in reading and spelling (Figure 17–2).
3. *Imaging Syllable Cards*—Students are shown single syllable cards, ranging from VC to CCVCC. The goal is to develop the students' ability to image, write, and decode nonwords and real words for *phonological and orthographic* processing.
4. *Imaging and Sequencing Syllables on the Syllable Board*—Using the tips of their fingers, students "write" imaged letters and syllables on the syllable board, which has placeholders for the imaginary letters.
5. *Imaging and Sequencing Syllables by Air-writing*—Students write imaged letters in the air, writing in a medium-sized print so as to facilitate a shadow-effect—an image—for them to visualize and decode (Figure 17–3).

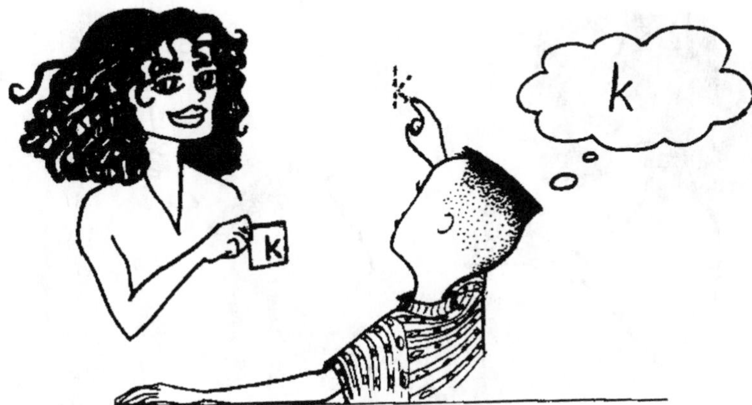

Figure 17–2. Students are shown consonant and vowel letter cards to develop their ability to image, say, and write single letters by name and sound.

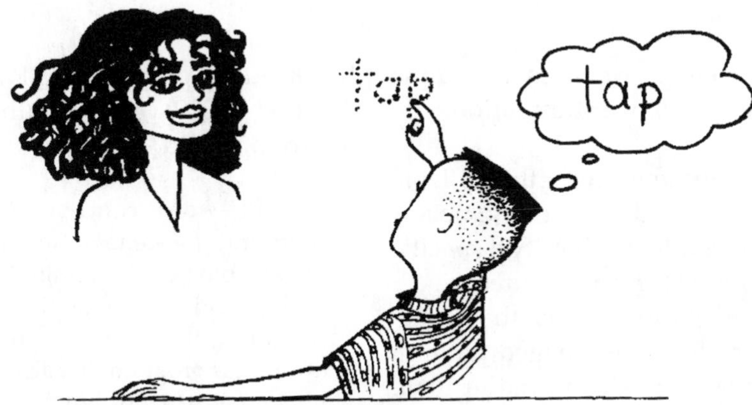

Figure 17–3. Students write imaged letters in the air to develop symbol imagery for sounds and letters in syllables.

6. *Imaging Sight Words and Spelling*—Students develop an extensive sight word base by accessing their new symbol imagery skills. Up to 1,000 sight words may be established for instant recognition and spelling, reinforced by questioning the students' symbol imagery for orthographic patterns.
7. *Imaging, Reading, and Spelling Multisyllables*—Students develop symbol imagery for two- through five-syllable words. Basic affixes are imaged, decoded, and encoded and applied to reading and spelling multisyllable words to ensure that phonological, as well as orthographic, processing is established (Figure 17–4).
8. *Contextual Application*—Students read in context to apply phonological and orthographic processing and improve paragraph reading fluency. To extend their sight word base, symbol imagery is continually questioned for newly encountered words.

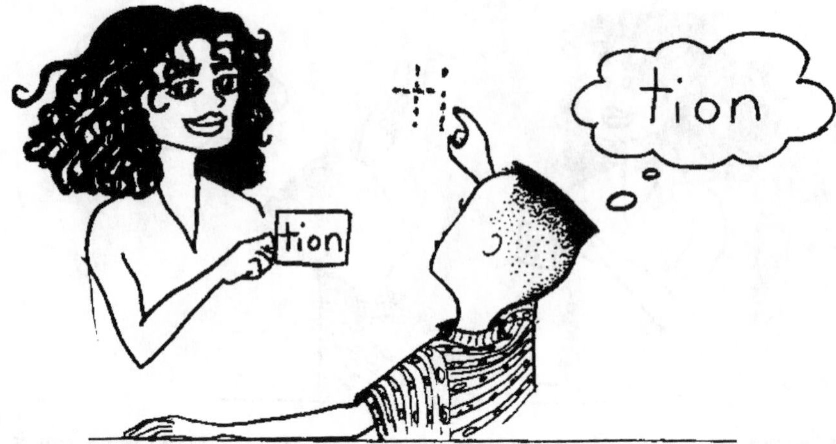

Figure 17–4. Students develop imagery for two- through five-syllable words to ensure that phonological, as well as orthographic, processing is established.

Symbol imagery exercises are done throughout the above stimulation:

- Decode: Students read the syllable from the imaged pattern (memory).
- Identify: Students identify a specific letter from the imaged pattern.
- Backward: Students say the letters backward from the imaged pattern.
- Manipulate: Students manipulate letters in the imaged pattern and then read the syllable from the new imaged pattern.

The Lindamood Phoneme Sequencing (LiPS) Program

Although both the *Seeing Stars* and *LiPS* programs develop reading and spelling skills, the two programs differ in sensory focus. The primary sensory focus of the *LiPS* Program is the development and application of articulatory feedback to reading, spelling, and speech.

The *LiPS* program was formally known as the *Auditory Discrimination in Depth* (*ADD*) program. As Patricia Lindamood (2000), the coauthor of the program, stated,

> The PH-word concepts (phonics, phonemic awareness, and phonetic or phonological processing) provide background for categorizing the *LiPS* program. It is truly a phonemic awareness program that also includes phonics instruction and application of phonemic awareness to phonetic processing in both reading and spelling. Before addressing letter symbols, the *LiPS* program engages students in discovering the articulatory gestures that differentiate phonemes so they can use oral-motor feedback to concretize, track, and prove the identity, number, and order of phonemes in words. Second, *LiPS* engages students in a variety of 'phoneme tracking' experiences that directly require application of the newly developed awareness of articulatory feedback. Then, as they learn the letter symbols that represent phonemes, students have only a half step to take into reading and spelling (p. 59).

LiPS moves from phonemic awareness activities to single syllable, multisyllable, and contextual reading levels in which phonemic awareness and orthographic expectancies are applied.

The Steps of the LiPS Program

The following sequential steps develop articulatory feedback for sounds within words and apply that feedback to reading, spelling, and speech.

1. *Setting the Climate*—Students are helped to understand what they will be doing and why: learning to *feel* as well as see and hear speech sounds.
2. *Consonants and Vowels*—Students discover how each of the consonant and vowel sounds are articulated and use that sensory information to organize the sounds into pairs and groups. Simple, descriptive labels are attached to each category such as "lip poppers" for /p/ and /b/. The labels enable the teacher and the student to communicate about sounds within words in subsequent steps.
3. *Tracking*—As students gain awareness of articulatory gestures, they begin using their oral-motor awareness to track the identity and order of phonemes in spoken words. They first use mouth pictures to show what they feel for phonemes in words. Then they move to colored blocks to show sounds in words (Figures 17–5 and 17–6).

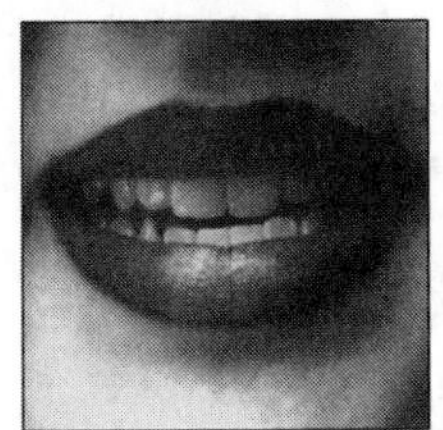
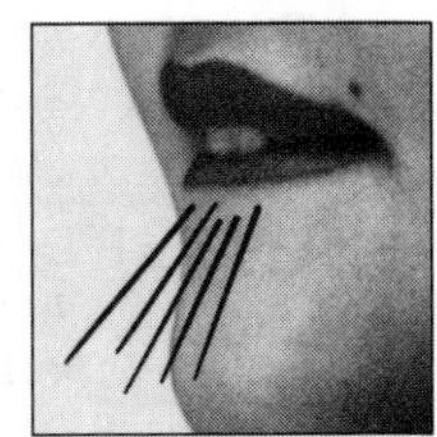

"Show me.../if/."

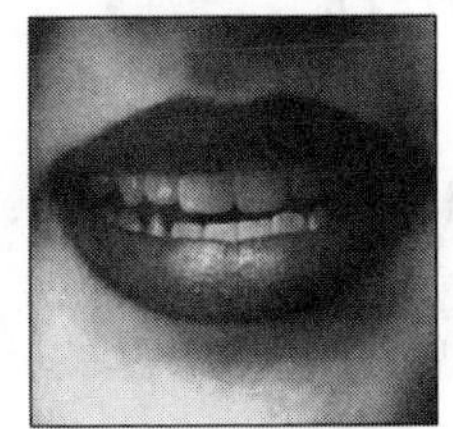
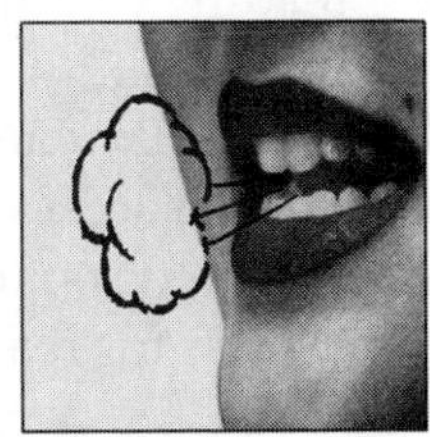

"That says /if/, now show me /it/."

Figure 17–5. Students use mouth pictures to track the identity, number, and sequence of sounds within words.

"If that says /snip/..."

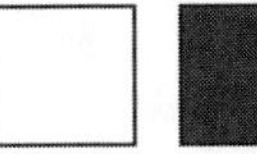

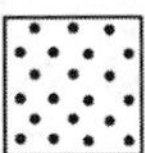
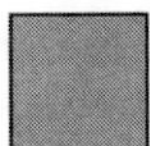

"...show me /skip/."

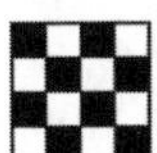
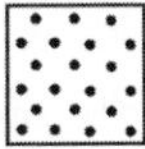

Figure 17–6. Students use blocks to track the identity, number, and sequence of sounds within words.

4. *Decoding and Spelling Single and Multisyllable Words*—Conscious attention to articulatory feedback for tracking phonemes in words is applied to reading and spelling. As Patricia Lindamood (2000) stated, "For decoding, 'Since I see an L right after the smile vowel, I will have to make my tongue do a lifter there.' As phonetic processing emerges, orthographic expectancies are introduced so that students begin to integrate phonetic processing with an ability to predict how words will be spelled or read" (p. 592). Tracking, spelling, and reading are kept synchronized as work progresses from single to multisyllable words. Sight words are also stimulated for contextual reading (Figure 17–7).

The *Seeing Stars* and *LiPS* programs are often used successfully together, or each may be used separately as the primary instruction for reading and spelling.

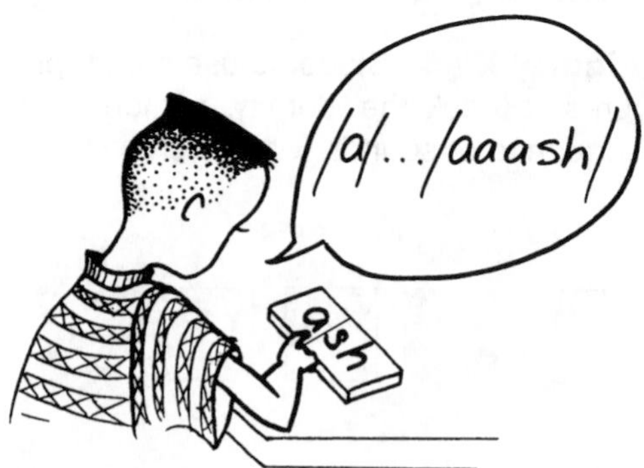

Figure 17–7. Conscious attention to articulatory feedback for tracking phonemes in words is applied to reading and spelling.

The Visualizing and Verbalizing for Language Comprehension and Thinking (V/V) Program

In contrast to the *Seeing Stars* program, which stimulates symbol imagery (parts), the *V/V* program stimulates concept imagery (wholes) with the goal to develop oral and written language comprehension, higher order thinking skills, the ability to follow directions, and expressive oral and written language. Where *LiPS* and *Seeing Stars* develop the students' ability to process the smallest parts of language (words), *V/V* develops the students' ability to visualize and process gestalts of meaning.

The symptoms of weakness in concept imagery extend to those of hyperlexia and autism:

- A tendency to process parts more than, or rather than, wholes. Students may get details rather than big pictures, and may attend to facts more than concepts.
- Difficulty with conceptual, critical, logical, and/or abstract thinking. Students may get stuck on details and parts and enjoy facts rather than concepts. They may appear to be "concrete thinkers" because they are processing specific part-images.
- Difficulty grasping oral language, whether in stories, conversation, or lectures. Students may not be interested in listening to stories, and they may seem unable to pay attention. They may miss the point of a lecture or conversation, or appear to process irrelevant and incidental parts of what they heard. They may often ask and re-ask the same question,

and may be labeled poor listeners or inattentive.

- Weak reading comprehension. Although oral vocabulary and decoding may be sufficient, these students may only get a few facts rather than the gestalt from what is read. They may have trouble answering higher order thinking skills questions, which relate to the main idea, conclusions, inferences, and predictions. They may read sentences, paragraphs, and chapters more than once and still not get the big picture or point. They may do poorly on tests that measure more than just facts.
- Difficulty following directions, oral or written. Students may get confused with more than one or two directions. Language may appear to go in one ear and out the other, without a connection. They may seem unable to pay attention.
- Weakness in expressing language orally. Their language expression is a random array of parts, facts, and details. They may talk about irrelevant parts or issues. They may tell stories out of sequence. Whether they talk very little or talk a lot, their language seems scattered and disconnected.
- Difficulty expressing language in writing. They often write in unrelated parts. They don't easily connect thoughts and make a point, a whole. They may have difficulty answering a question due to missing the point of the question.
- Difficulty understanding humor. Students may take language literally and not see the imagery in humor. They miss the joke. They may respond to physical humor, such as pie in the face, but they don't comprehend language-based humor. They may laugh at inappropriate times.
- Difficulty reading social situations. They may be primarily only able to grasp parts of an expression or situation. Based on that part, they may make inappropriate expressions or take inappropriate actions. They may have difficulty understanding cause and effect.
- Appear to find language and social interaction a confusing mix of disconnected parts. Students may prefer their own company. The communicating world seems to them a puzzling, disconcerting, and meaningless array of parts.

The firm "earth" of experience was the basis for the initial hypothesis of two types of imagery (symbol and concept imagery). Working in a clinical environment, instructing individuals of all ages who were experiencing language processing weaknesses, several insights were gained on the sensory-cognitive functions that underlie language processing:

- Individuals must be able to process a conceptual whole, not just parts, from language.
- Imagery is a sensory-cognitive tool that connects language and creates this whole.
- Individuals show different levels of ability in imaging conceptual wholes.

These insights eventually led to the instructional procedures of the *V/V* program. Clearly it wasn't enough to just *tell* someone to create mental images for language concepts. College students and adults with weak language comprehension often made comments such as, "I don't see anything. It is just dark up there." Sometimes they saw vague images that didn't have movement or color. Their imagery was not dynamic, but static, and they often had good symbol imagery, reading and spelling words easily. Specific steps were needed that would sequentially develop their dynamic imagery for concepts.

The Steps of the V/V Program

The *V/V* program develops concept imagery from the smallest unit of language—a word—and extends the imagery to sentences, paragraphs, and pages of content as a base for higher order thinking skills and problem solving.

1. *Climate*—Students learn what they are doing and why. They come to understand that by making pictures in their minds and by learning to talk about those pictures, they will better understand and remember what they read and hear.
2. *Picture to Picture*—The goal is to develop fluent, detailed verbalization from a given picture prior to requiring the detailed verbalization of a generated image in the next step. The students describe a simple picture using *structure words—what, size, color, number, shape, where, when, background, movement, mood, perspective,* and *sound*—as concrete descriptive elements that will help concretize the language experience. The teacher asks questions to specifically stimulate verbalization and visualization, such as, "What should I picture for the boy's hair?" (Figure 17–8).
3. *Word Imaging*—The goal is to develop detailed visualization (and verbalization) for a single word. Beginning with a high-imagery known noun, such as *boat*, the students are questioned for imagery and use the structure words to help them verbalize details, such as whether they pictured a yellow boat or a red boat (Figure 17–9).
4. *Phrase and Sentence Imaging*—The goal is to extend the imagery and language from one word to a phrase and then to a single, simple sentence. As the steps overlap, the students use a previously imaged known noun as the subject of a sentence to be visualized. For example, the boat that the individuals previously imaged with vivid, colorful mental representations is now the imagery to which action, a verb, is attached. "What do you picture for *The boat sailed past the beach*?" Again, the now-familiar structure words are used to assist the students with vivid, detailed, expansive imagery.
5. *Sentence by Sentence Imaging*—Sentence by sentence is the heart of the *V/V* program as it is here that imagery is used to *connect* language to a whole. Beginning receptively, the students create mental representations for each sentence in short, self-contained paragraphs. They visualize and verbalize each sentence, using a colored square to concretize sentence-imagery. At the completion of the paragraph, with approximately four to five colored

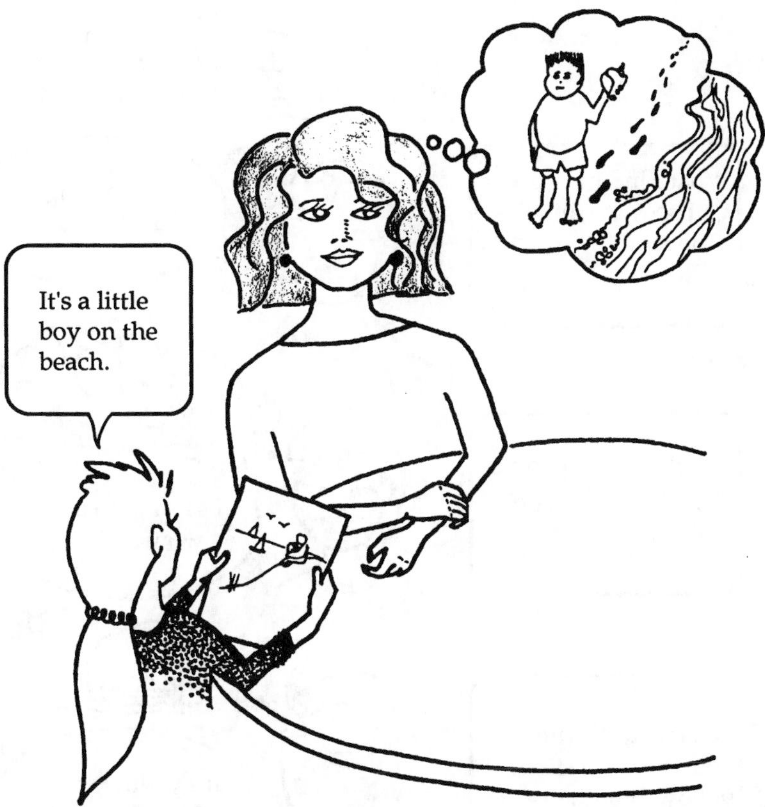

Figure 17–8. Students describe a simple picture using *structure words—what, size, color, number, shape, where, when, background, movement, mood, perspective, and sounds*—as concrete descriptive elements that will help concretize the language experience.

squares representing the sentences, they give a Picture Summary. Touching each colored square, they say, "Here I saw . . . " At the completion of the Picture Summary, the colored squares are collected and put away. The students then give a Word Summary using their own imagery to paraphrase the paragraph.

6. *Sentence by Sentence with Higher Order Thinking Skills (HOTS)*—The goal is to develop critical thinking from the imaged gestalt. Using the same Sentence by Sentence procedure described above, the students are asked main idea, conclusion, inference, and prediction questions based on the imaged gestalt. "What was the main thing you *pictured*?" "From your *images*, why do you think . . . ?" "What do you *picture* might happen if . . . ?" (Figure 17–10).
7. *Multiple Sentence, Paragraph, and Whole Page Imaging with HOTS*—The goal in each of the above steps is to increase and extend the language input, either receptively or expressively, to develop the imaged

What kind of boat do you see? A canoe? A battleship? A sailboat?
I see a big sailboat.
Are there any people in your boat? How many?
I see a man and a woman.
What color is the boat you see? Red, yellow, blue...?
It's yellow with a big white sail.

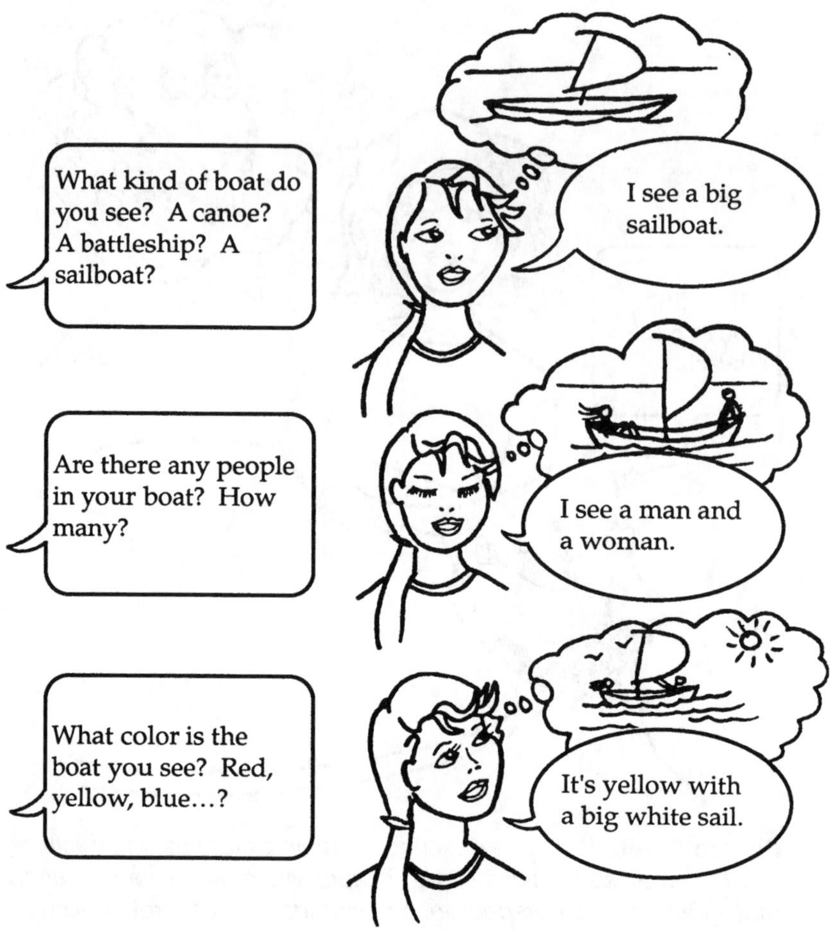

Figure 17–9. Beginning with a high-imagery known noun, such as *boat*, the students are questioned for imagery and use the structure words to help them verbalize details.

gestalt and apply that cognitive base to critical thinking, problem solving, and interpretation.

The above steps develop the students' ability to bring parts to a whole with imagery as a sensory tool. As the sensory tool is brought to consciousness, it becomes a cognitive tool for language comprehension, problem-solving, logical thinking, following directions, mathematics, play, and interpreting and responding appropriately to social situations.

Effects of a Theoretically Based Large-Scale Reading Intervention in a Multicultural Urban School District

For many years, clinical and classroom research has validated the efficacy of the *LiPS*, *Seeing Stars*, and *V/V* programs. As critical as all the research has been, it is more important to know if instruction based on the premise of dual coding can be implemented on a large scale to affect thousands of children in a school

What are you picturing when I read this: "Some spiders go fishing when they get hungry."
I see a spider by a river.

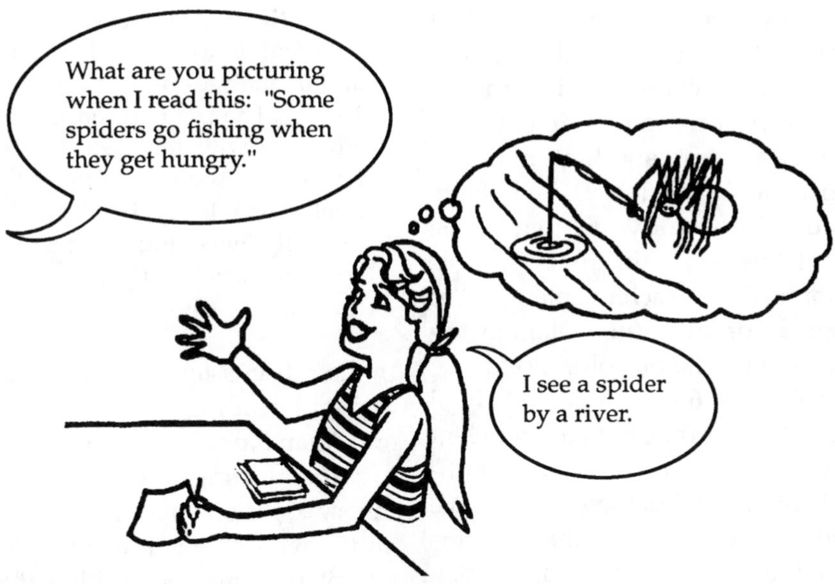

Figure 17–10. Students visualize and verbalize each sentence in a paragraph, using a colored square to represent each sentence.

district. Could Lindamood-Bell's programs—that bring imaginistic multisensory processing to a conscious level to be integrated with language—be scaled up for large numbers of children?

The importance of bringing instruction to scale cannot be overstated given the following statistics facing America's schools:

> 20,000,000 school-age children suffer from reading failure.
>
> 75% of students who drop out of school report difficulty learning to read.
>
> 38% of fourth graders in our nation cannot read at a basic level—that number reaches nearly 70% in many low-income school districts.

The last figure, that nearly 70% of fourth graders in low-income school districts cannot read at a basic level, has given rise to damaging discussion. Some believe, as Dan Seligman stated in *Forbes* magazine, that, "It is not possible to close the achievement gap . . . The poor and the disadvantaged have less cognitive ability than those of higher-status families" (p. 122).

The above statement is not true. A study published in the Spring 2006 issue of the *American Educational Research Journal* (AERJ) shows that children in a high-minority *urban school district* closed the achievement gap and outperformed the state of Colorado. Those children were taught to consciously process imaginistic multisensory information with the *Seeing Stars, LiPS,* and *V/V* programs. Lindamood-Bell's programs were implemented to teach children in special education classrooms and regular classrooms to dual code with imagery and verbal processing, especially for reading comprehension.

Drs. Mark Sadoski and Victor Willson of Texas A&M University wrote the *American Educational Research Journal* article. They conducted an independent longitudinal evaluation and comparative analysis to examine Lindamood-Bell's reading programs implemented in the high-poverty and high-minority Pueblo School District 60 in Pueblo, Colorado. The study compares the scores of Pueblo's elementary schools on Colorado's state achievement test to the scores of all other elementary schools in the state of Colorado.

In 1997, only 67% of Pueblo School District 60 third graders were proficient in reading. By 2006, 83% were proficient. Though the Pueblo schools have over 60% minority status, they outperformed the state of Colorado, which has only 30% minority status. Perhaps more importantly, Pueblo District 60's average scaled score on Colorado's state achievement test was 579, compared to 530 for a comparable district and 564 for the state. This revealed a statistically significant, favorable shift in the distribution of scores for children in Pueblo. Not only did the mean performance score increase, but also the lower scores shifted toward the mean, indicating even the lowest readers in Pueblo were reading substantially better. Drs. Sadoski and Willson (2006) stated that:

> Despite the ongoing national debate about improving reading achievement in schools, reading research has produced very few studies of the effects of specific instructional programs on student achievement scores on current large-scale assessments (p. 137). . . . The LBLP materials represented the centerpiece of this intervention; teacher training was exclusive to these materials, and the materials were used in providing corrective instruction (p. 153). . . . Statistically significant and increasing gains favoring the Lindamood-Bell reading intervention were found both overall and in analyses of Title I Schools (p. 137). . . . The emphasis on associating language with multisensory mental images . . . is a direct application of dual coding theory (i.e., instruction in mentally encoding information in both linguistic and imaginistic forms) (p. 140).

In their discussion of Dual Coding Theory and reading, Drs. Sadoski (2000) and Allan Paivio wrote, "Unifying reading and writing under the aegis of a theory of general of cognition is a timely and inevitable scientific step. Any theory of reading and writing that does not eventually align with a broader theory of general cognition will not endure. Reading and writing are cognitive acts" (p. 1).

Summary

Sensory processing—and specifically the dual coding of verbal and nonverbal information—is the heart of good language processing, and its absence is the root of many language problems. Lindamood-Bell's language intervention programs specifically develop the imaginistic sensory processing of (1) symbol imagery and articulatory feedback for reading, spelling, and speech, and (2) concept imagery for language comprehension.

We believe intensely that every individual of every age, race, and socioeconomic background has the potential to learn if he or she is given explicit instruction in processing sensory information, especially when the focus is to bring imaginistic multisensory information to consciousness for dual coding. Specific levels of sensory-cognitive processing may be as critical to learning as specific levels of sensory acuity.

Stimulating dual coding through specific and directed attention to sensory information can prevent language and literacy disorders in the first place. Furthermore, successful remediation for children and adults who do not have the advantage of such preventive action, or the genetic gift of the functions, can help them learn to their potential.

For all of us making a difference in the lives of children and adults, remember, the brain is not broken; it just needs help perceiving and integrating sensory information with language.

Key Points Learned

- Dual Coding Theory states that cognition relies on an interplay between verbal and nonverbal (imagery) coding systems.
- Discussion of the role of imagery in cognition has a long history, from Aristotle to Aquinas to Einstein.
- Two kinds of imagery (symbol imagery and concept imagery) underlie the discrete skills of decoding/encoding and comprehension/critical thinking.
- Symbol imagery is the ability to create mental representations for sounds and letters within words, the parts of the whole. Individuals with weak symbol imagery have difficulty sounding out words, self-correcting reading and spelling errors, and reading fluently.
- Concept imagery is the ability to create an imaged gestalt from oral and written language. Individuals with weak concept imagery have difficulty understanding and remembering what they have read and heard. They also have difficulty with critical thinking skills.
- There are three Lindamood-Bell programs that develop dual coding by bringing sensory information to consciousness, each program having its own primary sensory focus.
- Both the *Seeing Stars* program and the *LiPS* program develop phonemic awareness for reading and spelling.
- The *Seeing Stars* program focuses on the sensory development of symbol imagery for phonemic awareness, reading, and spelling.
- The *LiPS* program focuses on the sensory development of articulatory feedback for phonemic awareness, reading, and spelling.
- The *Visualizing and Verbalizing* program develops concept imagery for comprehension and critical thinking.

- Evidence from a longitudinal study on Lindamood-Bell instruction in a public school district demonstrates that large-scale implementation of the instruction was effective. The study was conducted by independent reviewers from Texas A&M University.

References

Arnheim, R. (1969). *Visual thinking*. Los Angeles: University of California Press.

Bell, N. (1991) *Visualizing and verbalizing for language comprehension and thinking*. San Luis Obispo, CA: Gander Publishing.

Bell, N. (1998). *Seeing Stars an integrated reading and spelling program: Kit and materials guide*. San Luis Obispo, CA: Author.

Bell, N. (2000). *Seeing stars: Symbol imagery for phonemic awareness, sight words and spelling*. San Luis Obispo, CA: Gander Publishing.

Bell, N. (2000). Imagery and the language processing spectrum. *Clinical practice guidelines: Redefining the standards of care for infants, children, and families with special needs*. Bethesda, MD: The Interdisciplinary Council on Developmental and Learning Disorders.

Bell, N. (2006). *The role of imagery and verbal processing in language processing: A dual coding model for language and literacy development*. Anaheim, CA: Lindamood-Bell International Conference.

Bleasdale, F. (1983). Paivio's dual-coding model of meaning revisited. In J. C. Yuille (Ed.), *Imagery, memory and cognition*. Hillsdale, NJ: Lawrence Erlbaum Associates.

Kosslyn, S. M. (1975). Information representation in visual images. *Cognitive Psychology*, *7*, 341–370.

Kosslyn, S. M. (1976). Using imagery to retrieve semantic information: A developmental study. *Child Development*, *47*, 434–444.

Kosslyn, S. M. (1983). *Ghosts in the mind's machine*. New York: W. W. Norton.

Kosslyn, S. M., & Koenig, O. (1992). *Wet mind: The new cognitive neuroscience*. New York: Simon & Schuster.

Lindamood, P. (1985). *Cognitively developed phonemic awareness as a base for literacy*. San Diego, CA: National Reading Conference.

Lindamood, P., Bell, N., & Lindamood, P. (1997). Sensory-cognitive factors in the controversy over reading instruction. *Journal of Developmental and Learning Disorders*, *1*(1), 143–182.

Lindamood, P., & Lindamood, P. (1998). *The Lindamood phoneme sequencing program for reading, spelling, and speech* (3rd ed.). Austin, TX: Pro-Ed.

Lindamood, P., & Lindamood, P. (2000). Speech-language development: Oral and written. *Clinical practice guidelines: Redefining the standards of care for infants, children, and families with special needs*. Bethesda, MD: The Interdisciplinary Council on Developmental and Learning Disorders.

Paivio, A. (1969). Mental imagery in associative learning and memory. *Psychological Review*, *76*, 241–263.

Paivio, A. (1979). *Imagery and verbal processes*. Hillsdale, NJ: Lawrence Erlbaum Associates.

Paivio, A. (1986). *Mental representations: A dual coding approach*. New York: Oxford University Press.

Piaget, J., & Barbel, I. (1969). *The psychology of the child*. New York: Basic Books.

Piaget, J., & Barbel, I. (1971). *Imagery and the child*. New York: Basic Books.

Pribram, K. (1971). *Languages of the brain: Experimental paradoxes and principles in neuropsychology*. New York: Brandon House.

Sadoski, M., & Paivio, A. (2000). *Imagery and text: A dual coding theory of reading and writing*. Mahwah, NJ: Lawrence Erlbaum.

Seligman, D. (2005, December 12). Gapology 101. *Forbes* [Online]. Retrieved Oct. 23, 2006 from http://www.forbes.com/business/forbes/2005/1212/120.html

Sorabji, R. (1972). *Aristotle on memory*. Providence, RI: Brown University Press.

18

Utilization of Computer Software as a Management Tool for Addressing CAPD

Larry Medwetsky

Overview

Computer applications for addressing processing related deficits have been implemented in a wide range of settings, including school districts, clinics, and, even within the home setting. Although the developers of the various products have touted the significant benefits of their programs in promoting various language-related skills, and, in turn, academic performance, there still remain many questions relative to their actual efficacy. This chapter reviews three different computer programs: (1) Fast ForWord family of products (Scientific Learning Corporation); (2) Earobics (Cognitive Concepts); and (3) Captain's Log/Sound Smart/Smart Driver (BrainTrain). The rationale, description, intended populations, and skills targeted for each of the programs are presented. In addition, clinical efficacy data from the product's developers as well as peer-based research are included. The chapter concludes with a critical analysis of the research as well as questions that need to be addressed in the future.

Introduction

Although there remains no uniform consensus regarding central auditory processing disorders, it is clear that the ability to process spoken language effectively as well as establishing the underlying phonemic representations critical for reading and related skills involves numerous intertwined skills (Medwetsky, 2006). It is also clear that a significant percentage of individuals, ranging from 3 to 8%, experience some sort of deficit impinging on normal development of these skills (Burlingame, Sussman, Gillam, & Hay, 2005; Cohen et al., 2005; Hartley, Hill, & Moore, 2003;). Depending on the specific deficit encountered, this may take the form of a central auditory processing disorder (CAPD), specific language impairment (i.e., difficulty with some aspect of language in the absence of any hearing loss, neurologic/cognitive deficit, or behavioral disorder) or dyslexia (reading-related difficulty, which may encompass spelling and/or writing difficulties as well). The assessment of CAPD has shifted from its initial focus of site-of-lesion testing to the use of test batteries for delineating the specific processing difficulties being encountered (Tillery, in press). In turn, this shift has served as an impetus for developing management strategies to assist individuals with defined deficits.

Management strategies for CAPD can be defined in three broad areas, described as the Tripod Approach (Ferre, 2002). These include: (1) *Compensatory Strategies* (e.g., clear speech such as good elocution and increased insertion of pauses between grammatical clauses, previewing of concepts/vocabulary before material is taught in class, extended time for tasks/tests, etc.); (2) *Environmental Enhancement Strategies* (such as acoustic modifications of classroom settings, use of overheads/Power Point presentations, preferential seating, and assistive listening systems); and (3) *Specific Therapeutic Approaches* (depending on the deficit identified, these may include training phonological awareness skills, improving lexical decoding speed, enhancing attentional allocation to reduce the occurrence of fading-memory, working on sequencing/organizational skills, increasing the ability to perceive/utilize suprasegmental information, etc.).

The advent and increased sophistication of computer technologies has recently allowed for the development of computerized, interactive approaches to the treatment of various developmental delays, be it at school, home, and so forth. Much has been invested, both in time and dollars, in the utilization of these programs within schools as well as by consumers within clinics and/or the home setting. Reports from the developers of these products indicate that hundreds of school districts have incorporated these programs as either part of their curriculum or for addressing special educational needs. The widespread usage of these programs leads us to a critical question. Are these products delivering on their claims and producing positive results?

In this chapter, three of these product families are reviewed. The rationale behind each product family, the target populations, intended goals, as well as research concerning their efficacy are presented. The goal is to provide sufficient information so that the reader can be better informed regarding the various issues and better able to provide objective information to others when asked.

Fast ForWord Family of Products (Scientific Learning Corporation)

Product History and Development

The Fast ForWord family of products can trace its origin to the early work by Paula Tallal and colleagues in the 1970s and 1980s (Tallal & Piercy, 1973a, 1973b, 1975; Tallal et al., 1981). Tallal and her colleagues conducted a series of experiments with children identified with language-learning impairments, often referred to as specific language impairment, "SLI." Children with SLI have normal intelligence (at least on tasks of nonverbal ability), normal hearing ability, no neurologic impairments, no history of behavioral or emotional problems, yet, exhibit language delays. The impact may be solely in the receptive/expressive language domain or may also involve poor literacy skills (such as poor phonological awareness and reading skills), and delayed academic progress. Tallal's research led her to conclude that the mechanisms giving rise to SLI lie in perceptual processing difficulties in the temporal domain. That is, children with SLI require longer processing times to discriminate, sequence, and remember stimuli of short durations or rapid transitions. Tallal (2000) has proposed that children who exhibit typical language and reading abilities are capable of integrating orally presented information within a more fine-grained (tens of msec) time window, whereas individuals with SLI integrate information across longer time windows (hundreds of msec). In turn, this does not allow SLI children to segment the complex acoustic information contained in speech effectively into the smaller units of speech, internally represented as phonemes. It is this difficulty that results in the language and/or reading impairments (especially in the areas of phonological awareness/phonics) exhibited in these individuals.

To better understand the key components of Fast ForWord, one needs to be aware of the research that led to Tallal's conclusions and, in turn, the development of the program itself. Tallal and Percy (1973a, 1973b) designed a task to measure the perception of rapid tonal sequences. The studies examined both frequency discrimination and temporal order judgment (via what was referred to as the Auditory Repetition Test). The subjects consisted of children (6–9 years old) who had been identified with developmental dysphasia as well as children who served as Performance IQ-matched controls. In one study, identical sets of stimuli were presented in both the temporal order judgment (TOJ) and frequency discrimination tasks (Tallal & Percy, 1973a). Stimuli consisted of two 75-msec duration complex tones. These consisted of four sinusoids of which the second through fourth were identical in both complex tones, but differed in the fundamental frequency (Low F_0 = 100 Hz; High F_0 = 305 Hz). All possible combinations of these complex tones were presented in pairs. The two tones in the pair were separated by silent intervals of varying durations (interstimulus interval: ISI). In the TOJ task, children were instructed to press two response buttons to indicate the order of the two tones. If the same tone was presented twice, then the button representing that tone was pressed twice. If two different tones were presented, the child was trained to indicate which came first or second using the two button method. In the discrimination task, children were trained to push one button if the two tones were the same and the other button if they were not the same. Tallal and Percy found that even for these brief, 75-msec stimuli both groups performed well on either task when the ISIs were fairly large (300 msec). However, when these brief stimuli were presented rapidly in succession (i.e., the ISI durations were in the tens of msecs), it was determined that the developmental dysphasic group performed poorly whereas the control subjects were still able to perform above chance levels with ISIs as brief as 8 msec. In a separate experiment (Tallal & Percy, 1973b), the duration of the tones were manipulated, being either short (75 msec) or long (250 msec) with ISI being held constant (i.e., interval of 150 msec). Tallal and Percy found that the SLI children performed significantly better on the TOJ and discrimination tasks for the longer duration tones, whereas the matched controls exhibited no difficulty at either duration. The results from these studies suggested that the processing difficulties of the SLI children were due to difficulty processing and discriminating brief, rapidly successive acoustic stimuli.

In a subsequent experiment by Tallal and Percy (1975), the researchers examined discrimination between two synthetic, consonant-vowel pairs /ba/ and /da/. Both of these stop-release consonants are characterized by brief onset bursts (approximately 25 msecs in duration), followed by rapid formant transitions to the steady-state vocalic portions. In the experiment, the formant transitions within these syllables were extended from 40 to 80 msec, whereas the duration of the following-steady-state portion representing the vowel portion was reduced from 210 to 170 msec (thus, maintaining the same overall syllabic duration). The results revealed that for the brief formant transitions typical of everyday speech, the SLI children performed significantly poorer than their matched controls. When formant transitions were lengthened, the SLI subjects improved significantly in their discrimination ability, to the point that they performed as well as their matched controls.

The research described above was then extended to children with reading disability (Tallal, 1980). Tallal hypothesized these children might also have a general perceptual deficit in the processing of rapidly, changing acoustic information, and, in turn, lead to impairment of phonological processing, whose importance to reading acquisition has been well established (Cornwall, 1992; Mann, 1993). In this study, Tallal compared good and poor readers on both the Auditory Repetition Test and the Discrimination task. The stimuli consisted of the 75-msec complex tones, presented at interstimulus intervals (ISI) ranging from 8 to 305 msec. Approximately half of the poor readers (8 out of 20 children) revealed significant difficulty when the ISI were of short duration but did somewhat better as ISI were lengthened. When children were presented with an even longer ISI than was initially targeted in the study, (i.e., 428 msec), no differences were observed between the two groups of readers. Please note that although this study shows the influence of ISI intervals on performance, not all poor readers evidenced this difficulty. This indicates that there are different subgroups of impaired readers with different underlying causes.

In addition to the work done by Tallal, Merzenich and his colleagues elsewhere were investigating learning-induced, neural plasticity in monkeys. Through the use of electrophysiologic measures from the neocortices of monkeys, Merzenich et al. (Merzenich et al., 1993; Merzenich et al., 1995) found that adult animals could be trained to make finer distinctions of both temporal and spectral features of complex inputs through a period of intensive behavioral training. The experimental findings obtained by Tallal regarding temporal processing deficits and Merzenich's work on plasticity led the two researchers to conduct a series of experiments to investigate if they could substantially alter the deficient temporal processing capacities of young, school-aged SLI children. This resulted in two highly publicized papers (Merzenich et el., 1996; Tallal et al., 1996) on results obtained from SLI children who were trained to make distinctions about fast and rapidly sequenced acoustic inputs presented in the format of computer games. Modification of the speech input involved two stages: (1) the duration of the speech signal was prolonged by 50% (while preserving spectral content and natural quality); and (2) the transitional elements of speech were differentially enhanced by as much as 20 dB. The researchers felt that amplifying the fast elements would render them more salient, and, thus, less likely to be subject to forward or backward masking by the neighboring, slowly modulated speech elements. Seven SLI children participated in a 6-week study aimed at evaluating the effects that exposure to acoustically modified speech had on speech discrimination and language comprehension. Training exercises were conducted for 3 hours a day, 5 days a week at the laboratory and 1 to 2 hours a day at home over a 4 week period. Children rotated through 10 different listening exercises involving acoustically modified speech as well as involvement in two audiovisual (AV) computer games.

The first AV game (prototype of what is now known as the Circus Sequence game) was a perceptual task involving nonverbal stimuli in which a correct response involved the correct ordering of two-stimuli sound sequences by touch screen, button-press sequences. The stimuli were 16 octave-per-second upward- or downward-gliding (U and D, respectively) frequency-modulated (FM) tonal pairs (U-U, U-D, D-U, D-D). Stimuli in each pair swept across the same frequency range. The authors indicated that these stimuli were in the range of sweep frequencies and speeds for formant transitions of speech sounds that SLI children typically have difficulty recognizing.

The second game was a phonetic element recognition exercise, presented within a two-alternative forced choice task (prototype of the Phonemic Identification game). For each item, children were presented with two consonant-vowel (CV) stimuli with contrasting consonants (e.g., /ba/ or /da/) in rapid sequence. The child's task was to identify the sequence position of the target CV for that item (in this example, either the precued /ba/ or /da/). The main variables were: (1) the durations of the synthetically produced consonants (and, reciprocally of the following vowels, thus ensuring total duration of the CVs were constant); (2) the magnitude of the amplification of the consonant portions relative to the vocalic segments; and (3) the ISIs between the CV pairs.

Both games commenced with stimuli that the SLI children could easily distinguish and recognize: (1) long tonal stimuli (60 msec) or consonant transition (65 to 70 msec) durations; (2) long ISIs (500 msec); and (3) for the CV stimuli, maximal amplification of the consonant portion (+20 dB). These variables were altered adaptively in training to drive each child in the direction of normal performance levels. The seven subjects were assessed pretraining and at 6 weeks post-training with natural, unprocessed speech through a series of standardized speech, language, and auditory temporal tests. A comparison of the pre- and post-training test scores revealed that the subjects improved significantly in their ability to recognize and sequence tonal and CV stimuli of shorter durations and shorter ISIs. In addition to the perceptual task scores, the SLI subjects revealed significant gains in speech and language skills. The SLI subjects were initially 1 to 3 years behind their chronologic age in speech and language. Post-training test measures showed that the speech and language test scores improved by approximately 2 years, with each SLI child approaching or exceeding normal limits for their age in speech discrimination and language comprehension.

A second study examined the extent to which the significant improvements were replicable in a larger SLI group, as well as examined the extent to which those improvements were derived specifically from training with acoustically modified speech coupled with temporal processing training. Twenty-two children between the ages of 5 and 10 years of age with severe receptive and expressive language impairments served as subjects. These individuals performed the same training exercises used in the first study (though the exercises were revised to enhance attention and reliability) as well as two additional Fast ForWord game prototypes (Old McDonald's Flying Farm and Phonic Match). To assess the efficacy of the processed speech and temporal training, the children were divided into two matched groups (on the basis of age, nonverbal intelligence, and receptive language skills). Half of the children were trained with computer games that adaptively trained temporal processing as well as language exercises that incorporated acoustically modified speech (Group A). The other half received essentially the same training but with computer games that were not temporally adaptive (i.e., used natural speech) as well as the same language exercises but with natural, unmodified speech (Group B). Results revealed that the performance of both groups improved significantly from pretraining to post-training but the improvements for Group A were significantly greater.

The success obtained in these studies led to large scale examinations of the benefits of these computerized adaptive approaches involving temporal processing. In 1996, a multisite study was conducted in collaboration with over 60 independent professionals at 35 sites (primarily clinics and private practices) in both the United States and Canada (Tallal et al., 1997; Troia & Whitney, 2003; Scientific Learning Corporation Web site at http://www.scilearn.com). At each site, independent speech and language professionals or educators selected the participants and administered the FFW program. Over 500 children with listening or language comprehension deficits between 4 and 14 years of age participated in this field study. The children varied in their diagnoses and severity of impairment. Subject participation varied from 4 to 8 weeks, depending on the length of daily participation and how quickly subjects were able to reach criterion on the various Fast ForWord programs. According to Tallal et al. (1997), approximately 90% of the participants achieved a gain of about one standard deviation on one or more norm-referenced tests of auditory perception and discrimination, and oral language development. Most made significant gains in multiple areas, including phonemic awareness, listening, attention/ability to follow directions, oral language, and grammar, with gains on average from 1 to 2 years in the tested areas.

In a separate school field study held in the fall of 1997 (Miller et al., 1999), 452 at-risk students for failure in reading and language in grades K through three in 19 schools (9 school districts in a number of states) participated in a stratified, randomized group experiment. Classroom teachers selected students who were "at risk" for reading and language difficulties. The children were randomly assigned to an experimental group that used Fast ForWord (FFW) or a comparison group (matched to the experimental group by age and gender) who remained in the regular classroom and received non-Fast ForWord instruction. Data from the school based trial reveal that the majority of children (67%) who received FFW training over a period of about 40 school days, demonstrated significantly greater progress (average of 1.8 years in growth) in language comprehension and phonological awareness than their comparison group peers who did not receive FFW training (cited in Troia & Witney, 2003).

Description of Fast ForWord Products

Based on their research, Drs. Tallal and Merzenich, among others, formed the Scientific Learning Corporation to distribute and train others on the Fast ForWord line of products. Initially, there was one product (now known as Fast ForWord Language) but there is now a family of products that are available. These include:

1. Fast ForWord Core series (computerized adaptive training programs involving acoustically modified speech): (1) Fast ForWord Language; (2) Fast ForWord Middle/High School; (3) Fast ForWord Language to Reading; (4) Fast ForWord Literacy and (5) Fast ForWord Advanced Literacy;
2. Fast ForWord to Reading: (1) Fast ForWord to Reading Prep;

(2) Fast ForWord to Reading 1;
(3) Fast ForWord to Reading 2;
(4) Fast ForWord to Reading 3;
(5) Fast ForWord to Reading 4;
(6) Fast ForWord to Reading 5.

Fast ForWord to Reading products comprise a series of computerized programs that have been developed to assist students who have successfully completed one of the Fast ForWord Core products and who are at risk for reading failure. These programs differ from the Fast ForWord Core series in that the stimuli encompass natural speech without any acoustic modifications. The goal of these programs is to help these students establish key reading skills that are commensurate with their peers. The selection of a particular program and component skill is based on an individual's age/level of difficulty and deficit area. Skills that can be worked on include sound-symbol associations, word attack, word clustering, sight vocabulary, listening and reading comprehension, and so forth.

In terms of addressing auditory processing-related difficulties, the signature series from Fast ForWord involves the Fast ForWord Core product line. Fast ForWord for Language was the first of the products developed. The product was initially developed for use with 4- to 12-year-olds, but recently products have been added to provide exercises more specific to the age groups involved in the intervention.

Fast ForWord Language Middle/High School incorporates a core of five exercises, four of which were developed in Fast ForWord Language but with different graphics. In addition, a fifth exercise was added that includes narrative language comprehension, following directions, and syntax skill building with language content and concepts that are more appropriate for middle and high school-age students.

Fast ForWord Language and Fast ForWord Language Middle/High School programs are based on the same computerized delivery/adaptive techniques for acoustically modifying the linguistic stimuli and utilize similar exercise formats. For the purpose of this chapter, only the exercises that encompass Fast ForWord Language are described (for a description of the various programs in Fast ForWord Middle/High School as well as the other Fast ForWord Core programs, the reader is referred to the scilearn.com Web site). Appendix 18-A describes the seven exercises used in Fast ForWord Language.

Fast ForWord Language (FFW-L) is commercially available, on a fee per child basis, via the Internet using CD-ROM software. The FFW-L program has been advertised as a comprehensive language training program to train children with language impairment to process sounds and words at increasing rates of presentation until they are able to differentiate and process language at the typical rate of speaking. An additional purpose of several of the games is to build phonological awareness (i.e., the awareness of the speech sounds that make up words and the ability to manipulate these sounds, Griffith & Olson, 1992), a skill that the National Reading Panel (2000) has deemed necessary for children when learning to read. Clients are identified as candidates for FFW-L if they have difficulty in any one of the following areas: phonological awareness, reading or spelling, language comprehension, understanding concepts and directions, discriminating words, or displaying age-appropriate language abilities (Veale, 1999).

The FFW-L program is offered through providers that have been trained through a self-paced tutorial that is available on-line. The training covers the theory, research, and technical aspects of program administration. At the conclusion of the on-line tutorial, prospective providers take a test on the material covered in the tutorial. Following successful completion of the test and signing of a certified professional agreement, SLC provides the individual with an Organization ID that permits him or her to be a provider of Fast ForWord. Educators can alternatively be trained to provide the Fast ForWord family of products through on-site professional development instruction through their schools or school districts.

Children can go through the program exercises at a school or clinic that has obtained a license through Scientific Learning Corporation or in the convenience of their home (as long as there is a trained individual coordinating the implementation/utilization of the program with the child's parents). As mentioned earlier, Fast ForWord Language consists of seven sets of computer exercises. Originally, students were required to participate in five of the seven games each day, with a total of 100 minutes of actual computer time being required. This schedule has recently been altered to provide some flexibility, whereas students can now use the software following one of three schedules:

- 50 minutes each day, 5 days/week for 8 to 12 weeks (3 exercises/day)
- 75 minutes each day, 5 days/week, for 6 to 10 weeks (4 exercises/day)
- 100 minutes each day, 5 days/week for 4 to 8 weeks (5 exercises/day)

Children wear headphones to hear the instructions or stimuli, and use the computer mouse to respond. An adult monitor is available during exercises to observe and supervise each child's progress. Points are generated as correct responses are made, which can be used for reinforcement.

Each exercise begins with training at a level that most of these children can perform successfully. The difficulty level is continuously adapted so that the child will get the majority of responses correct (depending on the program, varying from 80 to 90% correct). When the child has demonstrated mastery at a particular level (according to the algorithms entered for that particular exercise), the software is automatically advanced to the next level. The child's performance is continually monitored and saved on the computer or network and uploaded at the end of the day, via the Internet, to the SLC Web site. Measures are obtained regarding the progress made on each exercise (% successful completion) and reported by Fast ForWord Progress Tracker. The participation day is indicated on the x-axis and the percent complete is indicated on the y-axis. This analysis is automatically delivered to the provider with specific recommendations for instructional intervention. A student participates in FFW-L until he or she has reached a criterion of 90% completion on a majority of the exercises and/or successfully participates for at least 6 to 10 weeks of training, depending on the protocol used. Percentage completion indicates the percentage of computer exercises the children have mastered or how far they have advanced through the adaptive training levels. The intervention period varies depending on the relative difficulty of the individual exercises for any given student.

Fast ForWord: Peer-Related Research

Results of Fast ForWord Intervention on Language and Reading Performance

Before describing the research, please note that subjects included in the various studies were determined to have normal hearing, normal or near normal nonverbal IQ, and no history of neurologic or significant behavioral disorders.

Friel-Patti, DesBarres, and, Thibodeau (2001) reported a case study of five children with language learning difficulties who were enrolled in FFW-L. The purpose of the case studies was to obtain independent objective data and identify patterns of performance with FFW-L relative to the children's preintervention language profiles. In addition to assessing progress on FFW-L, the children were assessed on a number of language measures and conversational language samples, pre and post-FFW-L intervention. In reviewing the findings, Friel-Patti et al. observed that the three participants with the poorest language before intervention were the same individuals who progressed least and did not meet dismissal criteria. In examining their performance on FFW-L, these three participants had not met the 90% completion criterion on five of the seven exercises. They were observed to have exhibited very poor performance on the Circus Sequence (CS) exercise; even at dismissal, these three individuals had attained percent completion rates of 4%, 0%, and, 2% (recall that the CS test involves the individual to recognize and indicate the sequential order of two rapidly changing complex tones). The authors postulated that children who exhibit severe difficulty on the CS test may be less likely to perform well on the other FFW-L exercises that require the child to segment and distinguish phonemes, follow directions, or match pictures with increasingly complex morphologic and syntactic demands. A second pattern that the authors noted was that the same participants who performed so poorly on the Circus Sequence test revealed a significant drop-off in performance on the other two sound exercise games, (a) Phoneme Identification (identifying which one of two characters' utterances matches the initially presented target CV or VCV syllable, the two choices differing in one phoneme) and (b) Old MacDonald's Flying Farm (participants hear a rapid succession of a particular syllable and must identify when a different syllable occurs, differing in the initial phoneme). Yet, these same individuals continued to show progress on the word exercises. The authors theorized that the auditory stimuli (nonverbal) may have resulted in increasingly stressed resources. On the other hand, because of the varied cognitive and linguistic aspects on the other tests (i.e., on the games comprising the word exercises), the authors wondered if the children may have continued to improve on aspects related to cognitive and linguistic demands.

In a study by Loeb, Stoke, and Fey (2001), language changes were examined in four children who received FFW-L within the confines of their homes. Because of the costs associated with on-site mentoring, the authors presumed that implementation of FFW-L in home settings would be appealing, and thus wanted to assess its viability. Second, the authors wanted to assess FFW-L on children's speech, language, and reading performance, and determine which of these measures may be most sensitive to the program's effects. Four children who had been diagnosed with a speech-language impairment and scored below 1 SD on at least one test of language development participated in the study. The four subjects were assessed before and after intervention (immediately after intervention and 3 months postintervention) on a number of measures. One set of measures used the same instruments that had been administered by Merzenich et al. (1996). Loeb et al. also assessed grammatical structures in spontaneous language, measures related to reading skills, as well as the children's pragmatic use of language. In examining the data, three of the four children reached 80% completion criteria on five out of seven of the exercises, whereas all of the children made some gains on the standardized measures. Of a total of 115 scores, 37 (32%) were a positive change and 7 (5%) were negative changes. However, only 11 (9%) positive scores were maintained 3 months after discontinuing FFW-L. Although positive changes were noted, they were far less dramatic than those reported by Merzenich, Tallal, and colleagues. There was no consistent pattern of performance observed across the four children, nor did reaching 80% completion criteria predict language gains. For example, one child who improved on nine of the 18 test measures did not reach completion criteria. The authors wondered whether this may have indicated a strengthening of word and language skills in the continued presence of impaired auditory perception skills. The other three children revealed milder language impairments and all had reached completion on five out of seven of the exercises on FFW-L, even though they did exhibit temporal auditory deficits from the outset. However, in analyzing their change in language performance, the children differed greatly and no pattern was evident that could predict a priori which skills were likely to improve following FFW-L intervention. In addition, the children who revealed gains in standardized measures in syntax did not reveal it in their spontaneous language.

Gillam, Crofford, Gale, and, Hoffman (2001) reported on a study of four children examined for functional language change following computer-assisted language intervention. They compared the results obtained for FFW-L training with two children with another type of language intervention software—that produced by Laureate Learning Systems (LLS), for two other children. The authors selected seven LLS programs that focused on vocabulary, memory, syntax, morphology, and narration, thus targeting somewhat different language skills than FFW-L. Like FFW-L, each exercise has multiple levels of increasing difficulty. Unlike FFW-L, the LLS programs do not use modified speech. Although none of the children reached the mastery criteria, all four children achieved significantly higher scores on two of the scales of the OWLS (Oral and Written Language Scales:

Carrow-Woolfolk, 1995), with the children making very similar gains. The fact that FFW-L and the LLS programs focus on listening exercises and none require the children to talk would lead one to expect that language comprehension would increase more than oral expression, which, in fact, did occur; however, for two of the children, the degree of improvement in language comprehension was not statistically significant. The authors also evaluated the extent to which training with either of these programs generalized to measures of language form, content, and use in conversational contexts. The results suggest that both FFW-L and LLS did lead to observable improvements in spontaneous language production, with similar results being obtained. Yet, it must be recalled that FFW-L uses an adaptive program involving acoustically modified speech versus the natural speech stimuli employed by LLS; in addition, the programs targeted very different aspects of speech/language. It may be that even though LLS targeted different behavioral changes, both programs required the children to attend carefully to repetitive stimuli, and encouraged children to respond at faster rates. Both programs also targeted a variety of higher order language processing/cognitive skills, such as working memory and sequencing. Given the similar outcomes obtained, the authors questioned whether specialized acoustic modification or adaptive practice was necessary for the improvements noted.

Hook, Macaruso, and Jones (2001) sought to examine the efficacy of FFW-L training on facilitating the acquisition of reading skills in children with reading difficulties. Tallal and colleagues have posited that difficulties in temporal processing can significantly impact on the development of accurate phonemic representation (Tallal, 2000). In turn, phonological awareness is considered a core component of learning to read (Share & Stanovich, 1985; Torgeson, Wagner, & Rashotte, 1995). Because a number of structured language techniques also focus on improving phonemic awareness, Hook et al. set out to examine the efficacy of FFW-L as compared to a phonemic/orthographic based approach—the Orton Gillingham (OG) program (Gillingham & Stillman, 1997; www.orton-gillingham.com). Subjects involved children with reading disability. Phonemic awareness and reading skills as well as receptive/expressive spoken language skills were assessed. Both short- and long-term gains over a 2-year period were examined. In addition to the FFW-L and OG subjects, a longitudinal control group (LC) of children were also included in the study. Children in the three groups were matched on the basis of age, full-scale IQ, phonemic awareness ability, and reading level. FFW-L treatment consisted of the standard procedures/time frame (5 exercises for a total of 100 minutes/day, 5 days a week for 2 months), whereas OG treatment involved 1 hour a day, 5 days a week for 5 weeks. Children in both the FFW-L and LC groups also participated in multisensory structured language programs through their school districts. The FFW-L and OG groups were assessed before and after treatment, whereas the LC group was assessed initially at the time of FFW-L and OG intervention completion. The FFW-L and LC groups were also assessed 1 and 2 years post FFW-L intervention. Results reveal:

- FFW and OG subjects made similar statistical improvements in phonemic awareness; word identification did not improve significantly for either group over the intervention period; the OG group did improve in word attack skills, whereas the FFW group did not.
- In comparing the results from the FFW-L to the LC group, both improved in phonemic awareness and reading-related skills over time (typically more than 1 year of gain per year) but there was no statistical difference between groups.
- Regarding receptive/expressive language and a verbal working memory measure, there were no significant differences between the FFW-L and LC groups at 1 or 2 years postintervention.

The results reveal that both intervention groups improved similarly in phonemic awareness but only the OG group improved in the area of word attack (i.e., combining phonemic awareness with direct instruction in the alphabetic code). Since this is an area explicitly taught by the OG approach but not in FFW-L, this result was not surprising. The fact that word identification did not significantly improve in either group is likely a reflection of the short period of training time. In comparing the long-term gains made by the FFW-L and LC groups, both exhibited improvements in phonemic awareness and a number of language-related areas (suggesting that the multisensory approach used in both groups was beneficial) but FFW did not result in additional or faster improvement.

Another study examining the effect of FFW-L training and reading skills was conducted by Agnew, Dorn, and Eden (2004). The study had a number of goals, one of which was to determine if the original findings from a laboratory setting (Tallal et al., 1996) could be reproduced in a clinic setting. A second goal was to determine whether training with acoustically modified speech results in reading gains. Tasks included (1) a visual processing measure to determine if processing changes occurred across modalities, or if intensive training in auditory processing was restricted to the auditory modality; (2) independent measures of auditory duration judgment not specifically trained by FFW-L, thus avoiding an outcome measure that was similar to the task involved; that is, is the improvement related to learning a specific task or is the learning more generalized? (3) assessment measures of nonword decoding as well as phonemic awareness skills related to reading acquisition. Seven individuals who were about to engage in FFW-L were recruited for the study (mean age being approximately 8 years). Subjects were given two measures of phonological awareness (a word attack subtest and a phoneme deletion subtest) before and after intervention. In addition to these measures, subjects were evaluated also on a judgment of duration task in the auditory and visual domains. In the auditory task, for each trial an 800-msec tone was followed by an interstimulus interval of 500 msec and then a tone of variable duration (differing from the first tone by 10 to 2,000 msec). The subject's task was to indicate whether the first or second tone was longer. All tones were presented at 1 kHz. An analogous visual task was also conducted. Results indicate that subjects performed more accurately on this task after training; however, this improvement only occurred in the auditory modality, and, thus, was not due to a supramodal benefit (such as in overall attentional ability). However, the data concerning the phonological awareness tasks revealed that subjects did not exhibit any significant improvement on either the word attack or phoneme deletion tasks; thus, gains in the ability to perceive auditory durations did not generalize to skills related to reading. One problem with the latter conclusion is that it is not clear if any of these subjects exhibited any reading difficulty as no mention of this was included in the article.

Another study regarding the implementation of FFW-L and its efficacy concerning language and reading ability is by Rouse and Krueger (2004). In a field trial discussed earlier in this chapter (Miller et al., 1999), SLC reported significant treatment effects not only in language related skills but also on a number of reading related measures. One problem as reported by Rouse and Krueger is that SLC researchers appear to have excluded data from those students who did not complete the FFW-L program, which may have introduced sampling selection bias into their estimates. In addition, a number of students required an extension of their treatment duration to complete the program, which may have resulted in a longer time interval than their control counterparts. In an attempt to parallel the target population for the FFW programs, the authors recruited individuals who scored in the bottom 20% on a state's standardized reading test. Subjects consisted of individuals from grades three to six, with a total sample size of 512; approximately one-half were assigned to the FFW-L group and the other half served as a control group. This study used an "intent-to-treat" model, meaning that (1) students were randomly assigned to one of the two groups and (2) regardless of whether students completed the study, their results, or estimations of their results, were included in the appropriate group. Note that FFW-L was primarily an add-on to regular reading instruction; thus, in actuality this resulted in these individuals receiving more language/reading related-instruction than their matched peers. Test measures included: (1) a computerized test called the Reading Edge (measuring skills in phonological awareness, decoding, and processing); although the test has been specifically designed to assess various aspects of the FFW-L program, the authors indicated that it is unclear if the capabilities examined in Reading Edge, in fact, are associated with language acquisition and/or literacy skills; (2) receptive portion of the Clinical Evaluation of Language Fundamentals—3 as well as the Listening to Paragraphs subtest; (3) assessments administered from the Success for All school district curriculum regarding examining students' progress in reading; and (4) students' scores on a state criterion-referenced standardized test.

Results show that there was a small effect of training on performance on the Reading Edge (statistically significant at the .10 level); however, no benefit of FFW-L training was observed on the CELF-3 language measures. The authors also found no statistically detectable effect of the program on reading skills as reflected in the reading measures of the Success-for-All and the state standardized reading assessments. The authors concluded that although FFW-L may have improved a few aspects of language skills, it did not appear that these gains translated into a broader measure of language acquisition or into actual reading skills. An important caveat to these findings is that there was a great variability in the time spent in Fast ForWord training among subjects and a significant percentage of individuals did not complete the requisite number of exercises; in addition, results from one or more tests were not always available and had to be estimated, possibly limiting the opportunity to detect effects.

The last study mentioned here regarding the effectiveness of FFW-L and its efficacy is a study by Cohen et al., (2005). Seventy-seven children with a diagnosis of severe mixed, receptive-expressive language deficits participated. Subjects were separated into three groups: (1) children trained on FFW-L; (2) children trained on six commercially available, educational software packages designed to encourage language development; and (3) a control group. The two treatment groups received similar training on a daily basis and overall length of intervention (6 weeks); note that all of the children were also receiving ongoing language training through their schools. All of the groups were matched on a number of criteria, with no significant differences being noted on a number of selection measures. The results show that although not all of the children in the study made progress, all three groups made statistically significant gains on both receptive and expressive language measures at both the 9-week and 6-month follow-up points. However, the results also revealed that there was no additional benefit for either of the treatment conditions involving computer-assisted intervention. Thus, the findings from this study did not support the efficacy of FFW-L as an intervention method for this population. However, proponents of Fast ForWord point out that this study used an "intent-to-treat" model, with all results being included in the final analysis. This means that even students whose participation in Fast ForWord Language fell far short of the recommended protocols were considered as having participated fully. It appears in these cases that the time spent (e.g., less than 4 full days for two of the students) or progress through the content was so limited that potential benefit was reduced, and their inclusion likely negatively affected the evaluation of Fast ForWord's efficacy. Furthermore, the authors replaced test scores from missing post- and follow-up tests with scores from a prior test. In addition, in some cases estimated scores rather than actual scores were included in the final analysis. This essentially added zeros into the average improvement observed and decreased the study's ability to detect change over time or between groups. The use of these artificial replacement scores thus caused a watering-down effect and possibly minimized the assessed impact of Fast ForWord intervention.

Psychoacoustic and Electrophysiologic Performance in Individuals with Language Learning or Reading Impairments

As discussed earlier, Tallal and colleagues have proposed that temporal processing deficits are causally related to language learning impairments or to reading disorders in some children via the mediating effects of phonological processing deficits subsequent to difficulty perceiving sounds of short duration/rapidly changing speech segments such as formant transitions involving plosives (Tallal, 2000; Temple et al., 2000). A number of researchers have explored the relationship between impaired temporal processing and language impairment with the goal of ascertaining if (1) the temporal processing abilities of those with language impairment are, in fact, poorer than their normally functioning peers, and (2) if so, establish its causal relationship. Wright et al. (1997) evaluated temporal processing through masking tasks in which detection of a brief tone was measured when presented with another signal, known as the "masker." The masker could occur before, simultaneously, and after the target tone, and are referred to as forward, simultaneous, and, backward masking. When a tone occurs simultaneously with a masker, this is a form of figure-ground task that involves the ability to selectively attend and filter out the tone from the embedded noise. The occurrence of a masker prior to or after a target tone involves two aspects: (1) the ability to separate the acoustic events in time to perceive the brief tone; and (2) the strength of the memory trace and continued processing in light of the interfering stimulus (for example, a strong vowel subsequent to the presentation of a weak consonant may cease processing of the prior consonant, such as evident in individuals with high-frequency hearing loss). In the Wright et al., study, the masker was a narrow-band noise with a center frequency corresponding to the target tone. Participants in the study included eight children with specific language impairment (SLI) and eight control children. Two identical narrow band noises (300 msec in duration) were presented in two intervals, one after another. A 20-msec, 1-kHz tone served as the target stimulus. In the simultaneous masking (SM) paradigm, the subjects had to indicate which interval contained the tone. The level of the tone was adaptively varied to estimate the listeners' tone threshold. In the forward masking (FM) task, the tone was presented immediately after the noise, whereas in the backward masking (BM) task the tone was presented immediately before the masker. Subjects revealed similar performance on the SM and FM paradigms but the SLI children were significantly impaired on the backward masking task; that is, compared to the control subjects they required the tone to be of significantly greater intensity in this condition (in general, SM thresholds were significantly higher than the BM and FM thresholds; however, for a number of SLI children the BM thresholds were almost the same as their SM thresholds). This suggests that compared with control children, children with SLI required a longer sample of an auditory stimulus in order to detect it, and this process was disrupted if a noise stimulus began before identification had been achieved. Wright et al. concluded that such deficits could interfere with the ability to perceive the rapid elements of speech.

In examining previous research, Bishop, Carlyon, Deeks, and Bishop (1999) noted there appeared to be conflicting findings regarding SLI children's performance on psychoacoustic tasks. For example, under certain experimental conditions, language-impaired children revealed adequate discrimination of brief or rapidly changing auditory stimuli (Sussman, 1993). Bishop et al. also noted that questions had been raised about the validity of auditory temporal processing tasks, since children's performance in some studies showed marked variations across testing sessions (Wightman & Allen, 1992; Wightman, Allen, Dolan, Kistler, & Jamieson, 1989) and possibly were subject to systematic influence of practice on the task, rather than actual change in processing (Tomblin & Quinn, 1983). Taken together, these findings indicated that performance on measures of auditory temporal processing could be dependent on the test method as well as possibly reflecting (a) attentional differences between subjects, (b) failure to adapt to specific task demands, or (c) slow learning of a novel task by SLI children rather than a more fundamental perceptual limitation. To distinguish between these possibilities, Bishop et al. felt that it was important to test children across a range of different auditory measures, including incorporating repeated testing to minimize learning effects. For inclusion in the Bishop et al. study, subjects had to score below the 10th percentile on at least two of five language measures. There were 11 children in each of the SLI and matched "normal" control groups. For the purpose of this chapter, only two of the four auditory temporal processing tasks administered are discussed: (1) simultaneous masking (SM) threshold estimation using a two-interval forced-choice method (the child was instructed to indicate which interval they heard a tone) as well as an easier three interval, two-alternative forced choice task (the child heard just noise in the first interval but was asked to indicate whether the second or third intervals contained a tone embedded in the noise, thus, involving notice of a change in one of the intervals relative to the first—just noise—interval); (2) backward (tone presented immediately prior to one of the maskers) and forward masking (signal ended after offset of a masker). Subjects were assessed in each task a number of times over the course of a number of test sessions (for example, BM threshold estimation was assessed five times). The findings show that regarding SM thresholds, the effect of grouping was not significant; however, the effect of test session was highly significant. Thresholds for the initial test session were much higher than those obtained in the second test session, without any further improvement. When the effect of the two versus three-interval forced choice task was examined, children who performed the most poorly on the two-interval task improved significantly when the easier three-interval task was used. This finding suggests that some of the difficulty children exhibited had more to do with the different encoding demands entailed by the different tasks. Thus, intellectual demands of psychophysical procedures and training can exert important effects on performance. When backward and forward masking were examined, the effect of interstimulus interval was not significant, although there was a trend toward poorer performance by the SLI group in the backward masking task (but this did not reach statistical significance). A point to consider in examining the results, especially in light of the different findings obtained by Bishop et al. relative to those obtained by Wright et al., is that SLI children are heterogeneous. It is possible that Bishop et al. may have included a greater number of individuals whose difficulties had a nonauditory basis. Bishop et al. also noted that a number of the control children performed poorly on some of the temporal processing measures. Bishop et al. argued that the finding of children with normal language but with poor auditory processing poses difficulty for any theory that regards auditory deficits as a necessary and sufficient cause of language impairment.

In subsequent studies, McArthur and Bishop (2001) and Bishop and McArthur (2004) further explored some of these early findings using auditory event-related potentials (ERPs). Importantly, different results and conclusions were reached based on electrophysiologic (ERP) data than those that had been observed using psychoacoustic data. Specifically, most of the subjects with SLI had aberrant ERPs, despite their frequency discrimination performance on psychoacoustic measures. For example, McArthur and Bishop's study found that only a subgroup of individuals with SLI (approximately ⅓ of the subjects) were less able to discriminate between the frequencies of sounds regardless of their rate of presentation than their control peers. These individuals tended to be the younger participants, and were characterized by relatively poor nonword reading. However, an examination of the auditory-event related potentials of the same group to unmasked tones found that most of the listeners with SLI tended to have age-inappropriate waveforms in the N1-P2-N2 region regardless of their auditory discrimination scores. These results suggest that SLI may be characterized by immature development and may not always be identified by performance on psychoacoustic tasks, especially in older children. In a follow-up ERP study by Bishop and McArthur (2005), in which the authors aimed to directly reassess the original findings of Tallal and Piercy (1973a), their ERP results demonstrated that children with SLI were significantly different from controls in their physiologic response to tone sequences. This result was in contrast to previous behavioral results obtained with the same subjects. In addition, an interesting age effect was found across groups, with older participants (>14 years) showing less deviant ERP responses than younger subjects.

In 2000, Hartley, Hogan, Wright, and Moore examined age-related improvements in auditory backward and simultaneous masking in 6- and 8-year-old children as well as adults without any evidence of language impairments using the identical masking tasks and procedures of Wright et al. (1997). Hartley et al. found that tone thresholds improved with age in both the backward and simultaneous masking conditions; however, improvements in the backward masking paradigm was much greater than in the simultaneous masking condition. A negative exponential decay function indicated that simultaneous masking reached adult-like performance by 8 to 9 years of age, whereas backward masking only reached adultlike performance between 11 and 15 years of age. The importance of this finding relates to the age of subjects involved in any research of psychoacoustic performance, age of subjects at the time of intervention, any analysis conducted after a lengthy time interval postintervention, and, in turn, possible interpretation of the findings.

Because of concerns that conclusions regarding temporal processing deficits were being generalized to SLI/reading disordered populations as a whole, yet, being based on between-group comparisons likely involving heterogeneous populations, Heath and Hogben (2004) examined the reliability and validity of tasks measuring the perception of rapid sequences in children with dyslexia. Subjects consisted of a good reader group (22 children) and Dyslexic group (30 children) between the ages of 8 to 11 years. Criteria for inclusion in the Dyslexic group included reading accuracy level of at least 18 months below chronologic age with a Performance IQ of at least 85. In one task, stimuli were constructed to match those in Tallal's Auditory Repetition Test (Tallal, 1980). Two complex tones consisting of four sinusoidal components were synthesized, the first sinusoidal component being different and the three remaining sinusoids being identical. The child's task was to identify the sequence of the complex tones (e.g., hi-hi, or low-hi) as a function of interstimulus interval (ISI) duration. The results revealed a significant group mean difference, with the dyslexic children performing more poorly. However, further analysis revealed that (1) there was large variability within the groups; (2) most dyslexic children performed within the same range as the good readers; and (3) a subset (20% of the dyslexic children) revealed extremely high ISI thresholds. A second experiment examined reliability of individual measurements across time and practice. Ten dyslexic and 10 good readers from the pool of children assessed in the first experiment served as subjects. Subjects were assessed on the same task 3 to 4 months later (Time 2) and on four more occasions within a 2 week period after Time 2. Results revealed that both groups had improved significantly by Time 2, with no significant difference between groups in the amount of improvement. Thus, just aging rather than practice "per se" was sufficient to result in enhanced performance; note that the distribution of performance remained the same (i.e., the overall pattern of performance among the subjects remained essentially the same). Performance continued to improve over the four practice sessions, with no significant differences between groups being apparent by the last of the four practice sessions. In examining the data, the greatest learning occurred between the initial (Time 1) and second session (Time 2), which agrees with other researchers' findings that the greatest proportion of learning on psychoacoustic tasks tends to occur in the early sessions.

Fast ForWord Intervention and Psychoacoustic Findings

Thibodeau, Friel-Patti, and Britt (2001) examined psychoacoustic performance in children completing Fast ForWord-Language (FFW-L). Subjects consisted of five individuals who comprised an experimental group (receiving language therapy for over a year) and five of whom comprised a control group (no history of speech and language difficulties). Testing was conducted weekly over a 5 to 6 week period and coincided with FFW-L training sessions for the experimental group. The key results from this study were:

- SM thresholds were more similar across the control and experimental groups than BM thresholds;
- BM thresholds were generally lower than the SM thresholds, with two exceptions (both from the experimental group); in examining the case profiles, these two individuals were those who had the severest language impairments;
- frequency sweep thresholds were not significantly different between groups nor did they change significantly over session for either group;
- two of the five experimental group children met FFW-L dismissal criteria at the end of the 5 weeks of intervention; these two children were also the ones who performed most like the normal children on the masking and frequency-sweep discrimination tasks, revealed the greatest improvement in BM thresholds over time, and, had the least language impairment.

The authors indicated that the variability exhibited (primarily in the backward masking task) may speak to the heterogeneity of language-impaired children. Based on the findings, the authors suggested that intensive auditory training may be most productive if tailored to the individual temporal processing abilities of the child and that psychoacoustic tasks may be a useful way to predict benefit from intensive auditory training.

One study by Marler, Champlin, and Gillam (2001) examined auditory temporal processing in children who received FFW-L and in children who received training with computer programs published by Laureate Language Systems (LLS). (Recall that the LLS programs are not designed specifically to improve auditory perceptual skills.) The primary goal of this study was to investigate changes in auditory processing abilities of children subsequent to training from either of the programs. Seven children participated in the study. Two received FFW-L training, two received training using the LLS software, and three individuals with typically developing language served as a control group. Measures were obtained at the onset of treatment (baseline testing) and at weekly intervals thereafter until computer-assisted training was completed

In general, SM and BM thresholds tended to improve across test sessions; however, the normal listeners exhibited their best thresholds at the final session, whereas the SLI subjects exhibited great variability. In examining the overall data, most of the subjects' improvement was achieved within the first week training period, leading to the question as to whether the improvement was due primarily to a practice effect. The decrease in BM thresholds was independent of the type of treatment the SLI subjects received. In comparing the findings from Marler et al. to those obtained by Thibodeau et al. (1999), it appears that the SLI subjects in this study were more language impaired.

In concluding this section, it seems likely that some of the variable findings in the psychoacoustic research in individuals with language learning or reading impairments result from methodologic differences across studies, subject characteristics, auditory stimulus characteristics, and differential sensitivity of assessment measures at different ages.

Analysis of the Research Concerning Fast ForWord-Language

Regarding the benefits derived from the application of Fast ForWord for Language (FFW-L), peer-based studies have not found effects as dramatic as those obtained by Scientific Learning Corporation (SLC). These could be due to:

- The difference in intensity of the remediation (Gillam, 1999);
- Biasing the results by using language measures similar to the FFW exercises, thus favoring a positive effect (Veale, 1999);
- In some studies, there may have been sample selection bias and students who received treatment beyond the recommended treatment period, thereby possibly receiving more intervention time than control students (Rouse & Krueger, 2004);
- The initial studies by Merzenich et al. (1996) and Tallal et al. (1996) included only children with SLI, whereas many subsequent studies included children with other disorders (e.g., dyslexia);
- The degree of success obtained from FFW-L intervention appears to depend on the severity of the disorder. Because of the small samples usually included in any of these studies, results could be easily impacted by subject selection.

When children have been trained on FFW-L versus curricular based approaches (such as Orton Gillingham (Hook, Macaruso, & Jones, 2001) or the Lindamood Phoneme Sequencing Program—discussed in the Earobics section (Pokorni, Worthington, & Jamison, 2004), gains derived have been similar, although for some skills subjects performed better when they were trained on the curricular-based approaches—such as on word attack (Hook et al., 2001) and phonemic segmentation and blending (Pokorni et al., 2004).

There is an extremely important caveat before one can draw any conclusions regarding FFW-L's efficacy, and it is one that goes to the original proposition for developing the FFW-L program. That is, this program was based on the premise that SLI children have a temporal processing deficit that underlies their difficulties. As discussed further in the Earobics section, it is clear that most learning disabled children (and likely SLI children) do not have a temporal processing deficit. Thus, rather than administering FFW-L to all children with a language or learning related disorder, some form of psychoacoustic testing involving various aspects of temporal processing (or possibly even better, electrophysiologic procedures such as those involving speech stimuli, as discussed later on) should be administered. By restricting research to those with confirmed temporal processing deficits, one could then better compare the clinical efficacy of FFW-L with control groups. This will confirm the beneficial aspects of FFW-L, at least for the population for which this product was initially intended. For those individuals who have been determined to have phonologic/phonemic processing, reading, or language related deficits in the absence of any temporal processing deficits, it appears that other approaches specifically targeted to the deficit areas may be more appropriate. This may be one reason why Scientific Learning Corporation (FFW-Reading series), as well as Earobics (Literacy Launch) have developed accompanying curricular based approaches for addressing reading related deficits.

Earobics Family of Products (Cognitive Concepts, Incorporated)

We now turn our attention to another popular computer-assisted program for improving language processing skills.

Product History and Development

The stated purpose of Earobics is to "develop the auditory and phonemic awareness skills that are critical for speech and language development and academic success" (Wasowicz, 1998; cited on p. 109 of Diehl, 1999). It should be noted that there have been few papers or independent studies written regarding Earobics. Therefore, the overview of the product and review of the research is significantly less than for Fast ForWord.

The Earobics software program focuses on phonological encoding (converting sensory input about sound structure into a representational form that can be stored in memory) and phonological awareness/phonics (awareness, manipulation, and representation of the speech sounds making up words). The perceptually based programs in Earobics target auditory processing abilities, whereas the more linguistically based activities are intended to target phonological awareness skills. As cited by Dr. Joseph Torgesen (member of Cognitive Concepts Strategic Advisory Board; citation from The Scientific Foundation of Earobics, p. 1)," Research has repeatedly demonstrated the important role of phonemic awareness in learning to read and spell. Earobics effectively incorporates many of the activities that have been used in research to stimulate phonemic awareness."

The Earobics line of software was designed by a team of literacy and language specialists. As stated by Cognitive Concepts, the software was based on decades of research and clinically proven techniques, resulting in a highly effective method for systematically developing the key skills that drive the ability to read and spell. According to Diehl (1999), based on references provided from the author of the Earobics program, its conceptual base is based on: (1) the auditory processing perspective, including research on temporal processing; and (2) the phonological awareness perspective. Earobics provides individuals with systematic and explicit phonological/phonemic awareness instruction following a systematic hierarchy based upon the principles of speech acoustics and speech perception. Among the goals of Earobics is to teach individuals to recognize and identify nonverbal sounds, syllables, and phonemes when presented in isolation or when embedded in words, and to recognize the position of sounds in words.

Description of Earobics Products

Similar to Fast ForWord, there is now a family of Earobics products. These consist of two product lines:

I. Earobics Computer Assisted Software: (1) Earobics Step 1 (4–7-year-olds); (2) Earobics Step 2 (7–10-year-olds); and (3) Earobics Step 1 for Adolescents and Adults
II. Earobics Literacy Launch Step 1 and Step 2

Earobics Literacy Launch combines the Earobics software with manipulatives, classroom activities, take-home books and materials, and parent activity guides to provide instruction in the full range of phonological awareness skills, including: phoneme identification, blending, segmentation, rhyming, and, phoneme manipulation. In addition, these materials and activities provide instruction in phonics and the alphabetic principle, vocabulary development, reading fluency, and comprehension.

In terms of working directly on auditory processing skills and phonological awareness, the Earobics computer-assisted software programs provide interactive instruction via a game-style multimedia format. Each of the three Earobics Step programs (Step 1, Step 2, and Step 1 for Adolescents and Adults) consists of a number of games focusing on different aspects of processing, in which the level of difficulty is automatically adjusted based on the individuals' success at a current level. Appendix 18-B describes the games, target skills worked on, and general adaptive principles used in Earobics Step 1. For information concerning Earobics Step 2, and, Earobics Step 1 for Adolescents and Adults, the reader is directed to the Earobics Web site (link is http://www.earobics.com/products/ad_ad.cfm).

Earobics-Related Research

There has been little published research regarding the efficacy of Earobics software. A number of internal reports from Cognitive Concepts describe results obtained from various school district pilot studies conducted throughout the United States (see http://www.earobics.com). These reports describe the reading performance of large groups of children before and after the introduction of Earobics Literacy Launch. In all of the reports listed, overall performance greatly improved. However, it should be noted that these studies included second language learners and children at risk for reading difficulties. Thus, the effectiveness of Earobics Literacy Launch in addressing the specific needs of language learning-disabled children cannot be determined. Second, one cannot partial out the beneficial effects of the Earobics software from all of the accompanying activities in Earobics Literacy Launch.

Recently, a number of studies have been published from Northwestern University by Nina Kraus and her colleagues on the beneficial effects of Earobics software training on the neural encoding and perception of speech (Kraus, McGee, Carrell, King, & Tremblay, 1999); Nicol & Kraus, 2005; Russo, Nicol, Zecker, Hayes, & Kraus, 2004; Warrier, Johnson, Hayes, Nicol, & Kraus, 2003). Kraus et al. (1999) examined the effects of auditory training in 13 normal adult subjects on mismatched negativity (MMN). MMN is an attention independent metric of the physiologic detection of acoustic change that occurs approximately 170 to 200 msec post-stimulus onset. It is obtained by comparing the electrophysiologic response to a series of frequently occurring stimuli and the response that occurs when there is some change introduced by a randomly inserted stimulus. The two responses are subtracted from each other, the so-called mismatched negativity. The 13 subjects who participated in the study underwent speech-sound discrimination training. Prior to training, the subjects' discrimination of two similar /da/ stimuli was at chance levels. Subsequent to six, 1-hour training sessions, not only did the subjects' discrimination ability improve but the mismatched negativity increased in duration and amplitude in nearly all of the subjects. Similar findings with other speech stimuli were replicated in other studies (Tremblay, Kraus, Carrell, & McGee, 1997; Tremblay, Kraus, & McGee, 1998). These findings revealed that training not only could result in behavioral changes but also could be reflected in auditory evoked measures as well.

Recently, a new electrophysiologic procedure known as the BioMAP (Biological Marker of Auditory Processing) has been developed by Northwestern University Auditory Neuroscience Laboratory, in partnership with Natus Company's Bio-logic Systems division (see http://www.communication.northwestern.edu/brainvolts/clinicaltechnologies for more information). Unlike traditional brainstem evoked response recordings using clicks or tone bursts, the BioMAP uses a complex speech syllable (/da/) that reflects the acoustic and phonetic characteristics of speech sounds that present difficulties for language-disordered populations. Timing measures obtained from the speech ABR response provide insight into (1) the accuracy with which the brainstem nuclei are synchronously responding to acoustic stimuli (e.g., peak latency, interpeak interval, and slope), and (2) the fidelity with which the response mimics either the stimulus or another response (e.g., stimulus-to-response correlations, and inter-response correlations). Magnitude measures provide information about (1) the robustness with which the brainstem nuclei respond to acoustic stimuli and (2) the size of a given spectral component within the response.

A growing body of literature from the Northwestern University Neuroscience lab has produced findings regarding speech-evoked brainstem responses obtained from normal children and children with learning problems. Warrier et al. (2004) and Johnson, Nicol, and Kraus (2005) among others have found that about one-third of children with language-based learning problems exhibit a unique pattern of auditory neural activity that easily distinguishes them from the larger population of children with learning problems. These findings indicate that brainstem measures relating to the encoding of linguistic information can serve as a biological marker for auditory function in children with language-based learning problems, such as dyslexia. As a result, BioMAP may help to separate learning-impaired children whose underlying cause of their difficulty may be due to ineffective temporal processing/encoding of speech patterns from those SLI individuals whose learning difficulties may be due to other causes.

Kraus and colleagues have also examined the effect of auditory training with SLI children. In one study (Russo et al., 2004), 19 children of 8 to 12 years of age participated. The experimental group consisted of nine SLI children, whereas the control group consisted of both normal (n = 5) and SLI (n = 5) children. Children in the experimental group participated in 35 to 40, one-hour sessions of Earobics over an 8-week period, whereas the control group did not participate in the training program. Brainstem measures to the /da/ stimulus (both transient responses—the traditional ABR peaks elicited by clicks/pips and evident within the first 10-msec poststimulus onset, and sustained ABR responses—consisting of peaks elicited 11.5 to 46.5 msec after post-stimulus onset) were obtained in quiet and in the presence of noise, pre- and post-training. In addition, a number of behavioral test measures were also administered; these consisted of a number of measures of auditory language processing as well as academic achievement. The results show that the transient evoked responses did not change after training and, thus, were resistant to the effects of training. However, auditory training did alter sustained response timing in the experimental group (i.e., coinciding with formant transitions and peak formant energy), especially in their neural encoding ability in the presence of background noise. Just as importantly, after training the children in the experimental group revealed significantly enhanced performance on the behavioral task measures and performed similarly to their control group peers. It should be noted that not all of the SLI children who received auditory training exhibited changes in their electrophysiologic measures. However, the authors noted that it was possible that these children's learning-related problems may not have stemmed from an auditory encoding deficiency at the brainstem level but from other causes.

A separate study by Warrier et al. (2004) compared the results for SLI children who received Earobics training (experimental group) to those who did not (a control group consisting of both SLI and normal subjects). In this study, the speech evoked ABR responses of the experimental group were further analyzed; based on the ABR morphology, the authors determined that there were two subgroups. One subgroup had similar evoked responses to the normal controls, whereas the other group's pretraining evoked responses revealed poor encoding of the speech stimuli, especially in their evoked response to the speech stimulus /da/ when presented in noise. Subsequent to Earobics training, the latter group's speech evoked responses improved to resemble the evoked responses of those of the normal subjects. This was also accompanied by significantly improved scores on the behavioral measures administered.

The results from these two studies show that for a subportion of individuals with SLI (i.e., for those exhibiting an abnormal evoked response to a fast-changing speech stimulus such as /da/, especially when presented in the presence of background noise), subsequent to undergoing auditory training using the Earobics Step 1 or Step 2 program, typically show clinical improvement as well as changes in their BioMAP response after training is completed.

In addition, the studies also show that Earobics training can benefit LD children without an observed audiologic basis to their difficulties. Thus, it can be inferred that the Earobics program works not only on bottom-up (auditory based perceptual) skills such as enhancing speech-sound discrimination but also on higher order cognitive-based skills (e.g., phonological awareness) thus benefiting children whose learning difficulties are more cognitively based. These findings provide support for the effectiveness of the auditory perceptual and phonological awareness aspects which served as the basis for development of Earobics.

To date, there has been only one published study (Pokorni, Worthington, & Jamison, 2004) that has compared the benefits derived from Earobics training to those obtained utilizing other approaches; this study also examined the benefits derived from Fast ForWord training. In the Pokorni et al. study, the authors examined the benefits derived from three intervention programs: Earobics Step 2, FFW-L, and the Lindamood Phoneme Sequencing Program (LiPS: Lindamood & Lindamood, 1998) on phonemic awareness, and language and reading-related skills. In contrast to the two auditory-based computer interventions, LiPS incorporates an articulatory based approach, in which a trained instructor works individually or within groups. The LiPS program divides auditory processing into five general processes: sensory input, perception, conceptualization, storage, and retrieval. Children are first trained on becoming aware of sounds in their environment. They are then taught to identify, classify, and label speech sounds by place and manner of articulation. This is followed by training on tracking and labeling speech sound changes (initially of consonants, followed by vowels) and subsequently through the use of letter associations.

Subjects in the Pokorni et al. study consisted of 62 children between 7.5 to 9 years of age, receiving school-based speech/language services, reading more than one year below grade level, and, scoring more than one standard deviation below the mean on at least one language measure. The children were randomly assigned to one of the three intervention programs, which consisted of three 1-hour intervention sessions per day over a 20-day period. The study incorporated measures of (1) phonemic awareness (two measures of the Phonemic Awareness Test, Robertson & Salter, 1997); (2) language-based skills (three subtests of the Clinical Evaluation of Language Fundamentals—3, Semel, Wiig, & Secord, 1995); and (3) reading-related skills (four subtests of the Woodcock Language Proficiency Battery—Revised, Woodcock 1991). Subject performance was examined pretest (4–6 weeks before intervention) and post-test (6–8 weeks after intervention ended). The results show that the students receiving Earobics and LiPS made gains only in the area of phonemic awareness, whereas the Fast ForWord group did not show gains. The Earobics group improved in their ability to segment phonemes, whereas the LiPS group improved in their ability to segment and blend phonemes. There was no transfer of any benefits from intervention to reading or language-based skills for any of the groups. The authors concluded that training programs that focus narrowly on phonemic awareness with little or no application to decoding are relatively ineffective in remediating reading deficits; however, they did note that it is possible that the intervention period was too short to see transfer to reading or language. The fact that LIPS resulted in the most improved performance on the phonemic awareness measures may be due to it being the intervention program that most directly targeted the phonemic awareness skills assessed in this study. The authors also pointed out that the intervention period of 4 weeks did preclude most of the students from reaching criteria on any of the interventions administered, which could have been a factor in the number of students achieving significant gains on the posttest measures administered.

Going forward, studies need to be conducted to assess: (1) which aspects of phonological/phonemic awareness are enhanced through Earobics training, (2) which aspects of Earobics training are correlated with and best address underlying auditory perceptual and/or cognitive bases in different groups of LD children, and (3) the optimal training schedule.

BrainTrain

Although not traditionally thought of as a product that can assist individuals with central auditory processing related disorders (CAPD), there are a number of skills addressed that may improve spoken language processing skills, including: attention, memory, and, sequencing. Although there has been no published research concerning the effectiveness of BrainTrain products with learning disabled children or children with CAPD, there has been some research, be it limited, on the program's efficacy for individuals with ADHD and in neurologically impaired populations. The following is meant to provide a brief overview of this program and its possible utilization with CAPD populations.

Rationale

Dr. Joseph Sandford (Clinical Neuropsychologist, President of BrainTrain) developed the BrainTrain family of computer interactive products to improve an individual's capability to accurately and efficiently identify, discriminate, and process relevant ongoing information is his or her environment. The operating principle is that by working systematically on deficit areas that impair aspects of information processing, individuals will improve their overall ability to learn and retain new information and concepts important to academic success (www.braintrain.com; Captain's Log Training Manual, available through BrainTrain). The target populations include individuals with ADHD, learning disabilities, brain injuries, developmental delays, and psychiatric disorders (note that even though LD children are considered a target population, no research concerning this population has been published).

Description of BrainTrain Products

BrainTrain products consist of three different programs: (1) Captain's Log, (2) SoundSmart, and (3) SmartDriver. SmartDriver focuses specifically on various aspects of visual attention and is not reviewed in this chapter. Captain's Log and SoundSmart consist of a number of modules designed primarily to address attention, working memory, and sequencing, although related skills such as phonemic awareness and processing speed are also trained in the SoundSmart program. The products have been designed for individuals, for ages 6 to adult (though there is a module in SoundSmart that goes down to the age of 4). The programs are adaptive and increase in difficulty as tasks are mastered. One can obtain trial CD versions of each program by contacting BrainTrain. Each of the trial CDs allows the reviewer to try out the various programs and derive a better understanding of the exercises employed and skills that are trained. The following provides a general overview of Captain's Log and SoundSmart programs.

Captain's Log

Captain's Log consists of three training tracks: (1) Silver (6 years up to age 11), (2) Gold (12 to 16 years of age), and (3) Diamond (17 and older). Each of these tracks differ in the type of stimuli and visual images presented. Determination of the track employed is automatically selected by the software subsequent to the individual's age being entered upon initial registration. The exercises contained within each track consist of 15 different stages although in one exercise—the Maze Learning program—there are 30 stages. The first 5 stages are conceptualized as beginner level, stages 6 to 10 as intermediate level, and stages 11 to 15 as an advanced level. Increasing the level of difficulty results in the introduction of new concepts, likely more stimuli being presented at any one time, stimuli that are more complex, and presented at a faster pace.

There are currently 35 training exercises available within Captain's Log, bundled within six different modules. These include: (1) Attention Skills: Developmental, (2) Visual Motor Skills; (3) Conceptual/Memory Skills; (4) Numeric Concepts with Memory Skills; (5) Attention Skill: The Next Generation; and (6) Logic Skills. Each of the modules and exercises contained have been carefully organized and systematized to train specific cognitive skills and meta-concepts. According to BrainTrain, over 22 different types of cognitive skills can be trained using the Captain's Log system, such as auditory/visual processing speed, selective/alternating/divided/sustained attention, immediate and working memory, response inhibition, visuospatial sequencing, and so forth. The Captain's Log program also provides what has been coined as a "Personal Trainer Wizard," which allows the trainer to select which of the cognitive skills he or she would like the player to work on. In turn, this guides the Captain's Log software in selecting the specific exercises administered to that trainee. BrainTrain recommends a minimum of 2 hours of training per week if progress is to be made and maintained, but for greater progress they recommend more intensive training. It appears that training is conducted over a 9 week time frame but this is determined by the level of mastery achieved within the various modules. The average grade for each individual is automatically recorded and visible in each of the Captain's Log programs.

SoundSmart

The exercises contained within SoundSmart are presented in the form of a Bingo game (http://www.BrainTrain.com; readme file from trial CD version of SoundSmart). Within any game, the "player" follows the spoken instructions until he or she gets four correct answers in a row, across, down, or diagonally. Success is reinforced by the reward of BrainTrain bucks, which the player may exchange for actual prizes at the trainer's discretion. Similar to Captain's Log, SoundSmart automatically adapts its presentation to the age of each player. At the end of each session, the program automatically generates a summary data report.

SoundSmart consists of three modules: (1) Attention Coach, (2) Math and Memory Coach, and (3) Sound Discrimination Coach. The Attention Coach and Sound Discrimination Coach are each divided into Beginner, Intermediate, and Advanced Levels, whereas the Math and Memory Coach is divided into five levels (Levels A, 1–4) correlated with math levels kindergarten through fourth grade. Each module constitutes a self-contained program and may be purchased separately or as part of an entire set. Thus, if one wanted to work on skills more directly related to spoken language processing, one could choose to order levels from just the Attention Coach and Sound Discrimination Coach. Each level within each module contains 100 stages, with advancement from one stage to the next being controlled automatically by the computer. In addition to being trained on discriminating, sequencing, retaining various stimuli, as well as following directions, SoundSmart also employs four training tracks, any of which can be simultaneously deployed with one of the SoundSmart modules:

- *The Patience Track.* The goal is to develop the ability of the trainee to wait until all directions are presented, thus decreasing the prevalence of impulsive responses. A traffic light is used, with the listener being instructed not to respond until the green light has been flashed. The manner in which instructions are provided are varied during the course of training. This is accomplished by varying instruction speed, varying the amount of time in which the yellow light is displayed, or by the instructor changing her mind and restarting the instruction.
- *The Listening Track.* When employed, this track incorporates various distracting sounds and figure/ground discrimination exercises.
- *The Speed Track.* This track encourages faster processing speed by limiting the amount of time for the player to select an answer. In this interactive track, the computer automatically adjusts its speed of presentation based on the trainee's responses.
- *The Challenge Track.* This track combines all of the types of training just listed, with completion of this track leading to the highest level of mastery.

Please note that, although BrainTrain indicates that trainees receive phonemic awareness and phoneme discrimination training within the SoundSmart Discrimination Coach, the program does not really accomplish this. For example, within the phonemic awareness exercises the trainee hears a particular sound (vowel or consonant) and is asked to point to the letter that represents that sound or to represent a sequence of sounds by the various letters representing them. Thus, the program actually works on sound-letter correspondences (i.e., phonics). In addition, there does not appear to be a hierarchal sequence in terms of the auditory complexity in which the speech sounds are presented within the phonemic awareness/discrimination exercises. Rather, it is the scanning, sequencing, and memory requirements that are adjusted in complexity.

BrainTrain-Related Research

As mentioned in the introduction section on BrainTrain, there has been no published research concerning the use of BrainTrain with learning disabled populations. Most of the research has examined the use of BrainTrain products with populations such as those with traumatic brain injury, multiple sclerosis, schizophrenia, or early stage Alzheimer's. However, there have been published studies regarding the use of cognitive training via BrainTrain products in individuals with ADHD. The goal of these studies has been to examine whether the implementation of cognitive therapy could result in improved attentional, behavioral, and working memory skills as compared to the provision of medications and behavioral interventions. Some small scale studies (Hall & Kataria, 1992; Klingberg et al., 2005; Kotwal, Burns, & Montgomery, 1996) have shown that individuals who have undergone training with the Captain's Log system improved in their attentional skills as well as in a number of processing-related skills, such as processing speed and working memory.

It remains to be seen if children with central auditory processing disorders can benefit from either the Captain's Log or SoundSmart program. For example, with its strong emphasis on selective attention, working memory, and sequencing skills it may be that these products can greatly enhance cognitive/language-based skills, as compared to traditional classroom/home intervention. Research with learning disabled populations with BrainTrain matched with various control groups (such as those receiving only school-based instruction and/or those receiving computer-assisted instruction) may reveal if any cognitive enhancements ensue subsequent to BrainTrain training over and above any other treatment regimen. In addition, the various exercises in the SoundSmart program involving sound-letter representations may be beneficial in developing phonics skills; however, that needs to be explored.

Thus, in discussing the BrainTrain program in this chapter, I have tried to bring attention to a program that has shown promise with related populations and to mention some of the program's aspects that may be beneficial when working with children with central auditory processing deficits.

Summary

This chapter reviewed two commercially available, computer-assisted adaptive programs touted as innovative interventions for children with auditory and language-based deficits (Fast ForWord-Language and Earobics) as well as one program used with related populations (BrainTrain). Although Fast ForWord and Earobics are widely used, there has been surprisingly little research regarding their clinical efficacy. In the studies that have been published, the results have generally been mixed. The literature seems to indicate that employment of Fast ForWord (FFW-L) or Earobics for significantly improving reading and language skills is not definitive. The few studies that have compared FFW-L or Earobics to curricular-based approaches (such as the Orton Gillingham approach, Gillam et al., 2001; or the LiPS program, Pokorni et al., 2004), have shown similar gains, and, for some reading-based skills individuals trained on the curricular based approaches have actually derived better results (it should be noted, however, studies that have examined the effectiveness of FFW-L and Earobics in enhancing reading and language performance may not have permitted enough time for adequate transfer of the trained skills to the reading and language domains, a factor that should be explored in future research). It appears that both Scientific Learning Corporation (SLC) and Cognitive Concepts have recognized the need to expand their respective computer products' limitations to address the reading and language domains, and thus, launched FFW—Reading and Earobics—Literacy Launch, respectively.

In regard to addressing temporal processing deficits, the purported goal of Fast ForWord, the results are mixed at best. Although the research conducted by SLC indicated significantly enhanced temporal processing abilities (Merzenich et al., 1996; Miller et al, 1999; Tallal et al., 1996), subsequent peer-based studies (e.g., Thibodeau et al., 2001) have revealed far less dramatic results. However, in a number of studies, many of the subjects did not complete the targeted percentage completion of exercises. It is possible that had training been extended, subjects would have revealed improved language and/or related reading performance (however, this could be true for any treatment regimen that is extended in time). It is also possible that for a number of individuals, their temporal processing abilities were so poor that the acoustically modified speech used in Fast ForWord training may not have been sufficient for them to distinguish between the stimuli, and consequently they did not benefit from FFW-L training. This should be explored further in future studies, and if this is indeed the case, then possibly even greater acoustic modifications within the FFW-L program may be beneficial for some individuals.

Regarding the general premise that temporal processing deficits underlie language learning-related impairments, some studies have shown that SLI children exhibit poorer temporal processing skills (e.g., Wright et al., 1997), whereas others have shown little difference between the temporal processing abilities of SLI children versus those without a language disorder (e.g., Bishop et al., 1999). Many factors may have contributed to the discrepancy in findings among studies:

- *Subject selection:* for example, in psychoacoustic studies that have involved dyslexic populations, only a certain percentage may have actually had an underlying temporal processing deficit (Heath & Hogben, 2004);
- *Time of assessment:* some studies have shown the greatest improvement in performance to occur very early on, gains that were possibly due to a practice effect rather than from the intervention;
- *Age of subjects:* Hartley et al. (2000) showed that psychoacoustic performance improves with age up to 11 years of age; thus, any assessment of intervention over a relatively long interval (such as 6 months) may be influenced by the aging process; this is supported by McArthur and Bishop's (2001) findings whereby the younger SLI subjects tended to reveal poorer psychoacoustic performance than their control peers;
- *Test parameters* and varying cognitive load introduced.

Based on the recent data from Kraus and colleagues (Nicol & Kraus, 2005; Russo, Nicol, Zecker, Hayes, & Kraus, 2004; Warrier, Johnson, Hayes, Nicol & Kraus, 2004), it appears that only a certain percentage of learning disabled children reveal an underlying temporal auditory processing deficit (approximately 33%), a finding that supports the conclusions obtained by Heath and Hogben (2004). Thus, the presence of a heterogeneous SLI population could explain much of the variance among studies. In turn, this stresses the need of partialing out individuals via either psychoacoustic measures or speech evoked response measures when conducting research on the effectiveness of any intervention program. As suggested by Thibodeau et al. (2001), intensive auditory training may be most productive if tailored to the individual temporal processing abilities of the child, and that psychoacoustic tasks (and possibly an electrophysiologic procedure such as BioMAP) may be a useful way to predict benefit from intensive auditory training. A natural extension of the work of BioMAP relative to Earobics training would be to extend the BioMAP research to those receiving FFW-L.

Future research should continue to address whether these programs are any more effective than a speech pathologist or related professional using a curricular-based approach as well as further studies comparing the effectiveness of Fast ForWord to Earobics. Also, in answering these questions, one needs to conduct a cost/benefit ratio.

Last, none of the computer-assisted programs effectively employ the teaching of metacognitive strategies as the various skills are taught; rather, they rely on practice/drilling. To address this, the companies could (a) incorporate meta-cognitive strategies into the software that the trainee could use as they practice the various skills, or (b) encourage the active involvement of specialists (such as a speech-language pathologist) in teaching metacognitive skills that the child could employ when receiving training on the computer program.

In conclusion, much remains to be done before we can determine if any of these computer-assisted programs offer more than traditional, curricular-based approaches. Future research will require a carefully chosen subject selection process and well-matched control groups if we are to better correlate treatment aspects to clinical needs. The employment of psychoacoustic and electrophysiologic measures not only offers hope in this subject selection process but also in evaluating changes and efficacy resulting from any intervention program.

Key Points Learned

- The research indicates that temporal processing deficits underlie language learning impairments for only a segment of the population.
- Although touted as a tool to significantly improve the language skills of children with specific language learning deficits, research regarding Fast ForWord reveals mixed results.
- Much of the research concerning Fast ForWord is difficult to interpret because the subjects have included heterogeneous populations, some of whom may have been more or less amenable to the training parameters included with Fast ForWord; in cases where benefits have been reported, these may have been due to factors (cognitive, linguistic) other than the acoustical modifications and adaptive training program employed by Fast ForWord.
- Findings differ widely among studies, factors contributing to the discrepancies include: subject characteristics, age at time of testing or intervention, task characteristics, intellectual demands of the task, and test measures used.
- Psychoacoustic and electrophysiologic measures offer tools for better controlling subject selection as well as measuring the benefits derived from intervention.
- Much research remains to be done in examining the clinical efficacy of Fast ForWord, Earobics, and BrainTrain software and for whom these programs may best benefit.

References

Agnew, J. A., Dorn, C., & Eden, G. F. (2004). Effect of intensive training on auditory processing and reading skills. *Brain and Language, 88*(1), 21–25.

Bishop, D. V. M., Carlyan, R. P., Deeks, J. M., & S. J. Bishop. (1999). Auditory temporal processing impairment: Neither necessary nor sufficient for causing language impairment in children. *Journal of Speech, Language, and Hearing Research, 42*(6), 1295–1310.

Bishop, D. V. M., & McArthur, M. (2004). Immature cortical responses to auditory stimuli in specific language impairment: evidence from ERPs to rapid tone sequences. *Developmental Science, 7*, 11–18.

Bishop, D. V. M., & McArthur, M. (2005). Individual differences in auditory processing in specific language impairment: A follow-up study using event-related potentials and behavioral thresholds. *Cortex, 41*, 327–341.

Burlingame, E., Sussman, H. M., Gillam, R. B., & Hay, J. F. (2005). An investigation of speech perception in children with specific language impairment on a continuum of formant transition duration. *Journal of Speech, Language, and Hearing Research, 48*(4), 805–816.

Carrell, T. D., Bradlow, A. R., Nicol, T. G., Koch, D. B., & Kraus, N. (1999). Interactive software for evaluating auditory discrimination. *Ear and Hearing, 20*, 175–176.

Carrow-Woolfolk, E. (1995). *Oral and written language scales*. Circle Pines, MN: American Guidance Service.

Cognitive Concepts. (2003). *The scientific foundation of Earobics: How proven techniques for developing phonological awareness and auditory processing skills are built into Earobics software*. Article obtained directly from Cognitive Concepts, Inc.

Cohen, W., Hodson, A., O'Hare, A., Boyle, J., Durrani, T., McCartney, E., et al. (2005). Effects of computer-based intervention through acoustically modified speech (Fast ForWord) in severe mixed receptive-expressive language impairment: Outcomes from a randomized controlled trial. *Journal of Speech, Language, and Hearing Research, 48*(3), 715–729.

Cornwall, A. (1992). The relationship of phonological awareness, rapid naming and verbal memory to severe reading and spelling disability. *Journal of Learning Disabilities, 25*(8), 532–538.

Diehl, S. F. (1999). Listen and learn? A software review of Earobics. *Language, Speech, and Hearing Services in Schools, 30*, 108–116.

DiSimoni, F. (1978). *Token Test for Children*. San Antonio, TX: Psychological Corporation.

Dunn, L. & Dunn, L. (1981). *Peabody Picture Vocabulary Test*—Revised. Circle Times, MN: American Guidance Service.

Elliot, L. L. (1962). Backward and forward masking of probe tones of different frequencies. *Journal of the Acoustical Society of America, 34*, 1116–1117.

Ferre, J. (2002). Behavioral therapeutic approaches for central auditory problems. In J. Katz (Ed.), *Handbook of clinical audiology* (5th ed., pp. 525–531). Philadelphia: Lippincott Williams & Wilkins.

Friel-Patti, S., Desbarres, K., & Thibodeau, L. (2001). Case studies of children using Fast ForWord. *American Journal of Speech-Language Pathology, 10*(3), 203–215.

Friel-Patti, S., Loeb, D .F., & Gillam, R. B. (2001). Looking ahead: An introduction to five exploratory studies of Fast ForWord. *American Journal of Speech-Language Pathology, 10*(3), 195–202.

Gillam, R. B. (1999). Computer-assisted language intervention using Fast ForWord: Theoretical and empirical considerations for clinical decision-making. *Language, Speech, and Hearing Services in Schools, 30*, 363–370.

Gillam, R. B., Crofford, J. A., Gale, M. A., & Hoffman, L. M. (2001). Language change following computer-assisted language instruction with Fast ForWord or Laureate Learning Systems. *American Journal of Speech-Language Pathology, 10*(3), 231–247.

Gillingham, A., & Stillman, B. W. (1997). *The Gillingham Manual* (8th ed). Cambridge, MA: Educators Publishing Service, Inc.

Griffith, P., & Olson, M. W. (1992). Phonemic awareness helps beginning readers to break the code. *The Reading Teacher, 45*, 516–523.

Hall, C. W., & Kataria, S. (1992). Effects of two treatment techniques on delay and vigilance tasks with attention deficit hyperactive disorder (ADHD) children. *The Journal of Psychology, 126*(1), 17–25.

Hartley, D. E. H., Hill, P. R., & Moore, D. R. (2003). The auditory basis of language impairments: Temporal processing versus processing efficiency hypotheses. *International Congress Series, 1254*, 215–223.

Hartley, D. E. H., Hogan, S. C., Wright, B. A., & Moore, D. R. (2000). Age related improvements in auditory backward and simultaneous masking in 6 to 10 year old children. *Journal of Speech, Language, and Hearing Research, 43*, 1402–1415.

Heath, S. M., & Hogben, J. H. (2004). The reliability and validity of tasks measuring perception of rapid sequences in children with dyslexia. *Journal of Child Psychology and Psychiatry, 45*(7), 1275–1287.

Hook, P. E., Macaruso, P., & Jones, S. (2001). Efficacy of Fast ForWord training on facilitating acquisition of reading skills by children with reading difficulties—a longitudinal study. *Annals of Dyslexia, 51*, 75–106.

Jenkins, W. M. (1998). *Stimulus and adaptive characteristics of FFWD training components*. Internal document from Scientific Learning Corporation.

Johnson, K. L., Nicol, T. G., & Kraus, N. (2005). Brainstem response to speech: A biological marker of auditory processing. *Ear and Hearing, 26*(5), 424–434.

Klingberg, T., Fernell, E., Oleson, P. J., Johnson, M., Gustafsson, P. Dahlstrom, K., et al. (2005). Computerized training of working memory in children with ADHD—a randomized, controlled trial. *Journal of American Academy of Child Adolescent Psychiatry, 44*(2), 177–186.

Kotwal, D. B., Burns, W. J. & Montgomery, D. D. (1996). Computer-assisted cognitive training for ADHD. *Behavior Modification, 20*, 85–96.

Kraus, N., McGee, T. J., Carrell, T. D., King, C., & Tremblay, K. (1999). Central auditory system plasticity associated with speech discrimination training. *Journal of Cognitive Neurosciences, 7*, 27–34.

Lindamood, C. H., & Lindamood, P. C. (1998). *Lindamood Phoneme Sequencing Program* (LiPS). Austin, TX: Pro-Ed.

Loeb, D. F, Stoke, C., & Fey, M. E. (2001). Language changes associated with Fast ForWord-Language: Evidence from case studies. *American Journal of Speech-Language Pathology, 10*(3), 216–230.

Mann, V. (1993). Phoneme awareness and future reading ability. *The Journal of Learning Disabilities, 26*(4), 259–269.

Marler, J. A., Champlin, C. A., & Gillam, R. B. (2001). Backward and simultaneous masking measured in children with language-learning impairments who received intervention with Fast ForWord or Laureate Learning Systems software. *American Journal of Speech-Language Pathology, 10*(3), 258–268.

McArthur, G. M., & Bishop, D. V. (2001). Auditory perceptual processing in people with reading and oral language impairments: current issues and recommendations. *Dyslexia, 7*, 150–170.

Medwetsky, L. (2006). Spoken language processing: A convergent approach to conceptualizing (central) auditory processing. *ASHA Leader, 11*(8), 13–17.

Medwetsky, L. (in press). Mechanisms underlying central auditory processing. In J. Katz (Ed.), *Handbook of clinical audiology* (6th ed.). Philadelphia: Lippincott Williams & Wilkins.

Merzenich, M. M., & Jenkins, W. M. (1995). In B. Juliesz & I. Kovacs (Eds.), *Maturational windows and adult cortical plasticity* (pp. 242–272). New York: Addison-Wesley.

Merzenich, M. M., Jenkins, W. M., Johnston, P., Schreiner, C., Miller, S. L., & Tallal, P. (1996). Temporal processing deficits of language-learning impaired children ameliorated by training. *Science, 271*(5), 77–81.

Merzenich, M. M., Schreiner, C. S., Jenkins, W. M., & Wang, X. (1993). In P. Tallal, M. Galaburda, R. R. Lindas, & C. V. Euler (Eds.), *Temporal information in the nervous system: Special reference to dyslexia and dysphasia* (pp. 1–22). New York: New York Academy of Sciences.

Miller, S. L., Merzenich, M. M., Tallal, P., Devivo, K., LaRoosa, K., Linn, N., et al. (1999). Fast ForWord training in children with low reading performance. *Proceedings of the 1999 Netherlands Annual Speech-Language Association Meeting*.

The National Reading Panel. (2000). *Teaching children to read: An evidence-based assessment of the scientific literature on reading and its implications for reading instruction.* Washington, DC: The National Institute of Child Health and Human Development.

Nicol, T., & Kraus, N. (2005). How can the neural encoding and perception of speech be improved? In J. Syka, & M. M. Merzenich (Eds.), *Plasticity and signal representation in the auditory system* (pp. 259–270). New York: Kluwer Plenum.

Pokorni, J. L., Worthington, C. K., & Jamison, P. J. (2004). Phonological awareness intervention: Comparison of Fast ForWord, Earobics and LiPS. *The Journal of Educational Research, 97*(3), 147–157.

Robertson, C., & Salter, W. (1997). *The Phonological Awareness Test*. East Moline, IL: LinguiSystems.

Rouse, C. E., & Krueger, A.B. (2004). Putting computerized instruction to the test: A randomized evaluation of a "scientifically based" reading program. *Economics of Education Review, 23*(4), 323–338.

Russo, N. M., Nicol, T. G., Zecker, S. G., Hayes, E. A., & Kraus, N. (2004). Auditory training improves neural timing in the human brainstem. *Behavioral Brain Research* (available online at http://www.sciendirect.com).

Scientific Learning Corporation. http://www.scilearn.com/results/science/articles

Semel, E., Wiig, E. H., & Secord, W. A. (1995). *Clinical Evaluation of Language Fundamentals, CELF-3* (3rd ed.). San Antonio, TX: The Psychological Corporation.

Share, D. L., & Stanovich, K. E. (1995). Cognitive processes in early reading development: A model of acquisition and individual differences. *Issues in Education: Contributions from Educational Psychology, 1*, 1–57.

Sussman, J. E. (1993). Perception of formant transition cues to place of articulation in children with language impairments. *Journal of Speech, Language, and Hearing Research, 36*, 1286–1299.

Tallal, P. (1980). Auditory temporal perception, phonics, and reading disabilities in children. *Brain and Language, 9*(2), 182–198.

Tallal, P. (2000). Experimental studies of language learning impairments: From research to remediation. In D. V. M. Bishop & L. B. Leonard (Eds.), *Speech and language impairments in children: Causes, characteristics, intervention, and outcome* (pp. 131–155). Hove, UK: Psychology Press.

Tallal, P., Merzenich, M. M., Burns, M., Gelfond, S., Young, M., Shipley, J., & Polow, N. (1997, November). *Temporal training for language-impaired children. National Clinical trial results.* Paper presented at the American Speech-Language-Hearing Association Annual Convention, Boston, MA.

Tallal, P., Miller, S. L., Bedi, G., Byrna, G., Wang, X., Nagarajan, S. S., et al. (1996). Language comprehension in language-learning impaired children improved with acoustically modified speech. *Science, 271*(5), 81–84.

Tallal, P. & Piercy, M. (1973a). Defects of non-verbal auditory perception in children with developmental aphasia. *Nature, 241*(5390), 468–469.

Tallal, P., & Piercy, M. (1973b). Developmental aphasia: Impaired rate of non-verbal processing as a function of sensory modality. *Neuropsychologia, 11*(4), 389–398.

Tallal, P., & Piercy, M. (1975). Developmental aphasia: The perception of brief vowels and extended stop consonants. *Neuropsychologia, 13*, 69–74.

Tallal, P., Stark, R., Kallman, C., & Mellits, D. (1981). A reexamination of some nonverbal perceptual abilities of language-impaired and normal children as a function of age and sensory modality. *Journal of Speech and Hearing Research, 24*(3), 351–357.

Temple, E., Poldrak, R. A., Protopapas A., Nagarajan, S., Salz T., Tallal, P. et al. (2000). Disruption of the neural response to rapid acoustic stimuli in dyslexia: Evidence from functional MRI. *Proceedings of the National Academy of Sciences of the United States of America, 97*(25), 13907–13912.

Thibodeau, L. M., Friel-Patti, S., & Britt, L. (2001). Psychoacoustic performance in children completing Fast ForWord training. *American Journal of Speech-Language Pathology, 10*(3), 248-257.

Tillery, K. (in press). Auditory processing evaluation: A test battery approach. In J. Katz (Ed.), *Handbook of clinical audiology* (6th ed.). Philadelphia: Lippincott Williams & Wilkins.

Tomblin, J. B., & Quinn, M. A. (1983). The contribution of perceptual learning to performance on the repetition task. *Journal of Speech, Language, and Hearing Research, 26*, 369–372.

Torgesen, J. K., Wagner, R. D., & Rashotte, C. A. (1997). Approaches to the prevention and remediation of phonologically based reading disabilities. In B. Blachman (Ed.), *Foundations of reading acquisition and dyslexia: Implications for early intervention* (pp. 387–304). Hillsdale, NJ: Lawrence Erlbaum Associates.

Tremblay, K., Kraus, N., Carrell, T. D., & McGee, T. (1997). Central auditory system plasticity: generalization to novel stimuli following listening training. *Journal of the Acoustical Society of America, 102*, 3762–3773.

Tremblay, K., Kraus, N., & McGee, T. (1998). The time course of auditory perceptual learning: Neurophysiological changes during speech-sound training. *NeuroReport, 9*, 3557–3560.

Troia, G. A., & Whitney, S. D. (2003). A close look at the efficacy of Fast ForWord Language for children with academic weaknesses. *Contemporary Educational Psychology, 28*(4), 465–494.

Veale, T. K. (1999). Targeting temporal processing deficits through Fast ForWord: Language therapy with a new twist. *Language, Speech, and Hearing Services in Schools, 30*, 353–362.

Warrier, C. M., Johnson, K. L., Hayes, E. A., Nicol, T., & Kraus, N. (2003). Learning impaired children exhibit timing deficits and training-related improvements in auditory cortical responses to speech in noise. *Experimental Brain Research, 157*, 431–441.

Wightman, F., & Allen, P., (1992). Individual differences in auditory capability among preschool children. In L. A. Werber & E. W. Rubel (Eds.), *Developmental psychoacoustics* (pp. 113–133). Washington, DC: American Psychological Association.

Wightman, F., Allen P., Dolan T., Kistler D., & Jamieson, D. (1989). Temporal resolution in children. *Child Development, 60*, 611–624.

Woodcock, R. W. (1991). *Woodcock Language Proficiency Battery—Revised.* Itasca, IL: Riverside.

Woodcock, R. W. & Johnson, M. (1989). *Woodcock-Johnson Psycho-Educational Battery—Revised.* Tests of Cognitive Ability. Allen, TX: DLM Teaching Resources.

Wright, B. A., Lombardino, L. J., King, W. M., Puranik, C. S., Leonard, C. M., & Merzenich, M. M. (1997). Deficits in auditory temporal and spectral resolution in language-impaired children. *Nature, 387*, 176–178.

Appendix 18-A
Description of the Seven Programs that Encompass the Fast ForWord Language Intervention Program[1]

The stimuli and general principles (algorithms) used in modifying the stimulus acoustic parameters are discussed.

Sound Exercises

Circus Sequence (CS)

The CS game is designed to train a child to process nonverbal sounds more quickly and accurately. Taking place inside a circus tent, the game requires the child to reproduce a two-sound sequence by clicking on one or two buttons, each of which corresponds to a specific sound. The stimuli are frequency-modulated (FM) tonal sweeps. They start at a particular frequency and either move up to higher frequencies (corresponding to the "Up" button) or move down to lower frequencies (corresponding to the "Down" button). The child's task is to reproduce the order of a two-tone sequence of the "Up" and/or "Down" presentations by clicking on the corresponding buttons.

All FM sweeps change frequency at the rate of 16 octaves per second; this rate of change reflects the average rate of change found in normal speech within the formant transitions of stop consonants. There are three frequency ranges: (1) 0.5 kHz; (2) 1 kHz; (3) 2 kHz. Within each frequency range, upward-moving stimuli always start at 0.5, 1, or 2 kHz, whereas downward-moving stimuli always end at 0.5, 1, or 2 kHz.

Within each frequency range, there are six stimulus durations: 80 msec, 60 msec, 40 msec, 35 msec, 30 msec, and 25 msec. Within each stimulus duration, there are 45 different interstimulus intervals (ISI): 500 msec, 400 msec, 300 msec, 250 msec, 250 msec, and 195 to 0 msec decreasing in 5-msec steps. Thus, there are three frequency ranges × 6 durations × 45 ISI, which result in a total of 810 training levels.

The CS game starts at the easiest level (i.e., at 80-msec tonal duration and 500-msec ISI). The CS game uses three correct responses in a row to advance to the next ISI level (in this case to 400 msec), while one error retreats to the previous level (in this case, remains at 500 msec ISI). The 3-to-1 rule produces about 80% correct when a child is working near the limits of his or her ability. Advancement across ISI levels and duration categories occurs independently within each frequency range. Note that multiple duration categories can be open simultaneously. That is, a new shorter duration category is added to the stimulus list once the immediately shorter duration category reaches 150 msec ISI. For example, an individual can initially commence at 80 msec duration at 0.5 kHz, 1kHz, and 2kHz with an ISI of 300 msec. If the individual were to reach 150 msec for 0.5 kHz, then a new duration category at

[1]Jenkins, 1998; Veale, 1999; Freil-Patti, Loeb, & Gillam, 2001; Miller et al. (1999). Available at the http://www.scilearn.com Web site.

0.5 kHz would be introduced (e.g., the next durational step would be 60 msec). At this point, the individual would not only be working on stimuli at 0.5, 1, and 2 kHz of 80 msec duration but also stimuli at 0.5 kHz of 60 msec duration. A stimulus duration category is closed once the 5-msec ISI level has been successfully reached and completed for that particular duration.

Old MacDonald's Flying Farm (OMFF)

This game requires a child to use the computer to "capture" and hold a flying animal. While holding the mouse down, the child hears a rapid succession of nonsense syllables. When the child hears a different nonsense syllable (i.e., differing in the initial phoneme) in the sequence, the child is required to release within 150 msec of the presentation the captured farm animal which then flies into a designated hiding place.

The OMFF game contains five phoneme contrast categories associated with 10 syllables. These are /gi/-/ki/, /chu/-/shu/, /si/-/ti/, /ge/-/ke/, and /do/-/to/. The phonemes differ in voice onset time (e.g., /gi/ versus /ki/) or in the fricative–vowel gap time (e.g., /si/ versus /sti/). In OMFF, the target syllable is presented in natural speech, whereas the initial consonant of the differing syllable is modified by extending the voice onset time (VOT) for the stops or by expanding the silent period between the fricative and vowel for the fricatives. There are 18 levels in each of the phoneme contrast categories, two of the acoustic parameters being systematically varied across these 18 levels. These parameters are the intersyllable presentation and either the voice onset time (VOT) or fricative-vowel gap time. First, the intersyllable interval is reduced from 500 msec to 300 msec in five steps. Second, the VOT times or fricative-vowel gap times for the foil stimuli which are initially expanded, are reduced ultimately to normal values.

Phoneme Identification (PI)

PI trains the child to distinguish single phonemes. The game takes place in an Olympic stadium in which a turtle presents a specific phoneme within the context of a target CV or VCV syllable (e.g., /bi/. The child then sees two animals side-by-side: one which says the target phoneme and another which says a distractor phoneme (e.g., /di/). The stimuli choices are presented in random sequence. The child's task is to identify the character that produced the target sound.

PI features five phoneme contrast pairs that differ by one phoneme: /va/-/fa/, /aba/-/ada/, /ba/-/da/, /be/-/de/, and /bi/-/di/. There are 26 levels for each of the five phoneme contrast categories. Three acoustic parameters are systematically varied across these 26 levels. These parameters are the (1) interstimulus-interval (ISI) which varies from 500 msec to 10 msec; (2) formant transition duration; and (3) intensity enhancement of the formant transitions. First, the ISI between the target phoneme and its foil is reduced. Then the formant transition duration is reduced from an initial 80-msec duration, ultimately to a normal duration of about 40 msec. Then the formant intensity enhancement (initially + 20 dB) is gradually reduced to normal. Finally, the ISI is reduced further.

Word Exercises

Word exercises comprise four games, each described below. Each word exercise contains words or sentences that have been digitally recorded and then acoustically modified using digital signal processing technology. The modification is of two forms, one is time expansion and the other is restricted intensity enhancement. The restriction refers to the fact that the intensity enhancement centers around the second formant frequency and is limited to the rapidly changing acoustic information within this region. Each of the word exercises contains four types of modified speech as well as normal speech. The five processing levels are:

i. Level 1 Characteristics: 150% expansion; 20 dB enhancement
ii. Level 2 Characteristics: 125% expansion; 20 dB enhancement
iii. Level 3 Characteristics: 100% expansion; 20 dB enhancement
iv. Level 4 Characteristics: 100% expansion; 10 dB enhancement
v. Level 5 Characteristics: 100% expansion; 0 dB enhancement (normal speech)

Fast ForWord uses a so-called 90% correct rule for determining when to shift processing levels for all games comprising the word exercises. Each of the exercises differs in the use of the 90% rule, described below.

Word Exercises Games

Phonic Words (PW)

Using a word discrimination paradigm, PW requires the child to distinguish between minimal pair words that differ either by an initial consonant (such as *bat* versus *pat*, or a final consonant (such as *pat* and *pack*). First, the child is instructed to "point to" followed by the word. The child then chooses between the two pictures presented, one of which represents the target word. The game is intended to provide the child with practice in making correct phonetic distinctions between sounds presented in word contexts.

Performance is evaluated each time after one full round comprising all word contrasts has been presented. If performance is at or above 90% correct, the program adjusts to present the same words at the next modified level. If performance is below 90% correct for the entire stimulus set, the entire stimulus set is presented again until the 90% criterion is reached.

Phonic Match (PM)

Although PM is classified as a word exercise, it features both sounds as well as words. PM contains a grid of "crazy animal creatures" in 2 × 2, 3 × 3, or 4 × 4 formats. Each tile has a corresponding single word or nonsense syllable (e.g. /ra/, /la/), in a CV or CVC syllable format that differ in either initial or final consonants. Within a particular game, all stimuli contain the same vowel sound.

PM stimuli consist of 96 sounds and words. When the child selects a tile, he or she hears the word or nonsense syllable corresponding to that tile. The child must find the other tile in the grid that produces the same word/syllable, thus adding a memory component. When the child selects two tiles with matching words in successive order, the two tiles disappear. The child is given a limited number of matching attempts on each board, with extra points being awarded if he or she clears the board with fewer match attempts. The number of tiles in the next grid increases if the child clears the game board quickly.

Block Commander (BC)

BC is a three-dimensional board game that consists of familiar colored shapes that the child selects and manipulates. The game is related to the increasingly challenging commands of the Token Test for Children (DiSimoni, 1978). BC increasingly forces the child to use his attention, comprehension, memory, and, sequencing skills by asking him or her to follow increasingly complex commands.

The child receives instructions to point to or move different colored geometric shapes on the computer monitor. BC consists of 58 commands (within five cognitive categories) of increasingly longer sentences/syntactic difficulty that range from simple, one-step instructions to multistep commands that require understanding of prepositional phrases. Across training sessions, the amount of speech processing is systematically decreased. Processing level change from levels 1 to 3 require 90% performance on the easiest three cognitive category items. If performance is below 90% correct, then items from all of these levels are presented again until the 90% criterion is reached. Modification level movement from level 4 to 5 requires 90% performance on all of the five cognitive category items. If performance is below 90% correct on all items, then the items from all of the cognitive categories are presented again until the 90% criterion is reached.

Language Comprehension Builder (LCB)

The objective of LCB is to train a child to make appropriate grammatical distinctions in a sentence context. LCB presents children with pictures depicting actions and complex relational themes to build a child's phonologic, morphologic, and grammatical comprehension skills. Children must match the spoken sentences with the correct picture. Using 200 sentences that describe actions and relational themes, LCB trains participants on 40 specific areas of language comprehension including increasingly complex phonologic, syntactic, and morphologic structures, spread over seven approximate age-level groups (2, 3, 4, 5, 6, 7, and 8). The child must click on one of two to four picture choices corresponding with the production heard auditorily. Processing level movement requires 90% performance on the items. If performance is below 90% correct, all items are repeated again until 90% criterion is reached, at which point the program moves to the next processing level.

Appendix 18-B
Description of the Six Programs that Encompass Earobics Step 1 (Cognitive Concepts, Inc.)

An overview of the skills worked on and stimuli used, as well as a description of the general principles used in adjusting the level of difficulty are discussed.

Phonemic Recognition and Identification Skills

Overview

Phonemic recognition and identification is taught following a systematic hierarchy based upon the principles of speech acoustics and speech perception. Children are taught to recognize and identify phonemes when presented in isolation or when embedded in words, and to recognize the position of sounds in words. The phonemes are carefully ordered based on their acoustic and phonetic properties with the most distinct, acoustically and phonetically salient, sounds presented first, progressing systematically to sounds that are more difficult to hear.

Game: CC Coal Car Game (74 levels of play)

The CC Coal Car pulls into the station instructing the child to listen for a target sound (e.g., "Long vowel 'a' says 'a'. Click on the letter 'a' when you hear the 'a' sound."). Thus, the child is presented with an auditory and visual representation of the target speech sound. A series of subsequent sounds are then presented. If the child hears the target sound, she or he is instructed to click on the letter representing that speech sound. If the child does not hear that sound, then the child clicks on a symbol signifying that she or he heard a different sound. If the child is correct, the car fills with coal, and, the child receives an engine in the score box. If the child is incorrect, she or he is reminded of the target sound, the coal train fills with dust, and train tracks appear in the score box.

After the child masters phoneme identification for sounds presented in isolation, phonemes are presented within the context of a word. For example, the child is instructed to listen for the long vowel 'e' sound. The child hears a word (e.g., "bike" or "bee") and identifies whether or not the word contains the target sound. The training progresses through various levels, teaching children to identify long vowels, short vowels, and consonant sounds. Once the child can identify phonemes in words, she or he learns to identify the position of a phoneme in a word. This time, the CC Coal car pulls into the station with three cars—an engine, a coal car, and a caboose. The child is instructed to click on the engine if the target sound is at the beginning of the word, on the coal car if the sound is in the middle of the word, or the caboose if the sound is at the end of the word. The child listens to words containing consonant sounds, ordered based on their acoustic and phonetic saliency.

Phonemic Blending

Overview

Sequential training of phonologic blending skills is provided following a developmental hierarchy including blending words into compound words, syllables into words, and phonemes into words. Factors such as the perceptual similarity of response choices and the timing between sound segments are carefully controlled. Note that in addition to working on blending skills, auditory discrimination of vowels and consonants, attention, and memory are also worked on.

Game: Caterpillar Connection (56 levels of play)

Training begins by teaching the child to blend words into compound words. The child hears two single syllable words such as "dog . . . . house" and is asked to click the corresponding picture from a choice of three. If the child is correct, Katy caterpillar turns into a butterfly and the child receives a rewarding caterpillar in the score box. If the child is incorrect, she or he is corrected and a stick appears in the score box. Once the child masters blending words into compound words, the child blends two syllables into words ('butter," and then two phonemes into words (e.g., "m-e"). Once mastery has been achieved for these tasks, the child is asked to blend three syllables, then three phonemes, and finally four phonemes into words.

As the training proceeds, auditory memory is increasingly taxed as the time interval between the segments gradually increase from 0.25 to 2 seconds. Additionally, after the child is able to blend the segments at the various time intervals, the perceptual similarity of the response choices becomes more challenging. Initially, the three response choices are not perceptually similar but as training progresses, the response choices become increasingly similar (e.g., "nose, rose, hose") requiring the child to make finer-tuned discriminations among the response choices.

Segmentation

Overview

Segmentation is taught following a developmentally appropriate hierarchy. Skills worked on include auditory temporal processing, auditory short-term memory, and phoneme segmentation. Training begins with counting nonspeech and speech sounds, and progresses to segmenting words into syllables and words into phonemes. Variables including the time interval between sounds and the amount of auditory feedback are systematically controlled across the various levels.

Game: Rap-A-Tap-Tap (16 levels of play)

Training begins by teaching the child to count drum beats. A number of drum beats are presented (up to a maximum of four beats) and upon cessation, the child is asked to click on the mouse once for each beat heard. If the child responds correctly, the band plays music and a musical note appears in the box. If the response is incorrect, an empty musical staff appears in the score box. The training teaches the child to process sounds more quickly by providing practice at time intervals varying from 1.0 to 0.25 seconds. Auditory feedback is initially provided, allowing the child to hear the beats on the drum as she or he clicks on the mouse. As the child progresses, the auditory feedback is removed, requiring the child to recall and count the drum beats independently.

After achieving mastery with the drum beats, the child learns to count speech sounds. The child hears one to four speech sounds and is asked to click on the mouse once for every sound heard. For example, if the child hears "s," "b," "d," the child would click on the mouse three times. The program automatically controls the timing between the sounds as well as auditory feedback as in the previous set. Once the child can successfully count speech sounds, she or he learns to break words into syllables. The child is asked to click on the mouse for each syllable in a one- to four-syllable word. Initially, when responding the child hears each syllable when she or he clicks on the mouse, but eventually when the child has shown that she or he can segment the words successfully into its component syllables, the software program removes the auditory feedback.

After the child is able to successfully segment the word and count the number of syllables contained, the child learns to segment words with two or four phonemes. For example, for the word "dog," the child would click the mouse three times representing the three phonemes (d-o-g). The game progresses as above, controlling the number of phonemes as well as auditory feedback.

Rhyming

Overview

Rhyming skills are taught in two ways: (1) selecting rhyming words from a group of nonrhyming words and (2) selecting nonrhyming words from a group of rhyming words. Skills taught include rhyming, auditory performance with competing skills, and auditory sequential skills.

Game: Rhyme Time (11 levels of play)

Training begins by asking the child to identify the nonrhyming word from a set of three words. Three frogs sit on lily pads, and each says a word (e.g., "hop, top, dog"). The child clicks on the frog that says the nonrhyming word. If correct, the frog leaps into the score box but if the child is incorrect the frog leaps into the water and the child receives a lily pad in the score box. Training increases in difficulty by increasing the number of choices from three to five words.

Once the child can identify a nonrhyming word from a set of five words, figure-ground discrimination training begins. Low level background noise is introduced, requiring the child to attend and complete the rhyming task in the presence of the noise. The level of the noise is increased after the child masters the task at the particular level of noise being presented. After the child is able to select the nonrhyming word from a set of two to five words with a high level of background noise, the format changes and the child is asked to select the rhyming words from a set of two to five words. The software systematically increases the number of words and level of background noise as the child progresses through the levels.

Auditory Discrimination

Overview

Earobics incorporates extensive speech discrimination activities that develop vowel and consonant discrimination skills in a systematic, adaptive training format. The software has been designed to acoustically modify the speech signal, making certain parts of the speech sounds more distinctive, thus facilitating the development of discrimination skills. In addition, pattern recognition, sequential memory, and temporal memory are worked on.

Game: Basket Full of Eggs (114 levels of play)

Training begins by pairing vowels that are separated by four or more steps on the acoustic continuum or those vowels that sound the most different (e.g., "ee" versus "oo"). The child is asked if the two vowel sounds are the same or different. If correct, an egg falls in Farmer Fardell's basket, but if incorrect the egg drops and cracks. Training progresses in difficulty by presenting pairs of vowels that are more and more perceptually similar. (e.g., "hood" and "who'd"). Once the child masters vowel discrimination, the training progresses to teaching discrimination of consonants in CV syllables. It is at this level of play that computer-generated, acoustically modified speech is used. Acoustic speech characteristics such as onset formant frequency (for liquids, nasals, and plosives) are also carefully controlled across levels of play.

The training begins with a pair of sounds that have a relatively large difference in formant onset frequency or voice onset time (VOT). As the child progresses, the acoustic difference (i.e., degree of acoustic modification) is gradually reduced in single steps along an 8-step continuum, challenging the child to make finer distinctions between the two sounds in the pair. When successful, a pair of sounds that have less of a difference in formant onset frequency or VOT are presented and the steps repeated.

Auditory Sequential Memory

Overview

Earobics uses individualized adaptive training to develop and extend sequential memory. Tasks gradually increase in the number and complexity of different sounds, with fading visual cuing to develop auditory sequential memory. In addition, auditory and phoneme discrimination, phoneme identification, sound-level correspondence, and auditory performance with competing signals are worked on.

Game: Karloon's Balloons Game (38 levels of play)

Four stimulus types are used to develop sequential memory: environmental sounds, words, digits, and speech sounds. Karloon the clown asks the child to click on the picture of what she or he hears. Initially, the child hears one environmental sound and clicks on the corresponding picture from a set of two pictures. If the child is correct, Karloon's balloon floats to the top of the screen; if incorrect, the balloon pops and the child is shown the correct response. If the child responds correctly three consecutive times, the program automatically adjusts and presents the child with two sounds to recall in order. After the child can correctly recall the sequence of two environmental sounds, the child hears three sounds and must recall them in order. If two items are missed in a row, the program adjusts backward for additional training. Initially, pictures display simultaneously with the auditory presentation of the sounds. This allows the child to use visual cues to complete the task. As the child progresses, the visual display of the response choices is delayed, requiring the child to complete the task without the benefit of visual cuing.

After the child has been successful in sequencing three environmental sounds with and without a simultaneous visual display, the game progresses to teaching sequential memory for words. The child works through sequences from one to four words in order, with and without visual cuing.

After the child has successfully sequenced words with a delayed visual display, auditory figure-ground training begins. At this level, the child learns to focus his or her attention and process environmental sounds, and subsequently words, in the presence of competing noise. First, low level circus noise is introduced, and when the child is successful the intensity of the background noise increases.

Once the child masters auditory sequential memory for four words without visual cuing in the presence of background noise, the child is presented with number stimuli (from one to four digits), with and without visual cuing, with low and high-level background noise. After mastering sequential memory for digits, the stimulus type changes to phonemes, requiring the child to match sounds to letters (sequence increasing from one to four phonemes) with the same adaptive paradigm described for the other stimuli.

19

Application of Neuroscience to Remediation of Auditory Processing, Phonological, Language, and Reading Disorders

The Fast ForWord Family of Products

Martha S. Burns

Overview

The acquisition of language in young children occurs easily and effortlessly in most cases and follows the same developmental sequence despite native language and culture. Yet, for a number of children, despite normal intelligence and exposure to language, this process does not unfold smoothly. For these children, language acquisition is a struggle, violating predictable patterns of acquisition and affecting later learning.

Psycholinguists, acousticians, and neuroscientists have shared in the struggle to determine how the normal language acquisition process evolves and why. These researchers have uncovered certain aspects of auditory perceptual development, namely, categorical perception, speech sound categorization, and statistical strategies that guide this process (Dehaene-Lambertz et al., 2006). Adding another dimension to our understanding of language development, is emerging evidence from electrophysiological and brain imaging research that highlights the neural resources required for language development to proceed normally. Patricia Kuhl (2004) has highlighted this scientific expansion of our understanding of language acquisition in her recent review of the research in the area:

> Early in development, learners commit the brain's neural networks to patterns that reflect natural language input. So, early learning promotes future learning that conforms to and builds on the patterns already learned, but limits future learning of patterns that do not conform to those already learned (p. 831).

For several decades, intervention for language-impaired children has focused on determining the developmental level at which acquisition has broken down and applying known timetables of normal language development to restructure language exposure to conform to known hierarchies of phonologic, syntactic, and semantic skills. The evidence that perceptual skills underlie the neurocognitive processes of language learning, and later reading, although understood for several years, has been harder to apply to therapeutic intervention. Nonetheless, several systematic intervention approaches have been developed to address the perceptual element of language and reading intervention (see especially Chapters 13 [Katz] and 17 [Bell] in this volume).

The application of our understanding of the neural resources that underlie language acquisition has also taken time to be applied to language and reading interventions. Over three decades of research in neuroscience have clarified our understanding of the neural processes in the cerebral cortex that underlie the human capacity to learn (Merzenich & Jenkins, 1995). In the last decade, much of this research has been specifically applied to the neural processes involved in acquisition of speech and language (Dehaene-Lambertz et al, 2006; Kuhl, 2004) as well as the neural constraints, both acquired and inherited, that might negatively affect acquisition in language-impaired children (Benasich et al., 2006; Tallal & Gaab, 2006). To date, only one compilation of neuroscience derived programs has been developed that applies this research to intervention with auditory, linguistic, and reading impairment: the Fast ForWord family of products. The purpose of this chapter is to specifically address the neuroscience that underlies all of the Fast ForWord computer interventions and review the neurophysiologic and behavioral evidence of their efficacy.

Twelve Fast ForWord Interventions

Fast ForWord refers to a family of interventions developed and distributed by Scientific Learning Corporation for auditory processing, language, and reading disorders in children and adults. At this writing, nearly 750,000 individuals worldwide have completed at least one of these interventions since they were introduced in 1997. There are five core products that were designed by neuroscientists to enhance the underlying cognitive skills of auditory processing, attention, and memory. These intensive interventions each contain approximately 60 to 100 hours of exercises that adapt to each keystroke a participant makes in such a way that every participant ends up with a unique intensive practice on core discrimination, memory, and language activities. The five core products include:

Fast ForWord Language

Fast ForWord Language to Reading

Fast ForWord Middle School and High School

Fast ForWord Literacy

Fast ForWord Literacy Advanced

In addition to the five core products, Fast ForWord also has six reading products that continue to build cognitive skills, but in the context of curriculum-based reading activities. These products include Fast ForWord to Reading Prep and Fast ForWord to Reading 1, 2 ,3, 4, and 5. There is an introductory product, Fast ForWord Language Basics, which provides necessary practice on computer and phonological awareness skills to prepare for the core products. Finally, there are supplemental products that can be used in addition to the core and reading products: Fast ForWord Bookshelf Volumes I and II and The Reading Edge, a screening test for children at risk for reading problems.

The Neuroscience Behind Fast ForWord Products

Although much has been written about Paula Tallal's rapid auditory processing theory of language impairment that was fundamental to the design of Fast ForWord Language (compare this chapter with chapter 18 for two different perspectives on this component of the Fast ForWord Language program), the actual exercises themselves evolved from standard auditory training, speech discrimination, and language comprehension tasks that have been components of aural rehabilitation as well as speech and language intervention for decades. The fact that the auditory speech signals in some of the exercises in Fast ForWord Language had been acoustically enhanced drove a great deal of debate and discussion about whether auditory processing problems cause language delay and, conversely, whether auditory modification of speech signals is useful or necessary in remediation of language delay. As only two of the 12 Fast ForWord products are specifically designed to address rapid auditory processing, this chapter briefly updates readers on current research relevant to this debate under Other Views toward the end of this chapter.

The 12 Fast ForWord products actually all share a common foundation in their design and methodology: neuroscience principles of learning and brain plasticity. It is this foundation that provides the power in the products and has been the basis of more current research designs of product efficacy (Temple et al., 2000; Temple et al., 2003; Troia, 2004). The contribution of neuroscience to the study of learning is the clarification of how auditory processing, and the learning dependent on it (language and reading), is a dynamic and modifiable neurological capacity.

Neuroplasticity: Methodological Remodeling of Distributed Brain Responses for Learning

For almost a century, neuroscientists believed that the human brain was "hard wired" and that after an early critical period of development it was incapable of dramatic growth or change. Neurologists were taught that brain damage in an adult was irreversible and changes that occurred as the result of therapy were either due to a reduction in swelling and resumption of "shocked" connections (diaschisis) or compensatory adaptations (Harvey, 2003). In the 1980s however, research with animals was beginning to suggest that there were neurological mechanisms that allowed for central nervous system repair of damaged connections (for an excellent review, see Kolb, 2003). At about the same time, neuroscientists in other labs were showing that sensory maps in the primary somasthetic and auditory brain regions could be dramatically altered in adult animals by specific kinds of training (Merzenich et al., 1988). By the 1990s views of the inalterable human brain were changing and researchers across disciplines began to realize that, far from being "hard wired," the human brain is a remarkably plastic organ: constantly changing to meet the demands of an ever changing organism in an ever changing environment (Benasich et al., 2006; Merzenich & Jenkins, 1995; Sterr et al., 1999). With the advent of functional imaging procedures in the late 1980s and 1990s, it became possible to actually chart the changes in human brain processing schemes after specific kinds of environmental stimulation (Fiez, 1995; Mintun et al., 1989).

Enter, Fast ForWord Language (originally called HAILO and later Fast ForWord I). Two of the most influential researchers in brain plasticity in those early days were Dr. Michael Merzenich and Dr. William Jenkins at the W. M. Keck Center for Integrative Neurosciences at the University of California at San Francisco. They applied research from two decades of study on basic cerebral cortex neural processes of learning to a methodology for perceptual and language enhancement in language-impaired children. The neuroscientific research pointed to six principles that Merzenich and Jenkins (1995) believed could be applied to rehabilitation and learning:

- *Attention*—little or no enduring changes are driven in the cerebral cortex if stimuli are delivered when an individual is not responding or attending; underlying the human ability to focus and maintain attention to a task is the neurotransmitter acetylcholine which can be enhanced by the nature of tasks used (Kilgard & Merzenich, 1998).
- *Memory*—changes in the cortex fade when a well-learned behavior does not have to be held in memory, most likely because the cognitive relevance assigned to the task decreases; thus practice alone, without requirements for retention do not drive brain changes.
- *Reinforcement and novelty*—behavioral scientists had understood the power of timely reinforcement in learning since research on classical conditioning in the 1950's; more recently neuroscientists began to understand why—specific reinforcement schedules and intermittent novelty drive neurotransmitters like dopamine and norepinephrine which are critical to creating permanent new neurological connections. (Bao et al., 2001).
- *Frequency and Intensity of stimulation*—in animals it took thousands of repetitions of new stimuli to effect neurological changes; clinicians often refer to this as the "practice effect."
- *Adaptability*—the brain builds skill upon skill; by carefully grading stimuli to tasks that increasingly stress the brain to process faster or more efficiently, exercises can adapt to each individual's unique gains in skill.
- *Cross-training*—the brain processes in networks of distributed neuronal clusters that develop simultaneously (Mesulam, 2000); effective rehabilitation of language (a complex cognitive skill) would benefit from cross-training all components of the language network.

None of these principles were new to educators or therapists although the neurological bases had been unknown; but integrating all of them at one time was possible with technology in ways that could not be managed even in one-on-one rehabilitation. Computer exercises could be programmed to provide thousands of stimuli every hour. They could be developed to time reinforcement for correct responses so that dopaminergic systems are enhanced. They could build novelty into the exercises so that when a person mastered a skill he or she not only received new stimuli but might periodically have novel activities or characters. And, they could be designed to cross-train a variety of sensory and cognitive skills so that entire networks are stimulated. Finally, computer programs could control attention and thereby enhance neuroplastic changes by controlling stimulus presentation depending on participant readiness.

So, Michael Merzenich and William Jenkins set out to develop computer-based exercises based on these underlying principles that could enable any child or adult with auditory processing, language, or reading problems to cross-train cognitive skills like memory, language comprehension, and speech-sound discrimination to enhance the capacity of cognitive skills required for language and reading. They intended that the products they developed would be an adjunct to other types of intervention: neuroscience-derived software that could augment and enhance a child or adult's capacity to learn.

How the Neuroscience Methodology Is Applied

All of the Fast ForWord products combine a depth of content designed to develop perceptual, memory, language, and reading skills. It is beyond the scope of this chapter to review the research behind the selection of content for each of the Fast ForWord core and reading products. However, much of that information is available on the Web site at http://www.scientificlearning.com

The discussion that follows describes how each of the six principles of neural processing and neuroplasticity discussed above are realized in all 12 core products and reading products with research results that support the value of that feature on language or cognitive skills.

Attention

A feature of all of the exercises in the Fast ForWord family of products is that attention is controlled to maximize learning. Prior to an individual receiving a stimulus on any of the exercises he or she must indicate a readiness by clicking a starter item (this varies on each exercise but is usually located in the lower left-hand corner of the exercise graphic) or click a stimulus item of the task itself. On most of the tasks, stimuli are only presented one time, not repeated, so that a participant must learn to pay attention to a stimulus the first time it occurs. The combination of requiring a readiness response prior to providing a stimulus as well as restricting the ability to receive a repetition enhances attention to each stimulus and increases the availability of acetylcholine for learning, thereby enhancing the probability that the stimulus and response will result in more lasting behavioral changes. A national field trial of 405 children conducted with Fast ForWord Language supported the value of this attentional control. Children with diagnoses of ADD made gains nearly equivalent to those without this diagnosis on language and processing skills (Agocs, 2006).

Memory

One of the advantages of technology over many paper and pencil educational tasks is that stimuli can be presented and then removed so that a participant cannot "look back" or review previous material to find answers. This feature is maximized in all the Fast ForWord products. When retention is a goal of the exercise, the information to be retained is removed from the screen prior to introducing stimuli to probe that retention. In some of the memory exercises, the participant actually loses points for guessing. These two features encourage a participant, over multiple stimuli, to increase their concentration on the task at hand and to develop memory strategies for learning.

To some extent, all of the exercises on the Fast ForWord core products and the

Fast ForWord Reading products have features that require retention. In some cases the exercises are designed specifically to drive auditory or visual working memory in the short term. Some of the exercises require short-term memory for phonological distinctions, others for matching words according to semantic categories, other for holding words in mind while other words flash across the screen. As the products progress in complexity and difficulty, long-term retention is required for completing sentences using closure tasks, demonstrating comprehension of sentences both auditorily and through reading, memory for spelling and punctuation, and finally, comprehension of extended narrative and later comprehension of extended written text.

Research on specific memory improvements after use of Fast ForWord products were reported using the Token Test for Children on 150 children during the National Field Trial of Fast ForWord Language. Ninety-one percent of the participants for whom Token Test data were available, both pre- and post-test, showed improvement, with an average gain of 1.7 standard deviations (Agocs et al., 2006). Other research reported from 14 schools, a university-based learning center, and a clinic, as provided on the scientific learning Web site showed significant phonological memory gains ($p<.05$) on the C-TOPP of 59 students who used Fast ForWord Middle School & High School compared to 35 controls.

Reinforcement and Novelty

A feature of all neuroscience-based research that demonstrates training-induced changes in local cortical wiring patterns is the use of strict classical conditioning paradigms (Merzenich & Jenkins, 1995). Newer research has pointed to the role of dopaminergic systems that act as the "save" button of the brain's computer. Dopamine released during carefully timed reinforcement increases the likelihood that a stimulus-response pattern will be retained permanently. This effect is so profound that several researchers whose research was used to develop the reinforcement protocols specifically as they apply to features of the Fast ForWord exercises have patented the technologic innovations and methodologies (Kilgard, Merzenich, & Bao, 2006, United States Patent 7,024,398.).

Frequency and Intensity of Stimulation

Neuroscience research consistently emphasizes the necessity for a high degree of stimulus-response frequency in an intense format delivered over several weeks or months to effect permanent neurologic changes in the cortex of humans (Karni & Sagi, 1993; Merzenich & deCharms, 1996). For this reason, all Fast ForWord products require intervention protocols of at least 50 minutes per day, 5 days a week, for up to 10 to 12 weeks. In the early implementations of Fast ForWord Language, the protocols required a minimum of 100 minutes per day and completion was established by criteria that participants would reach 80% completion of the product content in at least five out of seven of the product exercises. However, subsequent research showed that the duration of training is as important, if not more so, than content completion. In fact, it was the failure of many studies of Fast ForWord products conducted in schools and some in clinics, comparing Fast ForWord products with other interventions, to adhere to recommended protocols that appear to have accounted for variances in results (see Agocs et al., 2006). For this reason, content completion is no longer viewed as the most important criteria for exiting use of a product. Of more importance is the amount of time and consistency in use of each product. Because in recent years the value and importance of intensity of intervention has been supported by several research studies, most of the recent comparative studies of Fast ForWord products with other interventions have attempted to adapt interventions to the intense schedule recommended for all Fast ForWord protocols (Gillam et al., 2005).

In addition to the intensity of the Fast ForWord protocols, all Fast ForWord products utilize an extremely high frequency of stimulus presentations; hundreds of repetitions of stimuli each session. For this reason, on average, Fast ForWord products provide approximately 625 stimulus-response opportunities per 50 minutes of exercise. The combination of intensity and frequency of stimuli available with use of the Fast ForWord Language has been shown, along with other similarly intensive computer-based and one-on-one treatment-based interventions, to result in greater language gains among language-impaired youngsters than 3 years of conventional school-based speech and language therapy provided twice weekly in schools (Gillam et al., 2005).

Adaptability

Generally, the advantage of conventional classroom instruction or one-on-one individual therapy over "canned" intervention products is the ability of a teacher or therapist to individualize instruction to the specific needs of each student. The Fast ForWord products, through the development of complex computer models, have been developed to adapt to each keystroke a participant makes on each exercise. Some of the exercises in the products have hundreds of adaptive levels. This feature of the Fast ForWord core and reading products enables each product to individualize to the specific student's needs in ways that even the best classroom teacher would find difficult. The individual progress of each student on each exercise is collected during use of the product and the raw data accumulated into progress graphs that depict completion levels, historical progress over time, errors made, response rate, and percentage of correct responses by category. These progress graphs, called Progress Tracker, enable a teacher or therapist to directly observe the student's progress in whatever degree of detail they deem appropriate and structure additional educational or therapeutic interventions around the specific needs of each student.

This power of Fast ForWord products to adapt to each response a participant makes, and through Progress Tracker to reveal individual differences in progress by participant or groups (such as classrooms or schools), to directly measure every student's compliance with the protocol, and to derive supplemental educational or therapeutic materials based on each participant's unique learning needs, substantially increases the power of the products and has led to their adoption by hundreds of school districts nationwide. As of the date of this writing, the Scientific

Learning Web site provides data from 104 school districts nationwide and seven international schools and clinics that have provided independent research data on the effectiveness of the Fast ForWord core and reading products in their settings.

Cross-Training

The availability of functional brain imaging technology has resulted in revisions of older theories of brain processing which suggested that individual brain regions independently regulate specific cognitive functions. The newer view is that distributed cortical networks cooperate in cognitive skills (Mesulam, 2000). Functional imaging research has demonstrated that regions that serve as critical parts of cognitive networks often overlap and contribute to other cognitive networks (Hirsch et al., 2001). In this way, stimulation of a single cortical region may enhance other, seemingly unrelated, related regions. At the same time, simultaneous stimulation of several regions shown to contribute to a specific cognitive skill such as language or reading should have more profound therapeutic and educational effects than stimulation of a single cognitive domain.

All Fast ForWord products were designed to cross-train many cognitive domains including memory, sequencing, auditory processing, language, and reading simultaneously, depending on the specific product. The result has been that at the time of this writing, 15 states (Georgia, Oklahoma, South Dakota, Pennsylvania, Connecticut, Delaware, North Carolina, Florida, Idaho, Mississippi, Maryland, Ohio, Texas, California, and Tennessee) have provided independent results showing significant gains on statewide standardized achievement tests including DIBELS, FCAT, ISAT, SAT-9, and others. Several of the studies reported by school districts even include evidence of significant improvements on nonlanguage or reading standardized assessments such as math. Although Fast ForWord products do not promote their products for use in increasing these other academic areas, the results do speak to the value of cross-training large neural networks for improved generalized academic outcomes.

Independent Neuroscience-Derived Outcomes

Two independent controlled research studies employing functional magnetic resonance imaging (fMRI) were conducted using Fast ForWord Language to measure cortical changes attributable to the intervention by Elise Temple and her colleagues at Stanford University (Temple et al., 2000; Temple et al., 2003).* The research was based on earlier findings that children with developmental dyslexia have problems with language processing as well as demonstrating a

*Although Michael Merzenich and Paula Tallal are listed as co-authors of this published research, it should be noted that they did not participate in subject selection, assessment, or analysis of results. They were included as authors because of their contributions to the development of the Fast ForWord Language program that was used as an intervention in these two studies.

neural deficit in temporoparietal regions associated with phonological processing of written language (Snow, Burns, & Griffin, 1998; Temple, 2002, respectively).

The results of the two investigations of individuals with developmental dyslexia, one with three adults and the other with 20 children in the experimental group, showed that overall both groups of dyslexic subjects showed improved auditory language comprehension after use of Fast ForWord Language. In the adult study, where three subjects participated in the Fast ForWord Language program, two of the three subjects showed significant improvement on both rapid auditory processing and auditory language comprehension. Those two subjects, but not the third, also showed increased fMRI activity in the left prefrontal cortex on responses to rapid nonspeech analogues after training. The other subject, who showed no behavioral changes also did not show neurologic changes.

In the pediatric investigation, rapid auditory processing changes were not specifically assessed. Rather, a correlation between fMRI temporoparietal activation during phonological processing was evaluated before and after Fast ForWord in the experimental group and correlated with pre- and post-test comparisons on language (Clinical Evaluation of Reading Fundamentals—3 [CELF-3]) and reading tasks (Woodcock Reading Mastery Tests—Revised [WRMT-R]). The research revealed that there was a significant positive correlation between oral language improvement and increased activity in the auditory association (phonological) region of the temporo-parietal cortex. Furthermore, the experimental group, who participated in Fast ForWord Language, showed significantly greater improvement on word attack and word identification subtests than the control subjects. Both groups showed significant gains on reading comprehension. Temple (2003, 2007) in later publications of the results summarized her findings as follows: "that it is possible to study the brain effects of training in human children . . . [and] that a specific remediation program, Fast ForWord Language, resulted in changes in brain function in children with dyslexia while improving their reading ability" (p. 47, 2007).

Other Views

Fast ForWord Language may be one of, if not the most, researched language interventions ever developed. Although the studies reported above demonstrated largely significant outcomes associated with use of Fast ForWord Language, there have been other studies with less dramatic outcomes. Not all of the published research on Fast ForWord is discussed here because some of the studies involved used very small sample sizes or less conventional research designs. For example, a few school-based studies published in the educational literature used an "intent-to-treat" design. This may be considered an interesting design for looking at whether an intervention might be effective when used in unstable school situations where not all students are able to complete an intervention because they move out of district or have attendance problems. However, from a scientific perspective, because the intent-to-treat research design includes missing data and uses pretest scores for post-test data when post-test results are not available; this research is not considered in this chapter.

Some carefully constructed independent scientific research has been conducted on Fast ForWord Language where the outcomes were not as dramatic as other studies. For example, Fast ForWord Language showed significant improvements on some language assessments but not others in several studies (Friel-Patti et al., 2001; Loeb et al., 2001; Troia & Whitney, 2003). There also have been some comparative studies of Fast ForWord Language where the subject selection or implementation methodology varied considerably from the other studies referenced above. For example, in a Hook et al., 2001 study, which compared an Orton-Gillingham-based intervention with Fast ForWord Language, the authors found Fast ForWord more effective in remediation of phonological skills than for improvement of reading. Many independent controlled studies have not reported this difference. But, in the Hook article, the subject selection varied considerably from the other research studies on reading referenced in this chapter. Other published research (Agnew, Dorn & Eden, 2004; Beattie 2001; Pokorni, Worthington, & Jamison, 2004) vary with respect to number of subjects and methods of implementation. It is more difficult to show significant changes in behavior with small subject groups. It is also difficult to see patterns of improvement on case studies. However, as new research continues to be published, it is hoped that the findings will shed light on characteristics of Fast ForWord products that need to be considered for successful implementation. It is possible, for instance, that Fast ForWord products will be most effective for reading-impaired individuals whose underlying auditory perceptual or language skills contribute significantly to their reading difficulties. Some of the above research also suggests that Fast ForWord products are not as effective when adherence to the recommended protocol of at least 50 minutes a day, 5 days a week, for 6 to 10 weeks is not observed. This would not be unexpected, as one of the primary neuroscience principles upon which Fast ForWord products were developed is the importance of stimulation intensity. For this reason, the developers of the Fast ForWord products now include warning flags in their Progress Tracker to alert administrators to groups or individual participants who are not adhering to the recommended protocol.

A second area of conflicting results can be found in studies addressing the temporal auditory processing component of Language and Reading problems (Tallal, Miller, & Fitch, 1993; Tallal & Piercy, 1973) and by extension the use of temporal auditory processing design components in the Fast ForWord Language intervention. Although, for the most part not directly related to the efficacy of Fast ForWord Language in treatment of language and reading problems, this debate has been argued continuously over 10 years, since Fast ForWord Language was first introduced, with theoreticians essentially lining up on one side of the debate or the other. As with any scientific theory, the issue appears to be predominantly one of theoretical perspective rather than one of scientific evidence or evidence-based clinical outcomes (Thomas & Karmiloff-Smith, 2002). Nonetheless, the issue warrants review in a discussion of Fast

ForWord interventions to enable the reader to follow and form unbiased decisions regarding the continuing research and discussion on this topic.

Some of the earlier contrary research (McArthur & Bishop, 2001; Mody et al., 1998; Rosen & Manganari, 2001) concerning Tallal and Piercy's (1973) temporal auditory processing hypothesis of language and reading problems stemmed from a debate about the "causal" connection between auditory processing deficits and phonological deficits. As Tallal and Gaab (2006) discuss in a recent review of the issues, these research studies for the most part contend that even though individuals with language or reading problems have some general auditory processing limitations, they do not indicate that temporal auditory processing deficits necessarily cause problems with the phonological representation of language that we see in children with language learning impairment (LLI) or dyslexia.

Subject selection variances and differences in definition of language and reading impairment appear to be primary factors in conflicting findings of some studies. For example, one of the most commonly cited challenges to the view that temporal auditory processing deficits might contribute to language and reading problems was made by Mody et al. (1998). In this study, the researchers looked for evidence of temporal processing deficits in children with "reading problems." However, for the purposes of their study the authors chose as "reading problems" second-grade students whose standardized reading scores fell within the expected (second grade) level for their age. Their control group tested with reading levels substantially above second grade level. As a result, the Mody et al. definition of "reading problem" varied substantially from the definition commonly employed in clinics and school systems. Denenberg, (1999) provides a very thorough critique of this influential study.

There are also several methodologic factors that seem to have contributed to some contradictory auditory processing results from older studies of Fast ForWord Language. First, data using different types of test stimuli that are not equivalent are often combined and compared. Temporal auditory processing is not a unitary function (Tallal & Gaab, 2006), yet variable, nonequivalent paradigms (e.g., simple gap detection, central gap detection, backward masking, and frequency and amplitude modulation) have been applied in most studies where discrepant findings are reported. (See especially the paradigms used in older studies reviewed by Medwetsky in Chapter 18.)

It is equally important, in addressing potentially conflicting evidence, to note that significant differences have been found between individuals with language and reading problems and control subjects when electrophysiological measurements were used that were not found with behavioral measurements, even in the same study population. This is true of studies by McArthur and Bishop, who initially (2001) used frequency discrimination and backward recognition as their auditory temporal processing tasks when studying 10- to 19-year-olds with language and reading problems. They found that their masking task did not differentiate between their experimental group and controls.

This finding led to their conclusion that the data failed to support a role for auditory temporal processing in language impairment in agreement with other critics of this theory such as Mody et al. (1997). However, McArthur and Bishop did find that a subset of their younger experimental subjects performed significantly more poorly than controls on frequency discrimination.

In later studies (Bishop & McArthur, 2004, 2005), these authors looked again at the issues of subject age and reported results from auditory event-related potentials (ERPs) in response to tones with the same subjects. When the electrophysiological (ERP) data were used, although the authors predicted that they would see abnormal ERPs only in those subjects with poor frequency discrimination, they reported that the majority of the language-impaired subjects had aberrant ERPs. This finding occurred irrespective of the earlier reported frequency discrimination performance.

In an ERP study by Bishop and McArthur (2005) the authors also sought to directly test the original finding of Tallal and Piercy (1973) that children with SLI require a longer silent interstimulus interval between two tones to process them correctly. In contrast to the previous behavioral results with the same subjects (McArthur & Bishop, 2001), electrophysiological results revealed that the language and reading-impaired children were significantly different from their control group in their ERP to tone sequences.

Again, an age effect was found across groups. The older subjects showed less deviant electrophysiological responses than the younger subjects. McArthur and Bishop have held that auditory processing is likely a maturational skill and that some children may mature more slowly than others, but that it does not necessarily represent an impairment nor does it suggest that auditory processing causes language or reading problems. This perspective is not necessarily at odds with Tallal and her colleagues (Tallal & Gaab, 2006), who appear to agree that maturation is an important variable in manifestations of temporal auditory processing. The issue, as they see it, appears to be that when some children have immature auditory processing capabilities this, at least in part, may interfere with subsequent development of the phonological system.

Although it will require continued research into causation to finally begin to put the temporal auditory processing controversy to rest, and that research does appear to be emerging (Tallal & Gaab, 2006), to date the contradictory findings that fail to find specific temporal processing deficits in language and reading-impaired subjects commonly result from methodological differences in research design: especially subject selection, age, auditory stimulus characteristics, and the way that age affects the processing of the experimental stimuli. Thomas and Karmiloff-Smith (2002) noted in their review a few years ago that some studies that appear to provide conflicting results use psychoacoustic tasks that require considerable attention and cognitive demands. These authors concluded that, to a great extent, most of the controversy and conflicting results surrounding the rapid temporal processing theory of language and reading impairment appear to derive from a failure to take a developmental neuroscience perspective.

Summary

The Fast ForWord family of products was developed by a team of neuroscientists to drive dramatic changes in neural-based cognitive skills including attention, auditory processing, and memory, which have been shown to underlie language and reading. Independent research to date has generally corroborated the initial lab-based and field trial research findings of significant improvements in auditory processing, language, and reading skills following use of these products when there is adherence to recommended intervention protocols. These products were designed to be used as part of comprehensive intervention and educational programs for children and adults with specific language impairment and reading disturbances. To date, although not all research studies show identical results, those studies published in scientific journals generally support the contention that technological methodologies do provide an avenue for enhancement of those neural-based cognitive capacities that underlie language and reading. Further research elucidating which individuals benefit most from specific software interventions should shed additional light on the application of neuroscience to learning.

Key Points Learned

- Researchers have uncovered certain aspects of auditory perceptual development, namely, categorical perception, speech sound categorization, and statistical strategies, that guide the process of language acquisition.
- To date, only one compilation of neuroscience-derived programs has been developed that applies this research to intervention with auditory, linguistic, and reading impairment: the Fast ForWord family of products.
- The 12 Fast ForWord products all share a common foundation in their design and methodology: neuroscience principles of learning and brain plasticity.
- The contribution of neuroscience to the study of learning is the clarification of how auditory processing, and the learning dependent on it (language and reading), is a dynamic and modifiable neurological capacity.
- Although not all research studies with the Fast ForWord products show identical results, those studies published in scientific journals generally support the contention that technologic methodologies do provide an avenue for enhancement of the neural-based cognitive capacities that underlie language and reading.

References

Agnew, J. A., Dorn, C., & Eden, G. F. (2004) Effect of intensive training on auditory processing and reading skills. *Brain and Language*, *88*(1), 21–25.

Agocs, M. M., Burns, M. S., DeLey, L. E., Miller, S. L., & Calhoun, B. M. (2006). Fast ForWord Language. In R. J. McCauley & M. E. Fey (Eds.), *Treatment of language disorders in children* (pp. 471–508). Baltimore: Brookes.

Bao, S., Chen, V. T., & Merzenich, M. M. (2001) Cortical remodeling induced by activity of ventral tegmental dopamine neurons. *Nature*, *432*, 79–83.

Beattie, K. K. (2001). The effects of intensive computer-based language intervention on language functioning and reading achievement in language-impaired adolescents. *Dissertation Abstracts International*, *61*(08), 3116A.

Benasich, A. A., Chowdhury, N., Friedman, J. T., Realpe-Bonilla, T., Chojnowska, C., Dehaene-Lambertz, G., et al. (2006). Nature and nurture in language acquisition: Anatomical and functional brain-imaging studies in infants. *Trends in Neuroscience*, *29*(7), 367–373.

Bishop, D. V. M., & McArthur, M. (2004). Immature cortical responses to auditory stimuli in specific language impairment: Evidence from ERPs to rapid tone sequences. *Developmental Science*, *7*, 11–18.

Bishop, D. V. M., & McArthur, M. (2005) Individual differences in auditory processing in specific language impairment: A follow-up study using event-related potentials and behavioural thresholds. *Cortex*, *41*, 327–341.

Dehaene-Lambertz, G., Hertz-Pannier, L., & Dubois, J. (2006), Nature and nurture in language acquisition: Anatomical and functional brain imaging studies in infants. *Neuroscience*, *29*(7), 367–373.

Denenberg, V. H. (1999). A critique of Mody, Studdert-Kennedy, and Brady's "Speech perception deficits in poor readers: Auditory processing or phonological coding?" *Journal of Learning Disabilities*, *32*, 379–383.

Dubois, J., Mériaux, S., Roche, A., Sigman, M., & Dehaene, S. (2006). Functional organization of perisylvian activation during presentation of sentences in preverbal infants. *Proceedings of the National Academy of Sciences*, *103*(38), 14240–14245.

Fiez, J. A., Raichle, M. E., Miezin, F. M., Petersen, S. E., Tallal, P., & Katz, W. F. (1995). PET studies of auditory and phonological processing effects of stimulus characteristics and task demands. *Journal of Cognitive Neuroscience*, 7(3), 357–375.

Friel-Patti, S., Des Barres, K., & Thibodeau, L. (2001). Case studies of children using Fast ForWord. *American Journal of Speech-Language Pathology*, *10*(3), 203–215.

Gillam, R., Loeb, D. F., Friel-Patti, S., Hoffman, L., Brandel, J., Champlin, C., et al. (2005, June). *A randomized comparison of language intervention programs*. Presented at the Symposium on Research in Child Language Disorders, University of Wisconsin-Madison.

Gou, Z. (2006). The infant as a prelinguistic model for language learning impairments: Predicting from event-related potentials to behavior. *Neuropsychologia*, *44*, 396–411.

Harvey, R. L. (2003) Preface: Motor recovery after stroke. In G. H. Kraft (Ed.), *Physical Medicine and Rehabilitation Clinics of North America: February 2003, Supplement*. Philadelphia: W. B. Saunders.

Hirsch, J., Moreno, D. R., & Kim, K. H. S (2001). Interconnected large-scale systems for three fundamental cognitive tasks revealed by functional MRI. *Journal of Cognitive Neuroscience*, *13*, 389–405.

Hook, P. E., Macaruso, P., & Jones, S. (2001). Efficacy of Fast ForWord training on facilitating acquisition of reading skills by children with reading difficulties: A longitudinal study. *Annals of Dyslexia*, *51*, 75–96.

Karni, A., & Sagi, D. (1993). The time course of learning a visual skill. *Nature, 365*, 250–253.

Kilgard, M. P., & Merzenich, M. M. (1998) Cortical map reorganization enabled by nucleus basilis activity, *Science, 279*(5357), 1714–1718.

Kilgard, M. P., & Merzenich, M. M. (2002) Order-sensitive plasticity in adult primary auditory cortex. *Proceedings of the National Academy of Sciences, 99*(5), 3205–3209.

Kolb, B. (2003) Overview of cortical plasticity and recovery from brain injury. In G. H. Kraft (Ed.), *Physical Medicine and Rehabilitation Clinics of North America: February 2003, Supplement* (pp 8–25). Philadelphia: W. B. Saunders.

Kuhl, P. (2004). Early language acquisition: Cracking the speech code. *Nature Reviews Neuroscience, 5*, 831–843.

Loeb, D. F., Stoke, C., & Fey, M. E. (2001). Language changes associated with Fast ForWord Language: Evidence from case studies. *American Journal of Speech-Language Pathology, 10*(3), 216–230.

McArthur, G. M., & Bishop, D. V. (2001) Auditory perceptual processing in people with reading and oral language impairments: Current issues and recommendations. *Dyslexia, 7*, 150–170.

Merzenich, M. M., & deCharms, R. C. (1996). Neural representation, experience and change. In R. Llinas & P. Churchland (Eds.), *The mind-brain continuum*. Cambridge, MA: The MIT Press.

Merzenich, M. M., & Jenkins W. M. (1995) Cortical plasticity learning and learning dysfunction. In B. Julesz & I. Kovacs (Eds.), *Maturational windows and adult cortical plasticity: SFI Studies in the Sciences of Complexity* (Vol. 23). Boston: Addison-Wesley.

Merzenich, M. M., Recanzone, G. M., Jenkins, W. M., Allard, T., & Nudo, R. J. (1988). Cortical representational plasticity." In P. Rakic & W. Singer (Eds.), *Neurobiology of neocortex*. New York: Wiley.

Mesulam, M. (2000) Behavioral neuroanatomy: Large-scale networks, association cortex, frontal syndromes, the limbic system, and hemispheric specializations. In M. M. Mesulam (Ed.), *Principles of behavioral and cognitive neurology* (2nd ed., pp. 1–120). Oxford: Oxford University Press.

Mintun, M. A., Fox, P. T., & Raichle, M. W. (1989). A highly accurate method of localizing regions of neuronal activation in the human brain with positron emission tompography. *Journal of Cerebral Blood Flow and Metabolism. 9*, 96–103.

Mody, M., Studdert-Kennedy, M., & Brady, S. (1997). Speech perception deficits in poor readers: Auditory processing or phonological coding. *Journal of Experimental Child Psychology, 64*, 199–231.

Pokorni, J. L., Worthington, C. K., & Jamison, P. J. (2004) Phonological awareness intervention: Comparison of Fast ForWord, Earobics and LIPS. *Journal of Educational Research, 97*(3), 147–157.

Rosen, S., & Manganari, E. (2001). Is there a relationship between speech and nonspeech auditory processing in children with dyslexia? *Journal of Speech Language and Hearing Research, 44*, 720–736.

Snow, C. E., Burns, M. S., & Griffin, P. (1998) *Preventing reading difficulties in young children*. Washington, DC: National Academy Press.

Sterr, A., Muller M., Elbert, T., Rockstroh, B., & Taub, E. (1999). Development of cortical reorganization in the somatosensory cortex of adult Braille students. *Electroencepalography: Clinical Neurophysiology Supplement, 49*, 292–298.

Tallal, P., & Gaab, N. (2006). Dynamic auditory processing, musical experience and language development. *Trends in Neuroscience, 29*(7), 382–390.

Tallal, P. S., Miller, S., & Fitch, R. H. (1993). Neurobiological basis of speech: A case for the preeminence of temporal processing. *Annals of the New York Academy of Sciences, 682*, 27–47.

Tallal, P., & Piercy, M. (1973). Defects of nonverbal auditory perception in children with developmental aphasia. *Nature, 241,* 468–469.

Temple, E. (2002). Brain mechanisms in normal and dyslexic readers. *Current Opinions in Neurobiology, 12,* 178–183.

Temple, E. (2007) Changes in brain function in children with dyslexia after training. In J. Hirschbuhl & J. Kelley (Eds.), *Computers in education* (12th ed). Dubuque, IA: Contemporary Learning Series. (Copied with permission from *The Phonics Bulletin* [2003] IRA Phonics SIG.)

Temple, E., Deutsch, G. K., Poldrack, R. A., Miller, S. L., Tallal, P., Merzenich, et al. (2003). Neural deficits in children with dyslexia ameliorated by behavioral remediation: Evidence from functional MRI. *Proceedings of the National Academy of Sciences, 100*(5), 2860–2865.

Temple, E., Poldrack, R. A., Protopapas, A., Nagarajan, S., Salz, T., Tallal, P., et al. (2000). Disruption of the neural response to rapid acoustic stimuli in dyslexia: Evidence from functional MRI. *Proceedings of the National Academy of Sciences, 97*(25), 13907–13912.

Thomas, M., & Karmiloff-Smith, A. (2002). Are developmental disorders like cases of adult brain damage? Implications from connectionist modeling. *The Behavioral and Brain Sciences, 25,* 727–750.

Troia, G. A. (2004) Migrant students with limited English proficiency. Can Fast ForWord make a difference in their language skills and academic achievement? *Remedial and Special Education, 25*(6), 353–366.

Troia, G. A., & Whitney, S. D. (2003). A close look at the efficacy of Fast ForWord Language for children with academic weaknesses. *Contemporary Educational Psychology, 28,* 464–495.

20

The Use of Assistive Technology for Students with Auditory Processing Disorders

Thomas Rosati

Overview

There are a variety of "technology tools" that can be used with a person with (central) auditory processing disorder ([C]APD). The specific items can range from highly specialized equipment to simple things found in most households. There is first a need to understand how these tools can impact each individual client and then to appreciate that there is no universal quick-fix machine. However, there are terrific aids and items that can greatly enhance and improve the richness of the *educational* experience for a person with (C)APD.

This chapter addresses the following questions: (1) What is assistive technology? (2) How does one get assistive technology for a client? (3) How is assistive technology evaluated? and (4) What are good technology tools for helping a client with a (central) auditory processing disorder?

What Is Assistive Technology?

To begin discussing assistive technology, we need to define what it is, as well as what it is not. Under the Revised Individuals With Disabilities Educational Act (I.D.E.A)., the definition of Assistive Technology is *"any item, piece of equipment, or product system, whether acquired commercially off the shelf, modified, or customized, that is used to increase, maintain or improve functional capabilities of children with disabilities"* (29 U.S.C. Sec 2202[2]).

This definition is purposely made broad to encompass virtually anything. So how does that fit in when creating a profile for a student with (C)APD and how does *assistive technology* aid them within their classroom?

Included with the definition of assistive technology in the I.D.E.A. document are definitions of what assistive technology service is: *"any service that directly assists an individual with a disability in the selection, acquisition, or use of an assistive technology device"* (29 U.S.C. Sec 2202[2]).

Again, this is a broad all-encompassing definition by the Federal government. So, it's helpful to add some detail to this picture. First, the discussion can be limited by the typical population characteristics of (C)APD. Second, it is necessary to look at specific student needs. Third, where are the students using these tools, and fourth, what assistive technology would be appropriate for a particular student? This is the basic philosophy compiled by Joy Smiley Zabala, which is called the SETT Model, the Student, the Environment, the Task, and the Tools (http://sweb.uky.edu/~jszaba0/SETT2.html)

The SETT Model contains four areas that require consideration when evaluating the potential use of assistive technology. Note that the technology (tools) is the last point of consideration in the process of evaluating for assistive technology. Regarding the term "tool," one should recognize that low-tech is often just as practical a solution as most high-tech. The goal is that, whatever technology is used, it be considered an aid or a tool to accomplish a task. Specifics about the SETT model will appear later in the chapter in the evaluation section.

For the purposes of this chapter, the student or client is primarily school-aged and the setting is the classroom, or possibly the therapy or home environment. Generally, the task is related to improving comprehension and retention of information by the student. Most professionals, educators, and parents are not well versed in the field of assistive technology, yet every student with an Individualized Education Plan (IEP) can have assistive technology considered for use. If the reader is more sophisticated about technology, then he or she should skim to the latter portion of the chapter.

Assistive Technology Primer

What Is an Assistive Technology Service?

Further clarifications have been developed by federal legislation that is reported in the most recent version of I.D.E.A.

An assistive technology service is described as any service that directly impacts a child with a disability in the selection, acquisition, or use of an assistive technology device which can include:

1. Evaluation
2. Purchasing
3. Selecting
4. Coordinating and using other services
5. Training of the client
6. Training of the professionals

Each of these services is discussed in greater detail later in this chapter. However, this listing helps to demonstrate the specific areas that should be considered during an evaluation. This listing also highlights the need to have evaluations completed by a knowledgeable and trained clinician in Assistive Technology.

Laws

Although I.D.E.A. covers the assistive technology needs of school-age children, assistive technology also has specific special legislation which is commonly known as the Tech Act. The most recent revision contained in Public Law (PL) 108-364 provides coverage for people with all disabilities of all ages, in all environments.

Two other federal laws have an impact on assistive technology. They are commonly known as Section 504 and Section 508. Section 504 is part of the Americans with Disabilities Act (ADA), and impacts access and compensations that can allow people to interact and work as normally as able-bodied individuals whenever possible. This also has been applied in public school settings for students who may have a handicapping condition, but need assistance that is not primarily academic. Authorizing the use of an elevator for a person in a wheelchair because of an automobile accident would be a classic example of making accommodations under Section 504 for physical, not academic needs.

Section 508 deals with the Internet and having federal Web sites accessible for people using screen readers and other sensory impairment aids to access these sites. Although not always obliged to comply with this law, many state, local, and business Web sites are now constructed to meet these federal standards.

Laws and regulations are powerful, but are also open for *interpretation*. Much of the interpretation has been left to three entities: governmental agencies, insurance carriers, and the legal community.

Governmental Agencies

Agency Policy Statements, position papers, and mandates have shaped the types of assistive technology eligible for funding. These can range from members of the U.S. Department of Education, down to the local Pupil Personnel Director in a local school district's Committee on Special Education (CSE). Although every student's I.E.P. is supposed to have a consideration of possible assistive technology, there is wide fluctuation in interpretation and spirit, with a common conclusion resulting in the student's ineligibility for assistive technology. This results in a major disparity between the students who do and those who do not get services, based on the skills of advocates and district representatives.

Insurance Carriers

The arena of insurance carriers is an area where assistive technology equipment and service can vary greatly. If a clinician is working in a clinical setting offering evaluation, training, and therapy for (C)APD, billing for assistive technology should or can be accommodated in the typical office billing practices. If a clinician is working within a public school setting, decisions relating to caseload placement and qualifying for services for (C)APD are determined by the school district's criteria for inclusion. However, getting assistive technology products for a student may not be simple. Decisions regarding the use of the most appropriate hardware and software during the school day by a child with (C)APD should be determined by the results of the assistive technology evaluation. Should the results identify a need for an expensive piece of equipment and a school district is not willing to approve its funding for educational use, there are private and governmental funding sources that may still allow the student to have access to a specialized technology tool.

For the client with benefit of good medical coverage, private insurance is typically the first source to look for funding. Insurance carriers typically require that service providers state a medical necessity in order for funding to take place. However, for (C)APD, it can be difficult to prove a medical necessity or identify a specific piece of equipment that will "correct" the identified auditory processing problem. These are examples of the litmus tests that most insurance carriers will pose before funding assistive technology. In many cases, a physician prescription stating that a person has a particular medical need is enough for an assistive technology item to be approved for funding. There is also a precedent that a comprehensive auditory processing evaluation report by a speech-language pathologist may be sufficient to acquire the desired assistive technology equipment. Clinicians with skills and expertise in assistive technology typically can justify the need for special equipment when the purpose is not obvious to the provider (insurance carrier).

It is typically more difficult to gain approval or clarity regarding coverage for assistive technology equipment through Medicaid and Medicare. Most assistive technology is not a covered benefit unless it meets the criteria for a Durable Medical Expense. This usually means that the item can have little practical purpose outside its original intent and most likely is not useful to anyone but the client for whom funding was approved.

There is a national network of Assistive Technology centers within the United States. Professionals with an interest in assistive technology equipment may find these centers to be a source for equipment rentals or lending. Assistive technology equipment manufacturers often have a preview policy which, for a nominal fee, allows a client to use a specific piece of equipment for a short period of time to determine if the equipment is appropriate for his or her use. Professionals are urged to look for computer software demos or 30-day trials that often can be downloaded from the Internet to determine if a product is right for a client.

Legal Issues

The third area that can impact assistive technology utilization can be a penchant for bureaucratic or due process proceedings to mire the process. Although the laws and regulations have a solid base of information and precedent, a client can often be made to feel as if he or she does not have an opportunity. Legally, items are not supposed to be denied because of cost or whim, but it has become standard practice in many districts and agencies to deny the request and challenge the client to go through an appeal process in order to get the desired assistive technology equipment or services. This is primarily due to the fact that the legislation is so new that there have been few court challenges directly involving assistive technology equipment and services. Those that have taken place at the state and occasional federal level have offered mixed results and little definitive light on what can and cannot be done. As a result, being informed and being legally correct may not always get the items one may want. There have been instances of public school districts or agencies spending $100,000 in court and legal fees to avoid spending $2,000 on a piece of assistive technology equipment. The rationale is to try to not set a precedent that would open up the floodgates for everyone to want a piece of assistive technology equipment. In reality, it is often from ignorance of assistive technology benefits, and failure to realize that a change made for the entire system, rather than for an individual, would reap a much larger benefit for all. This is why the initial evaluation, and the manner in which it is conducted, can be critical for getting the proper equipment and training.

How Do You Get Assistive Technology for a Client?

Assistive Technology decisions are strongly influenced by how to pay for it. Technology itself can be quite an expense, but assistive technology can run four to five times as much for products with a switch interface installed, or other minor alterations. Fortunately, there are times when a savvy buyer, or a person with enough vision or mechanical know-how to make some minor modifications, can find products at affordable prices. It also opens up the concept of "horse trading" at a local level if possible. Trading an additional group session for a client, or getting something that could help a classroom of students instead of just one, can more often cover the cost of adapted equipment and software.

For assistive technology it is suggested that the clinician attempt to convince the decision-making committee to agree that a student would benefit because of a particular need or type of remediation suggested rather than by pitching for the acquisition of a particular software title. General terms like "graphic organizers" and "voice input" are more "user friendly" than saying that the student needs Inspiration and ViaVoice on a G5 Mac. One should go in to negotiating situations knowing the specific names/titles of suggested software for which one would like approval. It is further suggested that one not give the impression that they are "married" to a specific product.

Many CSEs want to know if a low-tech method is sufficient to do a task instead of jumping right to a high-tech solution. Before a recommendation to use a keyboard-based system is considered, it is necessary to determine if a student's handwriting abilities are sufficient to convey their thoughts in most writing tasks. A major reason assistive technology is sometimes rejected is that there is no demonstration that a low-tech solution has been first attempted and determined to be insufficient. There are also perceptions and practical considerations regarding assistive technology. For example, there is an expectation that unless a student is having a significant problem with his or her writing skill ability, that using a pen or pencil is the most desirable way for most students to put information "to paper."

Assistive technology does not all have to be high-tech. There are many items that can be purchased at a Radio Shack or found at a local Salvation Army store that one might consider, at least as a way to test if a more expensive commercial product will work with a particular student. If used items are selected, be prepared to open, fix, and clean these bargains if necessary.

It is important to know how the funding for the technology was provided to the client. Furthermore, it is important to know how a clinician, therapist, or evaluator is compensated for providing an assistive technology service. With many sophisticated products being priced at over $3,000, who is responsible to fund an item quickly becomes an important decision. At this juncture, there needs to be some distinction made between assistive technology, educational technology, and rehabilitation technology.

Assistive technology refers to any item that can be used to aid an individual. Differences happen when the focus is placed on how to utilize the assistive technology. This is usually categorized into one of these areas: home, work, or school. In order to use funding of any type beyond out-of-pocket funding, these questions must be answered. Quite often, where and how the technology is utilized determine where to go and even what to write in an evaluation in order to obtain the necessary funding. Because of this, knowing who is responsible for paying for an item, funding costs associated with preparation of a written report or repair or modification work performed, becomes a critical factor. For our purposes, the difference between *educational technology* and *rehabilitation technology* is being made primarily for this funding difference. *Rehabilitation technology* is a technology that is primarily therapeutic and utilized in a clinical or nonschool setting in most cases. Rehabilitative services allow a client to work on the skills that are missing. *Educational technology,* on the other hand, is designed to aid an individual's educational development within curricular-based learning environments. Educational technology supports the classroom. This is a broad category that encompasses use of the computer and multimedia into the educational process. The use of assistive technology is supposed to be considered for every I.E.P. based student. It does not have to be designed for special needs populations, but can be very appropriate for a special needs student. The I.E.P. should reflect *adaptation* or *modification* of existing classroom technology.

Of greater importance is modification of the teaching process and classroom practices to take advantage of educational technology. Teachers may have some coursework in educational technology, but rarely take courses in teaching in an inclusion classroom, or learn how to implement Universal Design practices into their teaching. Trends in education are making classrooms more inclusive, but training in how to make, modify, and utilize assistive and regular educational technologies are optional, if available at all, for new teachers.

A profound way to offer this type of training is to create experience for teachers to be exposed to how instruction needs to be modified by experiencing the classroom dynamics as a student and as a teacher. My graduate students are offered an opportunity to have simulated handicapping conditions based on real student profiles. In class they assume the role of a student in an inclusion classroom, another week they are a caregiver or support "push in" teacher for a classmate, and a third week they assume the role of the teacher and must modify their presentations to best enable their multidisabled "students" into their educational practices. They quickly learn the value of making modifications for special needs students and learn to recognize the body language, and nonverbal cues that are typical of students having impairments like (C)APD when they are having difficulty listening and learning in a traditional lecture based learning experience.

Assistive technology can straddle these two genres and requires expertise in understanding products that may not be common in general educational or rehabilitative settings. This is why the person(s) responsible for evaluating and making decisions pertaining to assistive technology must be proficient in understanding all aspects, know how to utilize the best practices, and know what is currently available.

How Do You Evaluate a Client with CAPD for Assistive Technology?

The process of assistive technology evaluation assessment can be overwhelming given the range of testing instruments that can be utilized during an assistive technology evaluation. There is no specific tool or instrument that has been standardized for the evaluation of assistive technology. There is an excellent assessment checklist that has been developed for school-age children by the Wisconsin Assistive Technology Initiative (http://www.wati.org).

This organization has been in the forefront of assistive technology and their work serves as the basis of many educational assistive technology assessments. Optimally, the evaluation for assistive technology should be performed by an individual with extensive training in assistive technology, and if the results are to be used for determining educational uses, the evaluator should also be versed in curriculum and methods of integrating technology seamlessly into educational settings.

Augmentative and Alternative Communication

There is often confusion about the difference between Augmentative and Alternative Communication (AAC) and assistive technology (AT). The terms are not interchangeable. AAC is a subset of AT. Augmentative and alternative communication refers to a device that is primarily used to be substituted for the "voice" of an individual who is not capable of utilizing appropriate linguistic strategies. For example, if the client can adequately ambulate independently throughout the day then he does not need to have a wheelchair for mobility. Similarly a person, who can carry on a conversation and speak in sentences, will have little need for a device that speaks for him. Historically, Lyle Lloyd (1985), offered a description of AAC:

> *Augmentative is defined as a process of augmenting existing speech abilities.*
>
> *Alternative is the process of providing a substitute for speech.*
>
> *The utilization of professional services which is that the professional is not merely augmenting or providing alternatives to individual speech, but instead working to improve an individual's communication* (Zangari et al., 1994).

AAC falls under all of the requirements of I.D.E.A. in the updated regulations and is often tailored to meet the requirement as a durable medical expense. Therefore, the discussion in this chapter refers to assistive technology rather than augmentative and alternative communication. For the reader who is interested to learn more about augmentative and alternate communication, the following excellent texts are recommended:

1. *Handbook of Augmentative and Alternative Communication*, by Sharon L. Glennen and Denise C. DeCoste (1997);
2. *Augmentative and Alternative Communication: The Management of Severe Communication Disorders in Children and Adults*, by David R. Beukelman and Pat Mirenda (1998);
3. *Assistive Technologies: Principles and Practice* by Albert M. Cook and Susan Hussey (2002).

For individuals or organizations who may be seriously considering implementing assistive technology assessment, it is highly recommended that they read *Fundamentals in Assistive Technology Guide* (Herman, 2000), created for Rehabilitation Engineering and Assistive Technology Society of North America (RESNA). This guide discusses assessment team formation, qualifications for professionals performing the assessment as well as the assessment process in much greater detail. The assessment process detailed by Janice Hunt Herman in this guide is particularly appropriate for gaining a greater understanding of assistive technology.

Who Provides the Evaluation?

Before individuals or group organizations make decisions about how to evaluate for assistive technology, it is necessary that decisions concerning who will conduct the evaluation be made. Currently, anybody who wishes to do so can. There are no federal guidelines for qualifications for assistive technology assessment, but there are professional standards. Legally, there have been few challenges to assistive technology in general and these challenges are virtually nonexistent relating to qualifications of individuals performing assistive technology evaluations. In most settings, it is valuable to create a collaborative team of professionals who are able to evaluate the overall performance and capabilities of the student and match specific technology to the student's capabilities.

There is a national and international organization that has examined the field of assistive technology and established best practices, standards, and certifications appropriate for assistive technology assessment. National certification as an Assistive Technology Practitioner is currently issued from Rehabilitation Engineering and Assistive Technology Society of North America (RESNA), the only source for certification to date. RESNA offers rigorous qualification exams and provides technical assistance through their National Assistive Technology Technical Assistance Partnership (NATTAP). RESNA also provides and maintains a comprehensive listing of universities that offer assistive technology programs.

AT Evaluation

Assistive Technology evaluation has typically involved three professionals within a setting. These professionals include the school technology coordinator, the speech-language pathologist, and the occupational therapist. All of these specialized fields have had very little teaching on the subject of assistive technology in their formal university training or clinical practicum.

For a (C)APD auditory processing evaluation, the other licensed and certified professional typically involved in the evaluation process is an audiologist with specific training in auditory processing disorders. The evaluation and use of assistive technology with auditory processing disorders includes a speech-language pathologist and audiologist who may or may not be experienced with assistive technology. Conversely, a district technology coordinator or administrator may understand technology well, but may not understand the use of assistive technology for auditory processing. So, reaching a meeting of the minds is a critical step in the assessment process.

Optimally, the assessment team should comprise a group of professionals directly involved with the student in an educational setting. Team members would be encouraged to shed the particular "hat" they wear when they enter the room and discuss the whole student and not just how they view the student filtered through their specific area of expertise. This type of approach can provide an open forum where all stakeholders can share their knowledge and expertise as well as brainstorm ideas.

Although we would all like to see this evaluation process implement best practices, fiscal and human resource restrictions may make this nearly impossible. The difficulty with an assistive technology evaluation is that it tends to be a generalist practice performed in specialized areas (e.g., audiology, speech-language pathology, etc.) thus the need for a team approach to assess AT. When team assessments are practiced within an organization, the team has to think in a transdisciplinary manner. Doing so requires cross-training.

Additional Training

There are company-based trainings that are offered by many manufacturers of assistive technology equipment.

For independent training in assistive technology as a field of study, many companies offer conferences for training seminars such as: "Closing the Gap Conference" held each fall in Minnesota and the California State University, Northridge Conference held each spring and providing the latest news in assistive technology.

What Should Be Included in an Assistive Technology Evaluation?

Local assessment teams or Assistive Technology Providers (ATP) can find guidance for the evaluation process from a well-coordinated statewide project in the state of Wisconsin, known as the Wisconsin Assistive Technology Initiative (WATI), (http://www.wati.com). They have developed exceptional checklists and materials as part of an assistive technology assessment. WATI also offers assessment forms and position papers helpful to teachers, administrators, and parents.

The Wisconsin Assistive Technology Checklist assesses the "whole" student in both their school and home environments. Although some of the areas being assessed are less relevant for the (C)APD student, all areas should be assessed as a part of the overall profile of a client. The Wisconsin Checklist includes the following:

1. Computer access
2. Motor aspects of writing
3. Composing written material
4. Communication
5. Reading
6. Learning/studying
7. Math
8. Recreation and leisure
9. Activities of daily living
10. Mobility
11. Positioning and seating
12. Vision
13. Hearing

The Wisconsin Checklist provides practical and functional information relative to daily activities performed and accomplished by the individual in his or her natural environment. With the information gathered, the evaluator should be able to prepare a "whole" student review. This review should be compiled as a report that builds a case about what exists, what has been tried, and what should be considered. It is recommended that this analysis be conducted first.

The questions listed in Table 20–1 should be asked in gathering information.

Using the Information from an Evaluation

When an assistive technology evaluation has been performed and completed, it is necessary to focus on target needs of that particular student. Any evaluation should also assess the student's specific profile for strengths and weaknesses, as (C)APD is often not a "pure" disorder. Although there are typical problem areas with auditory processing, decisions and recommendations should address the specific individual needs of the student. Once (C)APD has been determined, then the evaluation summary report should build a convincing case that there is an educational need. It is necessary to demonstrate

Table 20–1. Analysis of AT Needs

What are the special needs, educational needs, and communication needs of the student?
• What are the student's current abilities?
• What materials and equipment are currently available that have been tried, including low-tech or training devices, and how well did they meet a client's needs?
• What is the physical structure of the instructional environment?
• How could activities be modified to accommodate the student's needs?
• What options could be considered (no-tech, low-tech, or high-tech) to develop a system for the student with (C)APD?
• Does the student have the motor ability and muscle tone necessary to use AT?
• What strategies can be used to increase the student's level of performance and interaction with the assistive technology?
• What support is available in the school and at home for acceptance and usage of any equipment?
• Is all the assistive technology being considered socially, personally, and developmentally, appropriate for the student?
• What are the student's learning styles?

(C)APD as an area of difficulty that is significantly impaired to the extent to which the student needs compensatory skill development.

A thorough Assistive Technology assessment typically includes more information than might be needed and should examine and consider all other areas such as environmental control units, computer access, AAC, aids to daily living (sometimes known as ADL), or electronic aids to daily living (EADL). At the same time, the need for different modifications for home, school, or work environments, as well as the effects on positioning, vision, and hearing skills should be determined.

When a more rehabilitative solution has been determined, there needs to be a solid justification to gain approval from a school district being asked to fund the hardware and software. To do this, it is necessary to answer the following list of questions:

What Are Good Technology Tools for Helping a Client with (C)APD?

The evaluation should allow the evaluator to confidently answer the following questions:

- Is there an AT item that can benefit the student in his or her particular setting?

- Is the AT item primarily for skill development or compensation?
- Is it expected that the AT item will be funded by an agency or school district, or will it be purchased by the individual?

Using the **SETT Model** these pointed questions can be addressed:

The STUDENT
- What does the student need to do?
- What are the student's special needs?
- What are the student's current abilities?

The ENVIRONMENT
- What materials and equipment are currently available in the environment?
- What is the physical arrangement? Are there special concerns?
- What is the instructional arrangement? Are there likely to be changes?
- What supports are available to the student?
- What resources are available to the people supporting the student?

The TASKS
- What naturally occurring activities take place in the environment?
- What is everyone else doing?
- What activities support the student's curricular goals?
- What are the critical elements of the activities?
- How might the activities be modified to accommodate the student's special needs?
- How might technology support the student's active participation in those activities?

The TOOLS
- Which no-tech, low-tech, and high-tech options should be considered when developing a system for a student with these needs and abilities doing these tasks in these environments?
- What strategies might be used to invite increased student performance?
- How might these tools be tried out with the student in the customary environments in which they will be used?

Procedures for conducting short trials with potential software and hardware products can be arranged at this stage. This may also be the point when specific plans of action regarding paperwork processing should be done to ensure proper funding. Reporting and carryover activities and specific goals and objectives could also be established at this juncture.

Hardware, Software, and Fitting for (C)APD

For the student with (C)APD there are two primary considerations for hardware use. The first consideration is a method designed to improve the use of auditory channels with poor signal to noise ratios. The second consideration would be the use of computer-driven software programs for auditory comprehension, temporal skill development, and auditory discrimination tasks.

Assisted Listening

For the average student the noise of a typical elementary classroom can be a true cacophony of sound. Such sound is distractible to a typical child. However, this same type of sound can totally eliminate the ability to process auditory information in a meaningful way for the child with (C)APD. For years, public schools have determined that they can improve their students' phonic and auditory comprehension skills with the addition of an FM system in the classroom. This improved listening accuracy has been deemed helpful to all students. However, the use of FM systems can still leave the student with (C)APD distracted by all of the other noise and activity in a classroom. In addition, if the child has preferential seating in the front of the class with a speaker attached to the rear wall, he will get little if anything out of a system. A better solution would be a personal FM-capable system. Personal systems may be used by others with a wireless headset enhanced to the additional 10 to 15 dB recommended for the (C)APD student.

See Chapter 11 for a discussion of assistive listening devices.

Computer Hardware

Today it is more of a preference than a need to be on one operating system. Unix, Windows, and Macs can all communicate with each other over the Internet and, in many cases, with each other directly. The choices concerning hardware are more about whether a classroom system is sufficient to meet IEP goals and objectives, or not. Selecting classroom technology is not as simple as acquiring many computers and dropping them into a classroom. A computer without a printer located in the back of the classroom and facing away from the teacher should not be considered as computer access if that is a key element to the assistive technology intervention. The changes in the classroom to accommodate assistive technology do not have to be significant if what is currently in place can be incorporated into the intervention plan. Modern computers have entire accessibility suites of built-in adaptability from print magnifiers to having vocal feedback for certain tasks. Voice input may even be incorporated into the version of Microsoft office on the school server. Microsoft VISTA operating system has voice recognition built into the operating system

Knowledge of what exists in a specific setting, instead of just knowing if Macs or Windows computers are used, can be very valuable for making final recommendations. Assistive technology does not have to be new equipment or stand-alone equipment. It does, however, need to be appropriate for a specific student. For some students, what the assistive technology provider has implemented may seem like magic. The real magic, however, is to weave the changes seamlessly into the existing location.

If the placement or flexibility of a classroom or networked system is not sufficient to meet a student's assistive technology needs then a laptop offers flexibility and portability between classes or from home to school. Knowing the student's assistive technology profile may direct the evaluator toward examining specialized laptops. If there is a concern concerning breakage problems, putting the laptop in a Toughbook-style casing or getting an extended warranty that includes damage protection is a good solution. If there are dual platform needs between home and school then consider Apple's new Powerbook duo which allows the user to work in Mac or Windows format, requiring a simple reboot to make the necessary switch.

Two other portable systems can also be considered. There are many benefits offered by using a convertible tablet PC computer, which is both a laptop and a writing tablet. There are also keyboard-based stand-alone systems like the Neo or Alphasmart, (http://www.alphasmart.com/neo), which are self-contained, light to carry, and less expensive. The drawback of these stand-alone systems are small monitors that are difficult to read and the inability to load any additional software program beyond those that have been included in their preselected inventory.

Computer Software

There is not a wealth of good computer software that has been specifically developed for the education market and less for the special education market. This gap in software development has been reduced to a trickle primarily because of the "drying up" of software development due to the advent of the Internet and its popularity. Very few companies are now willing to undergo the cost and expense of creating multiple platforms and updating software so that it fits into the operating systems of various computers. It appears that these software companies have opted primarily to work through the Internet and create software packages that work from a distance and in a much more generic manner. What does this mean for the person looking to use assistive technology? It means that the skill development desired for use may have to be more generic. There are also products that are appropriate for working on targeted concepts and skills but may not have been originally developed and marketed for that purpose. When looking for appropriate software for the (C)APD client, it may be necessary to be creative in selection.

One note about buying software: assistive technology providers can find closeout and bargain rack software that are terrific. Be aware that one might be taking a chance with some software if it was only designed for working in the Windows 95 environment. It may not run on later computer systems. The same notion applies to hybrid CDs that were designed to run on Macs and Windows machines. This bargain software may not run on either if one is working on a computer purchased in the last 3 years. Some Mac systems actually have the ability to run as if they were using an earlier operating system. For Windows systems, there is a back-door way to "trick" the system. Find the .exe file by exploring the folder that contains the program. One can right click and should find a choice for properties. Clicking here should give one a choice of compatibility. Now you can tell the system to treat the program as if it were a Windows 95 system. It will not work for all programs, but one just might find a great program on the closeout rack that is worth the gamble. A collection of these discount rack gems is listed in the software section.

Tools, Transparency, and Time

Tools should always be considered as tools. In the same way that a pen and paper may aid a person in taking notes, writing, or drawing, the technology needs to have a similar acceptance and fluidity to make it not seem intrusive and more trouble than it is worth. For a therapy situation the primary goal should be getting the student comfortable with the chosen technologies.

Transparency is the utilization of a technology so that it becomes secondary and the training and the "how to use a product" become less and less apparent to a person observing. For example, a student who can touch-type is not concentrating on the act of typing. They are listening and transcribing material directly into text without having to look at it. That is an optimal situation and the level of transparency of that product can be described as very good. However, when this is not happening, the person is thinking about the process of writing. This can be a serious problem for a student with (C)APD.

What is an appropriate level of typing speed for a person to have typing considered a transparent skill? It would be at the point at which an individual can put down his thoughts in a way not constricted by the technology he is using. So, a student on the elementary level should probably be able to type about 5 to10 words a minute without a significant need to look at keys or not think about how to write any more than if he or she were using a pencil to perform a similar task. A high school student or an adult should probably be at about 15 to 20 words per minute with that same level of comfort noted. There are a variety of "teaching typing" software programs available for commercial use. This is an area that will benefit a student in many areas including the amount of time spent on test-taking mechanics. A series of common typing programs and commentary about each are presented later in this chapter.

The Time Element

There are a few features that contribute to time and its effect with regard to assistive technology. Initially one must consider the amount of time that will be needed just to learn how to use the technology itself. If a student has many support people (e.g., resource specialist, speech therapy, occupational therapy, or physical therapy) there leaves very little room for adding assistive technology into his or her schedule. What was initially intended to provide support may, in fact, create more problems because of the time factor.

Components of a System Designed for Aiding a (C)APD student

What areas are typically deficit for a student with (C)APD?

- They have sound localization and lateralization difficulty

- They have trouble with auditory discrimination and pattern recognition
- They have inconsistent temporal comprehension including temporal resolution, temporal integration, and temporal ordering
- Their ability to understand auditory information is compromised with competing or degrading acoustic signals.

One for All and . . .

Anthropologists bemoan the vast learning that had been lost through the centuries before there was the written word. A reliance on the oral tradition to teach should have waned once Gutenberg bound his first book. Yet, it continues to flourish in today's modern classrooms. Creating environments where instruction can be enhanced for every student has a far greater impact on student learning. These are changes that would allow many students to benefit, especially the student with (C)APD.

A far greater benefit than any assistive technology program will be garnered by systemic changes to the training and presentation styles of the teaching staff. Persuading teachers to depart from lecture-based instruction with limited use of visual aids and transition to instruction that uses multimodality and learning style modifications would be a huge benefit for students with (C)APD.

Assistive technology can help through greater use of multimedia, and enhanced classroom design. A teacher working in a facility that incorporates a computer projection system, a SMARTBoard, and a classroom FM system could potentially improve the learning and test scores for every student in his or her class if he or she actively uses these systems in his or her teaching style. Creating an individual learning styles profile and developing cooperative learning activities through Web quests and portfolio assessment can impact on the quality of comprehension found in a student's educational program. All of these modifications fall under the conceptual framework of Universal design most notably championed by the Center for Applied Special Technology (http://www.cast.org). The changes listed above would cost an average classroom approximately $4,000 in equipment but will have a great benefit to overall student learning. Most classrooms have at least one computer, yet the majority of these computers are used far more for student record keeping than as an educational tool.

A technology tool that is perceived to be great and wonderful may be very inappropriate for a particular situation. An example of this would be the use of voice input for word processing, which is wonderful in a quiet home environment, but impossible to use in a noisy classroom. Determining both the technology and where and how it is going to be used has to be part of the process of accepting and utilizing appropriate assistive technology.

In a school setting, there are two critical factors affecting assistive technology decisions. The first factor has to do with the student and his or her ability to accept and use a device for technology intervention and the second has to do with the school and the teachers involved and how willing and able they are to accept and use the technology.

If an evaluator has taken the time to methodically profile a student to this point in the process and can answer the questions that have been posed then he or she should have a satisfactory understanding relative to the student's skill deficits and his or her assistive technology needs. Having gained this critical information, the evaluator has arrived at the point where hardware and software can be considered for use.

The following lists commercial products that are appropriate to review for the (C)APD target population whose needs include language, reading, processing speed, comprehension, writing, and organization. The product areas are grouped using a cognitive skill categorization system developed by the Adaptive Technology Center for New Jersey Colleges. The groupings are followed by a list of additional titles that should be available in any classroom, as well as others that are simply great bargain finds.

Reading Solutions

Scan/Read Systems. Scan/read systems combine software and a flatbed scanner to read aloud any printed text. Textbook pages, class handouts, and tests can be scanned in and then read aloud by a computer. A clear visual display highlights the text as it is being read. A built-in talking dictionary, a study skills tool bar, and a writing tool bar are additional helpful features.

Kurzweil 3000
http://www.kurzweiledu.com

WYNN
http://www.freedomscientific.com/LSG/products/wynn.asp

SOLO
http://www.donjohnston.com

Graphic Organizers. These programs are used in the prewriting stage to help students organize their thoughts. With the click of the mouse, a concept map can be turned into a text outline.

Inspiration Kidspiration
http://www.inspiration.com

Draft:Builder
http://www.donjohnston.com

Software Playback Systems. Software playback systems are the latest addition to the digital books software product line. These are full-featured software packages designed to play AudioPlus CD books on a desktop or laptop computer. They are specially designed with the blind and visually impaired community in mind and have a well-designed user interface for individuals with learning disabilities. Appropriate for classroom reading labs or for home use, the software playback systems are geared toward students at the middle level and up.

eClipseReader
http://www.eclipsereader.com

Victor Reader Soft
http://www.visuaide.com

Digital Book Readers. Digital book readers are portable CD players that read DAISY-compatible audiobooks. They provide CD navigation functions and playback features. These portable players are recommended for students and adults in grades 7 and up as an easy way to transport their players between school, work, and home.

Telex Scholar
http://www.telex.com

Victor Vibe
http://www.visuaide.com

Electronic Text Readers. Electronic text readers also read aloud and highlight text, but they can read only text that is already in an electronic format; for example, Internet sites or word processing files. E-readers do not contain the optical character recognition software that is needed to scan in printed text, but they are low-cost solutions for reading aloud text.

eReader
http://www.cast.org

PDF Aloud
http://www.texthelp.com

Premier Assistive Technology Suite of Products
http://www.premier-programming.com

TextAloud
http://www.nextup.com

ReadPlease
http://www.readplease.com

Reading Bar 2 for Internet Explorer
http://www.readplease.com

WordQ
http://www.wordq.com

Natural Reader
http://www.naturalreaders.com

Writing Solutions

Talking Word Processing. Word processing programs with text-to-speech features read text aloud as students type. This helps students edit and proofread their written work.

Read & Write
http://www.texthelp.com

Write:OutLoud
http://www.donjohnston.com

WordQ
http://www.wordq.com

SOLO
http://www.donjohnston.com

Microsoft OneNote
http://www.office.microsoft.com

Portable Note-takers. These sturdy, lightweight keyboards are a more affordable option than a laptop computer for taking notes in class. They interface with a student's computer and printer, so files can be transferred and/or printed easily.

AlphaSmart 3000
http://www.alphasmart.com

Dana

Neo

Word Prediction. Word prediction software helps students who have significant spelling and/or word finding problems. As a student starts to type a word, the software presents a list of predicted words from which the student can choose. Clicking on the word adds it to the sentence, and typing final punctuation transfers the sentence into an open word processing document. Topic dictionaries can be set up with specialized vocabulary for specific course work.

Co:Writer
http://www.donjohnston.com

Read & Write
http://www.texthelp.com

WordQ
http://www.wordq.com

SOLO
http://www.donjohnston.com

Speech Recognition. Students dictate into a microphone and their words appear on the computer screen. Speech recognition software requires very powerful computers with a lot of memory, adequate time to train both the computer and the user, and users who are very comfortable with computers. SpeakQ is a new product that has an easier interface with a shorter training time.

Dragon Naturally Speaking Professional
http://www.dragonsystems.com

ViaVoice
http://www.nuance.com/viavoice/

QPointer
http://www.commodio.com

SpeakQ
http://www.wordq.com

Test Taking. These programs provide students with electronic versions of tests. Questions and answers can be highlighted and read aloud for students who struggle with reading; answers can be typed on the computer for students who have difficulty with handwriting. The completed test is then printed out for submission.

Test Talker
http://www.freedomscientific.com

Kurzweil 3000
http://www.kurzweiledu.com

Audio Books. Many titles are now being released on tape. Textbook manufacturers are also required to make their books available in alternative formats. Large libraries of titles are also available from these sources.

National Library Service for the Blind and Physically Handicapped
http://www.lcweb.loc.gov/nls/

Recording for the Blind and Dyslexic
http://www.rfbd.org

Great Things for Any Classroom

Smartboards Classroom whiteboards that hook directly into the computer. Mimio can be used on any wall or chart the same way.	http://www.eduscapes.com/sessions/smartboard http://www.mimio.com
Classroom Amplification	http://www.phonak.com/professional/productsp/fm.htm
Boardmaker **Picture This** Graphic programs with libraries of associated programs for creating classroom graphics like P.E.C.S. symbols, listening lotto cards, and A.A.C boards	http://www.mayer-johnson.com http://www.autismshop.com

RosettaStone Designed for language instruction, this extensive series comes in many languages and uses structured real world language identification, speaking and writing with strong listening and memory skills development activities	http://www.rosettastone.com
Fast ForWord An intensive language and reading development series with listening and phonic awareness skill development	http://www.scilearn.com/
Earobics A popular series of arcadelike programs for developing listening and phonic listening acuity	http://www.superduperinc.com

Great Software Gathering Dust, or on a Discount Rack

These titles might not be easy to find or might not be designated to run on Windows 95 or earlier Macs. Sometimes you can find similar titles that will do similar things like the typing tutors. They may be designed for populations other than CAPD but can be useful.

Timon and Pumbaa Teach Typing	One of many Disney Software titles that mimic many of the skill-based drill and practice that clients may need. They work in game formats or are palatable to be used by a person who may need earlier skill development but may be older and not ready for Mavis Bacon Teaching Typing.
Beginning Sounds with the Muppets	Brighter Child created many titles with recognizable characters that are fun and have listening and easy interaction. Creative Wonders and Sesame Street Software have similar titles.

Arthur's Computer Adventure	Living Books has great children's literature programs where almost everything on the screen does something (and not always the same thing) when you click on it. Most are also available with additional languages that can be used with a setting change.
Arthur's Thinking Games	The Learning Company has produced numerous titles that are educational in nature but do not necessarily fit a grade level or particular skill area.
Jump Start Spelling	Knowledge Adventure has a large consumer-friendly series of titles that are still available at numerous locations with most of their software able to run on newer machines.
My First Amazing Dictionary	Written to accompany the book series are numerous Dorling Kindersley titles in their DK Interactive Learning Series.
Tonka PowerTools	A series that does not work easily on systems beyond Windows 2000 because it has special interfaces or keyboard overlays. Easy to use, multistep following directions in real-world simulations.

Summary

A large variety of assistive technology products can aid the student with (C)APD. "Techies," however, tend not to be well versed in assistive technology issues. Teachers and clinicians, without experience and training, often give little consideration to practices that take advantage of technology for special populations. C.S.E.s need to be aware of the range of assistive technology that is available and be willing to knowledgeably make decisions that have the potential to transparently help many students.

This knowledge should be derived from the results of the assistive technology evaluations performed by certified assistive technology professionals and transdisciplinary teams that are skilled in assistive technology integration as well as the dynamics of classroom instruction. There are evaluation tools that can offer systematic approaches for enhancing the "teachable moments" during a student's day in the classroom.

Planning and coordination with regular and special education decision-makers that examine and consider individual student learning styles, yet encourage multimedia instruction through universal design trends are needed in educational settings. Training and awareness of these components by all stakeholders will make systemic changes that are practical and economic for all students.

Key Points Learned

- Assistive Technology is a field of study that combines aspects of many other fields and has its own terminology and specialized training.
- Funding is a major consideration for getting some assistive technology. Determination of the type of equipment and the purpose for its need can impact the type of funding source available.
- The SETT Model for evaluating assistive technology provides information cross-modality. A qualified professional or collaborative cross-discipline assessment team is needed to evaluate assistive technology needs and generate solutions.
- Numerous commercial products are appropriate for aiding students with (C)APD. The use of products will vary depending upon the situation in which they will be utilized and should be selected based on individual needs. Low-cost assistive technology alternatives are available to evaluate a product's appropriateness and success.
- Commercial software programs not developed specifically for students with (C)APD, may be effective in improving auditory processing skills.

References

Adaptive Technology Center of New Jersey. *Assistive technology fact sheets.* Retrieved October 1, 2006 from http://www.adaptivetech.tcnj.edu/resources.html

Beukelman, D., & Mirenda, P. (1998). *Augmentative and alternative communication: Management of severe communication disorders in children and adults.* Baltimore: Paul H. Brookes.

C.A.S.T. Center for Applied Special Technology. *Universal Design for Learning.* Retrieved Oct. 1, 2006 from http://www.cast.org

Cook, A. M., & Hussey, S. (2002). *Assistive technologies: Principles and practice* (2nd ed.). St.Louis, MO: Mosby.

Glennen, S. L., & DeCoste, D. (1997). *Handbook of augmentative and alternative communication.* San Diego, CA: Singular Publishing Group.

Herman, J. H. (2000). Assistive technology. *Fundamentals in assistive technology guide* (3rd ed.). Arlington, VA: RESNA Publications

Lloyd, L. (1985). *Augmentative and Alternative Technologies, 1*(3).

Reed, P., & Lahm, E. A. (Eds.). (2004). Assessing students' needs for assistive technology: A resource manual for school district teams. Madison: Wisconsin Assistive Technology Initiative.

United States Department of Education. (2006). *I.D.E.A. definitions*. Retrieved October 1, 2006 from http://idea.ed.gov/explore/view/p/,root,statute,I,A,602

United States Department of Education. (2006) *I.D.E.A. regulations* Retrieved October 1, 2006 from http://www.ed.gov

Wisconsin Assistive Technology Initiative. *Assistive technology considerations*. Retrieved October 1, 2006 from http://www.wati.org/news/whatsnew.html

Zabala, J. (2006). *Update of the S.E.T.T. framework*. Retrieved October 1, 2006 from http://briefcase.yahoo.com/joyzabala@sbcglobal.net

Zabala, J. (2006). *The SETT framework revisited.* http://sweb.uky.edu/~jszaba0/SETT2.html

Zangari, C., Lloyd, L., & Vicker, B. (1994). Augmentative and alternative communication: An historic perspective. *Augmentative and Alternative Communication,* 10(1), 27–59. Retrieved October 1, 2006 from http://www.acsu.buffalo.edu/~duchan/new_history/overview.html

Internet Resources

Closing the Gap: http://www.closingthegap.com

U.S. Department of Education-IDEA: http://www.ed.gov

S.E.T.T. Model: http://www.joyzabala.com

Wisconsin Assistive Technology Initiative: http://www.wati.org/news/whatsnew.html

Universal Design: http://www.cast.org

Adaptive Technology Center of New Jersey: http://adaptivetech.tcnj.edu

Rehabilitation Engineer and Assistive Technology Society of North America: http://www.resna.org

21

Use of Medication with Auditory Processing Disorders

Kim L. Tillery

Overview

The professional concern over medication use and APD has continued, resulting in four published conflicting studies regarding the effectiveness of central nervous system (CNS) medication on auditory processing (AP) abilities of children with Attention-Deficit Hyperactivity Disorder (ADHD), auditory processing disorders (APD), or both (Cook, Mausbach, Burd, Generoso, Gascon, Slotnik, Petterson, Johnson, Hankey, & Reynolds, 1993; Gascon, Johnson & Burd, 1986; Keith & Engineer, 1991; Tillery, Katz, & Keller, 2000). Keller and Tillery (2002) introduced five probable causes related to these conflicting results. They noted that these four studies had one or more of the following problems: (1) small sample size, (2) no control for learning effects or medication peak periods, (3) use of descriptive rather than statistical analysis, (4) failure to clinically titrate CNS medication, and (5) use of different criteria for ADHD diagnosis.

This chapter outlines the four studies, with a focus on the differences seen among the studies, provides an explanation of mechanics of CNS medication, and concludes with clinical recommendations regarding APD and medication.

Introduction

In the early 1990s, psychologists requested our clinical service to administer central auditory processing (CAP) tests to clients being evaluated for ADHD on two occasions: once when the client was under the influence of the stimulant medication and again when nonmedicated. This request stemmed from a published investigation that concluded that CAP evaluations may be utilized as a tool to measure the treatment effect among those with ADHD (Gascon et al., 1986). The following questions may shed light on reasons that an audiologist may hesitate to administer CAP testing as a tool to assist with medication titration:

1. Which CAP test session should be administered first: the nonmedicated session, followed by the medicated session or the opposite? What length of time between test sessions would be appropriate to control for a possible learning affect?
2. What time of day should the client receive the medication and when should the CAP test battery be administered? Has the medication appropriately been titrated or would the test results be used for titration (the level and degree to which the medication is being ingested) purposes?
3. Would the client, in the nonmedicated state, receive a placebo or nothing? (A double-blind placebo controlled study controls for possible bias when compared to a study in which the client does not receive a placebo or medication at one test session and does receive medication at another test session).
4. Which session(s) would the insurance company reimburse: the first, second, or both?

The above concerns have persisted in the profession because of similar behavioral characteristics associated with auditory processing disorders (APD) and ADHD and the paucity of research regarding the effect of medication on auditory processing abilities. The growing need to understand the relationship of ADHD and APD was again brought to our attention in 1994 at the APD consensus meeting in Albuquerque, New Mexico, sponsored by the American Speech-Language and Hearing Association (ASHA, 1995). After individual presentations, ASHA panel members posed this question: "Should one administer a CAP test battery to the client when medicated with their CNS stimulant medication"?

The speaker responded with the following: "Do we withhold insulin when we test an individual with diabetes? Granted we may not be able to compare the affect of insulin and Ritalin, as insulin is associated with the endocrine system and a CNS stimulant medication is associated with the nervous system; however, they are both prescribed because of medical reasons; thus, why would we evaluate a client when nonmedicated? Furthermore, if a child receives medication to enhance attention, especially during academic instruction, then perhaps it is in the best interest of the child to receive the stimulant medication to control for inattention during CAP testing, thus enhancing the reliability of the CAP test performance."

CNS Medication

There are over 250 controlled studies investigating the effectiveness and safety among CNS stimulant medications in the treatment of ADHD, involving more than 6,000 children and adults, across all age groups (Wilens, Spencer, & Biederman, 2005). Stimulant medications probably potentiate the effects of norepinephrine (NE) and dopamine (DA) (Barkley, 1998; Lorys, Hynd, & Lahey, 1990; Zametkin & Rapoport, 1986). DA is related to anterior (motor) processing whereas NE is elated to posterior (sensory) processing (Barkley, 1998). Deficiencies in DA, NE, or both, may cause patterns of brain underactivity related to motivational learning and response to reinforcements (Barkley, 1998), giving rise to improvement in these areas when under the influence of stimulant medications.

Methylphenidate (Ritalin) is the most well-researched stimulant medication to the point that the pharmaceutical company (CIBA) that produces Ritalin does not manufacture placebos. Researchers wishing to use placebos must locate an available pharmacist able to make a placebo. (Ritalin is no longer under patent and is made by many drug companies.) The response to other medications is similar to the effect of methylphenidate (Pelham, Greenslade, & Vodde-Hamilton, 1990). Alternatives to methylphenidate are dextroamphetamine (Dexedrine), pemoline (Cylert), amphetamine compound (Adderall, made by SHIRA who also makes Daytrana Patch), and more recently newer long-acting stimulant medications such as Adderall XR, Ritalin LA, Metadate, Concerta (made by ALZA), and Focalin (manufactured by Novartis) are available to avoid several dosages in one day (Keller & Tillery, 2006).

All medications have a different onset and peak time of action. The short-acting medications, Ritalin and Dexedrine, have an onset of a 30- to 60-minute time period, peaking at 1 to 2 hours, with some form of lasting effect from 2 to 5 hours (*Physicians Desk Reference*, 2005; Wilens et al., 2005). Intermediate medications (amphetamine compound, sustained-release forms of methylphenidate and dextroamphetamine) have an onset time of 60 minutes, peaking at 1 to 3 hours and fading at 8 hours. A long-acting medication, Pemoline, has an onset time of 1 hour, peaking at 1 to 3 hours and fading at 12 hours (*Physicians Desk Reference*, 2005; Wilens et al., 2005). A long-acting amphetamine patch has been approved by the Food and Drug Administration (Keller & Tillery, 2006). Stratera is the first nonstimulant NE medication approved for treatment of ADHD, originally for adults, assisting those found with greater involvement of the NE versus the DA system (Keller & Tillery, 2006).

Researching Medication and APD

A review of conflicting studies regarding CNS stimulant medication in participants with APD/ADHD is needed to enhance the clinician's knowledge base. Three studies found some form of improvement in CAP test performance when under the influence of CNS medications (Cook et al., 1993; Gascon et al., 1986; Keith & Engineer, 1991), whereas a double-blind placebo controlled study (Tillery et al., 2000), found a medication effect for an attention measure and no medication effect for CAP abilities.

The first published study (Gascon et al., 1986) tested the CAP abilities of children (5 females and 14 males) with ADHD by administering a CAP test battery that included the Staggered Spondaic Word (SSW) test (Katz, 1968), and three tests in the Willeford (1977) test battery: a competing sentence test (CST), a filtered speech test (FST), and a rapidly alternating speech test (RAST). The participants, ages 5 years to 13.10 years, were diagnosed with ADHD by teacher and parent questionnaires, case history information, and neurological examination. Each participant received one of three different types of CNS stimulant medications (Dexedrine, Cylert, and Ritalin) in the sustained release (SR) form. Titration of the medication was complete in 2 to 3 weeks depending on the teacher and parental behavioral ratings of the effectiveness of the medication.

Findings revealed 15 participants with APD, based on failure of three of the five CAP tests. When the participants were retested, 13 of the 15 children showed improvement on two or more of the CAP tests. However, the reported test performance improvement was not based on statistical analysis and the authors did not indicate (1) the time the participants received the CAP test battery post-ingestion of the SR stimulant medication (as an indication of timing of the onset of the medication) and (2) the length of time between test sessions (as an indication of the potential for maturational affect). Gascon et al. (1986) concluded that CAP tests may assist in evaluating the effect of treatment, as 13 out of 15 participants improved on CAP test performance when retested in the medicated condition. These authors were the first to postulate that attention deficit disorders could be related to poor CAP test performance.

The researchers in the Gascon et al. (1986) study joined other colleagues (Cook et al., 1993) to address the methodological problems in their original study. Cook et al. (1993) evaluated the CAP abilities of 15 male children (ages 6 to 10 years) newly diagnosed with ADHD by physicians, in which Ritalin medication was titrated within 3 weeks. Twelve of the 15 participants were found to have APD. (Criterion for diagnosis of APD was not provided.) Another 10 participants (control group) were found without APD and ADHD.

The 15 original participants were divided into two experimental groups: one group ($N = 8$) received Ritalin for 3 days, followed by no medication for 2 days and then a placebo for 3 weeks. The other group ($N = 7$) received opposite conditions. All participants, physicians, and audiologists were blind as to whether the participant received a placebo or medication at test sessions. Time of CAP test administration, post-dosing, was not reported. The APD test battery consisted of speech discrimination (in noise and quiet), the SSW test, and three tests from the Willeford (1977, 1985) test battery including FST, RAST, and a competing sentence measure known as the Binaural Separation Test (BST).

Findings revealed an improvement in the medicated condition for the BST and RAST test results. The placebo condition revealed test improvement in the left ear BST score when the baseline test score with placebo condition test score were compared. The SSW and FST performances were not analyzed with the vague explanation that they did not "discriminate between subjects with and without ADD" (p. 133). The control group showed no change in test scores when comparing first and second test scores. The authors concluded that stimulant medication improved both APD and ADHD performance, based on the improvement of 3 of 13 dependent variables.

The third study (Keith & Engineer, 1991) found a medication effect for most of the measures administered to 20 participants (17 males and 3 females) who were previously diagnosed with ADHD by their physicians from 1 month to 4 years prior to their participation. All participants, ages 7 to 13 years, were first evaluated without medication and retested 1 to 3 months later while medicated. All participants received the tests 1-hour postingestion of Ritalin medication. However, six were medicated with the SR form of Ritalin, which would mean that peak performance is about 1 to 3 hours postingestion.

The test battery included the Auditory Continuous Performance Test (ACPT) (Keith, 1994), the Token Test for Children (DiSimoni, 1987), and three subtests in the SCAN: A Screening Test for Auditory Processing Disorders (Keith, 1986) including auditory-figure ground (AFG), competing words (CW), and filtered words (FW) subtests. This was the first study that utilized the ACPT, an auditory vigilance task, in which the client listens to a list of 96 monosyllabic words presented six times, and raises a thumb every time he or she hears the target word, dog. Impulsive scores are achieved when the thumb is raised to words other than the target word. Inattention scores are achieved when there is no response to the target word. The administration of all 576 words takes about 15 minutes. Findings revealed improved test scores on all measures except the AFG. The authors concluded that there is a need for further research employing a larger group of participants in blind studies.

The study by Tillery et al. (2000) investigated the effect of Ritalin on the CAP test performance of 32 children (3 females and 29 males) diagnosed with both APD and ADHD. The participants, ages 6.7 to 14 years, were obtained from an original sample of 66 children previously diagnosed with ADHD by psychological assessment (four to six sessions); each had never received a CAP test evaluation and showed improved ADHD behaviors when under the influence of their prescribed Ritalin dosage. The CAP test battery consisted of the SSW test, the Phonemic Synthesis (PS) test (Katz & Harmon, 1982), and the speech-in-noise test (Mueller, Beck, &, Sedge, 1987). CAPD diagnosis was based on test performance of at least two standard deviations below the mean on at least two CAP tests.

The participants received two test sessions separated by 30 to 52 days: one when medicated (Ritalin) and one when nonmedicated (placebo). All participants, the clinician, and parents were blind to the assigned randomized test condition, resulting in a double-blind method. To control for a learning or order effect, 16 participants received the Ritalin test session first and 16 participants received the placebo test session first. Morning test sessions were scheduled to control for fatigue and ensure the placebo condition was indeed without influence of the medication received from the prior day. Test sessions were administered 60 minutes postingestion of the capsule (Ritalin or placebo). The presentation order of tests was counterbalanced with the specific order maintained for each participant at both sessions.

Findings revealed a significant medication effect for the attention/impulsivity (ACPT) test performance, but no medication effect on the CAP measures that assessed a general dichotic speech test, phonemic skills task, or the ability to extract speech from noise. The authors concluded that Ritalin had a positive effect on sustained attention and impulsivity, but did not eliminate auditory dysfunction. They concluded also that ACPT may be a measure to assess the effect of medication, rather than CAP tests.

Methodological Concerns

Possible reasons why three studies (Cook et al., 1993; Gascon et al., 1986; Keith & Engineer, 1991) found a medication effect with CAP test performance, whereas one study (Tillery et al., 2000), did not find a medication effect on CAP test performance relate to sample size, manner in which the clients were diagnosed with ADHD, and lack of control for a learning effect (Keller & Tillery, 2002; Tillery et al., 2000). Understanding these differences is critical in ascertaining if CNS stimulant medication does or does not enhance APD.

The Keith and Engineer (1991) study had a large sample size ($N = 20$); however six of the children, those receiving Ritalin SR, were more likely controls (nonmedicated), due to the peak time of about 3 hours for Ritalin SR, and the CAP test battery was administered 1 hour postdosing of the medication. Gascon et al. (1986) provided one of three different types of SR medications to the 15 participants with APD and ADHD, thus it is questionable whether the medication peak time was congruent with the administration time of CAP tests. Therefore, the medication effect could have been confounded with the fact that the participants improved because of a learning effect rather than a medication effect.

Another methodologic concern for two of the studies (Cook et al., 1993; Gascon et al., 1986) was that the diagnosis of ADHD occurred just prior to participation in the studies. Keith and Engineer (1991), and Tillery et al. (2000), sought participants with an existing diagnosis of ADHD who were receiving medication treatment months to years prior to the study. Thus, the participants' titration may have been more reliable than when first diagnosed with ADHD as in the other studies.

Two studies maintained participant and clinician blindness to test conditions (Cook et al., 1993; Tillery et al., 2000). However, the sample size in Cook et al. (1993) was small ($N = 15$) with eight children in one group and seven assigned to the second group. In contrast, the Tillery et al. (2000) study, sample size was the largest ($N = 32$) in comparison to the other studies, assigning 16 participants to one group and another 16 participants to a second group.

The most critical issue concerns the use of a design that controls for learning. Keith and Engineer (1991) and Gascon et al. (1986) evaluated all of the participants first when nonmedicated and then when medicated, thus not controlling for a possible learning effect. Cook et al. (1993) tried to control for a learning effect by assigning eight participants to one group which first received the placebo condition and seven participants to the other group which received the medication condition. However, they used a small sample size. Tillery et al. (2000) randomly assigned the 32 participants to two groups: 16 children to Group 1 who first received the medication condition and 16 children to Group 2 who received the placebo condition; thus the participants were their own controls. The opposite test condition was applied in 30 to 52 days to further control for any learning effect. Furthermore, this was the only study to report on counterbalancing the administration of all CAP tests across all participants

Clinical Recommendations

Appropriate levels of attention and motivation are required for the clients to properly understand directions and test stimuli. The clinician should monitor the variables of attention, fatigue, and motivation to assist with the reliability of APD diagnosis. When clients with an attention or anxiety disorder are referred for APD testing it is recommended to administer the tests at morning appointments and provide breaks in order to assist with behaviors of inattention and distractibility (Tillery, 1998).

Clients, who receive successful medication treatment for the associated behaviors in attention deficits, should be evaluated under the influence of their medication regime (ASHA, 2005; Tillery, 1998) in order to decrease behaviors that could interfere with test taking (Keller & Tillery, 2002). Successful medication treatment includes appropriate titration (which may take several months) of medication associated with an improvement in observed behaviors by the client, school professionals, and family members. Psychologists and other mental health professionals may use continuous performance tests to monitor the appropriate titration of CNS stimulant medications. Because a clinician cannot assume that a client exhibits enhanced attention, based solely on the administration of medication, positive reinforcement should be used to maintain motivation and attention. Furthermore, extraneous visual or auditory stimuli (i.e., lights, mobiles, computer screen photographs, noise, music, etc.) should be removed from the testing area to avoid interference with test performance.

Summary

Four studies have investigated the effects of medication on APD test performance of children with APD and ADHD. Conflicting results may be related to the design of these studies due to (1) lack of control for learning effects, (2) small sample sizes, (3) weak titration of medication, (4) different peak times with administered medications, (5) the use of different diagnosis procedures for ADHD or APD, and (6) insufficient statistical analyses. Tillery et al. (2000) controlled for the above methodological concerns and found a significant medication effect on ACPT measures of attention and impulsivity; but did not find a significant medication effect for APD test performance. Because inattention can influence test performance, it is recommended that CAP tests be administered when the client is under the influence of his or her successful medication regime to control behaviors that may interfere with test-taking and the reliability of test performance.

Key Points Learned

- Clients with attention deficits should be evaluated under the influence of their successful CNS stimulant medication regime for attention deficits in order to control behaviors that may interfere with test-taking.
- CNS stimulant medication effectiveness on attention and impulsivity may be measured with the ACPT.
- Clinicians should control for inattention, fatigue, and motivation when CAP tests are being administered.

References

American Speech-Language-Hearing Association (ASHA). (1995). *Central auditory processing current status of research and implications for clinical practice. A report from the Task Force on Central Auditory Processing.* Rockville, MD: Author.

American Speech-Language-Hearing Association (ASHA). Task Force on Central Auditory Processing Consensus Development. (1996). Central auditory processing: Current status of research and implications for clinical practice. *American Journal of Audiology*, 5, 41–54.

American Speech-Language-Hearing Association (ASHA). (2005). *(Central) auditory processing disorders* (Technical report). Rockville, MD: Author.

Barkley, R. A. (1998). *Attention-deficit hyperactivity disorder: A handbook for diagnosis and treatment* (2nd ed.). New York: Guilford Press.

Cook, J. R., Mausbach, T., Burd, L., Gascon, G. G., Slotnick, H. B., Patterson, B., et al. (1993). A preliminary study of the relationship between central auditory processing disorder and attention deficit disorder. *Journal of Psychiatry Neuroscience*, *18*(3), 130–137.

DiSimoni, F. (1978). *The Token Test for Children.* Austin, TX: Pro-Ed.

Gascon, G. G., Johnson, R., & Burd, L. (1986). Central auditory processing and attention deficit disorders. *Journal of Child Neurology*, 1, 27–33.

Katz, J. (1968). The SSW test—an interim report. *Journal of Speech and Hearing Disorders*, *33*, 132–146.

Katz, J., & Harmon, C. (1982). *Phonemic Synthesis*. Allen, TX: Developmental Learning Materials.

Keith, R. W. (1986). *SCAN: A screening test for auditory processing disorders*. San Diego, CA: Psychological Corp.

Keith, R. W. (1994). *ACPT: Auditory Continuous Performance Test, Examiner's manual.* San Antonio, TX: Harcourt Brace.

Keith, R. W., & Engineer, P. (1991). Effects of methylphenidate on the auditory processing abilities of children with ADHD. *Journal of Learning Disabilities*, *24*, 630–636.

Keller, W., & Tillery, K. L. (2002). Reliable differential diagnosis and effective management for auditory processing and attention deficit hyperactivity disorders. *Seminars in Hearing*, *23*(4), 337–347.

Keller, W., & Tillery, K. L. (2006). Intervention for individuals with (C)APD and ADHD. In G. Chermak & F. Musiek (Eds.), *CAPD: From science to practice*, (Vol. 1, pp. 309–324). San Diego, CA: Plural Publishing.

Lorys, A. R., Hynd, G. W., & Lahey, B. B. (1990). Do neurocognitive measures differentiate attention deficit disorder (ADD) with and without hyperactivity? *Archives of Clinical Neuropsychology*, *5*, 119–135.

Mueller, G., Beck, G., & Sedge, R. (1987). Comparison of the efficacy of cortical level speech tests. *Seminars in Hearing*, *8*, 279–298.

Pelham, W., Greenslade, K., & Vodde-Hamilton, M. (1990). Relative efficacy of long-acting stimulants on children with attention deficit-hyperactivity disorder: A comparison of standard methylphenidate, sustained-release methylphenidate, sustained-release dextroamphetamine, and pemoline. *Pediatrics*, *86*, 226–237.

Physican's desk reference (55th ed.). (2005). Montvail, NJ: Medical Economics.

Tillery, K. L. (1998). Central auditory processing assessment and therapeutic strategies for children with attention deficit hyperactivity disorder. In G. Masters, N. Stecker, & J. Katz (Eds.), *Central auditory processing disorders: Mostly management* (pp. 175–194). Boston: Allyn & Bacon.

Tillery, K. L., Katz, J., & Keller, W. (2000). Effects of methylphenidate (Ritalin) on auditory performance in children with attention and auditory processing disorders. *Journal of Speech-Language and Hearing Research*, *43*, 893–901.

Wilens, T. E., Spencer, T.J., & Biederman, J. (2005). Pharmacotherapy of attention deficit/hyperactivity disorder. In T. Brown (Ed.), *Attention deficit disorders and comorbidities in children, adolescents and adults* (pp. 509–535). Washington DC: American Psychiatric Press.

Willeford, J.A. (1977). Assessing central auditory behaviors in children. In R. Keith (Ed.), *Assessment of central auditory dysfunction* (pp. 43–72). New York: Grune and Stratton.

Willeford, J. A. (1985). Assessment of central auditory disorders in children. In M. L. Pinheiro & F. Musiek (Eds.), *Assessment of central auditory dysfunction* (pp. 239–257). Baltimore: Williams & Wilkins.

Zametkin, A. J., & Rapoport, J. L. (1986). The pathophysiology of attention deficit disorder hyperactivity: A review. In B. Lahey & A. Kazdin (Eds.), *Advances in clinical child psychology* (pp. 177–216). New York: Plenum.

22

Alternative Therapies

Acoustic Self-Amplification in Auditory Training

Theresha Boomgarden-Szypulski

Overview

"Children and adults with (C)APD are a heterogeneous group of people who have difficulty using auditory information to communicate and learn. (C)APD is a set of problems that occurs in different listening tasks. It is a deficit in the processing of auditory input, which may be exacerbated in unfavorable acoustic environments and is associated with difficulty in listening, speech understanding, language development, and learning" (Jerger & Musiek, 2000).

This chapter describes the use of acoustic self-amplification combined with self-talk to enhance speech understanding, language development, and learning through prosody and phonemic training.

Introduction

Classrooms are notorious for unfavorable acoustic environments. Children, including those with deficits in the processing of auditory input, spend six or more prime hours of their approximately 14 waking hours, (over 42%) in this acoustic gymnasium (based on a child's day from 7 AM to 9 PM with 6.5 hours spent in school). It is in this environment that children must struggle to map the sounds and symbols for reading and writing, focus on understanding the speech of 20 to 30 other individuals, particularly the teacher, learn and retain subject matter primarily from listening and reading, and express their learning in speaking and writing. Additionally, children must accomplish all this throughout most of their grammar school years with a neurological system in which auditory brain structures will not be fully mature until approximately adolescence (Bhatnagar, 2002; Chermak & Musiek, 1997).

Humans learn to focus on the human voice above all other sounds by hearing their own voice repeated. The brain is experience expectant and experience dependent. Stimulation of the auditory centers of the brain is critical to the actual growth and organization of auditory brain pathways (Sharma, Dorman, & Spahr, 2002; Sloutsky & Napolitano, 2003). Because their brains are not yet developed, children need clear, distinct acoustic information. They need the primary signal, including their own voice, to be about 10 times louder than competing sounds (Flexer et al., 2006). In order to learn, all children need a quieter environment and a louder, clearer signal than adults (Anderson, 2001). Acoustic self-amplification improves the signal-to-noise ratio of the child's own speech, and supports the development and strengthening of the auditory feedback loop.

Adults describe the acoustic distraction and overload in noisy environments as "I can't hear myself think!" and if unable to move to a quieter environment will use ear plugging (fingers, plugs, headphones) to block the auditory onslaught. When trying to work in such an environment, it is not uncommon to observe adults using self-talk to increase their concentration and focus. Increasing the signal-to-noise ratio enhances self-talk and self-talk assists language processing and learning for all ages.

Theoretical Framework

Humans instinctively endeavor to hear their own speech more clearly by resorting to subvocalization or "self talk" to enhance the auditory feedback loop. The auditory feedback loop is the process of attending to and correcting one's own speech output. The only way to develop the auditory feedback loop is by hearing one's own voice or speech. Auditory feedback is foundational to speech and language development and the learning of language-based academic skills.

Subvocalization is an instinctive, natural, effective process for learners of all ages. Subvocalization involves actual movements of the tongue and vocal cords (Armstrong, 2006; Carver, 1990).

These actual movements of the tongue and vocal cords activate another feedback system, the tactile-proprioceptive-kinesthetic loop (T-P-K loop). The T-P-K loop is the body's continuous monitoring of touch, position, and movement of all its parts, including respiration, phonation, resonation, and articulation during speech production. Through the entwining of speech with language, these elements of speech production provide both specifics (e.g. morphologic endings) and nuances (e.g. prosody: pitch, duration, and intensity) to the role of auditory processing.

Along with the auditory feedback loop, the T-P-K loop provides information to train the brain and enables the brain to make automatic adjustments to speech as it is being fed back into the auditory system (Wilson, & Knoblich, 2005). Speech includes respiration, phonation, prosody (intonation, rate, and volume), articulation, and resonance, all of which are tweaked to convey specific meaning to a message in accordance with the individual's culture and language. When *people subvocalize to assist language processing, they activate* ***both the auditory and T-P-K loops (tactile, proprioceptive, kinesthetic)****, two powerful feedback systems for learning.* The caveat is, however, deficient auditory and T-P-K feedback and deficient speech and language production inhibit correct learning. The way the individual hears auditory input is how he or she will produce it and how he or she will produce it is how he or she hears it. More of the same input does not change the outcome. Enhanced acoustic signal strength is of benefit to all learners but critical for individuals with auditory or speech deficiencies.

Principles of Self-Amplification

Acoustic self-amplification is a non-electronic means of enhancing the signal strength of subvocalization in real-time auditory feedback as opposed to audio or video recording and subsequent playback. Devices to enhance auditory feedback vary, from sleek manufactured headsets to speaking into a bucket. Popular improvised tools have included phone receivers constructed of PVC-pipe, plastic echo microphones, plastic tubing bent into a phone-receiver shape, even plastic milk jugs cut and shaped into voice feedback apparatuses. Commercially available tools include the Tok-Bak®, Hear-Phones®, Toobaloo®, and WhisperPhone®. All of these items are designed to enhance the auditory feedback loop by channeling the user's voice directly into their ears. Of the commercially available products, the WhisperPhone headset appears to be the most esthetically acceptable to children and adults featuring hands-free use and a streamlined, less obtrusive design.

There are two basic premises of intervention underlying the use of acoustic self-amplification for treatment of auditory processing disorders. The first premise is that **behavior cannot be changed unless the individual is made aware of the behavior (at whatever level of awareness his or her cognitive skills support)**. This awareness may range on a continuum from survival level (stimulus-response) to higher order thinking levels (synthesis, application, and evaluation) but the clinician must first create and establish the individual's awareness of the behavior to be changed. Acoustic self-amplification facilitates instructing the client in awareness about the acoustic information the client is missing or not utilizing in his or her listening and speech. Once the individual is aware of the behavior, she or he can begin to comprehend and participate in the interventions designed to change it.

For example, during intervention, the client imitates from the model the subtle changes in vowel production, or the timing on the stressed syllables. The enhanced auditory feedback of self-amplification allows the client to more effectively monitor his or her explorations with speech and language production. Although the client first hears and observes the target production in the instructor's model, the most important aspect is that the client hears how his or her own production compares to the model. Acoustic self-amplification, by increasing the loudness and clarity of the client's speech, enables the client to better compare his or her production to the model. Once the client is aware of their speech-language behavior, he or she can begin to comprehend their speech different-ness and participate purposefully in the therapy designed to change it.

The second premise is that the **mind learns what the body does, whether it is accurate or inaccurate** (Flexer, Rasinski, & Szypulski, 2006). Practice does not make perfect, only perfect practice makes perfect! This is why it is so critical to reinforce accurate and correct perceptions and productions. As the client experiences the auditory feedback of his or her speech and language productions, the tactile-proprioceptive-kinesthetic feedback loop supports his or her discovery of production and modulation of prosodic features and phonemic distinctions. For example, semantic contouring of words and sentences uses the T-P-K feedback information about respiratory and laryngeal grading for pitch, loudness, and timing (prosody) to overlay vocabulary and syntax with connotation. Phonemic distinctions, likewise, depend on the T-P-K feedback from the oral cavity for shaping vowels and the placement of the articulators combined with management of the voice for cognates. The encoding and decoding patterns from the auditory feedback loop and the T-P-K feedback loop are reinforced through successful exchanges of receptive and expressive linguistic information.

It is this integration of the auditory feedback loop and the tactile-proprioceptive-kinesthetic feedback loop that enables the complexities of speech and language to become "automated." Automation reduces the need for the brain to be consciously vigilant in the mechanics of the message and instead can devote its attention to the message. The mind has learned what the body does.

Training the auditory system to take in, sort out, connect information, and formulate a response is, in part, a sensory process. It is typical of human nature that overwhelming sensory input that is too difficult to process, results in loss of interest, fatigue, or shutting down (e.g., visualize yourself experiencing a poor cell phone connection). Acoustic self-amplification, by increasing the signal-to-noise ratio, decreases the auditory sensory overload and clarifies the signal.

The following techniques are provided as starting points to generate creative therapy applications using acoustic self-amplification in prosody and phonemic training. Use a comfortable, well-fitting, acoustic feedback device (Figures 22–1 and 22–2) to derive optimum gain from each of these techniques.

Prosodic Training

Acoustic self-amplification is useful for instructing the client to recognize and produce the rhythm and intonation patterns (prosody) of Standard American English. Standard American English commonly uses four tones that combine with duration changes to form eight basic patterns of intonation (Sikorski, 1993). These basic patterns occur frequently and consistently to form the musical, even "jazzy," quality of Standard American English. Receptively, the ability to perceive stress and intonation patterns is essential to comprehension of denotative and connotative meanings in messages. Expressively, the ability to produce stress and intonation patterns is essential to being understood, and being able to repair communication that has been misunderstood.

Prosody is the collective term for the speech elements of pitch, intensity, duration, and rate of speech. These elements are combined to produce intonation and rhythm changes (stress) that influence the meaning of the grammar and lexicon of all languages. The prosodic elements of pitch, duration, and intensity regulate connotative meanings such as sarcasm and humor or contrastive stress for message specificity, clarification, or emphasis (Dauer, 1993). Discussion and dialogue are difficult for individuals with prosodic processing deficit and social exchanges are rife with misunderstandings.

One technique in prosody training is to guide the client to recognize and imitate the basic prosodic elements of pitch, duration, and loudness by providing models that contrast high-low pitch, long-short duration, and loud-soft

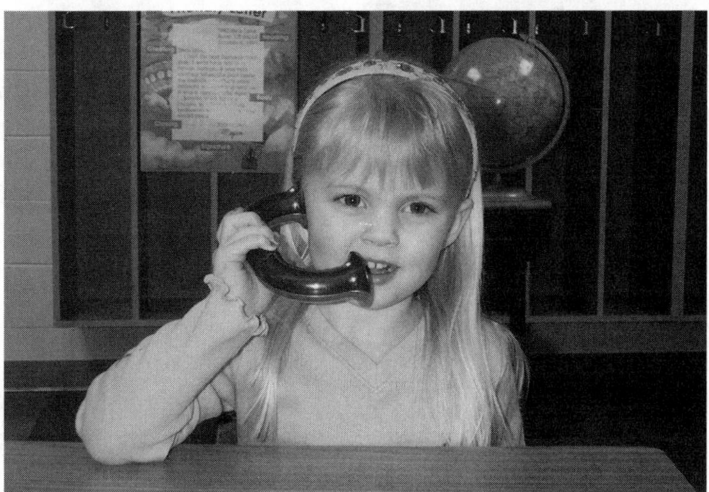

Figure 22–1. Toobaloo (see p. 455 for a description). (Photo courtesy of Toobaloo)

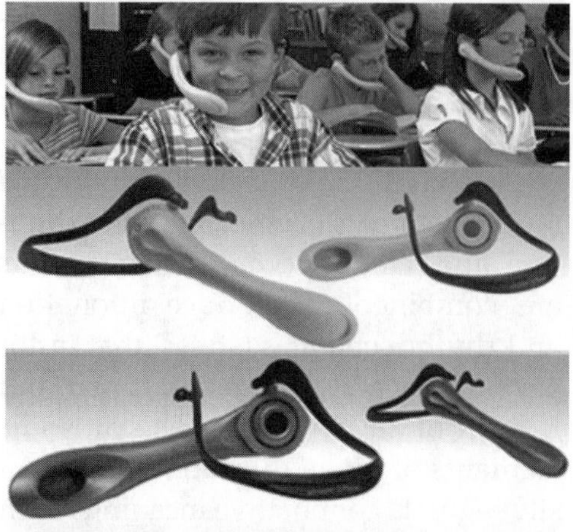

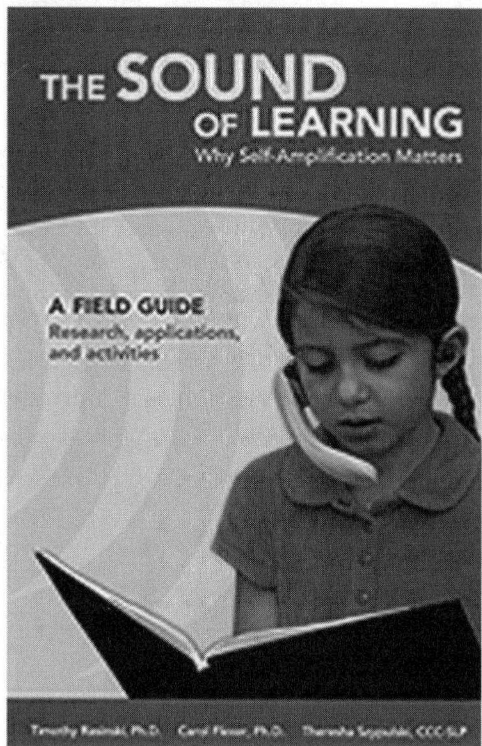

Figure 22–2. WhisperPhone (see p. 456 for a description). (Photo courtesy of WhisperPhone)

intensity (Ling, 1989). Initially, to avoid any semantic overload and focus *only* on basic prosodic elements, first use only tones (like those from an electronic keyboard) to discriminate high-low, long short, and loud-soft tones. Next, while wearing a self-amplification device, progress to recognition and imitation of vowels being modulated with rising and falling pitch, sustained and abrupt duration, and varying volume. A fun activity at this stage is to have short "conversations" using only vowels, and relying only on prosody, gestures, and facial expression to convey the dialogue. Use of role-playing themes with relatively closed-set vocabulary such as ordering food, getting a hair cut, and so forth, will ensure the most success. Most clients are amazed to discover how much meaning can be conveyed by these simple elements. Sikorski (1993) states many speech and language researchers report that at least 70% of our messages are conveyed to the listener by the intonation we use.

Accent modification materials, Mondegreen collections*, and Auditory Verbal Therapy materials are excellent resources for training prosody at the word, phrase, and sentence level while wearing a self-amplification device. (see Resources at end of chapter). This brief discussion demonstrates prosody training at the word level. However, bear in mind that this technique is also effective for prosody training at the phrase and sentence level.

Word Level

To address prosodic *duration* at the word level, instruct the client to detect, the syllables (segments) in a word.

*Named for the famous misheard lyric of a Scottish folk song: "and laid him *on the green*" misheard as "Lady Mondegreen".

Enhance the T-P-K loop in conjunction with the auditory feedback loop by use of physical cues to detect the syllables with longest duration (stressed) and shortest duration (unstressed). Use brief or sustained musical tones from an electronic keyboard, or tapping and gliding of the client's hand on a desktop to physically experience and hear the duration changes.

The stressed and unstressed syllables in words can be graphically depicted as dots, dashes, and lines to give visual cuing to the auditory rhythm of spoken language. Dots are used to depict short duration (weak stress), lines are used to depict longest duration (primary stress), and dashes are used to depict mid-length duration (secondary stress). For example: { _ . ___ . } is the graphic representation of the *rhythm* of the word "mac-a-ron-i." Acoustic self-amplification increases the client's opportunity to hear these duration changes in his or her own speech.

At the word level, it is very important to teach the client to perceive the unstressed syllable as well as the stressed syllable. The unstressed syllable occurs rapidly and is easily "lost" in words. Recognition of the unstressed syllable is parallel to recognition of unstressed words and word endings, which are easily "lost in" phrases and sentences. In American English, the *un*stressed portions of words, phrases, and sentences carry distinct and specific information such as verb tense and prepositions that are frequently missed by those with spoken language processing deficits.

To address prosodic *pitch* changes at the word level, instruct the client in detecting pitch jumps and pitch glides for each syllable. These pitch changes are superimposed on the rhythm, along with volume changes, to provide intonation patterns to words. These pitch changes can be depicted graphically by placing the dots, dashes, and lines in vertical relationship to each other, much like notes on a musical staff. For example, { – . ‾‾ . } is the graphic depiction of the *rhythm* **and** *pitch* changes of the word "mac-a-ron-i." Acoustic self-amplification increases the saliency of these intonation patterns in the client's own speech.

Phrases and Sentences

The stress contour of *phrases and sentences* can also be diagramed with dots, dashes, and lines, or as roof lines with peaks and valleys by depicting the stressed words on peaks and the unstressed words in valleys. Nouns and verbs predominate on the peaks, whereas smaller words such as prepositions, auxiliary verbs, articles (definite and indefinite), uncountable nouns (e.g. some) and so forth generally reside in the valleys. The stress in phrases impacts the semantics of the message. For example, in the well known Mondegreen; "the answer my friends . . . " with slight changes in pitch and duration becomes "the ants are my friends!"

For clients with auditory processing deficits, the importance of instructing them to detect the unstressed syllable in words from earlier auditory training is played out at the phrase and sentence level. Although the content words are the more obvious as peaks, the more differentiating words are "lost" in the valleys unless specific exaggerated or contrastive stress is used to specify, clarify, or repair the message. In the example "JOE must run **VERY** fast," where "VERY" receives primary stress and "JOE" receives secondary stress, note that the imperative action of the sentence is carried by a short, quick, unstressed word ("must") residing in the valley of the intonation contour. In this example, if the listener mishears the verb, he may substitute from his language experience his own possible words such as can, can't, did, does, doesn't, will, won't, all of which are all grammatically correct but not true to the message. In discussion, dialogue, test taking, and so forth, the misunderstood message can have consequences of varying degrees.

Clients with auditory processing deficits are prone to miss brief, unstressed, but significant words, causing them to misunderstand, answer incorrectly, or need frequent repetition. Acoustic self-amplification highlights prosody training and significantly improves the potential for the client to derive maximum benefit from intervention.

Phonemic Training

Acoustic self-amplification is particularly beneficial in phonemic training for developing speech to print (writing) and print to speech (reading) processing. Acoustic self-amplification intensifies isolating, blending, and sequencing of phonemes in minimal pairs, CV and VC syllables, and words. By enhancing the clarity of the client's voice, while the client produces and modifies phonemes, the T-P-K loop and auditory feedback loop are mutually reinforcing. Teach the client to hear, feel, and see (mirror work) the distinctive features of consonants (e.g., manner and place of production) and characteristics of vowels (tense-lax, round-spread, and high-low). This provides the client with an additional descriptive and visual reference (rounded, spread, bilabial, plosive, etc.) that can strengthen the perceptions of the T-P-K loop, improve the accuracy of phoneme productions, and increase the accuracy of the auditory input. Training the client to simultaneously hear, feel, see, and say phonemes accurately provides a multisensory self-monitoring scaffold for accurate discrimination, analysis, and automaticity of phonological processing.

Another approach is the Auditory-Verbal Therapy approach (AVT) which is the application and management of technology, strategies, techniques, and procedures to enable children who are deaf or hard of hearing to learn to listen and understand spoken language in order to communicate through speech. The children learn to use sound and speech through hearing aids or their cochlear implants to listen to their own voices, the voices of others, and the sounds of their environment to understand spoken communication and develop meaningful conversations. Through play and active involvement in everyday situations, listening can become a way of life (Estabroks & Samson, 1992; Pollack, 1985). The materials are well suited for instructing prosody and phonemic skills to clients with APD. The use of this approach has proven to be effective in literacy development (Robertson & Flexer, 1993). Although certain language curricula might be employed, these materials are designed for children with normal hearing abilities. The clients learn to use their amplified hearing to listen to their own voices, and attend to the voices of others and the sounds of their environment to understand spoken language; that is, to integrate hearing, language, and spontaneous speech.

Target Population

Acoustic self-amplification is an effective, affordable, and portable tool for treatment of auditory processing deficits, particularly phoneme and prosody training for children and adults in the therapy setting. Beyond the therapy setting, acoustic self-amplification in the classroom assists students with and without auditory processing deficits to train their ear to tune in to their subvocalizations and filter out competing stimuli without disturbing other classmates.

Case Study

History

B. A., a 23-year-old male with diagnosis of high-functioning Down Syndrome and Autism Spectrum Disorder—High Functioning. Comorbid autism was not diagnosed until age 22. B.A. received consistent speech therapy from infancy to present age. B.A. has ultraexcellent family support and community services.

Reason for Referral

In the workplace, when B.A. did not understand or could not be understood, he would go into "shutdown" frequently escalating to "meltdown." Job coach and parents were concerned that B.A. would lose coveted work opportunity due to communication breakdowns.

Speech and Audiometric Evaluation

Normal hearing APD audiometric testing was not available and client would not be appropriate due to cognitive deficits, yet behavioral symptoms strongly suggested APD prosodic deficit. B.A. frequently tuned out or misunderstood speech of others, and frequently said "huh?" even to familiar phrases and topics, suggesting that he heard, but did not comprehend. Informal assessments were used to sample auditory processing skills. B.A. exhibited monotone speech with Parkinson-like verbal rushes and mild articulation errors. Consistent with Autism Spectrum Disorder B.A.'s flat affect, lack of eye contact, and reduced facial expression increased the difficulty in understanding his speech.

B.A. showed decreased interest and reticence in social conversation, but was passionate about music, drums in particular. He had taken drum lessons for several years and also sang very well, even participating in school chorus. B.A. carried his drumsticks with him wherever he went, but would lay them aside if requested. B.A.'s passion for rhythm and lyrics provided opportunity for informal assessment and ruled out temporal patterning, and interhemispheric deficits. Informal assessment suggested auditory closure skills were commensurate with cognitive ability level. Auditory memory was reported by family to be "excellent." In fact, B.A. frequently served as the repository for family events and scheduling. Informal assessment of prosody confirmed receptive and expressive deficits. Receptively, client required consistent second or third repetitions to select correct response from spoken language stimulus. Expressively, client was unable to modulate pitch of speaking voice, yet could sing very well. Client was unable to segment words or phrases, yet could maintain song tempos by singing and drumming. Client could not tap rhythm of spoken phrases, but could replicate drum licks.

Intervention

Music and drumsticks were the keys to unlocking prosodic training for B.A. ! B.A.'s favorite band and obsessive topic was Fleetwood Mac. He would willingly engage in extensive discussion about this band, every CD they produced, band members names, profiles, and current news about their personal lives. B.A.'s lack of prosodic elements in his expressive language and speech rushes made comprehension of his favorite topic difficult to an unfamiliar listener. B.A. tolerated requests for clarification only because of his passion for this topic.

Prosody of speech was presented as the "music of speaking." Favorite band member's names, song titles, and so forth such as Lindsey Buckingham (5-syllable phrase) were diagrammed with dots, dashes, and lines with pitch-related vertical distances. Client was successful in using his drumsticks to "get the beat" of these phrases when spoken by the clinician. Client accepted an acoustic self-amplifier (WhisperPhone) and verbalized the words and phrases while tapping with the drumsticks. Use of the drumsticks was faded rapidly and B.A. delighted in saying these names and phrases "with the beat." Acoustic self-amplification provided immediate reinforcement of his verbal modifications and his superb auditory memory ensured retention after only a few repetitions. Client's mother stated B.A.'s learning pattern always was "once he got it—he GOT it !" This proved to be accurate, as B.A. quickly generalized his improved prosodic rhythm to all speaking environments.

Pitch modulation proved to be very difficult for B.A. B.A. held very strong gender identification boundaries. He was stuck in the perception that his low tones were a "guy voice" and although he could be coaxed to produce pitch modulation, he resisted any changes that he perceived were "not a guy voice." Progress on prosodic pitch changes was slowly emerging when the clinician changed jobs and B.A.'s therapy was transferred to another speech-language pathologist.

During intervention, the clinician held a team meeting with B.A.'s job coach, community services team, music instructor, and family members. The clinician gathered high-frequency vocabulary and phrases of the vernacular associated with each of these communication environments. These individuals were instructed in basic elements of prosody, B.A.'s deficits, and specific intervention strategies for B.A. The team members agreed to provide reinforcement and prosodic cuing to B.A., particularly when needed for clarification and communication repair strategy. Not only did all of the team members report a significant change in understanding B.A.'s speech, but also reported a near total reduction in shut downs and virtually no "meltdowns" over a 5-month period. Additionally, older siblings living in other states reported that B.A. was "so much easier to understand on the telephone!"

At the time of the clinician's job change, B.A. was continuing to make progress with spontaneous generalization of prosodic rhythm elements to all communication encounters. Pitch modulation was only accomplished during therapy. B.A. continued to prefer his low-pitch, monotone pattern.

Overall, the successful prosodic changes in his use of duration (even without pitch change) were enough to make a dramatic improvement in his day-to-day communication in all environments by reducing the frequency of his misunderstanding and miscommunicating. Social communication difficulties that previously led to shut down or meltdowns were reduced to instructive moments in which caretakers in his environment exaggerated their prosody for his understanding or cued B.A. to repair his communication by instructing him to "say it with a beat." Follow-up inquiry confirms that B.A. has continued to be a more successful communicator—even while maintaining his low monotone "guy voice!"

This case study demonstrates how an individual with complex, comorbid diagnoses of Down Syndrome and Autism Spectrum Disorder and (by behavioral assessment) Auditory Processing Prosody Deficit was helped with acoustic self-amplification and prosody training provided on the premises that:

1. Behavior cannot be changed unless the individual is aware of the behavior (at whatever level of awareness their cognitive skill supports).
2. The mind learns what the body does—whether it is accurate or inaccurate.

Summary

Using acoustic self-amplification combined with self-talk enhances prosody and phonemic training for speech understanding, language development, and learning. Along with the auditory feedback loop, the T-P-K (tactile-proprioceptive-kinesthetic) loop provides information to train the brain and enables the brain to make automatic adjustments to speech as it is being fed back into the auditory system. When people instinctively subvocalize to assist spoken language processing, they activate both of these powerful feedback systems for learning. Acoustic self-amplification increases the loudness and clarity of the client's speech, so that the client is better able to monitor and compare his or her production to the model. Once the client is aware of their speech-language behavior, he or she can begin to comprehend their speech different-ness and participate purposefully in the therapy designed to change it.

Key Points Learned

- Humans instinctively endeavor to hear their own speech more clearly by resorting to subvocalization or "self-talk" to enhance the auditory feedback loop.
- Subvocalization is an instinctive, natural, effective process for learning.
- Subvocalization involves actual movements of the tongue and vocal cords
- Subvocalization activates **both** the auditory feedback loop and the tactile-proprioceptive-kinesthetic loop, (T-P-K), two powerful systems for learning.
- It is the integration of the auditory feedback loop and the tactile-proprioceptive-kinesthetic feedback loop that enables the complexities of speech and language to become "automated" both receptively and expressively.
- Behaviors cannot be changed unless the individual is made aware of the behavior (at whatever awareness level his or her cognitive skill supports).
- The mind learns what the body does, whether it is accurate or inaccurate.
- Training the client to simultaneously hear, feel, see, and say phonemes accurately provides a multisensory, self-monitoring scaffold for accurate discrimination, analysis, and automaticity of phonological processing.
- Acoustic self-amplification is an affordable and portable tool for treatment of auditory processing deficits, particularly phoneme and prosody training for children and adults.

This approach is seen as an alternative one as no efficacy data are available. It is by clinical experience that this program is seen as effective.

References

Anderson, K. L. (2001, April). Voicing concern about noisy classrooms. *Educational Leadership*, 77–79.

Armstrong, D. (2006, April 10). *The silent speaker: NASA researchers can hear what you're saying, even when you don't make a sound.* Forbes.com Technology.

Bhatnagar, S. C. (2002). *Neuroscience for the study of communicative disorders* (2nd ed.). Philadelphia: Lippincott Williams & Wilkins.

Carver, R. P. (1990). *Reading rate: A review of research and theory*. New York: Academic Press.

Chermak, G. D., & Musiek, F. E. (1997). *Central auditory processing disorders: New perspectives.* San Diego, CA: Singular Publishing Group.

Dauer, R. M. (1993), *Accurate English: A complete course in pronunciation* Englewood Cliffs, NJ: Prentice-Hall.

Estabrooks, W., & Samson, A. (1992). *Do you hear that?* Washington, DC: A. G. Bell Association for the Deaf and Hard of Hearing, Inc.

Flexer, C., Rasinski, T., & Szypulski, T. (2006). *The sound of learning: Why self-amplification matters.* Minneapolis, MN: Harebrain.

Jerger, J., & Musiek, F. E. (2000). Report on the consensus conference on the diagnosis of auditory processing disorders in school-aged children. *Journal of the American Academy of Audiology, 11*, 467–474.

Ling, D. (1989). *Foundations of spoken language for hearing-impaired children.* Washington, DC: A. G. Bell Association for the Deaf and Hard of Hearing, Inc.

O'Sullivan, S. B., & Schmitz, T. J. (2006). *Physical rehabilitation* (5th ed.). Philadelphia: F.A. Davis.

Pollack, D. (1985). *Educational audiology for the limited-hearing infant and pre-schooler.* Springfield, IL: Charles C. Thomas.

Robertson. L., & Flexer, C. (1993). Reading development: A parent survey of children with hearing-impairment who developed speech and language through the auditory-verbal method. *Volta Review, 95*, 253–261.

Sharma, A., Dorman, M. F., & Spahr, A. J. (2002). A sensitive period for the development of the central auditory systems in children with cochlear implants: Implications for age of implantation. *Ear and Hearing*, 23(6), 532–539.

Sikorski, L. D. (1993). *Mastering the intonation patterns of American English.* Santa Ana, CA: LDS and Associates.

Sloutsky, V., & Napolitano, A. (2003, May–June). Auditory versus visual dominance in preschool children. *Child Development, 74*(3), 822–833.

Wilson, M., & Knoblich, G. (2005). The case for motor involvement in perceiving conspecifics. *The Psychological Bulletin, 131*(3), 460–473.

Recommended Materials and Resources

Accent Modification

Dauer, R. M. (1993). *Accurate English: A complete course in pronunciation.* Englewood Cliffs, NJ: Prentice-Hall.

Sikorski, L. D. (1993). *Mastering the intonation patterns of American English.* Santa Ana, CA: LDS and Associates.

Mondegreens

http://www.phrases.org.uk/meanings/mondegreen.html

http://www.sfgate.com/columnists/carroll/mondegreens.shtml

Auditory Verbal

www.agbell.org
A. G. Bell Association for the Deaf and Hard of Hearing, Inc., 3417 Volta Place, NW, Washington, DC, 20007

http://www.listen-up.org/oral/a-v.htm

http://www.learningtolisten.org/publications.php

Self-Amplification Devices

Toobaloo (see Figure 22–1)

What is a TOOBALOO? The TOOBALOO is a phonelike device that allows children to hear themselves clearly while speaking softly into it. The design of the TOOBALOO magnifies their voice causing them to hear their sounds and words distinctly.

- Students are able to listen more clearly to their reading rate, phrasing, and expression (sound, duration, pitch, and stress)

- The TOOBALOO can be used by speech pathologists to help clients with fluency disorders, monitor and regulate their speech
- The TOOBALOO provides auditory feedback to help the clients detect their errors (articulation, phonological), regulate vocal intensity, and self-monitor their fluency.

WhisperPhone—WhisperPhone.com (see Figure 22–2)

What is WhisperPhone? WhisperPhone is a hands-free acoustic self-amplifier worn on either ear to simply and effectively convey the user's voice directly into their ear so they can hear their own voice clearly.

- Research has proven that users can hear phonemes 10 times more clearly when they are wearing the WhisperPhone. This means users can hear themselves better over background noise for improved focus on what they are learning. WhisperPhone is affordable, is easy to use, and is available in adult and child sizes.
- WhisperPhone assists children and adults who struggle with articulation, auditory discrimination, dyslexia, CAPD, reading fluency, prosodic deficits, self-monitoring/correcting, and autism by permitting acoustical self-amplification in a variety of settings, without disruption to others.
- Hearing their own voice clearly encourages children to speak or read aloud softly and hear themselves without disturbing others. This results in a quieter classroom and an environment more conducive to learning.
- The large WhisperPhone (black) is designed for grade 5 through adult. It is beneficial for speech training, impacting literacy, refining one's singing voice, learning lines for a theater performance or speech, learning a new language, and more.

The *Sound of Learning* book includes practical applications of the WhisperPhone self-amplification device in the classroom and home. Included in the book are exercises to use in conjunction with WhisperPhone, whether you are a teacher or a parent. Authored by a literary expert, an audiologist, and a speech-language professional, this book offers compelling analysis, enjoyable, effective exercises, and other resources to utilize.

23

Alternative Therapies

Sound-Based Interventions

Dorinne S. Davis

Overview

Sound-based therapy uses sound vibration to impact the body using special equipment, programs, modified music, and/or specific tones/beats, the need for which is identified with appropriate testing (Davis, 2005). It is more than just listening to music. It also involves more than the ear's hearing and auditory processing abilities. However, because of sound's overall impact on the body, sound-based therapy can be considered as a treatment option for auditory processing issues. This chapter reviews many of the different sound-based therapies available, provides a rationale for them, and discusses their use and the order in which they should be considered as a possible treatment option for auditory processing deficits.

Introduction

Sound is vibrational energy. Vibrations have a frequency, and frequency is sound. Our ear picks up these frequency vibrations and sends the information to the brain. However, our body also "hears" the frequencies of the many sounds around us by responding to the vibrations received through our bone structure, our sense of touch, and our interconnected cell network. These responses are often at a subconscious level.

The ear, of course, is responsible for our "sense of hearing," yet it also houses our vestibular and balance center. The eighth cranial nerve is our "auditory/vestibular" nerve and sends information to the brain. Additionally, cranial nerves II through XI receive direct or indirect stimulation from sound vibration as it stimulates the ear. Through this indirect stimulation, all of the body's sensory systems are affected.

Sound-based therapies impact the total body response to sound vibration versus an auditory-based response. The key to understanding sound-based therapies is to understand the process of how they impact the entire body, not just the auditory sense. There is a developmental flow for the correct administration of the therapies (Davis, 2004). The answer for understanding if, when, how long, and in what order for any sound-based therapy can be conceptualized by *The Tree of Sound Enhancement Therapy®* (Davis, 2004).

Theoretical Framework

In 1957, Dr. Alfred Tomatis demonstrated his ideas to the French Academie of Science. They incorporated these ideas into *The Tomatis Effect*, a series of three laws demonstrating a connection between the voice, the ear, and the brain. Simply put, these laws state that "the voice contains the frequencies that the ear hears." Dorinne Davis-Kalugin (2004) demonstrated further connection between the voice, the ear, and the brain by adding two additional laws known as *The Davis Addendum to the Tomatis Effect*. These laws demonstrated that not only does the voice produce what the ear hears, but also that the ear emits the same stressed frequencies of the voice. Together these five laws state that if the voice is modified, the ear changes and vice versa; and that both the input to the brain and the response to the body will also change.

Having used these five laws, and evaluating the various sound-based therapies, *The Tree of Sound Enhancement Therapy®* was developed. There are many sound-based therapies. Each has the capacity to effect change.

Principles of Sound-Based Therapy

The analogy of a tree helps demonstrate both the body's response to sound as it pertains to the voice-ear-brain connection and the appropriate use of the individual sound-based therapies. The "Root System" refers to one's sense of hearing. The "Trunk" incorporates all general sound processing abilities of the ear and the body. The "Leaves and Branches" include specific auditory processing skills like auditory memory, auditory sequencing, auditory discrimination, sound identification, and more —many of the skills that are part of the deficit areas of auditory processing as defined in other chapters. The "Overall Maintenance of the Tree" refers to one's wellness or body support for maintaining change (Davis, 2005a).

The Root System

The "Root System" includes sound-based therapies that address the body's physiological response to sound, or one's "sense of hearing." To make a tree grow, the root system must be firmly in place. Can a tree grow with weak roots? Yes, of course, but it will not flourish or grow beautiful flowers. As humans, our hearing sense must be working appropriately so that we can process auditory and sound input well. Having a hearing loss does not preclude being able to process sound input well because a person with a hearing loss can still process sound vibration through their bone structure and/or cell network.

Auditory Integration Training

To date, there is one sound-based therapy that addresses the sense of hearing—Auditory Integration Training or AIT—specifically, the Auditory Integration Training established by Dr. Guy Berard, a French ear, nose, and throat physician (Berard, 1992). The name should not be confused with other sound-based therapies as all sound-based therapies are not the same.

Dr. Berard studied with Dr. Alfred Tomatis but created his own method, very different from the Tomatis Method. Dr. Berard used an audiogram, or hearing test, to test his patients. After reviewing over 8,000 of his patients' audiograms, he noticed similar patterns and irregularities in the configurations of the audiograms and connected them to combinations of hyper- and hypo-sound sensitivities that were also similar in these patients. He theorized that the quality of sound that one hears is equal to the behavior of the individual (Berard, 1992). He worked with people of all ages, but as he began to work with children with learning challenges, he noticed that he was making a significant change to their behavior as a result of his method.

He designed a device as a "hearing retraining device," which he called the Audiokinetron. He later gave approval for another device called the Earducator™. Both devices work similarly in retraining how one hears or responds to frequency specific information. The outcomes were improved eye contact, better clarity of sound input, decreased sound hypersensitivities, better comprehension of language input, and more. The result, as Dr. Berard saw it, indicated an improved behavioral response in each individual (Berard, 1992).

Davis began researching the acoustic reflex muscle pre and post the AIT program. This muscle helps attenuate loud sounds and was found to be over or underactive in people being helped with AIT. This muscle consistently demonstrated positive retraining after Auditory Integration Training (Davis, 2004). Porges (Edelson, 2003) found that both muscles in the middle ear played an important role for people who were hypervigilant to sound. The result as Davis reported suggests a physiological change that may result in a behavioral response.

For those with auditory processing issues, a repatterning of how the ear "hears" auditory and sound input can often provide comfort when listening in noisy situations, and improve clarity of the speech input, awareness of the surrounding environment, and comprehension. Much of the data based on outcomes from AIT are anecdotal and additional research is encouraged. For updated information, go to http://www.berardaitwebsite.com or http://www.AITInstitute.org.

It should be noted that the American Speech-Language-Hearing Association (ASHA) published a Technical Report/Position Paper on Auditory Integration Training in the ASHA Supplement Number 24 in 2004 (ASHA, 2004). This paper provided confusing information about AIT or Auditory Integration Training for its members as it lumped many sound-based therapies under the title of AIT. It did not provide for the differentiation between the many sound-based therapies as this chapter does. For example, it reported on Auditory Integration Training by Dr. Berard, but provided references for both Dr. Berard's equipment, the Clark method's equipment, and DAA equipment as offering similar results. Each provides a different input and listening response and therefore should not be equated but compared. As reported in the next sections, other methods such as the Tomatis Method and Samonas, which are also mentioned in the ASHA Position Paper, are also different methods from AIT and should not be labeled as such. The recommendation from the position paper was to discourage the use of AIT as a treatment, given its limited efficacy data, but to support research for the methodology to determine the effectiveness of such methods. It is very important to move forward as the new field of sound-based therapies evolves. It is also important that the groundwork for sound-based therapies should be established as well. The "Tree of Sound Enhancement Therapy" attempts to explain a foundation for establishing this basic research.

The Trunk

The "Trunk" incorporates the basic connections of the voice-ear-brain. Therapies that use these connections can be called Listening Training Programs, or therapies that address how sound energy and processing impacts all the responses that the ear stimulates either directly or indirectly. The "Trunk" is the foundation. When a tree has well-supporting roots to provide good growth and development to the part of the tree that sends nutrition to the leaves and branches, the branches are strong. If it is weak, the tree does not thrive.

The Tomatis® Method

The foundational method of the "Trunk" is The Tomatis Method, researched and established by Dr. Alfred Tomatis. It was the first sound-based therapy and incorporates all the components of the ear's sensory stimulation and connections. It works on more than hearing. Dr. Tomatis developed a "listening therapy"—one that used sound to repattern a person's listening responsiveness. This method typically has the greatest impact on the listener educationally and developmentally, especially when applied in the correct order of application (Davis, 2004).

There are three important concepts in this method. For the *first* concept, Dr.

Tomatis introduced filtered and gated music to achieve an awakening of the brain to what he called "cortical charge" (Tomatis, 1991). He wanted to wake up the brain to high-frequency sounds to keep the brain and body active. For the person with issues in auditory processing, the weaknesses may be seen as lack of attention and focus, poor organizational skills, and/or poor speech discrimination.

The importance of bone conduction in the listening process is a *second* concept of The Tomatis Method. Bone conduction often relates to our inner body response to sound and, for some, this can keep the person from being receptive and/or responsive to sound. For the person with auditory processing weaknesses, this is often seen as having difficulty with listening to long conversations, comprehending, listening in background noise, discriminating between certain speech sounds, and hypersensitivity with reverberant sounds, or with rhythmical patterns of speech.

A *third* concept of The Tomatis Method is the introduction of *active vocal production*. Because the voice produces what the ear hears, the voice becomes the stabilizer for the person in maintaining changes as they occur. Before dismissing someone from The Tomatis Method, the person must be able to listen to his own voice and modify it when necessary. When the listener is unable to monitor his own voice appropriately, the positive outcomes may decrease if the additional sessions do not occur.

Because of these three concepts, the method is an intensive one. The typical program includes listening through a device called the Electronic Ear, which, with programming established from a proprietary Listening Test, not a hearing test, and a Laterality Test, these concepts are incorporated. The sessions last for 2 hours per day for 15 days, followed by a 3 to 6 week break. Then another 2 hours a day of listening for 15 more days are required. Some centers use an 8-day schedule, 1-month break, and another 8 days, instead of the second 15 days. For the more severely challenged, additional 8-day sessions are needed so that the person can work toward allowing the voice to be stabilized. The person listens to Mozart music or Gregorian Chants. The program is considered educational in nature. The goal of a Tomatis program is to establish good functional use of the auditory/vestibular system by improving listening and communication skills.

The types of changes that occur with this method for those with auditory processing challenges are numerous. Davis reported on changes for individuals with autism, AD/HD, and Williams syndrome (Davis, 2005b). With just the basic Tomatis program of two sets of 15 days each, parents with autistic children reported that 87% of the subjects reported change with Interpersonal Growth, 85% change with Listening and Speech, 81% change with Thinking and Learning, (Figure 23–1) (Davis, 2005b), and parents of children with Williams syndrome reported that 100% of the subjects experienced change in Attention, 100% reported change in Thinking and Learning, and 80% reported change in Behavior, (Figure 23–2) (Davis, 2005b). Parents of children with AD/HD reported that 80% of the subjects experienced change in Attention,

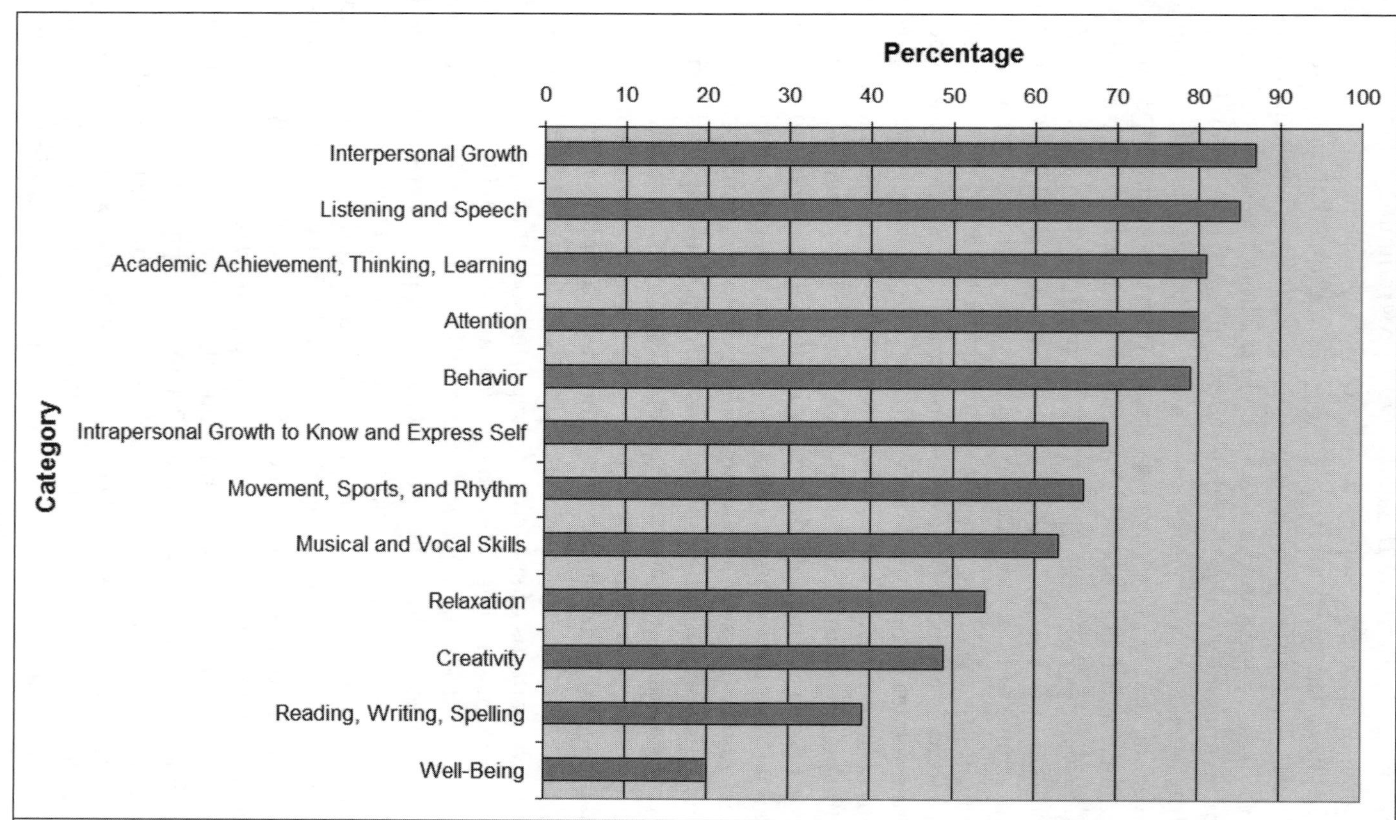

Figure 23–1. Changes pre- and post-Tomatis training with 100 autistic children.

Academic Achievement, Thinking, Learning	100
Attention	100
Behavior	80
Intrapersonal Growth to Know and Express Self	80
Musical and Vocal Skills	80
Creativity	60
Interpersonal Growth	60
Listening and Speech	60
Movement, Sports, and Rhythm	60
Reading, Writing, Spelling	40
Well-Being	20
Relaxation	20

Figure 23–2. Changes pre- and post-Tomatis training with five children with Williams syndrome.

and 91.25% had change in Thinking and Learning, Behavior, and Listening and Speech. (Figure 23–3) (Davis, 2005b). These changes were tabulated from an Abilities Improved Form provided to the parents by this author pre and post the listening sessions. Adolescents and adults who have used the method report other positive changes as well, such as improved sense of self, improved posture and balance, improved oral motor skills, improved tonal qualities, a feeling of being better connected with the world, and/or an improved sense of maturity (personal conversations with 50 Tomatis clients at The Davis Center, Mt. Arlington, NJ).

The Tomatis Method has been tested rigorously and found to be effective in the treatment of learning difficulties as well a behavior problems. Gilmore (1999) published a meta-analysis based on five studies involving 231 children. The results of the study demonstrated that the Tomatis Method significantly improved linguistic skills, psychomotor skills, personal and social adjustment skills, cognitive skills, and auditory processing skills. Stutt (1983) concluded that the Tomatis Method produces benefits beyond what could be expected by maturation or remedial education alone. Stutt's findings reported benefits that include:

- An increase in intelligence quotient
- Improved reading skills
- Improved perceptual processing skills
- Improvement in academic skills
- A general sense of adjustment
- Increase in the development of communication skills
- Improved expressive communication ability.

Swain (in press) examined auditory processing skills before and after the Tomatis Method of auditory stimulation. The retrospective study evaluated the results of the treatment on 41 randomly selected subjects. The effect of the treatment was measured using the Test of Auditory Processing Skills (TAPS) and The Token Test for Children.

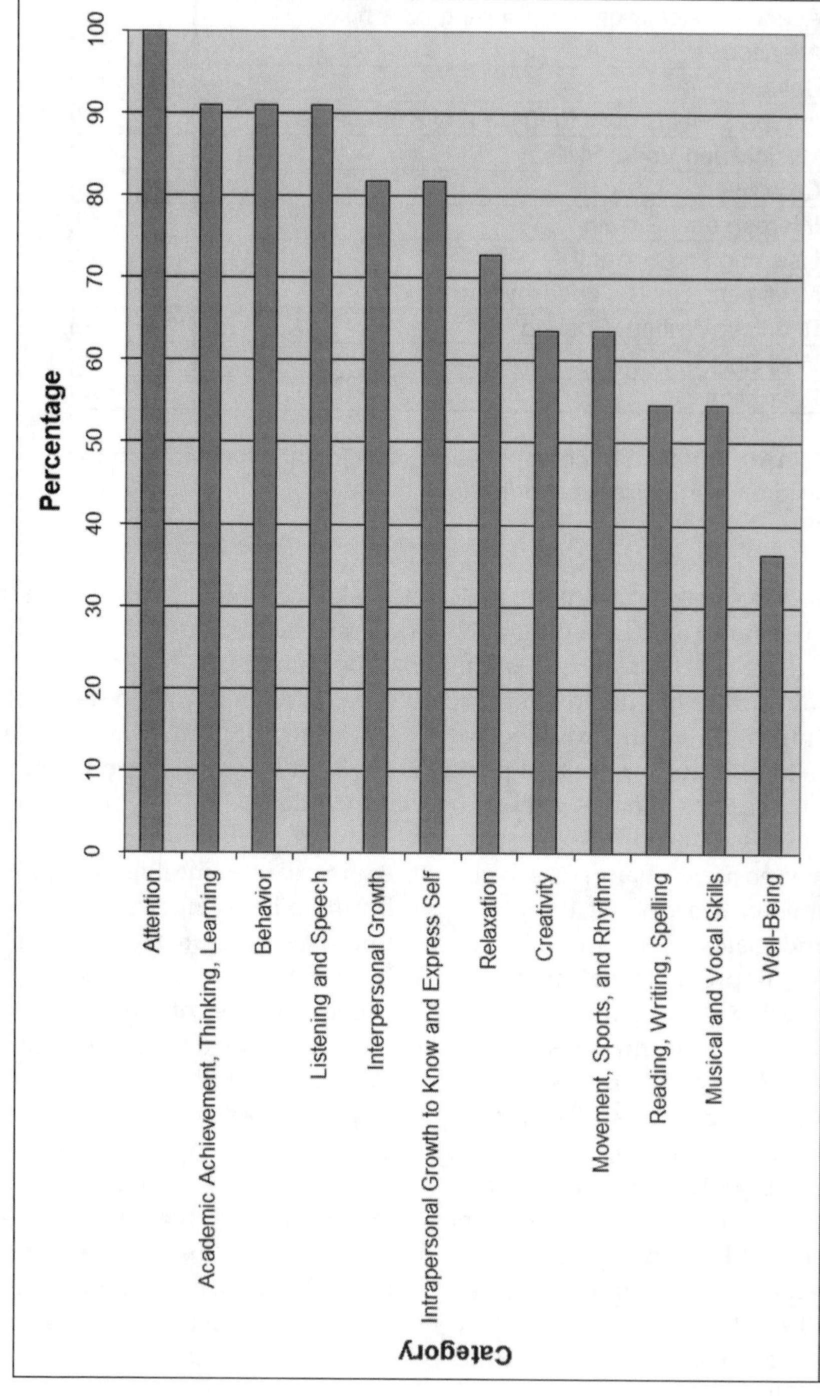

Figure 23–3. Changes pre- and post-Tomatis training with 11 children with AD/HD.

The findings revealed significant improvement with immediate auditory memory, interpretation and following directions, auditory discrimination, and auditory cohesion. Reductions in auditory latency were reported.

Neysmith-Roy (2001) conducted a study with six male subjects with a diagnosis of severe autism. The results of the study demonstrated that three of the subjects (50%) demonstrated significant benefit from the Tomatis Method of auditory stimulation. Of particular interest were changes that occurred in the prelinguistic areas of five of the six subjects. These changes included: adaptation to change, listening response, nonverbal communication, emotional response, and activity level. Neysmith-Roy suggests that the Tomatis Method may be helpful in making prelinguistic behaviors manageable and thus help prepare a child with autism to learn basic skills necessary for the development of language and learning.

Other Sound-Based Therapy Programs

Many people have tried to replicate or "copy" Dr. Tomatis' Method, but few have succeeded. However, over the past few years, some have become competitive. Each will receive a brief description.

Samonas Sound Therapy (SST)

Based on the theoretical framework of Dr. Tomatis, Samonas is the acronym for Spectral Activated Sounds of Optimal Natural Structure. Developed by a German engineer, Ingo Steinbach, Samonas Sound Therapy is used extensively in Europe, Australia, the United Kingdom, and the United States by occupational therapists, speech-language pathologists, physicians, psychologists and educators. This method uses prerecorded CDs that incorporate filtered and gated classical music and sounds of nature. Furthermore, the modulated music and nature sounds provide spectral activation. Samonas Sound Therapy offers a large array of different CDs so that listening programs can be individually tailored to an individual's needs. Professionals using Samonas Sound Therapy must participate in training and certification programs. For information, contact http://www.samonas. com.

Dynamic Listening System® or DLS

DLS was developed by Dr. Ronald Minson, a Tomatis practitioner of many years. His program modifies the program and listening time established by Dr. Tomatis, yet uses state of the art technology to bring high quality sound to the listener. It is not applicable for home usage. For information, contact http://www.dynamiclistening.com

The Listening Program®

This program conceptualized by Alex Doman, attempts to improve auditory processing skills through an auditory therapy program using CD recordings that require the person to listen with a set of quality headphones and a CD player. TLP is a prepackaged generic listening program containing eight

CDs in which the listener will undergo a listening protocol for an 8-week period of time. It was developed for children ages 2 through adults. The music is electronically altered to "help balance, strengthen and restore one's ability to listen and process sounds across the full auditory spectrum from 20 Hz to 20,000 Hz." They claim improvement in academic performance and emotional balance. Use of TLP attempts to exercise and tone the tiny muscles in the ear and build stronger multisensory pathways to the brain. The brain receives the auditory stimulation and improves its ability to process sound. It can be located through the Rocky Mountain Learning Systems in Parker Colorado, developed by the Center for Psychoacoustic Research.

Therapeutic Listening™

Founded by Sheila M. Frick, OTR, Therapeutic Listening is a part of Vital Links and is an AOTA-approved provider of continuing education opportunities that incorporates Therapeutic Listening, vestibular habilitation, and core development. The primary objective of all Vital Links courses is to provide innovative clinical tools and strategies that can be immediately implemented upon course completion in schools, clinics, and homes.

The concept of Therapeutic Listening is a highly individualized method of auditory intervention utilizing electronically altered compact discs in protocols specifically tailored by sensory integrative professionals to match client needs. Listening is a function of the entire brain; when we listen we listen with the whole body. There is a series of CD recordings that the client will listen to over a period of time to "exercise" the auditory muscles and brain.

JoEE® Products

The JoEE series of products were developed by a sound engineer, Chris Faddick who had been a Tomatis clinician for 15 years. Realizing the potential of the Tomatis Method, Mr. Faddick created a state of the art system incorporating all the concepts of Dr. Tomatis. The JoEE-Pro is a simple to use, clinic-based unit. The JoEE is a series of units—some designed for the home user. One unit does not include the voice, and the another does. This system could provide opportunities for people who are unable to locate a Tomatis center near them or want to only use a home-based unit. Information about these systems can be found at http://www.bigbangsoundworks.com

Earobics®

Earobics was developed by Jan Wasowicz, Ph.D., a speech-language pathologist. Dr. Wasowicz'z experience working with children with speech, language, and related disorders led to the development of this program. Earobics offers multilevel programs for various age groups ranging in age from 4 to 7 years, 7 to 10 years, and adolescents and adults.

The computer-based programs consist of multimedia games that host delightful animated characters and lively music used to captivate the user while making the experience of learning fun and pleasurable. The various levels throughout the programs provide extensive practice and comprehensive skill training. The user can work independently or with a trained provider. These programs use sophisticated techniques that include acoustic enhancement of the speech signal and adaptive training to facilitate the development of the auditory and phonologic skills critical for speech and language development and the development of written language skills.

The format of the Earobics programs is adapted to maximize learning by allowing the user to progressively move to more challenging levels of difficulty at their own pace. The program should be used at least once a week over an extended period. The length of time required for training and practice is determined by the length and duration of training sessions. For more information contact: http://www.earobics.com.

Interactive Metronome®

Interactive Metronome was developed by engineer and sound technician James Cassily. Previously having worked in the music industry as a sound mixer for record producers, he became curious about music-based technology. He was interested in developing a high-tech version of the metronome, in consideration of the relationship between motor skills, concentration, and cognitive abilities. Cassily theorized that if a person improved the ability to plan and sequence motor actions, then important learning, cognitive, and social skills could be influenced and possibly improved. Cassily tested his theory with 56 boys diagnosed with ADHD. Significant improvements were noted in attention, motor control, language processing, reading, and regulation of aggressive behavior. He applied this research to a study with people active in sports, as he found an improvement in motor control, focus, and performance in the golfers who were tested.

Interactive Metronome is a computer-based interactive version of the musical metronome. It provides real-time testing and teaching capabilities. The listener uses a tapping motion for each limb of the body, creating a motor skill catalyst. The purpose of the program is not simply to learn how to move our limbs, but how to develop precise control over basic mental functions through the use of the program's movements. The movements are simple and enhance the ability to consistently concentrate without interruption.

The listener uses either an arm or a leg to tap in time with the reference beat heard through the headphones. The trigger sends a signal to the computer, which analyzes when the tap occurred in relation to the reference beat. The information is translated into a sound that changes according to the response of early, late, or on-time sound. The responses are immediately analyzed by the computer and identified in millisecond accuracy averages, measuring the listener's ability to maintain focus over an extended period.

There are two stages of training. The first stage breaks existing deficient rhythmic patterns. The second stage instructs the listener to focus only on the steady beat and ignore the guide sounds, any internal thoughts, and any unrelated environmental stimuli. The listener learns to repeat their motions without deliberate adjustments. They entrain their brain to maintain a better beat, thereby having a positive effect on their overall functioning. The average program is composed of 15 one-hour sessions over a period of 3 to 5 weeks. For more information contact: http://www.interactivemetronome.com

Specific Auditory Skills

Specific auditory processing skills include memory, discrimination, sequencing, rhythmic patterning, pitch differences, and so forth. These skills typically are evaluated with a standard Central Auditory Processing Evaluation, as mentioned earlier in this book. Although many of the sound-based therapies suggested at this level can be stand-alone therapies, the results may not be maintained if the foundation is not sufficiently supporting it.

Body Maintenance and Support

Whereas Dr. Tomatis discovered that the voice produces what the ear hears and developed a program to address the foundation of "The Tree," a further connection is made between the voice, ear, and brain (*The Davis Addendum to the Tomatis Effect)* bringing "The Tree" together. According to Davis (2004), the voice represents the body's ability to process, use, and respond to sound. The concept has been around for thousands of years in yoga, mantras, and many native Indian traditions. Very few people can train their ear to self-correct, so the ability to collect and analyze the frequencies of the voice by vocal analysis is the last part of "The Tree." The "Body Maintenance and Support" is important to how well "The Tree" survives.

The science of BioAcoustics™ is the final piece of *The Tree of Sound Enhancement Therapy.* BioAcoustics is the study of the frequencies produced by all living systems. Through voice spectral analysis, this scientific method identifies and interprets the complex frequency interactions within the body.

Every cell in our body continuously absorbs and emits a sound (Davis, 2004). Every nutrient, biochemical, toxin, hormone, or pathogen also provides a unique vibration, defined as a Frequency Equivalent™. As a result, each person's body vibrates with its own combinations of frequencies which can be captured by the frequencies of the voice and demonstrated in a "voiceprint."

The science of BioAcoustics analyzes the voiceprint and identifies the frequencies that will help the person make change. BioAcoustics explores the potential that the body is a mathematical matrix of predictable frequency relationships (Davis, 2004). For example, when the Frequency Equivalents of calcium and magnesium are combined, the result is the Frequency Equivalent of phosphorus, an element that is necessary for calcium and magnesium metabolism.

For the person with auditory processing issues, the science of BioAcoustics may identify an imbalance of the frequency relationships that can be repatterned by introducing low-frequency analog sound of a "self-correcting" frequency. Such imbalances may be seen in behaviors as loss of attention, focus, and lethargy, or feeling like "being in a fog." BioAcoustics becomes an adjunct supportive therapy for those with biological issues that manifest as auditory processing weaknesses. For more information, go to http://www.soundhealthinc.com.

The Diagnostic Evaluation for Therapy Protocol (DETP®)

Sound Enhancement Therapy provides clarity for understanding the many existing sound-based therapies and new ones as they are developed. A problem that existed was how to know if a sound-based therapy was appropriate for a particular person; and if more than one therapy was possible, in what order the therapies should be administered. *The Diagnostic Evaluation for Therapy Protocol* (DETP®) (patent pending) was developed to solve this problem (Davis, 2006).

The DETP is a series of audiologic based tests that determine one's sense of hearing, general sound processing issues, specific auditory processing issues, and issues related to support of the body (Davis, 2006). This test battery takes the guesswork out of administering sound-based therapies and offers solutions to the many complexities of how, when, and how long the various therapies should be administered. For more information go to http://www.dorinnedavis.com.

It is recommended that the DETP be considered in a Central Auditory Processing Evaluation. The DETP is designed to determine what therapy should be initiated or whether other foundational sound-based therapies should be considered first.

Summary

Sound-based therapies provide foundational change for each individual based upon the anatomy and physiology of the ear, the voice-ear-brain connection, and the body's cellular response to sound. The entire field of sound-based therapies is in its infancy. More research is required before the specific outcomes can be determined.

Editor's Note. To date, evidence-based data have been sparse to render sound-based intervention a treatment of choice.

Key Points Learned

- All sound-based therapies are not the same. Each should be evaluated for both the physiological processes and learning and/or behavioral outcomes that may occur with each therapy.
- Sound-based therapies address issues of hearing, sound processing, and body process in different ways.
- One should not randomly suggest the use of a sound-based therapy without an appropriate diagnostic tool such as the *Diagnostic Evaluation for Therapy Protocol (DETP).*

- There are five laws that establish a connection between the voice, the ear, and the brain. Three were established in *The Tomatis Effect* and two were established in *The Davis Addendum to The Tomatis Effect.*
- The ear affects more than one's sense of hearing. It is key to balance and coordination; or vestibular function. Sound stimulation through the ear also impacts on the central nervous system.
- *The Tree of Sound Enhancement Therapy* provides an understanding of how all the sound-based therapies can be utilized appropriately.

References

American Speech-Language-Hearing Association. (2004). Auditory integration training. *ASHA*, (Suppl. 24).

Berard, G. (1993). *Hearing equals behavior.* New Canaan, CT: Keats.

Davis, D. S. (2004). *Sound bodies through sound therapy* (pp. 168, 246, 255–275). Landing, NJ: Kalco.

Davis, D. S. (2005a, June 24). *How sound-based therapy can help the isodicentric 15 individuals.* Paper presentated at Isodicentric 15 and Other Chromosomal Imbalances Conference, Schaumberg, IL.

Davis, D. (2005b, July) *A review of various abilities improved after the basic Tomatis Method Program for autistic, Williams syndrome, and AD/HD clients.* Presentation at 2005 Educational Audiology Association Summer Conference, Myrtle Beach, SC.

Davis, D. S. (2006). *Every day a miracle: success stories with sound therapy.* Landing, NJ: Kalco.

Davis-Kalugin, D. S. (2004, November). *The Davis Addendum to the Tomatis Effect*, Presented at the Acoustical Society of America Annual Conference, San Diego, CA.

Edelson, S. (2003). Dr. Stephen Porges' research may support Dr. Berard's and Tomatis' theory on middle ear muscle dysfunction. *The Sound Connection, 9*(4), 1–2.

Gilmor, T. (1999). The efficacy of the Tomatis method for children with learning and communication disorders. *International Journal of Listening, 13*, 12.

Neysimith-Roy, J. M. (2001). The Tomatis Method with severely autistic boys: Individual case studies of behavioural changes. *South African Journal of Psychology, 31*(1), 19–27.

Stutt, H. A. (1983). *The Tomatis method. A review of current research.* Montreal: McGill University.

Swain, D. (in press). The effects of the Tomatis Method on auditory processing skill weaknesses: A summary of findings. *The International Journal of Listening.*

Tomatis, A. (1991). *The conscious ear: My life of transformation through listening.* Barrytown, NY: Station Hill Press.

Tomatis, A. (1996) *The ear and language* (p. 87). Ontario, Canada: Moulin.

Wheeler, M. (2004, March) Signal discovery? *Smithsonian Magazine.*

24

Educational Implications

Rhandee Lipp

Overview

Students with Auditory Processing Disorders (APD) are at a great disadvantage in school, yet with proper interventions, they may experience successful academic outcomes. There are numerous laws in place to ensure that these students receive a free and appropriate education. The 2001 law, No Child Left Behind, ensures that all students are to be counted because all students count! The laws allow for numerous accommodations and modifications in addition to supplemental education services to enable students with APD to reach their full potential. Improving educational results for children with disabilities is an essential element of the United States' governmental policy to ensure equal opportunity to all children. Discriminatory practices that deny benefits or services, or provide an unequal benefit to any student with a disability are illegal in the United States. These Federal protections are applicable when the child has an impairment that substantially limits one or more major life activities. This chapter aims to provide the reader a basic understanding of these Federal laws, resources when more in-depth knowledge is desired, as well as practical suggestions with regard to classroom modifications and accommodations.

Evolution of Federal Laws for Disability Protection

Over the past 35 years, Congress has passed more laws to protect children with disabilities than most people could have ever imagined.

- 1965, Elementary and Secondary Education Act, Title I (ESEA)
- 1973, Section 504 of the Rehabilitation Act (Section 504)
- 1974, Family Educational Rights and Privacy Act (FERPA)
- 1975, Education for All Handicapped Children Act (Public Law 94-142)
- 1986, Handicapped Children's Protection Act (HCPA)
- 1990, Americans with Disabilities Act (ADA)
- 1997, revisions of the 1975 Public Law 94-142, enacted as Individuals with Disabilities Education Act (IDEA)
- 1999, revisions of the IDEA regulations
- 2001, No Child Left Behind Act
- 2004, Individuals with Disabilities Education Improvement Act; aligns IDEA closely to the No Child Left Behind Act (NCLB)
- 2006, August 14, IDEA Part B final regulations are published in the *Federal Register*

All public school districts that receive Federal funding have pledged to comply with all applicable Federal laws. Some school districts may refer exclusively to their state and local rules and regulations, but they are bound by law to comply with all Federal education laws. If a dispute arises with the school district, it is suggested that parents of children with APD ask, "Where is that in the Federal law?" Parents should make clear that they are advocating for their student's Federal rights under the IDEA, under Section 504, under the ADA, under FERPA, and under NCLB to be sure their student is not being shortchanged by state and local laws (Martin 2004).

Individuals with Disabilities Education Improvement Act 2004

The following information has been extracted directly from the IDEA Improvement of 2004 (Public Law 108-446):

Congress recognizes that disability is a natural part of the human experience and in no way diminishes the right of individuals to participate in or contribute to society. Improving educational results for children with disabilities is an essential element of our national policy of ensuring equality of opportunity, full participation, independent living, and economic self-sufficiency for individuals with disabilities.

Since the enactment and implementation of the Education for All Handicapped Children Act of 1975, this title has been successful in ensuring children with disabilities and the families of such children access to a free appropriate public education and in improving educational results for children with disabilities. However, the implementation of this title has been impeded by low expectations, and an insufficient focus on applying replicable research on proven methods of teaching and learning for children with disabilities.

Almost 30 years of research and experience has demonstrated that the education of children with disabilities can be made more effective by:

1. Having high expectations for such children.
2. Ensuring their access to the general education curriculum in the regular classroom, to the maximum extent possible, in order to—
   a. meet developmental goals and, to the maximum extent possible, the challenging expectations that have been established for all children;
   b. be prepared to lead productive and independent adult lives, to the maximum extent possible.
3. Strengthening the role and responsibility of parents and ensuring that families of such children have meaningful opportunities to participate in the education of their children at school and at home;
4. Coordinating this title with other local, educational service agency, State, and Federal school improvement efforts, including improvement efforts under the Elementary and Secondary Education Act of 1965, in order to ensure that such children benefit from such efforts and that special education can become a service for such children rather than a place where such children are sent.
5. Providing related services, and aids and supports in the regular classroom, to such children, whenever appropriate.
6. Supporting high-quality, intensive preservice preparation and professional development for all personnel who work with children with disabilities to ensure that such personnel have the skills and knowledge necessary to improve the academic achievement and functional performance of children with disabilities.
7. Supporting the development and use of technology, including assistive technology devices and assistive technology services, to maximize accessibility for children with disabilities. (Public Law 108-446)

2006 IDEA Part B Final Regulations

With the release of the final regulations for 2004 IDEA Part B, there are some important changes to the 1999 IDEA Part B regulations. The American Speech-Language-Hearing Association (ASHA) offers a detailed comparison in the *ASHA Leader* periodical, which can also be found at http://www.asha.org/about/publications/leader-online. Highlights of changes that may pertain to children with a diagnosis of APD include:

1. The final regulations removed the provision that requires state education personnel standards to meet the highest requirement for a profession or discipline in that state. The regulation allows the use of paraprofessionals and assistants who are appropriately trained and supervised. This does not permit the use of paraprofessionals as a replacement for

teachers or related services providers. Paraprofessionals are not directly responsible for the provision of services; rather they provide services only under the supervision of special education and related services personnel. ASHA encourages speech-language pathologists and audiologists to work with decision-makers in their state to ensure that personnel standards are maintained.

2. Free appropriate public education (FAPE) has been revised to clarify that a FAPE must be available to any individual child with a disability who needs special education and related services, even though the child has not failed or been retained in a course and is advancing from grade to grade. Additional language has been added to clarify that public agencies provide access to nonacademic and extracurricular services and activities and this includes the provision of supplementary aids and services determined appropriate and necessary by the child's IEP Team.
3. "Child Find" for parentally-placed private school children with disabilities is now determined by the geographic location of the private school, not the residence of the student. Even if the student resides in a different state, that student will be included in the local education agencies (LEA) Child Find, including evaluations and re-evaluations. This topic is reviewed in depth later in this chapter.
4. All the requirements included in IDEA 2004 for evaluations, eligibility determinations, individualized education programs, and educational placements apply to students suspected of having a specific learning disability. In addition, IDEA 2004 provides local education agencies (LEA) with alternative methods to use in identifying children with learning disabilities. In determining whether a child has a specific learning disability, the LEA is not required to take into consideration whether a child has a severe discrepancy between achievement and intellectual ability in oral expression, listening comprehension, written expressions, basic reading skill, reading comprehension, mathematical calculation, or mathematical reasoning. In hearings related to the reauthorization of IDEA, Congress found that:

   > There is no evidence that the IQ–achievement discrepancy formulas can be applied in a consistent and meaningful (reliable and valid) manner. In addition, this approach has been particularly problematic for students living in poverty or culturally and linguistically different backgrounds, who may be erroneously viewed as having intrinsic intellectual limitations when their differences on such tests really reflect lack of experience or educational opportunity.

5. IDEA 2004 also indicates that, in determining whether a child has a specific learning disability, a local

education agency may use a process that determines if a child responds to scientific, research-based intervention as a part of the evaluation procedures used to determine if the child is a child with a disability. Generically, this is known as Response to Intervention (RTI).

6. A member of the IEP team is not required to attend the IEP meeting if that member's area is not being discussed, or if the parent and local education agency agree in writing that the member may submit written input prior to the meeting in lieu of attendance.
7. Development, review, and revision of the IEP has been reworded to include "the academic, developmental, and functional needs of the child." Also, IEPs may be amended without a team meeting if the parent and LEA agree.
8. The wording for the definition of an IEP has been changed from "educational performance" to "academic achievement and functional performance," with the term functional being generally understood to refer to skills/activities that are not related to the child's academic achievement. Measurable annual goals have been clarified as "including academic and functional goals." Short-term objectives are now only required for children with disabilities who take alternative assessments aligned to alternative achievement standards. Special education services must now be "based on peer-reviewed research to the extent practicable."
9. The term "modifications" has been changed to "appropriate accommodations" and the phrase "how the child's parents will be regularly informed" has been changed to "when periodic reports . . . will be provided" (http://www.asha.com).

Response to Intervention

The reauthorization of IDEA 2004 provides an opportunity to address concerns about the appropriate identification of students with specific learning disabilities (SLD). The rationale for Response to Intervention (RTI) as part of an alternative approach to the identification process is to improve instruction and provide more immediate help to struggling students and to prevent over-identification of students as SLD. The Education Department urges states and school districts to adopt RTI models. The success of RTI will depend on whether it is appropriately implemented by highly trained professionals. Some experts embrace RTI whereas others are skeptical (http://www.wrightslaw.com).

After discussions with school district staffs and others, the National Research Center on Learning Disabilities (NRCLD) presents the following core concepts of RTI (funding for NRCLD is provided by the U.S. Office of Special Education):

- Students receive high-quality instruction in their general education setting
- General education instruction is research-based
- General education instructors and staff assume an active role in students' assessment in that curriculum

- School staff conduct universal screening of academics and behavior
- Continuous progress monitoring of student performance occurs
- Continuous progress monitoring pinpoints students' specific difficulties
- School staff implement specific, research-based interventions to address the student's difficulties
- School staff use progress-monitoring data to determine interventions' effectiveness and to make any modifications as needed
- Systematic assessment is completed of the fidelity or integrity with which instruction and interventions are implemented
- The RTI model is well described in written documents (so that the procedures and criteria used in schools can be compared to the documents)
- Sites can be designated as using a "standardized" treatment protocol or an individualized, problem-solving model.

Furthermore, the NRCLD reports RTI models have also been implemented with variations. Some attributes common to many RTI implementations include the following:

- The concept of multiple tiers of increasingly intense student interventions
- Implementation of a differentiated curriculum
- Instruction delivered by staff other than the classroom teacher
- Varied duration, frequency, and time of interventions
- Categorical or noncategorical placement decisions
- Severity levels for placement decisions
- Use of a problem-solving model or standardized treatment protocol for addressing students' difficulties.

The Center on Accelerating Student Learning (CASL) receives federal funding from the U.S. Office of Special Education Programs (OSEP) and has specifically investigated the nature of nonresponsiveness to generally effective instruction. The directors of CASL are Lynn Fuchs and Doug Fuchs of Vanderbilt University. With IDEA 2004, educators now can use RTI as a substitute for, or supplement to, IQ-achievement discrepancy to identify students with learning disabilities. CASL defines RTI by specifying a four-step process and distinguishes between what they deem are "acceptable practices" from more desirable "best practices." They emphasize that their "blueprint" for RTI is but one way to define RTI (Fuchs & Fuchs, 2005).

Blueprint for RTI

Step 1: Screening

In the first month of the school year, students are screened to identify those "at risk for school failure." *Acceptable Practices*: The previous year's state assessment scores are reviewed to identify any student scoring below the 25th percentile in reading or math; or an achievement test is administered to all children in a given grade, with at-risk children designated as those scoring below the 25th percentile. Students can also be identified by teachers or parents. *Best Practices:* Everyone is assessed using brief screening tools that demonstrate diagnostic utility for predicting performance on the reading and math state assessments or only those students who perform below the 25th percentile on the previous year's state assessment, or who perform below the 25th percentile on a more current achievement test are screened individually with tools that have diagnostic usefulness.

Step 2a: Implementing Classroom Instruction (Tier 1; Responsibility: General Education)

Students receive instruction in general education in conjunction with No Child Left Behind and the Adequate Yearly Progress provision. *Acceptable Practice:* School districts implement classroom instruction that reflects sound instructional design principles. *Best Practice:* School districts choose evidence-based curricula and instruction, and provide teachers with relevant and rigorous professional development. Teachers implement the curricula and instruction, and their fidelity of implementation is documented.

Step 2b: Monitoring Responsiveness to Classroom Instruction (Tier 1; Responsibility: General Education)

At-risk students are monitored for 8 weeks to identify a subset that responds inadequately to general education. *Acceptable Practice:* At the end of 8 weeks, at-risk students are administered a screening tool or brief standardized achievement test in the area of risk (e.g., reading or math). Adequate Tier 1 response is determined by a score above the 16th percentile. *Best Practice:* At-risk students are assessed every week for 8 weeks in the area of risk using brief monitoring tools. Adequate Tier 1 response is determined using (a) local or national normative estimates for weekly improvement OR (b) criterion-referenced figures for weekly improvement.

Step 3a: Implementing a Supplementary, Diagnostic Instructional Trial (Tier 2; Responsibility: General and Special Education)

Tier 1 nonresponders receive an 8-week supplementary, diagnostic instructional trial. *Acceptable Practice:* The special educator and colleagues (e.g., school psychologist, speech/language clinician) collaboratively problem-solve to design a supplementary, diagnostic instructional trial tailored to the needs of the student. This instruction may be implemented by the classroom teacher, but more likely by a specialist or an aide trained by the specialist. *Best Practice:* The Tier 1 nonresponder participates in small-group instruction with no more than two additional students who share similar needs. The group is taught 30 minutes per session, a minimum of three times per week by a certified teacher or aide using a scientifically validated, standard tutoring protocol.

Step 3b: Monitoring Responsiveness to a Supplementary, Diagnostic Instructional Trial (Tier 2; Responsibility: General Education and Special Education)

Response to the 8-week Tier 2 supplementary, diagnostic trial is monitored to identify the subset of students who respond inadequately (i.e., Tier 2 nonresponders). *Acceptable Practice:* At the end of 8 weeks, at-risk students are administered a screening tool or brief standardized achievement test in the area of risk. Adequate Tier 2 response is specified in terms of a score above the 16th percentile. *Best Practice:* At-risk students are assessed every week for 8 weeks in the areas of risk using brief monitoring tools. Adequate Tier 2 response is determined using (a) local or national normative estimates for weekly improvement OR (b) criterion-referenced figures for weekly improvement.

Step 4: Designation of LD, and Special Education Placement (Responsibility: General and Special Education)

The Tier 2 nonresponders receive an individualized, comprehensive evaluation that addresses all eligibility determination, evaluation, and procedural safeguards specified in the IDEA 2004 (Fuchs & Fuchs 2005).

Section 504 and the ADA

Section 504 of the Rehabilitation Act of 1973 and Title II of the Americans with Disabilities Act (ADA) are civil rights laws that prohibit discrimination on the basis of a disability. It is illegal under the Section 504 and ADA regulations for public school systems to use policies and practices that intentionally or unintentionally result in discrimination. The regulation for both Section 504 and ADA use the term "criteria and methods of administration." "Criteria" are written or formal policies; "methods of administration" are the school system's actual practices and procedures. This ban on discriminatory practices includes those that:

- Have the effect of discriminating against students with disabilities, or
- Have the effect of defeating or impairing accomplishment of the objectives of the education program in regard to students with disabilities.

Specifically, these laws make it illegal for public schools to discriminate on the basis of disability by:

- Denying a student the opportunity to participate in or benefit from a benefit or service,
- Providing an opportunity to participate or benefit that is unequal to that provided to others,
- Providing a benefit or service that is not as effective as that provided to others,
- Providing different or separate benefits or services, unless it is necessary to provide benefits or services that are as effective as those provided to others (http://www.wrightslaw.com).

Section 504 ensures that children with disabilities have equal access to an education. The ADA broadens the agencies and businesses that must comply with the nondiscrimination and accessibility provisions of the law. Unlike the Individuals with Disabilities Education Act (IDEA) which was last amended in 2004, Section 504 and the ADA do *not* ensure that a child with a disability will receive an Individualized Educational Program (IEP). The child who has a disability, such as auditory processing disorder, does not automatically qualify for special education services under the IDEA. To be eligible for protections under Section 504, the child must have a physical or mental impairment. This impairment must substantially limit one or more major life activities. Major life activities include walking, seeing, hearing, speaking, breathing, learning, reading, writing, performing math calculations, working, caring for oneself, and performing manual tasks. The key is whether the child has an "impairment" that "substantially limits one or more major life activities." Section 504 requires an evaluation that draws information from a variety of sources and it does not require a meeting prior to changing a child's placement. (http://www.wrightslaw.com).

Which Is Better: IDEA or Section 504 Advocacy?

Some parents and educators assume that protection under Section 504 is more desirable than protection under the IDEA. According to the Web site, http://www.wrightslaw.com, the child who receives Section 504 protections has fewer rights than the child who receives special education services under the IDEA. The child who receives special education services under the IDEA is automatically protected under Section 504. Section 504 protects a child from discrimination; however, if a child does not receive special education services under IDEA, this child does not have the procedural protections that are available under the IDEA statute. Section 504 ensures that a child has access to the same free appropriate public education that is available to children who are not disabled. Section 504 does not require public schools to provide an educational program that is individualized to meet the unique needs of the child with the goal of enabling the child to become independent and self-sufficient. The public schools obligation is only to provide an education that is equal to that provided to the non-disabled population. However, under Section 504 the child may receive accommodations and modifications that are not available to children who are not disabled (http://www.wrightslaw.com).

Additional procedural safeguards that are included with IDEA but not Section 504 deal with discipline issues and "Prior Written Notice" requirements. If a Section 504 child misbehaves and the school determines that the behavior is not a manifestation of the disability, the child can be expelled from school permanently. The IDEA child has the right to a Free Appropriate Public Education, even if expelled from school. Section 504 and the ADA do not provide these protections. The IDEA includes numerous procedural safeguards designed to protect the child and parents. These include prior written notice before any change of placement and the right to independent educational evaluation at public expense. Section 504 does not include these protections. For parents who disagree with identification, evaluation, or placement, both Section 504 and IDEA require school districts to conduct impartial hearings. Under 504, the parent has the right to participate and obtain representation by counsel, but other details are left to the discretion of the school district (http://www.wrightslaw.com).

Reed Martin, J.D. (2004) in his book, *"Section 504" How You Can Use It to Get Your Child What They Need,* makes a case for advocacy using Section 504. He states that he has been advocating for students with disabilities for over 30 years and Section 504 is the strongest tool available for advocacy. Martin claims that Section 504 provides for very specific protections for disabled children. The IDEA does not have such specific protections, but there is nothing in the IDEA that can restrict a parent from using Section 504 when advocating for their child. According to Martin, many local school districts and state education agencies know very little about Section 504. It is up to the parent to request the appropriate documents. Martin further claims that Section 504 covers more than simple accommodations in the regular classroom. All of a student's activities are covered including academics, nonacademics, extracurricular, preschool, post-school, transportation, and even a private educational placement. If a parent feels the school district is deliberately indifferent to their student's learning differences, Martin outlines 10 steps for making a successful complaint.

1. Notify in writing, school personnel about the problem(s). Be prepared to prove the date of notification, the person who was notified, and the nature of the complaint.
2. Indicate that the school district or state education agency is a recipient of Federal financial assistance.
3. Show that the person you complained to has the authority to investigate your complaint and has the authority to correct the wrong when they investigate.
4. State what the discriminatory activity against the child is or was.
5. State that the school district exercises control over the site where the discrimination occurred (or is occurring) and that the school district exercises control over the personnel who committed the discriminatory acts.
6. Explain that the discrimination was not a single act but was severe and pervasive.
7. Show that the discrimination excluded the student from continuing their participation in school, or denied the student the benefits of what the other students in school are able to access.
8. Indicate what the school needs to stop doing wrong and/or what the school needs to start doing right to stop this harm or to remediate its effects on the child.
9. Indicate that the school district or state education agency does not have the required "grievance procedures" available under Section 504 (even if the child has an Individual Educational Plan under the IDEA) that would allow "prompt and equitable resolu-

tion" of the complaint, with the result that the discrimination continued to harm the child.

10. State that if the recipient of this complaint letter does not investigate, it shows deliberate indifference to the discrimination. Furthermore, if the recipient of the complaint letter does investigate but takes no corrective action based on their findings, or takes action that is ineffective in ending the discrimination, this also shows deliberate indifference to the discrimination.

Martin provides a sample letter in his book that covers these key points (Martin, 2001).

According to Martin, a Section 504 plan is based on a three-pronged evaluation: first establish that the student has "a mental or physical impairment," second establish that it is substantially limiting the student, and three that it is limiting one or more major life activities (walking, seeing, hearing, speaking, breathing, learning, reading, writing, performing math calculations, working, caring for oneself, and performing manual tasks). To determine whether a student is *substantially limited*, compare the student to a typical child. A partial list of skills that are typically expected by the schools but may be challenging for the student with an auditory processing disorder includes:

- Understand and follow the school rules
- Respond appropriately to instructions from school personnel
- Ask for help when needed
- Receive information both orally and in writing
- Communicate effectively through speech or writing to teachers and classmates
- Participate in class as required by the teacher
- Work independently
- Work in groups
- Handle the volume of material introduced each day in the regular curriculum
- Handle the rate at which material is introduced in the regular curriculum
- Read and write at grade level
- Not require the use of assistive technology during the day
- Take tests without modifications such as extra time, oral administration, taking the test in a quiet place, or using assistive technology
- Copy down the homework assignments correctly in each class
- Do the required homework each night in a reasonable amount of time
- Take the homework and necessary materials back to school the next day
- Stay for the whole day
- Make up any work that is missed without any great difficulty
- Stay after school and participate in extracurricular activities if interested
- Pass each year and advance to the next grade
- Return to school each fall without substantial regression in skills over the summer
- Take all required exit exams or other tests
- Be on schedule to graduate with a regular diploma after 12 years of instruction.

The inability of a student to perform any of the above listed tasks (or other similar tasks) means they should be addressed in a Section 504 plan for the *conditions, manner, or duration under which they can be performed in comparison to most people.* The goal of a Section 504 plan is normative behavior. The measurement and evaluation of the plan would determine whether to move to the next step or keep the accommodation (Martin, 2001).

If a State Education Agency does not respond to a complaint or indicates that it has no responsibility under Section 504, the parents or child advocates must establish their school district and state education agency's duty under Section 504. State and local school agencies must swear that they are in compliance with Section 504 when they request Federal funding. Martin (2001) suggests that parents write to request a copy of the document sent to the U.S. Department of Education indicating that they are in compliance with Section 504. In effect, state and local agencies would be ineligible to receive Federal monies if they are not in compliance with Section 504. State education agencies are forbidden to pass Federal assistance to local education agencies if that would perpetuate discrimination. The state agencies are responsible for policing Section 504 compliance of all local education agencies. Both state and local agencies must have a designated employee to coordinate Section 504 compliance efforts (Martin 2001).

No Child Left Behind Act

In 2001 Congress passed the Federal law entitled No Child Left Behind (NCLB). The intent of this law was to ensure that even children who function so differently that they are hard to test, hard to teach, and almost impossible to compare with other children are counted. **All children will be counted because all children do count.** This law further ensures that no child is left out of the process. By adding this newest Federal statute (No Child Left Behind), to the other disability rights statutes parents and professionals can advocate even more strongly for their students. The Congress wants every child to be a successful reader by the end of third grade. In order to achieve this, Congress wants children found, identified, evaluated and placed earlier than ever before; therefore "Child Find" is highly emphasized in NCLB. The law wants children identified, evaluated, and placed in an appropriate program by age three (Martin, 2004).

Under NCLB, the evaluation of a student provides a comparison to where they should be on the grade level of a typical student, their age, and what the problems are that keep this student from being on grade level. Next it is important to determine the methodology that is "most suitable to the child's needs and it must be a proven methodology based on scientific research." Many schools argue that methodology cannot be discussed at the IEP meeting and that methodology is left up to the school district. If the evaluation results show the need for a specific methodology that is scientifically proven, then under NCLB, parents have a right to ask for that methodology. They further have the right to write and ask for a full written explanation of the teacher's credentials, training, and experience with that particular methodology. Furthermore, if the methodology does not seem to be working with that child, parents have a right to inquire whether the teacher is actually using it. If the desired result is not being accomplished with the student, there may be a need to explore other methodologies to meet that child's needs. If teacher training and retraining does not bring the child closer to grade level, then the parent can inquire about a Master Teacher being assigned to either teach the child or to supervise those teaching the child (Martin, 2004).

Many parents are told that their student has to be more than two grades behind academically before they can be considered for "identification" and "evaluation" that could lead to special help. This would obviously save schools a lot of dollars, but it prevents many school children from getting the help they need, when they need it, to be able to eventually perform at grade level. That is not in keeping with NCLB. But NCLB is not intended to stand by itself as a law; however, it can be added to other special education laws to advocate for children with special needs. Parents should make it clear that they are advocating for their student's Federal rights under the Individuals with Disabilities Education Improvement Act (IDEA), under Section 504, under the American Disabilities Act, (ADA), under Family Educational Rights and Privacy Act (FERPA), and under No Child Left Behind (NCLB) (Martin, 2004).

NCLB includes compensatory school services and extended school year services. However, there has been at least one major school district that decided not to take "Title I" funding. One of the arguments raised is that the Federal government did not fully fund all the costs associated with NCLB compliance. However, even if the school district does not take the Title I funding connected to NCLB, the school district is required to do much of what is in NCLB under IDEA, Section 504, and the ADA. Under the IDEA parents have a right to request a program carried on after school hours, a program carried on over the summer, a program carried on after the time that a student would typically have exited the secondary education program, compensatory services, and transfer to another school. Now with NCLB aligning with the IDEA, it should be easier to discuss these options with the school district (Martin, 2004).

Students with disabilities have the right to the full curriculum at school, including full academic, nonacademic, and extracurricular activities at school. Some students are given a shortened day because their behavior is too disruptive and they get less exposure to nonacademic activities because there are not adequate personnel available and trained to deal with students with disabilities. This is a violation of the IDEA, Section 504, and the ADA, as well as NCLB (Martin, 2004).

Children Placed by Parents in Private Schools

According to the Office of Special Education Programs of the U.S. Department of Education, the obligation of states and local education agencies (LEAs) to children with disabilities enrolled by their parents in private elementary schools and secondary school changed with the final regulations of IDEA of 2004. IDEA 2004 now requires that after timely and meaningful consultation with private school representatives, the LEA must conduct a thorough and complete child find process to determine the number of parentally placed children with disabilities attending private schools located in the LEA. (Previously, the responsibility to conduct child find rested with the LEA in which the children resided.) In addition, IDEA 2004 makes clear that the obligation to spend a proportionate amount to provide services to children with disabilities enrolled by their parents in private schools now refers to children enrolled by their parents in private elementary schools and secondary schools "in the school district served by a local education agency."

IDEA 2004 defines "consultation" as discussions between the LEA, private school representatives, and parents (or their representatives) of children with disabilities. The consultation should provide positive and productive working relationships and the opportunity for all parties to express their views. A unilateral offer of services by an LEA with no opportunity for discussion is not adequate consultation. The consultation process must include the following:

- The child-find process and how children suspected of having a disability can participate equitably, including how parents, teachers, and private school officials will be informed of the process;
- The determination of the proportionate share of Federal funds available to serve parentally placed private school children with disabilities, including how the proportionate share of those funds was calculated;
- How the consultation process among representatives of the agency, private school, and parents will take place, including how the process will operate throughout the school year to ensure that parentally placed private school children with disabilities identified through the child find process can meaningfully participate in special education and related services;
- How, where, and by whom special education and related services will be provided, including a discussion of types of services—including direct services and alternative service-delivery mechanisms, as well as how such services will be apportioned if funds are insufficient to serve all children—and how and when these decisions will be made;
- How, if the LEA representatives disagree with the views of the private school officials on the provision of services or the types of services whether provided directly or through a contract, the LEA will provide to the private school officials, a written explanation of the reasons why the LEA chose not to adopt the recommendation of the private school officials.

The intention of the "child find" process is to obtain an accurate count of the number of eligible private school children with disabilities in private schools in order to calculate the proportionate share of funds that the LEA must expend annually for services for parentally-placed private school children with disabilities. Furthermore, the child find activities carried out by the LEAs for private school children must be similar to activities undertaken for child find in public schools. These activities must be completed in a time period comparable to those activities for public school students; this includes individual evaluations. The amounts expended for child find, including individual evaluations, cannot be deducted from the required amount of funds to be expended on special education and related services.

Equitable services must be provided by employees of a public agency or through contract by the public agency with an individual, association, agency, organization or other entity. An LEA may use Part B funds (of the IDEA 2004) to make public school personnel available in other than public facilities to the extent necessary to provide equitable services for private school children with disabilities and if those services are not normally provided by the private school. An LEA may use Part B funds to pay for the services of an employee of a private school to provide equitable services if the employee performs the services outside of his or her regular hours of duty and the employee performs the services under public supervision and control.

Services offered to parentally placed private school children with disabilities may be provided on site at a child's private school, including a religious school, to the extent consistent with law, or at another location. In the interests of the child, efforts should be made to provide services as near as possible to the child's private school so as not to unduly disrupt the child's education experience. The phrase "extent consistent with law" is statutory, and is interpreted to mean that the provision of services on the premises of a private school takes place in a manner that would not violate the Establishment Clause of the First Amendment to the U.S. Constitution and would not be inconsistent with applicable state constitutions or law.

The location of services is one of the subjects discussed during the consultation process among LEA officials, private school representatives, and representatives of parents of parentally placed private school children with disabilities. The public agency makes the final decision, after this consultation process.

Private school officials may not obligate or receive Part B funds. The LEA must control and administer the funds used to provide special education and related services to parentally-placed private school children with disabilities, and maintain title to materials, equipment and property purchased with those funds. Part B funds for equitable services may not be paid directly to a private school.

The public agency may place equipment and supplies in a private school for the period of time needed for the program. The public agency must ensure that equipment and supplies placed in a private school are used only for Part B purposes and can be removed from the private school without remodeling the private school facility. The public agency must remove equipment and supplies from a private school if the equipment and supplies are no longer needed for Part B purposes or if removal is necessary to avoid unauthorized use of the equipment and supplies for other than Part B purposes.

Whether home-schooled children with disabilities are considered parentally placed private school children with disabilities is determined by the state. If the state recognizes home schools or home daycare as private elementary schools and secondary schools, children with disabilities in those home schools or home daycare must be treated in the same way as other parentally placed private school children with disabilities.

If the LEA where the private elementary or secondary school is located conducts an individual evaluation on a child and the parents disagree with the evaluation and wish to have an independent educational evaluation (IEE) conducted, the parents should file the request for an IEE with the LEA that conducted the evaluation with which the parents disagree. (U.S. Department of Education, Office of Special Education Programs).

Inclusion of All Students in Standards-Based Assessment

IDEA provides that the performance results of children with disabilities be reported to the public just as performance results are reported for all children, as long as the reporting method will not result in identifying the performance of individual children. IDEA places significant emphasis on ensuring that children with disabilities participate in general state and district-wide assessment programs, with appropriate accommodations if necessary as determined by the IEP team. IDEA also provides that alternate assessments be developed and provided for students for whom the regular assessment is deemed inappropriate.

Standards-based reform for all children is just one of many policy decisions facing educational decision makers. Tension exists between the traditional special education focus on individual student achievement and the corresponding general education focus on group achievement—with neither side in full agreement as to the whos, whats, and wherefores of standard-based reform. Many students continue to be excluded from accountability systems; in fact, some state policies encourage exclusions and exemptions. Within the education profession, some opposition to including students with disabilities in reform efforts is based on a belief that doing so would, in fact, be harmful to students.

A mindset of universal access to standards-based reform is necessary if students with disabilities are to be equally included in accountability systems. Including students with disabilities in standards-based reform initiatives requires that policies are coordinated and coherent. Academic and nonacademic results are clear for all students, individual student results are honored, and systems are held accountable for student progress.

On December 15, 2005, the Department of Education published a Notice of Proposed Rulemaking (NPRM) on the topic of permitting states to develop modified achievement standards and assessments based on those standards for certain students with disabilities. These assessments would be for students with disabilities who do not have the most significant cognitive disabilities and for whom assessments based on alternative achievement standards would be inappropriate. A copy of the proposed regulations has been posted on the Department's Web site at: http://www.ed.gov/legislation/FedRegister/proprule/2005-4/121505a.pdf.

Because many students with disabilities may not achieve grade-level proficiency within the school year covered by their IEP (or Section 504 plan) in spite of high-quality instruction, the Department of Education is permitting states to develop and implement modified achievements standards for this limited group of students. The proposed regulations require that states have in their guidelines for IEP teams certain key criteria to ensure that students with disabilities are not inappropriately held to modified achievement standards. The criteria are as follows:

1. The student's disability has precluded the student from achieving grade-level proficiency, as demonstrated by objective evidence such as—
   - State's Title I assessments; or
   - Other assessment data that can validly document academic achievement.
2. The student's progress in response to high-quality instruction, including special education and related services designed to meet the student's needs, is such that the student is not likely to achieve grade-level proficiency within a year. Progress must be measured by multiple indicators, over a period of time, and with valid assessments.
3. The student is receiving instruction in the grade-level curriculum for the subjects in which the student is being assessed.
4. Student eligibility for being assessed based on modified achievement standards is not limited to a particular disability category.
5. A student may be assessed based on modified achievement standards in one or more subjects assessed as part of the state assessment system.
6. A student's IEP team must review annually whether it is appropriate for the student to be assessed based on modified achievement standards

The proposed regulations would not require states to develop an entirely new assessment. A state could modify an existing grade-level assessment for this purpose. Out-of-level assessments will not meet the requirements of these proposed regulations, as they are not aligned to grade-level content standards. The basic requirements for the assessments are that they:

- Be aligned to grade-level content standards;
- Yield results in reading/language arts and mathematics separately;
- Meet the requirements for high technical quality including validity and reliability; and
- Fit coherently in the state assessment system.

Some schools may not make Adequate Yearly Progress (AYP) because students with disabilities did not score well on the state test. Only by holding schools accountable for *all* students will the spotlight of attention and necessary resources be directed to those children most in need of assistance and most often left behind academically.

With regard to state testing, accommodations are changes in testing materials or procedures, such as repeating directions or allowing extended time, that, by design, do not invalidate the student's test score. In other words, accommodations help students access the material but do not give students with disabilities an unfair advantage. These accommodations instead help level the playing field so that a test measures what the student knows and can do and not the effect of the child's disability. It is not unfair to allow valid accommodations during a test because these accommodations allow a test to measure the student's knowledge and skills rather than the student's disability.

The state is responsible for analyzing accommodations to determine which are acceptable on the basis of the test design. It is important for the state to make sure that students use only those accommodations that result in a valid score. For example, if the assessment is supposed to measure how well a student decodes text, reading the test aloud to the student would result in an invalid score.

For further information on this topic, contact the U.S. Office of Special Education Programs (OSEP).

School Accommodations and Modifications

The Families and Advocates Partnership for Education (FAPE) project is a partnership that aims to improve the educational outcomes for children with disabilities. (This acronym is not to be confused with *Free Appropriate Public Education*, also known as FAPE). This project links families, advocates, and self-advocates to information about the IDEA. The project is designed to address the information needs of the 6 million families throughout the country whose children with disabilities receive special education services. The FAPE project is coordinated by the PACER Center, Inc. Their website provides excellent information about accommodations and modifications. Although the IDEA does not define accommodations or modifications, there is some general agreement as to what they mean. An *accommodation* allows a student to complete the same assignment or test as other students, but with a change in the timing, formatting, setting, scheduling, response, and/or presentation. An accommodation does not alter in any significant way what the test or assignment measures. Examples would include a student taking a test alone in a quiet room or a student listening to a textbook on compact disc.

A *modification* is an adjustment to an assignment or a test that changes the standard or what the test or assignment is supposed to measure. Examples would include a student completing work on *part* of a standard or a student completing an alternative assignment that is more easily achievable than the standard assignment.

Accommodations and modifications should be chosen to fit the student's individual needs. A student who is protected by the IDEA will have an Individualized Education Program (IEP). Needed modifications and accommodations should be written into a student's IEP or Section 504 Plan. Once the IEP team writes the accommodations/modifications into the IEP or Section 504 Plan, they must, by law, be provided.

This comprehensive list of accommodations and modifications is offered by the Families and Advocates Partnership for Education (FAPE) project of PACER Center, Inc.

Textbooks

- Provide alternative books with similar concepts, but at an easier reading level.
- Provide audiotapes of textbooks and have the student follow the text while listening.
- Provide summaries of chapters.
- Provide interesting reading material at or slightly above the student's comfortable reading level.
- Use peer readers.
- Use marker to highlight important textbook sections.
- Use word-for-word sentence fill-ins.
- Provide two sets of textbooks, one for home and one for school.
- Use index cards to record major themes.
- Provide the student with a list of discussion questions before reading the material.
- Give page numbers to help the student find answers.
- Provide books and other written materials in alternative formats such as Braille or large print.

Curriculum

- Shorten assignments to focus on mastery of key concepts.
- Shorten spelling tests to focus on mastering the most functional words.
- Substitute alternatives for written assignments (clay models, posters, panoramas, collections, etc.).
- Specify and list exactly what the student will need to learn to pass. Review this frequently.
- Modify expectations based on student needs (e.g., "When you have read this chapter, you should be able to list three reasons for the Civil War.").
- Give alternatives to long written reports (e.g., write several short reports, preview new audiovisual materials and write a short review, give an oral report on an assigned topic).

Classroom Environment

- Develop individualized rules for the student.
- Evaluate the classroom structure against the student's needs (flexible structure, firm limits, etc.).
- Keep workspaces clear of unrelated materials.
- Keep the classroom quiet during intense learning times.
- Reduce visual distractions in the classroom (mobiles, etc.).
- Provide a computer for written work.
- Seat the student close to the teacher or a positive role model.
- Use a study carrel. (Provide extras so that the student is not singled out.)
- Seat student away from windows or doorways.
- Provide an unobstructed view of the chalkboard, teacher, movie screen, and so forth.
- Keep extra supplies of classroom materials (pencils, books,) on hand.
- Use alternatives to crossword puzzles or word finds.
- Maintain adequate space between desks.

Directions

- Use both oral and printed directions.
- Give directions in small steps and in as few words as possible.

- Number and sequence the steps in a task.
- Have student repeat the directions for a task.
- Provide visual aids.
- Show a model of the end product of directions (e.g., a completed math problem or finished quiz).
- Stand near the student when giving directions or presenting a lesson.

Time/Transitions

- Alert student several minutes before a transition from one activity to another is planned; give several reminders.
- Provide additional time to complete a task.
- Allow extra time to turn in homework without penalty.
- Provide assistance when moving about the building.

Handwriting

- Use worksheets that require minimal writing.
- Use fill-in questions with space for a brief response rather than a short essay.
- Provide a "designated note-taker" or photocopy of other student's or teacher's notes. (Do not require a poor note-taker or a student with no friends to arrange with another student for notes.)
- Provide a print outline with videotapes and filmstrips.
- Provide a print copy of any assignments or directions written on the blackboard.
- Omit assignments that require copying, or let the student use a tape recorder to dictate answers.

Grading

- Provide a partial grade based on individual progress or effort.
- Use daily or frequent grading averaged into a grade for the quarter.
- Weight daily work higher than tests for a student who performs poorly on tests.
- Mark the correct answers rather than the incorrect ones.
- Permit a student to rework missed problems for a better grade.
- Average grades out when assignments are reworked, or grade on corrected work.
- Use a pass-fail or an alternative grading system when the student is assessed on his or her own growth.

Tests

- Go over directions orally.
- Teach the student how to take tests (e.g., how to review, to plan time for each section).
- Provide a vocabulary list with definitions.
- Permit as much time as needed to finish tests.
- Allow tests to be taken in a room with few distractions (e.g., the library).
- Give progress reports instead of grades.
- Grade spelling separately from content.
- Provide typed test materials, not tests written in cursive.

- Allow take-home or open-book tests.
- Provide possible answers for fill-in-the blank sections.
- Provide the first letter of the missing word.

Math

- Allow the student to use a calculator without penalty.
- Group similar problems together (e.g., all addition in one section).
- Provide fewer problems on a worksheet (e.g., 4 to 6 problems on a page, rather than 20 or 30).
- Require fewer problems to attain passing grades.
- Use enlarged graph paper to write problems to help the student keep numbers in columns.
- Provide a table of math facts for reference.
- Tape a number line to the student's desk.
- Read and explain story problems, or break problems into smaller steps.
- Use pictures or graphics.

Other

- Use Post-it notes to mark assignments in textbooks.
- Check progress and provide feedback often in the first few minutes of each assignment.
- Place a ruler under sentences being read for better tracking.
- Introduce an overview of long-term assignments so the student knows what is expected and when it is due.
- Break long-term assignments into small, sequential steps, with daily monitoring and frequent grading.
- Have the student practice presenting in a small group before presenting to the class.
- Hand out worksheets one at a time.
- Sequence work, with easiest part first.
- Provide study guides and study questions that directly relate to tests.
- Reinforce student for recording assignments and due dates in a notebook or planner.
- Draw arrows on worksheets, whiteboard, or overheads to show how ideas are related, or use other graphic organizers such as flow charts.

Behavior

- Arrange a "check-in" time to organize the day.
- Pair the student with another student who is a good behavior model for class projects.
- Modify school rules that may discriminate against the student.
- Use nonverbal cues to remind the student of rule violations.
- Amend consequences for rule violations (e.g., reward a forgetful student for remembering to bring pencils to class, rather than punishing the failure to remember).
- Minimize the use of punishment; provide positive as well as negative consequences.
- Develop an individualized behavior intervention plan that is positive and consistent with the student's ability and skills.
- Increase the frequency and immediacy of reinforcement.
- Arrange for the student to leave the classroom voluntarily and go to a designated "safe place" when under high stress.

- Develop a system or a code word to let the student know when behavior is not appropriate.
- Ignore behaviors that are not seriously disruptive.
- Develop interventions for behaviors that are annoying but not deliberate (e.g., provide a small piece of foam rubber for the desk of a student who continually taps a pencil on the desktop).
- Be aware of behavior changes that relate to medication or the length of the school day; modify expectations if appropriate.

For further information, contact PACER Center, Inc., 8161 Normandale Blvd., Minneapolis, MN 55437 http://www.fape.org

According to Reed (2001), the U.S. Department of Education "Joint Policy Memorandum" lists 22 accommodations and modifications that must be available in regular classrooms for Section 504 eligible students. This memorandum indicates that this is not an exclusive list and other items could be added.

1. Providing a structured learning environment
2. Repeating and simplifying instructions about in-class assignments
3. Repeating and simplifying instructions about homework assignments
4. Supplementing verbal instructions with visual instructions
5. Using behavioral management techniques
6. Adjusting class schedules
7. Modifying test delivery
8. Using tape recorders
9. Computer-aided instruction
10. Other audio-visual equipment
11. Selecting modified textbooks
12. Selecting modified workbooks
13. Tailoring homework assignments
14. Consultation with special education
15. Reducing class size
16. Use of one-on-one tutorials
17. Use of classroom aides
18. Use of classroom note-takers
19. Involvement of a services coordinator to oversee implementation of special programs and services
20. Possible modification of nonacademic time such as lunch room
21. Possible modification of nonacademic time such as recess
22. Possible modification of nonacademic time such as physical education

Summary

Individuals with auditory processing disorders typically have normal intelligence yet they experience extreme difficulties in school. We are fortunate in the United States to have many educational laws and regulations that protect children and adults with disabilities. By referencing all of the laws designed to protect children with special needs, parents and professionals can advocate for a Free Appropriate Public Education that is truly appropriate, not simply a program that fits comfortably within the local education agency's budget. This includes students who are parentally placed in private schools. An appropriate education may include special services to students such as speech/language intervention, resource specialist programs, assistive listening devices, adaptive technology, as well as classroom accommodations and modifications to the curriculum. Furthermore, the No Child Left Behind law allows parents to ask for a specific methodology provided the evaluation results show the need for that methodology and the methodology is scientifically proven. The dilemma of course is that local education agencies are facing reduced funding at a rapid rate so there is likely to be strong opposition to requests that will incur additional costs. Nonetheless, Congress has enacted numerous laws to protect these children and it is the duty of each parent to advocate for their child and, when necessary, seek outside counsel.

Key Points Learned

- All public school districts that receive Federal funding have pledged to comply with all applicable Federal laws regardless of state and local rules and regulations.
- Parents should cite all pertinent laws when advocating for their child: Individuals with Disabilities Education Improvement Act (IDEA), Section 504 of the Rehabilitation Act, the Americans with Disabilities Act (ADA), Family Education Rights and Privacy Act (FERPA), and No Child Left Behind (NCLB).
- It is necessary to establish that the student with an auditory processing disorder has "a mental or physical impairment," that is limiting one or more major life activities as applicable to APD (hearing, speaking, learning, reading, writing, and performing math calculations).
- Congress found no evidence that the IQ–achievement discrepancy formulas can be applied in a consistent and meaningful manner and suggests use of response to intervention (RTI) as an alternative method. Although RTI is embraced by some professionals, others are skeptical. It will likely be a time-consuming process for local education agencies to adopt a RTI model, train staff adequately, and successfully implement the model.
- Key steps for making a successful complaint to a local education agency include but are not limited to: (1) written notification of the complaint to school personnel who have the authority to investigate, (2) a clear description of the discriminatory action that was severe and pervasive, (3) establish that the school district is a recipient of Federal funds, (4) show that the discrimination denied the student the

benefits of what other students in school are able to access, and (5) indicate what the school needs to stop doing and/or start doing to correct the discrimination.

- It is not unfair to allow valid accommodations during a test because these accommodations allow a test to measure the student's knowledge and skills rather than the student's disability. This may include repeating directions, allowing extended time, reading the test to the student (unless it is a reading test), and taking a test in a separate room that is free of distractions. This applies to state testing as well as classroom tests.

References

Fuchs, D., & Fuchs, L. S. (2005). Responsiveness-to-intervention: A blueprint for practitioners, policymakers, and parents. *Teaching Exceptional Children*, *38*(1), 57–61.

Martin, R. (2004). *No child with a disability left behind.* Available to purchase and download from http://www.matthewsmediallc.com

Martin, R. (2001). *Section 504: How you can use it to get your child what they need.* Morgantown, WV: Matthews Media, LLC (http://www.reedmartin.com).

Internet Resources

American Speech-Language-Hearing Association: http://www.asha.org

Families and Advocates Partnership for Education (FAPE); a project of PACER Center, Inc., 8161 Normandale Blvd., Minneapolis, MN 55437. http://www.fape.org

National Research Center on Learning Disabilities: http://www.nrcld.org

U.S. Department of Education, Office of Special Education Programs; 330 C Street, SW; Room 3531 Washington, DC 20202, Phone: 202-358-2849, Web site: http://www.ed.gov

Wrightslaw (http://www.wrightslaw.com) is a huge Web site that includes thousands of articles, legal decisions, and news items on different topics relating to educational law.

25

Sample Reports

Deborah Ross-Swain

Overview

Summary reports following comprehensive auditory processing evaluations or assessments are necessary to report the findings, present quantitative and qualitative data, interpret the results, form impressions, and make recommendations for treatment interventions, compensatory strategies, and environmental modifications. The summary evaluation/assessment report is one way to inform the reader of the nature and extent of the auditory processing areas of weakness and the effects on listening, communicating, and learning. However, there is no *one* report format that would be considered to be the *perfect* or *preferred* template for reporting testing findings. The report format is determined by the purpose of the report and who will be reading the report. For example, is the report for a physician who has been following the child for chronic ear infections? Perhaps the report will be submitted to a fiscal intermediary for authorization of services. Furthermore, the report may be prepared for a classroom teacher and an Individualized Educational Plan (IEP) team to make recommendations for educational placement, treatment interventions, and classroom modifications. This chapter offers the reader several types of sample reports that have been prepared by speech-language pathologists and audiologists following auditory processing assessments. These reports reflect different writing styles as well as different styles for interpreting the results.

Reports Prepared by Audiologists

Sample Report 1

The following sample report summarizes findings of an evaluation for auditory and language processing skills.

AUDITORY AND LANGUAGE PROCESSING EVALUATION

Statement of the Problem and Referral

XXX, a 7.8-year-old male, was seen for an auditory and language processing evaluation on 8/26/06, accompanied by his parents who acted as informants. The family was referred by Dr. XXX SLP, CCC who has been treating him for a speech problem. She suspects that an auditory processing deficit is interfering with his learning and attention. According to his mother, XXX has been slow to pronounce his Rs and has been in speech therapy for 6 to 9 months. His speech-language pathologist became increasingly concerned about his letter and number recognition, his ability to remain engaged, and ability to recall words. XXX's educational environment is very relaxed, unstructured, loud, and distractible. The parents have thought about whether this is the most appropriate educational environment for his specific learning needs. XXX is highly distracted, especially in noisy environments.

According to the father, reading skills are not good. XXX had difficulty from the onset and is just beginning to put sounds together. He is described as being organized, but easily distractible and cannot sit for more than 20 minutes. He has difficulty maintaining focus in noisy environments and does not enjoy birthday parties (if noisy). He has no real problems communicating, except for word retrieval difficulty.

Teleconference with XXX, Ph.D. took place on 8/26/06. Dr. XXX indicated difficulty with sound discrimination and blending, possible language processing issues, and attentional concerns.

Educational History

XXX is a regular education student entering the 2nd grade at the XXX School (a private school), receiving no special services. Speech therapy is provided privately by XXX, Ph.D. An oral motor screening was performed by XXX (Fall 2005) Grades are good, with reading ability reportedly below grade level. The Fast For-Word "Language" Computer program is being administrated by XXX.

Social History

XXX is the younger child (brother, XXX, age 10) in an intact professional family (father is a physician, mother a portfolio manager). Socially, he gets along well with others.

Medical History

Pregnancy history was unremarkable. Birth was via a cesarean section with no reported complications. There is no history of middle ear infections. Seasonal asthma is reported to be well controlled. Developmental milestones were reached within normal limits, including speech and language development. Currently, health is reported to be good.

Previous Evaluations (not presented)

The purpose of this evaluation is to determine if auditory and language processing deficits are contributing to XXX's learning and reading difficulties and to learn of any additional strategies or programs available to help him academically.

Direct Evaluation

XXX was cooperative. Attention and eye contact were good. Initially, his mother accompanied him into the sound booth, but he later separated. He was not on any medication for the testing session.

Audiologic Evaluation

Otoscopic examination was unremarkable bilaterally. Pure-tone air conduction audiometry indicated hearing to be within normal limits bilaterally. Speech Reception Thresholds were good (5 dB HL for each ear). Word Recognition scores (CID-W22) were good in quiet and in noise. Most Comfortable Listening Level was normal (55 dB HL). Most Uncomfortable Listening Level (MUCL) was normal (95 to 100 dB HL), with no indication of sound sensitivity.

Tympanometry testing revealed Type A tympanograms bilaterally (normal). Ipsilateral acoustic reflexes were elicited at normal levels (85 to 100 dB HL) at all frequencies. Distortion product otoacoustic emissions testing indicated a "pass" in each ear suggesting normal outer hair cell function of the cochlea. The peripheral system is intact.

Auditory Processing

Following an audiologic assessment to rule out pathology, it is important to administer a battery of different auditory tests to tap the central auditory system. The purpose of testing is to identify an **auditory processing disorder**, which is an inability to integrate auditory information and to recognize, discriminate, and understand the spoken message especially in competing conditions. Such a disorder contributes to poor social skills, language use, or academic performance and can have an impact on language, reading, retrieval, organization, and memory. Language processing testing is necessary to determine the impact of an auditory processing disorder on learning, language comprehension, and use.

General Tests of Auditory Processing

The SCAN C (Revised)—A Test for Auditory Processing Disorders in Children (Keith, 2000)

This test measures one's ability to process difficult stimuli. There are some individuals with normal hearing who exhibit difficulty processing auditory stimuli, presented in unfamiliar acoustic conditions, that is, distorted speech, speech in the presence of background noise, or listening to speech in a reverberant room. This test presents such adverse listening conditions.

Overall results on this test, according to test norms, XXX did not identify a deficit in auditory processing (21st percentile). However, difficulty in the area of auditory figure-ground listening was noted (16th percentile). An atypical left ear advantage was produced suggesting a right hemisphere dominance for language or a neurologically based learning disability.

Staggered Spondaic Word Test (SSW)

This test of central auditory processing requires the listener to respond to two spondaic words (two syllable words) that are presented in a staggered manner—that is, one reaches the right ear while the second reaches the left ear in a stagger. This test attempts to measure the cortical auditory pathways and taxes the skills of integration, decoding, organization, and memory. The pattern is based on percent of errors and on pattern of errors.

XXX's total error score (13) was within the criterion (22) for his age. However, his response to the dichotic listening task produced "Decoding" and "Tolerance Fading Memory" (TFM) patterns, associated with difficulties in reading accuracy, phonics. comprehension, distractibility, short-term, memory, figure-ground listening, receptive and expressive language, and attention. This TFM pattern is consistent with AD/HD.

Phonemic Awareness

This area of phonemic awareness measures ability to discriminate sounds in words and place sounds or blend sounds to make up a word. It is measured using two tests, the Phonemic Synthesis Test (Katz) and the Lindamood Auditory Conceptualization Test. This skill is inherent in decoding which is predictive of reading accuracy.

Phonemic Synthesis Test

This test of sound blending (g-i-f-t = gift) produced a below-criterion score (6); 17 would have been age appropriate, indicating significant difficulty blending sounds into words. This is consistent with Dr. XXX's findings.

The LAC-Lindamood Auditory Conceptualization Test

The test measures the dimension of auditory function judging the number, identity, and sequence of sounds in spoken patterns and conceptualization of sounds within patterns. If a child is unable to manipulate these sound patterns, he or she is at risk for decoding and reading problems. XXX had a score of 27, below the kindergarten level criterion (31–40), several years below his 2nd grade criterion (61–71). His phonemic awareness skills and decoding were not at grade level. He had particular difficulty discriminating, sequencing, and manipulating sounds within words, placing comprehension at risk. Right/left confusion was observed.

Temporal Processing

This is a measure of auditory processing that involves the timing of the spoken message, which is important in comprehension and response accuracy. It is assessed using acoustic cues not words.

The Random Gap Detection Test was used to measure the individual's ability to detect small differences in timing between two tones. It is a nonverbal test obviating the need for language interpretation. It also measures timing discrimination/resolution. In this task, XXX had to tell whether a tone presented was one or two tones. XXX was unable to accurately and consistently discriminate the gaps within the criterion of 2 to 18 msec, indicating temporal processing/resolution skills are not yet developed.

Language Processing Evaluation

Often when there are auditory processing difficulties, they are manifested in language processing problems, executive language dysfunction, such as organization, word finding difficulties, memory deficits, and struggles to formulate thoughts, and express them succinctly in an organized and sequenced manner. Receptive language and comprehension problems can be mistaken for an auditory processing problem. These problems often lead to academic difficulties and interfere with the individual's ability to communicate. Thus there is a need to assess language skills.

Assessment of language was performed using **The Clinical Evaluation of Language Fundamentals—Fourth Edition (CELF-4), 5–8 edition**.

Level 1 and 2 subtests were administered to assess his receptive and expressive language skills. Results are presented by subtest in percentile rank to determine strengths and weaknesses.

Receptive

Following Directions was assessed using the Concepts and Following Directions subtest. Here the student points to objects in response to oral directions of increasing difficulty.

Performance was average, in the 50th percentile. Where he did have difficulty, it (added it back) was in the area of understanding concepts of inclusion/exclusion (and), location (separated, left), sequence (first, last, second), temporal (after, before, then), serialization, and first and third level commands.

Auditory Comprehension

The Understanding Spoken Paragraphs section requires the student to answer questions about paragraphs read aloud by the examiner. The questions target the main idea, details, sequencing, and inferential and predictive information.

XXX scored in the 75th percentile, indicating good auditory comprehension.

Sentence Structure subtest evaluates the student's ability to interpret spoken sentences of increasing length and complexity and to select the pictures that illustrate referential meaning of the sentence. Performance was high average, 75th percentile.

Language Memory

Recalling Sentences

The student imitates sentences presented by the examiner. This is a short-term memory task. Performance was good in the 75th percentile.

Number Repetitions 1 and 2

The student repeats numbers forward and backward. Total performance was in the 84th percentile. For forward numbers, he scored in the 84th percentile and for backward numbers in the 63rd percentile (an organizational task).

Receptive and Expressive

Word Classes Receptive Ability

The subject is asked to select 2 out of 4 items that go together. His score was within average range (37th percentile). He had no difficulty recognizing relationships between words.

Word Classes Expressive Ability

The subject has to explain why the two items belong together. He scored in the 50th percentile. He was able to explain the relationship that linked the items.

Total Word Classes 1 and 2

The total composite score was within average range (37th percentile) for ability to select two out of four items that are related and identify the relationship between the two.

Expressive Language

Expressive Vocabulary

The student identifies an object, person, or activity pictured in the stimulus book. Performance was excellent in the 84th percentile.

In the Formulated Sentences subtest, the student formulates a sentence about the visual stimuli (picture) presented using target words or phrases. He scored average (50th percentile).

Word Structure

The student completes grammatically correct sentences by using correct morphology to mark inflections, deviations, and comparisons, and to select and use appropriate pronouns. Performance was average, 50th percentile.

Word Retrieval/Rapid Naming

The Rapid Automatic Naming (RAN) subtest of the CELF-4 was administered. Here the student names color/shape combinations as rapidly as possible. XXX had 15 errors, outside the criterion of 11 allowable errors and took 155 sec to perform the task, outside the criterion of 150 sec. Performance is described as slow and inaccurate, suggesting difficulty with rapid naming and word retrieval.

Word Associations

The student names words in specific categories within one minute.

XXX's performance did meet criterion (18 for his age). He had a raw score of 27, within age criterion for word knowledge, demonstrating no difficulty recalling names in specific categories.

Core Language Scores and Indexes

	Sum of Scaled Scores	Standard Score	Percentile
Core Language	42	102	55
Receptive Language	31	101	53
Expressive Language	32	103	58
Language Content	32	104	61
Language Structure	44	106	66

Summary

Overall language skills were good, with expressive language (58th percentile) slightly stronger than receptive ability (53rd percentile). Strength was observed in vocabulary (content), sentence structure (grammar), and understanding spoken paragraphs (auditory comprehension). Short-term memory was excellent. Understanding concepts and following directions, understanding and explaining word classes, word structure, and ability to formulate grammatically correct sentences (form) were within average range. Rapid naming was below criterion, suggesting word retrieval difficulty. Age equivalences ranged from 6.9 to 13;0 years. *For a specific error analysis, see the Appendix Item Analysis.

Informal Assessment

Speech and language were informally assessed in conversation. XXX was well related. He was fidgety with his hands and arms. An immature speech and language pattern was observed including poor motor planning (dyspraxic-like speech). Articulation errors consisting of substitutions of th/s, w/v and distortions of [l], [r], and [r blends] and [l] blends were noted.

Attention

McCarney Scale—Home Version

This questionnaire attempts to determine whether an inattentive or hyperactive type of attention deficit disorder exists. The parent completes questions pertaining to frequency of behavioral characteristics. This was completed by the parents.

XXX is not identified as having either an inattentive or hyperactive type of attention deficit on this scale by the parents.

Summary and Recommendations

XXX is an alert, well-related, and cooperative youngster who presents with good language skills but primarily a phonological processing disorder, word retrieval deficit, and a deficiency in auditory figure-ground listening. Given the finding that an auditory processing disorder has not been identified on two tests, he does not qualify as having APD. Hearing is within normal limits bilaterally, with good speech discrimination in quiet and in noise. On a formal test of auditory processing (SCAN-C), an auditory processing disorder is not identified (21st percentile); however, a specific deficiency in the area of auditory figure-ground listening is identified. This suggests that he will have difficulty hearing the message clearly in less than optimal listening conditions (i.e., a noisy classroom) and sorting relevant from irrelevant information. This is consistent with parent report. An atypical left ear advantage produced suggests possible learning issues. On another measure (SSW), the error score does not identify XXX, but auditory processing deficits are seen with "Decoding" and "Tolerance Fading Memory" patterns produced. These are associated with difficulties in reading accuracy, phonics, comprehension, figure-ground listening, distractibility, and attention. Phonemic awareness (decoding) is not at age level, with difficulty discriminating, sequencing, and manipulating sounds within words. His ability to decode is several grade levels below, putting him at risk for a reading disorder (dyslexia). Phonemic synthesis (blending) is deficient. Temporal processing skills (durational timing of acoustic tones) are not yet established and could underlie his speed of listening discrimination and decoding difficulties. Auditory comprehension is adequate.

Receptive and expressive language skills are good. Short-term memory is excellent. Categorization (word classes) is a relatively weak area. Word retrieval issues are observed on a rapid naming task. In conversation, he is well related, but motor planning and speech production errors (distortions and substitutions) affect intelligibility.

In summary, areas of deficit include: discrimination, figure-ground listening, phonemic awareness (decoding and synthesis), temporal processing, word retrieval, and speech production.

The following recommendations are being made to improve auditory and language processing:

1. Given XXX's performance on auditory processing tests and temporal processing, he would benefit from classroom accommodations to include: testing given in a quiet area or room with directions read and explained to ensure understanding, with extended time for testing; preferential seating up front, close to the teacher, away from doors, windows, and other distractions; assistance with note taking; study notes and outlines ahead of lecture. Information should be presented slowly, using pauses.
2. Earobics computer program, home version, for 7 to 10 year olds to improve auditory processing and phonemic awareness. Contact Earobics.com or Super Duper Publications at 1-800-277-8737.
3. Continue speech-language therapy (2 × week) to work on figure-ground listening, phonological processing, categorization, word classes, word retrieval, and speech production. Consider Jack Katz's Phonemic Synthesis Training program (Precision Acoustics). Speech therapy to work on the production of *s*, *th/s*, *v/w*, *l* and *r* blends.
4. Continue Fast ForWord "Language" Computer program and consider following up with "Language to Reading."
5. A specific reading program using a multisensory and phonemic awareness approach (i.e., Lindamood LiPS, Wilson Program or Orton Gillingham) is suggested.
6. Consider a personal FM system for normal hearing listeners to improve signal-to-noise ratio, discrimination, figure-ground listening, and attention. A sound enhancement classroom could be an alternative.
7. Monitor attention in the classroom. If attention becomes an issue, consider a medical evaluation by a pediatric psychiatrist, neurologist, or developmental pediatrician.

XXX should be taught, allowed and encouraged to ask for repetition, clarification, rephrasing, and reduced rate of speaking when necessary. With continued parental support, school accommodations, and specific intervention programs, prognosis for growth is positive.

Sample Report 2

This sample report summarizes the findings from an auditory processing evaluation on a young school-aged child performed by a dually certified professional.

Background Information

XXX is a 6 years, 8 months old, XXX whom Dr. XXX saw for a comprehensive auditory processing assessment on 03/2006. XXX was accompanied to the evaluation by her mother and father who provided background information. Additional background information was obtained from some records provided to this professional for review.

Based on the information provided, XXX is described as having problems in some academic areas in school. XXX's parents stated that math and reading are their daughter's most difficult subjects at school. Additionally, the parents reported that writing is an area in which XXX is not performing up to grade level expectations. They are especially concerned because XXX has an IEP, yet is still not performing well in all of these areas. The parents also described problems for XXX following multistep directions with their observation that she usually follows the last part of the direction and misses the beginning. (This suggests the possibility of a problem with auditory attention or memory that needs to be investigated.)

Because of difficulties with academics, the parents reported that XXX's self-esteem is being negatively impacted. For example, XXX makes statements about herself indicating that she feels she has a problem and she feels lost in class even though everyone else knows what is going on. Additionally, the parents report that homework time has become a problem because XXX breaks down crying, says, "I can't do this," and cannot do any of her homework independently.

Medical and developmental histories provided indicate only one significant issue that could be related to any hearing, auditory processing, or language problems. XXX had her hearing tested in the fall of 2005 because she failed a routine hearing screening at school. The doctor who saw her, Dr. XXX, suggested that there may be some auditory processing problems although hearing, itself, was normal. This indication along with continuing decreases in academic success led the parents to contact this professional and set up today's appointment for an auditory processing assessment.

In addition to XXX having failed the school hearing screening, the parents reported that XXX had chronic ear infections between 1 and 2 years of age.

Research has demonstrated that many children with histories of early, chronic middle ear problems often have auditory processing difficulties later, especially at school-age levels.

In order to obtain more specific information regarding listening problems that may be present, the parents completed the Children's Auditory Processing Performance Scale (CHAPPS). This scale asks the same seven questions relative to various listening conditions from ideal listening conditions (total attention, complete quiet) to listening when distracted or in the presence of noise and competition. Scores of –2 or lower are considered indicative of areas of concern for the person completing the scale.

Based on the parents' rating, XXX was identified as having problems both in quiet and ideal listening conditions related to following directions and listening when she is not fully attentive. Listening behaviors become more problematic with noise and multiple inputs. Thus, there are definite indications that there may be some underlying auditory processing problems present.

To obtain even more specific information regarding XXX's listening behaviors, the parents were asked to complete The Listening Inventory (TLI). TLI asks various questions related to observed behaviors with the parents and/or teachers rating whether the behavior has been noticed frequently or infrequently as well as not at all. TLI looks at listening and associated behaviors related to six categories including: language concerns, auditory processing concerns, auditory and language decoding concerns that could be related to early reading decoding skills, attention and organization concerns, social and behavioral concerns, and sensory-motor concerns. According to the results of TLI completed by the parents, concerns were identified in all six areas although only borderline concern was identified in the social and behavioral areas. Thus, there are many concerns raised and many interacting factors that could account for the observed issues questioning the possibility of some underlying auditory processing difficulties including possible underlying attention problems as well as auditory processing and/or language problems.

Further insights were obtained by having XXX's kindergarten teacher complete TLI. The teacher's findings were consistent with the parents relative to concerns regarding attention, auditory processing, and decoding. However, the teacher did not see any problems related to language, social, and behavioral concerns, nor in the sensory-motor area.

The parents also provided this professional with a copy of XXX's present IEP. The IEP identifies her as having a speech-language disability as XXX's only "educational disability." The IEP only offers XXX speech-language services 90 minutes a week with two 30-minute sessions being pull-out services with a small group and one 30-minute session having the speech-language professional go into the classroom for support. There was only one goal in the IEP relative to following directions. From what the parents reported and results of the CHAPPS, following directions is definitely an area of concern, but additional areas of concern seem to have "cropped up" since the IEP was written in the spring of last year when XXX was completing preschool.

One other important piece of data picked up in reviewing XXX's IEP was the results from the school psychologist's report. The school psychologist completed a cognitive assessment of XXX when she was in preschool identifying that cognitive areas both involving language areas (verbal) and visual-motor areas were within normal limits. Full-scale IQ was found to be very normal (92).

In view of the concerns raised by the parents, results of the CHAPPS and TLI indicating possible auditory processing problems as well as possible attention problems, the purpose of today's assessment was to identify whether XXX has any specific auditory processing deficits (APD) and, if so, in what specific areas of auditory processing such deficits exist. Additionally, a purpose was to identify whether the underlying factor accounting for any possible APD is due to primary auditory attention problems or some other specific category of APD (all categories described below). Last, a purpose of today's assessment was to identify what interventions may be needed to help XXX overcome and deal with any specific APD found.

Understanding the Auditory Processing Evaluation

Auditory processing is referred to in this report as those internal processes that a person uses to make sense out of auditory messages. As this professional describes in his model of auditory processing (2005, 2006), auditory processing are those things we do to obtain meaning from the information we receive through our auditory systems.

Auditory processing has been described as "What we do with what we hear" (Katz, Stecker, & Henderson, *Central Auditory Processing: A Transdisciplinary Approach,* 1992). Another description of auditory processing is "How the ear speaks to the brain." (Chermak & Musiek, *Central Auditory Processing Disorders: New Perspectives,* 1997). Lucker (2004, 2005) has defined auditory processing as the things the entire central nervous system does when it receives information through the auditory system and gets it into the higher cognitive levels of the brain where meaning is placed on that information so the listener makes sense out of and comprehends what he or she has heard.

For a long time, the term Central Auditory Processing was applied to this area. However, in view of recent concepts related to what is involved in auditory processing, and based on recent reports by professionals (Jerger/Musiek's report in the *Journal of the American Academy of Audiology*, 2000 and the technical report of the Working Group on Auditory Processing Disorders of the American Speech-Language-Hearing Association (ASHA, 2005), the term Auditory Processing Disorder or APD is used instead.

The approach taken by this consultant is one in which auditory processing is viewed as a series of steps (or processes) beginning after a person hears or "receives" the auditory signal at the ear and involves the entire central nervous system in the brain. In this approach, there are hypothesized to be six different areas of processing that interact with each other and lead to the final comprehension of the message. Furthermore, in each area are subcategories of processes that can be identified as normal or deficient during the comprehensive assessment of auditory processing abilities when taking into account various factors. These factors include a complex interaction of auditory abilities, language abilities, sensory factors, and cognitive abilities. Considering these factors, below is a summary of what today's auditory processing test battery indicates regarding XXX's abilities to process in each of these six areas and subcategories of auditory processing.

Auditory Processing Test Results

The first step in assessing XXX's auditory processing was to rule out the presence of any hearing loss that could contribute to auditory processing problems. Hearing thresholds were measured to determine if hearing was normal (less than or equal to 15 dB HL) for all frequencies (including interoctaves) from 250 through 8000 Hz. Additionally, thresholds for speech (SRT) and word recognition (WRS) in quiet were measured.

Results revealed normal hearing thresholds for both ears with normal thresholds for speech as well as normal word recognition at a normal conversational listening level of 50 dB HL. Thus, **hearing loss is <u>not present</u> and is not a significant contributing factor to any auditory processing problems found on today's auditory processing testing.** The findings of normal hearing are also in agreement with the hearing testing completed at Dr.XXX's office in fall 2005.

The first area of auditory processing, according to the approach taken by this consultant, is **auditory sensitivity** related to awareness and recognition of sound as well as to tolerance to loud and unwanted sounds (auditory hypersensitivity). Every task used in the APD assessment as well as informal observations of responses to verbal messages and sounds indicate that there are **no problems with auditory recognition and awareness.**

To obtain information regarding auditory sensitivity to loud sounds (i.e., auditory hypersensitivity), tolerance levels or UCLs for all frequencies tested for hearing thresholds were measured. UCL measures indicated that **XXX has no problems tolerating sounds at all of the frequencies tested in both ears** at the maximum level tested (110 dB HL). Therefore, today's results indicate **no problems with auditory sensitivity nor with any auditory hypersensitivities to sound**.

The second area of processing is **auditory extraction**. Extraction is the process by which the individual takes the entire signal (or code) and *extracts* the meaningful elements for that code to comprehend the message in the end. Tests using distorted speech, speech masked (covered up) by competing speech, and rapidly presented verbal messages were used to look at auditory extraction abilities.

Results of today's testing indicate that **auditory extraction is not an area of auditory processing deficit for XXX**. That is, no deficits were found for XXX extracting the meaningful information related to speech sounds (i.e., phonemic extraction), related to linguistic information (i.e., lexical extraction), and related to rapidly presented speech (i.e., temporal extraction).

The third area of auditory processing is **auditory attention**. This level involves a person's ability to focus attention to the relevant parts of auditory messages while filtering out the irrelevant pieces as well as dividing attention between two messages and being required to process only one relevant message. Tasks involving competing messages in which the listener would confuse the relevant message or be distracted by the irrelevant message are samples of the way this process is evaluated. Additionally, a task assessing sustained auditory focal attention (a process of general attention and self-regulation not specific to any APD) was presented.

What is important for the reader is to understand this professional's approach to auditory attention. This area is viewed as having two primary components: being distracted by the presence of external, competing sounds (**auditory distractibility**), and the ability for the listener to regulate his or her attention and sustain, auditory focal attention over time (**general, sustained, auditory focal attention**). Auditory distractibility is a problem in auditory processing. In contrast, general, sustained, auditory attention is related to internal regulation and general attention abilities such as might be seen in children diagnosed with attention problems such as AD/HD.

Results of the formal testing of sustained, auditory focal attention (a continuous performance test) indicated **no significant deficits in sustaining auditory, focal attention**. However, analysis of her responses indicated that she did have a lot of delayed, but correct, responses. From the analysis of all test findings and observations of XXX's behaviors, it is concluded that the delayed, yet appropriate, responses are due to possible planning issues or to XXX having problems making the decision to respond when she heard the target word on the continuous performance task. In the real world, this delayed responding could appear to be loss of attention, but may actually represent sensory-motor problems that need to be evaluated usually by an OT. What is interesting to note is that the parents' report on TLI indicated some concerns in the sensory-motor area.

As for the area of auditory distractibility, today's test findings indicate **no problems with auditory distractibility** for XXX. Thus, the reported observation by the parents that she seems to have more listening problems in the presence of background noise and competing messages is not due to any specific auditory processing problem or to any specific auditory attention problem. The problems reported with noise and competition are likely age-normal behaviors.

The fourth area of auditory processing is **auditory memory**. Although memory, itself, is felt to be a process beyond pure auditory processing, the present approach looks at how well a listener demonstrates responses relating to getting information into working memory and how well the person can retrieve information from working memory. Thus, the area of auditory memory is really more an area of how one processes auditory information during the storage phase of processing.

Results of today's testing indicate that **XXX has no problems getting information into or recalling information from short-term, auditory working memory**. Thus, no problems with auditory memory were found on today's testing. Actually, auditory working memory was found to be an area of strength for XXX (see Memory for Digits and Nonword Repetition subtests of the CTOPP).

The fifth area looked at is **auditory integration**. This process is felt to include how we take the pieces of the messages we hear and put the pieces together to form the unified whole needed to comprehend what we have heard as integration is highly related to comprehension. However, to test this factor, mere repetition of words is used as test stimuli, but listening is completed under an artificial, well controlled, standardized format known as dichotic listening. More specifically, tests looking at dichotic listening requiring multiple areas of the central nervous system to interact (i.e., integrate) correctly with each other, were used for assessing auditory integration.

Results of today's testing indicate that **auditory integration is a significant area of auditory processing deficit for XXX**. More specifically, the problem with auditory integration is at the speech sound or phoneme level. Such problems are part of what is often referred to as phonemic or phonological awareness in areas such as blending and segmenting and what this professional calls "sound play," that is, playing with words by removing sounds, substituting sounds, and reversing order of phonemes. (What must be remembered is that this area of auditory phonemic awareness specifically being referred to here is related to auditory-based processes.) Problems with auditory phonemic awareness can underlie problems in reading decoding and spelling. What is most interesting to note is that on TLI the parents identified auditory decoding as a problem area for XXX. Additionally, one major area of concern for the parents is XXX's poor development of early phonic skills. Today's test findings support their concern and identify a specific deficit in auditory processing related to the problems in this area of phonics.

In addition to the specific deficit in auditory phonemic integration, the overall pattern of findings on measures of auditory integration indicate that this entire area of auditory processing is weak and needs strengthening to mature and develop so that no further auditory integration problems will arise later. Thus, specific interventions into auditory phonemic integration are needed along with general practice to strength auditory integration at the linguistic (lexical) level as well.

The sixth, and final, area of auditory processing involves how we recognize the **organization and sequencing** of auditory information. Tasks that involved strings of verbal information needing to be processed in appropriate organized sequences were the stimuli used to evaluate this process. Results of today's assessment indicate that **XXX has no problems with organization and sequencing of auditory information**.

Conclusions and Recommendations

Results of today's auditory processing assessment are very surprising for XXX. Based on the presenting information and the parents' and the classroom teacher's responses on TLI, it was expected that XXX would have significant problems in auditory processing in many if not most of the specific areas of auditory processing as well as underlying attention problems. The surprising result was that only one area of auditory processing was found to be deficient. This area, auditory phonemic integration, could affect reading and writing, and could lead to XXX not being able to appropriately comprehend what is being said in class. This latter problem could relate to the problems reported understanding/following directions as well as the problems completing her homework. Additionally, a lack of comprehension could lead to a person losing his or her attention; thus, the problems with integration could lead to behaviors that might appear to be inattentiveness.

In addition to the specific deficit found in phonemic integration, a weakness was found in auditory lexical integration that could contribute to XXX having problems understanding the language used in oral messages. This also could contribute to inattention due to her inability to understand and follow verbal messages and, thus, getting lost and appearing to be inattentive.

In contrast to the problems found with auditory integration, no problems were found with auditory attention, no problems with auditory memory, and no problems in other areas of auditory processing. Thus, the one area needing intervention is the area of auditory integration.

Integration is the process by which we take the pieces we extract (or decode) from the auditory message and put them together to form the whole as well as take the whole and break it into its specific pieces. The necessity of performing normally in phonemic integration relates to reading decoding, reading accuracy, reading rate, and reading fluency. Additionally, without good reading decoding one cannot comprehend what one is reading. Thus, XXX needs specific, individualized instructional help in the area of auditory-based phonemic awareness skills related to sound blending, sound analysis in words, sound substitution, and what this professional calls "sound play."

Because the findings today indicate problems with auditory integration, the focus of intervention would be to improve XXX's auditory phonemic integration abilities in the areas of sound blending (not specifically related to reading as we want to remove the orthographic factors called letters), sound analysis (segmentation and deletion (sometimes called elision), and sound play (elision and phoneme reversals). To provide these skills for XXX, she would need individual treatment outside the classroom program from a professional, often a speech-language pathologist or reading specialist, who is knowledgeable and experienced in working on auditory phonemic awareness and auditory phonemic integration (mental manipulation of sounds in words).

Some examples of materials that can be used with XXX include the Earobics Step 1 (later, the Step 2) computer program for practice not for treatment (see www.earobics.com and www.superduperinc.com), the Lindamood-Bell LiPS program (www.lindamoodbell.com and www.ganderpublishing.com), and the Phonemic Awareness Training (PAT) program (www.linguisystems.com).

The second area in need of intervention is the linguistic or lexical integration area. This area relates to taking the pieces of the significant or key language information in messages and putting those pieces together to form the whole (often referred to as the mental image or visualization) as well as taking the whole and breaking it down into the individual pieces for analysis. One example of a commercially available program that provides exactly the type of work

XXX needs in this area is the Lindamood-Bell group's Visualizing and Verbalizing program.

In addition to these recommended programs, the professional working with XXX should play phonemic integration/sound play games and do phonemic awareness activities. These activities should begin purely at the auditory level and add other modalities such as visual cues such as speech-reading (how phonemes look when they are produced by another person) and practice identifying the motor elements of how phonemes are produced by XXX.

As stated above, a question arose during the auditory processing assessment as well as in the parents' TLI results that XXX may have some sensory-motor issues. Sensory-motor is an area typically evaluated and treated by OTs. Thus, XXX would benefit from seeing an OT who works on sensory-motor and sensory integration skills.

It is hoped that this report provides the reader with a better understanding of XXX's auditory processing abilities and needs. If there are any questions, feel free to contact Dr. XXX at (provide telephone number).

Test Data

Name: **XXX**

Date: **03/2006**

Age: **6.8**

Auditory Sensitivity: Pure Tone Hearing Thresholds

Frequency in Hz	250	500	750	1000	1500	2000	3000	4000	6000	8000
Right ear in dB HL	10	5	5	5	5	5	5	5	5	5
Left ear in dB HL	0	5	5	0	5	10	10	0	15	10

Auditory Hypersensitivity: Loudness Tolerance (UCL) Measures

Frequency in Hz	250	500	750	1000	1500	2000	3000	4000	6000	8000
Right ear in dB HL	>100	>110	>110	>110	>110	>110	>110	>110	>110	>100
Left ear in dB HL	>100	>110	>110	>110	>110	>110	>110	>110	>110	>100

Auditory Sensitivity: Speech Thresholds (SRT)

Measure	PTA	SRT
Right ear in dB HL	5	5
Left ear in dB HL	6.7	5

Auditory Sensitivity: Word Recognition (WRS) at 50 dB HL

Ear	WRS	Norm	Noise (S/N+5)	Q/N Difference	Norm
Right	100%	88%	88%	12%	22%
Left	96%	85%	80%	16%	23%

SCAN-C (Norms are standard scores between 7 and 13)

Subtest	Right ear	Left ear	Combined	Standard Score	Percentile
Filtered Words	18	17	35	14	91st
Auditory Figure-Ground	16	12	28	8	25th
Competing Words*	23	9	32	10	50th
Competing Sentences	10	1	11	12	75th

*Ear difference on Competing Words is *not* an age-appropriate finding

SSW Test

8CN

REF	RNC	RC	LC	LNC	LEF	LNC	LC	RC	RNC
	0	3	5	0		0	10	2	0

NOE

Condition	Value	Normal Cutoff at –2 SD	Normal Cutoff at –1 SD
RNC	0		
RC	5	13	10
LC	15	19	15
LNC	0		

RB

Effect	Value	Type	Difference	Normal Cutoff at 2 SD	Normal Cutoff at 1 SD
Ear	8/12	L/H	4	10	6
Order	13/7	H/L	6	12	7
Reversals	1			6	4
Type A	10/5	LC	5	7	
AYR	0				
All other areas	0				

Phonemic Synthesis Test (PST)

Analysis	Value	Normal Cutoff
Quantitative	16	17
Qualitative	15	12
Quick	1	2

Time-Compressed Sentence Test (TCST)

Percent Time Compression	Number of Errors	Z Score	Percentile
0%	0	Baseline	Baseline
40%	1	+0.4	66th
60%	4	+0.8	78th

Auditory Continuous Performance Test (ACPT)

Trial	1	2	3	4	5	6	Total
Target Words Missed	0	0	1	4	1	2	8
Non-Target Word Responses	1	1	1	2	3	1	9
Delayed Responses	1	1	2	1	2	0	7*

Auditory Continuous Performance Test (ACPT) *(continued)*

Analysis	Value	Normal Cutoff
Total Errors	17	37
Vigilance	2	4

Comprehensive Test of Phonological Processing

(Norms are standard scores between 7 and 13)

Subtest	Standard Score	Percentile
Elision	6*	9th
Blending Words	6*	9th
Blending Nonwords	<7*^	<16th^
Sound Matching	6*	9th
Memory for Digits	13	84th
Nonword Repetition	12	75th

^7/16th is the lowest standard score/percentile for her age level

*Indicates test results outside normal expected

The Listening Inventory (TLI)

Category	Parent^	Teacher^	Normal Cutoff
Linguistic Organization	76 (47)	42 (13)	29
Auditory and Language Decoding	67 (46)	65 (44)	21
Attention/Organization	119 (65)	90 (36)	54
Sensory/Motor	46 (26)	26 (6)	20
Social/Behavioral	38 (4)	26 (–8)	34
Auditory Processing	80 (48)	78 (46)	32

^Represents total value (deviation from the norm)

Reports Prepared by Speech-Language Pathologists

Sample Report 3

The following report summarizes the findings of an auditory processing and speech-language assessment on a young school-aged boy performed by a speech-language pathologist.

BACKGROUND INFORMATION

XXX was seen at his school on the above dates for an evaluation. His teacher, Mrs. XXX, expressed concern that XXX was having difficulty retaining information and focusing his attention. Pertinent history was provided by Mrs. YYY. XXX was the product of a full-term pregnancy and weighed 6 lbs. 14 oz. Prenatal, birth, and developmental history were not unusual. Health history is significant for chronic middle ear infections. XXX's hearing was evaluated at age 3 and his hearing acuity was reportedly very good. XXX was cooperative and attentive during the testing. Testing was conducted on 2 days in 45-minute sessions. Test results are felt to be valid.

Test Results and Interpretations

Tests Administered:

Illinois Test of Psycholinguistic Abilities—3, ITPA

Test of Language Competence—E, TLC-E

Comprehensive Test of Phonological Processing, CTOPP

SCAN-C: A Test of Auditory Processing in Children

Auditory Processing Abilities Test, APAT

Test of Auditory Processing Skills—3, TAPS-3

Test of Auditory Analysis Skills, TAAS

Listening Inventory, LI

The Illinois Test of Psycholinguistic Abilities—3 (Pro-Ed, 2001) is designed to assess performance in spoken and written language that is related to phonologic, morphosyntactic, graphophonemic, orthographic, and semantic competence. The subtests have a mean standard score of 10 with a standard deviation of 3; thus, according to the ITPA-3 manual, scores between 8 and 12 are considered average. The composite quotients have a mean standard score of 100 with a descriptive rating of average including scores from 90 to 110. XXX received the following scores:

SPOKEN SUBTESTS	Standard Score	Percentile	Rating
Spoken Analogies	9	37	Average
Spoken Vocabulary	11	63	Average
Morphologic Closure	12	75	Average
Syntactic Sentences	5	5	Below Average
Sound Deletion	7	16	Below Average
Rhyming Sequences	6	9	Below Average
COMPOSITE QUOTIENTS	86	18	Below Average
SPECIFIC QUOTIENTS			
Semantics	100	50	Average
Grammar	91	27	Low Average
Phonology	79	8	Below Average

Subtest Description and Discussion:

In the *Spoken Analogies* subtest, the examiner says a four-part analogy of which the last part is missing. The student tells the missing part. This subtest assesses verbal reasoning, listening comprehension, oral expression, and semantics. XXX's performance was average.

The *Spoken Vocabulary* subtest measures the ability to recall spoken words when provided with attributes of the words. XXX's score was average.

The *Morphological Closure* subtest measures the ability to complete a partially formed sentence by applying a final word that is correct grammatically. The subtest assesses morphology and listening skills. XXX's performance was average.

The *Syntactic Sentences* subtest requires the child to repeat semantically nonsensical but syntactically correct sentences. This subtest measures auditory sequential memory for spoken words, oral expression, and syntax. XXX's score fell below average. This may be secondary to mild weakness in auditory sequential memory and/or difficulty recognizing the words in unpredictable contexts.

The *Sound Deletion* subtest measures the ability to segment spoken words into smaller phonemic units by remembering and uttering the component of a word that remains after a portion is removed from the original stimulus word. This subtest assesses phonemic awareness. XXX's performance was below average.

The *Rhyming Sequences* subtest assesses phonology and phonemic sequential memory. The student repeats strings of rhyming words that increase in length. XXX's performance was below average.

The *Spoken Language Composite* is formed by combining the six subtests that measure oral language. It measures spoken language relating to semantics, grammar, and phonology. XXX's score was average.

The *Semantics Quotient* measures vocabulary and is the result of two subtests that measure the understanding and use of purposeful speech. Typically students who score high on this measure know a lot about word meanings. They know the dictionary meanings of words, are aware that words have multiple meanings, recognize the meanings of words they hear, and use words proficiently and accurately in speech. Children who do poorly on this measure often do not know the meanings of common words, and have trouble relating the words they know to abstract concepts. XXX's score fell in the average range.

The *Grammar Quotient* includes morphology (the patterns of word formation) and syntax (the patterns of sentence formation). Students who score high on this measure typically understand and correctly use grammatical inflections, such as plurals, possessives, and verb tenses, and are cable of generating complex sentences with a variety of dependent and embedded phrases. Students who score poorly on this measure often use short sentences that include many grammatical forms that are not characteristic of most English speakers. XXX's score was average.

The *Phonology Quotient* measures the student's knowledge of sounds within our words. Students who score high in this area are typically good at all kinds of phonemic awareness and will probably do well in phonics. Children who do poorly are likely to experience difficulty in learning to read and spell. XXX's performance was below average.

The *Test of Language Competence—Expanded Edition* is designed to measure metalinguistic competence in semantics, syntax, and pragmatics. The test consists of four subtests. Standard scores between 8 and 12 represent the average range from low to high. Composite scores between 90 and 110 represent the average range from low to high. XXX received the following scores:

	Standard Score	Percentile	Rating
Ambiguous Sentences	8	25	Low Average
Making Inferences	13	84	Above Average
Recreating Speech Acts	5	5	Below Average
Figurative Language	6	9	Below Average
Composite Summary			
Screening (Subtest 3+4)	73	4	Below Average
Expressing Intent (Subtest 1+3)	79	8	Below Average
Interpreting Intents (Subtest 2+4)	97	42	Average
TLC-E COMPOSITE (Subtests 1–4)	86	18	Below Average

The *Ambiguous Sentences* subtest first asks the child to tell two possible meanings for a given sentence, for example, "Look at that bat." XXX was only able to give one meaning per sentence. The child is then shown four pictures and asked to select two that could go with that sentence. XXX correctly identified both pictures for two of 13 trials. XXX's performance was low average.

On the *Making Inferences* subtest, the student is asked to determine why a particular scenario might have taken place, e.g., "Bob and Jane went to the park to play. Instead of playing, they came home and watched TV." The child then selects a yes/no response to four pictures that could be possible explanations. XXX's score was above average.

For the *Recreating Speech Acts* subtest, the student is shown a picture and asked to formulate a sentence using two given words. This task was difficult for XXX. He gave a sentence for the first item, "I'm now and hungry," but for the remaining items, he merely repeated the two target words, but did not use them in a sentence. His performance was significantly below average.

The *Figurative Language* subtest asks the child to explain the meaning of an idiom, e.g., "Let me give you a hand." The student then selects one of four pictures that match the phrase. XXX interpretations were often literal, e.g., "Go fly a kite," meant to literally go *and fly a kite. His score was below average.*

The *Comprehensive Test of Phonological Processing* (CTOPP) assesses phonological awareness, phonological memory, and rapid naming. A deficit in one or more of these kinds of phonological processing abilities is viewed as the most common cause of learning disabilities in general, and of reading disabilities in particular. In addition to their role in learning to read, phonological processing abilities also support effective mathematical calculation, listening, comprehension, and reading comprehension. The mean standard score is 10 with a standard deviation of 3; thus, according to the CTOPP manual, scores between 8 and 12 are considered average. XXX received the following scores:

	Standard Score	Percentile	Rating
Elision	7	16	Below Average
Blending Words	12	75	High Average
Sound Matching	9	37	Average
PHONOLOGICAL AWARENESS	96	39	Average
Memory for Digits	9	37	Average
Nonword Repetition	10	50	Average
PHONOLOGICAL MEMORY	97	42	Average
Rapid Digit Naming	10	50	Average
Rapid Object Naming	8	25	Low Average
RAPID NAMING COMPOSITE	94	35	Average
SUPPLEMENTAL SUBTEST			
Blending Nonwords	10	50	Average

The *Elision* subtest measures an individual's ability to say a word, then say what is left after dropping out designated sounds. The first two items ask the examinee to say a compound word, then say the word that remains after dropping one of the compound words (e.g., say "popcorn" without saying "corn"). The remaining items require deletion of a specific sound (e.g., say "bold" without saying "b"). XXX was unable to consistently delete syllables from compound words, but this skill appeared to be emerging. His performance was below average.

The *Blending Words* subtest measures an individual's ability to combine sounds to form words (e.g., What word do these sounds make: t-oy). XXX's performance was high average.

Sound Matching subtest requires the child to identify pictures that have the same initial sound and then pictures that have the same ending sound. XXX matched seven of 10 initial sounds. He was unable to match any final sounds. His overall performance was average.

The *Memory for Digits* subtest requires the examinee to repeat a series of numbers ranging in length from two to eight digits. XXX was able to repeat three digits consistently and up to five digits inconsistently. His performance was average on the day this test was administered.

The *Nonword Repetition* subtest measures the ability to repeat nonsense words that range in length from 3 to 15 sounds. XXX's performance was average.

The *Rapid Naming* subtests measure the speed with which an individual can name 72 items presented on two pages. XXX was given the subtests for digits and objects. His performance was average.

The *Blending Nonwords* subtest measures an individual's ability to combine speech sounds to make nonwords (e.g., What made-up word do these sounds make: nim-by). XXX's performance was average.

The *SCAN-C: Test for Auditory Processing Disorders—Revised* is administered via audio disc under earphones. The mean standard score is 10 with a standard deviation of 3; thus, scores between 7 and 13 are considered to reflect the average range from low to high. XXX achieved the following scores:

	SS	%
Filtered Words	4	2 Below Average
Auditory Figure-Ground	6	9 Below Average
Competing Words	7	16 Low Average
Competing Sentences	8	25 Low Average
SCAN Composite	75	5 Below Average
Typical Ear Advantage	YES	

The *Filtered Words* subtest contains 20 monosyllable words that are presented with a filter giving the effect of muffled speech. Poor performance on the Filtered Words subtest reflects difficulties in comprehending distorted speech. The student may have difficulty in understanding a person in another room, a person who is speaking with his or her back to the child, or a person who is speaking in a large auditorium. The child may have problems understanding someone who speaks rapidly, articulates poorly, or who has an unfamiliar accent or dialect. XXX's performance was significantly below average.

The *Auditory Figure-Ground* subtest contains 20 monosyllable words in the presence of multitalker speech babble; comparable to background noise of a party. Poor performance on the Auditory Figure-Ground subtest reflects difficulties in understanding speech in the presence of competing background noise. To enhance academic success, these children need preferential seating, reduction of ambient noise, and possibly even assistive listening devices. These types of listening difficulties can also contribute to misunderstandings in social situations. XXX's performance was below average.

The *Competing Words* subtest is made up of two lists of 15 monosyllable word pairs that are presented to the right and left ears with simultaneous onset times and the child repeats both words. The Competing Words subtest indicates a child's auditory maturation or developmental level of the auditory system. Standard scores below 7 are generally associated with delayed maturation of the central auditory nervous system. XXX's score fell at the first standard deviation, which is considered low average, but barely.

The *Competing Sentences* subtest contains 10 sentences, which are presented in the same fashion as the Competing Words subtest. The Competing Sentences subtest is another measure used to assess maturation of a child's auditory system. The expanded linguistic content of the Competing Sentences subtest provides additional data on how the student uses linguistic cues when interpreting speech. As the linguistic load increases, the speech signal engages the language-dominant left hemisphere more completely. With the additional linguistic information, XXX was able to improve his performance into the low average range. XXX's overall composite on the SCAN-C fell approximately one and one-half standard deviations below the mean.

The *Auditory Processing Abilities Test* is composed of 10 subtests that quantify a child's performance in various areas of auditory processing. The subtests have a mean of 10 with a standard deviation of 3. The indices have a mean of 100 with a standard deviation of 15. XXX achieved the following scores:

	Scaled Score	**Percentile Ranks**
Phonemic Awareness	9	37
Word Sequences	7	16
Semantic Relationships	12	75
Sentence Memory	9	37
Cued Recall	14	88
Content Memory, Immediate	10	50
Content Memory, Delayed	<7	<16
Complex Sentences	17	99
Sentence Absurdities	11	63
Following Directions	10	50
Passage Comprehension	10	50
COMPOSITE INDEX SCORES	**Standard Score**	**Percentile Ranks**
Global	107	68
Auditory Memory	91	27
Linguistic Processes	108	70

The *Phonemic Awareness* subtest measures awareness of sounds within word structures; these skills are necessary for the acquisition of written language skills. The student is required to identify sounds or sound sequences that are spoken, as well as to identify the first sound, number of sounds, and last sound in a nonsense word. XXX's performance was average.

The *Word Sequences* subtest measures auditory memory and auditory sequencing skills. The student is asked to repeat word sequences of increasing length. XXX was able to repeat up to two words consistently and three words inconsistently. XXX's performance was below average. This was in contrast to his performance for the same task using the TAPS-3 on a different day where he repeated four- and five-word series.

The *Semantic Relationships* subtest measures auditory memory and auditory cohesion. It requires the student to listen to three words spoken by the examiner, and to tell which words are related. This measures the ability to recognize common associations between words. XXX's performance was high average.

The *Sentence Memory* subtest measures auditory sequential memory and requires the student to repeat sentences of increasing length and complexity. XXX's performance was average.

The *Cued Recall* subtest measures auditory memory, auditory cohesion, and auditory attention. The examiner says five pairs of unrelated words. The student is presented with three recall trials with the order of the pairs being changed with each subsequent trial. XXX's performance was above average.

The *Content Memory* subtest assesses the ability to recall information contained in a brief story, immediately and after a delay. XXX's performance for immediate recall was average and his performance for delayed recall was below average.

The *Complex Sentences* subtest measures the ability to understand grammatically complex sentences and answer questions about the content. XXX's performance was superior.

The *Sentence Absurdities* subtest measures the ability to recognize incongruities in the sentence and to tell what is wrong with the sentence. XXX's performance was average.

The *Following Directions* subtest uses paper and pencil to measure the ability to follow oral instructions of increasing length and complexity. XXX's performance was average.

The *Passage Comprehension* subtest measures the ability to understand the main idea and recall details of passage-length material of increasing length and complexity. XXX's performance was average.

The *Test of Auditory Processing Skills*—3 (TAPS-3) is an assessment of auditory skills necessary for the development, use, and understanding of language commonly utilized in academic and everyday activities. Scaled scores for the subtests have a mean of 10 with a standard deviation of 3 and standard scores for the composite scores have a mean of 100 with a standard deviation of 15. XXX achieved the following scores for selected subtests:

	Scaled Score	Percentile Ranks
Number Memory Forward	6	9
Number Memory Reversed	1	<1
Word Memory	13	84
Auditory Comprehension	7	16

The *Number Memory Forward* subtest measures auditory sequential memory. XXX was able to repeat up to 3 digits. His performance was below average. However, on the CTOPP on a different day, XXX repeated 4 and 5 digit series.

The *Number Memory Reversed* subtest requires the student to be unusually attentive to auditory matter and to recall the digits as given, to reorganize and remanipulate the number structure, and finally to repeat the digits verbally in reverse sequence. This type of functioning taps a student's ability to concentrate and to perform an activity requiring mental control. XXX was unable to repeat any digits in reverse. His performance fell significantly below average.

The *Word Memory* subtest requires the student to repeat a series of unrelated words. XXX's performance was high average.

The *Auditory Comprehension* subtest measures how well a student understands spoken information that ranges in length from one to five sentences and increases in complexity. XXX's performance was slightly below average. However, on a different day using the APAT, his performance was in the superior range for a similar task.

The *Test of Auditory Analysis Skills* is designed to test a child's auditory perceptual skills. The TAAS starts at a relatively simple level by asking the child to analyze a two-syllable, compound word. He is told to say "baseball," then say it again, but don't say ball. The test progresses and requires the child to analyze a more refined unit, the phoneme, (single sound). For example, he is asked to say "meat," then say it again, but don't say the /m/ sound. XXX was unable to analyze any of the syllables. He received a raw score of 0 which is at the level of prekindergarten. This skill was tested using three instruments and XXX consistently had difficulty with this task.

The *Listening Inventory* is an informal child behavioral observation that can be completed by parents, teachers, and/or other education specialists. Mrs. YYY completed this inventory. Scores that fall below the cutoff score indicate adequate functioning in that area. Scores above the cutoff score indicate difficulty in that area.

Parent Rating	Score	Cutoff Score	Was Score Significant?
Linguistic Organization	40	32	YES
Decoding/Language Mechanics	21	25	NO
Attention/Organization	85	59	YES
Sensory/Motor	21	24	NO
Social Behavioral	51	37	YES
Auditory Processes	47	36	YES
OVERALL SCORE	265	223	YES

Linguistic Organization items reflect the student's ability to use, attend to, and organize expressive and receptive language. *Decoding and Language Mechanics* items tap the student's ability to decode receptive language and make phonological judgments, as well as their skill with conversational-spoken language to communicate perceptions, ideas, feelings, and intentions. *Attention and Organization* items refer to the child's ability to focus on and attend to stimuli with active awareness, initiative, judgment, and their ability to set and achieve goals. *Sensory-Motor Skills* reflect the student's integration of motor and sensory information, and the ability to use fine and gross motor skills. *Social and Behavioral Skills* reflect both internal self-regulation and external behaviors that may be problematic, the ability to interact, interchange ideas, relate to others, act appropriately in a given situation, and respond appropriately to stimuli, peers, and environment. *Auditory Processes* reflect behaviors commonly seen in children experiencing difficulty processing auditory information or listening to spoken language. This inventory suggests that XXX is experiencing difficulty in four of the six areas surveyed.

IMPRESSIONS AND RECOMMENDATIONS

XXX is a delightful little boy who was willing to work and always seemed to be trying his best. Interestingly, his performance was quite variable from day to day. For example, he was asked to repeat digits on the screening date and the second evaluation date. On the initial screening date, he repeated up to three digits and his performance was below average. On the second date, he repeated four digits and even one five-digit series. This second performance was average for his age.

The reverse happened for repeating series of unrelated words; on the screening date, XXX repeated four-word series and his performance was high average for that area, but on the subsequent date he could not consistently repeat three word series and his performance fell below average. I suspect this discrepancy has to do with a combination of auditory processing difficulties and auditory sequential memory. It is possible XXX did not clearly hear the words in order to repeat them accurately and/or he could not hold the sequence in his working memory. The difficulty XXX had on the Filtered Words subtest of the SCAN-C suggests he may have problems clearly understanding unpredictable words and information. Often a student who is experiencing auditory difficulties of this nature will have some days that are better than others. There was a significant discrepancy (16 points) between XXX's auditory memory skills and his linguistic processing skills on the APAT.

A third area that showed a marked discrepancy was for understanding complex sentences. XXX's performance on the screening date (using the TAPS-3) was below average but his subsequent performance (using the APAT) placed him in the superior range. One other area that was above average was cued recall (the examiner says five pairs of unrelated words, then the student is presented with three recall trials with the order of the pairs being changed with each subsequent trial).

XXX's performance for the following areas were average: spoken vocabulary, understanding word relationships (which word doesn't belong), grammar, correcting absurd sentences, immediate recall for a short story (content memory), auditory memory for sentences and for nonsense words, answering questions after listening to a short story, blending sounds into words, matching initial sounds in words, rapid naming, understanding ambiguous sentences, and making inferences.

Areas in which XXX's performance fell below average were: phonemic awareness for deletion of syllables and sounds from a word, repeating digits in reverse, recall of a short story after a 5 to 10 minute delay, sentence formulation with two specific words, figurative language, and processing auditory information under a variety of listening conditions. As mentioned earlier in this section, XXX's performance for repeating series of digits, repeating series of unrelated words, and for understanding complex sentences varied from below average to above average from day to day.

During the testing, XXX was working with the examiner on an individual basis and he was in a novel setting (new teacher and a new room). In this setting, he attended well to tasks. However, the ability to attend in a classroom setting can be much more challenging. The other factor that can make a child appear inattentive is auditory processing difficulties such as those in evidence by this testing. Attached is a list of suggestions for classroom modifications.

I recommend the following for XXX:

1. Classroom modifications, many of these will be more applicable to the primary grades than to kindergarten.
2. Individual therapy twice weekly in half hour sessions.

3. Participation in The Listening Program.
4. Earobics 2 software.

PROGRAM OBJECTIVES

1. Improve phonemic awareness for deletion of syllables and sounds from words.
2. Improve tolerance of background noise.
3. Improve delayed content recall of short stories.
4. Improve formulation of sentences with two specific words.
5. Improve understanding of figurative language (idioms).
6. Improve ability to hold information (both digits reversed and sounds in words) in working memory and manipulate the information accurately.
7. Improve sound/symbol correspondence using a multimodality approach.

It is a pleasure working with XXX and I appreciate the opportunity to participate in his care. Please call if I can answer any questions.

Sample Report 4

The following report summarizes the findings of an auditory processing assessment of a school-aged boy with a history of chronic otitis media that was performed by a speech-language pathologist.

Auditory Processing Assessment

XXX (XXX) XXX is a pleasant 10-year-old boy who was referred for a speech and language assessment by his physician, Dr. XXX, MD and parents, XXX and XXX XXX.They requested the assessment to determine if auditory processing deficits are contributing to the ongoing difficulty XXX is experiencing with written and spoken language, attention, focusing, and processing. The assessment was scheduled for July 2006.

Relevant Background Information

Background information was obtained through a client history form and during an intake interview with XXX's mother, XXX: Pregnancy was complicated by a tearing placenta and toxemia with Mrs. XXX confined to bed-rest during the first trimester. XXX was delivered full-term vaginally weighing 7 lbs. He was breast fed for 10 months. According to Mrs. XXX, XXX was a happy and talkative baby. Developmental gross motor milestones were considered to be within normal limits. Mrs. XXX reports that XXX spoke his first words at 5 to 6 months followed by two- to three-word phrases at 7 months, and complete sentences at 7 to 8 months. His history is significant for chronic otitis media, asthma, and food allergies.

His parents report that XXX is in good general health. He has had his adenoids surgically removed and ventilation tubes inserted. He is prescribed Albuteral, Claritin, Singulair, and Flovent for management of asthma and allergies. Vision has been evaluated with the results within normal limits. XXX's speech and language development is reportedly not an area of concern. Oral motor development is unremarkable.

Socially, XXX's parents describe him as being typical for his age. He is outgoing, talkative, and articulate. XXX is described as a caring person. He tends to be a worrier, fearing that something could be physically wrong with him. XXX can be easily frustrated which results in acting out in anger. He enjoys hockey and swimming. XXX lives at home with both of his parents and his younger brother, age 8.

With regard to XXX's auditory development, his parents report the following: His hearing acuity was evaluated this year with the results within normal limits. He has had approximately 10 ear infections resulting in insertion of ventilation tubes. Parents state he easily distracted, tends to "tune out" if background noise is present, and needs to have instructions repeated frequently. He often says "you know what?", "huh?" or "what?", needs an unusually long amount of time to process verbal information before responding, has difficulty remembering what has been said, and frequently loses his concentration. It takes XXX a long amount of time to explain things. In fact, others who work with XXX have commented on his poor listening skills.

XXX's parents reported the following about him academically: He is enrolled in the fifth grade at First Christian School in Napa. XXX has previously had an IEP, but one is not currently in place. Per parental report, specific areas of weakness are in comprehension; following directions from the teacher; spelling; writing sentences that are not dull or repetitive; attention; getting homework completed without assistance; learning new vocabulary; sequencing; misunderstanding what to do on projects or assignments; and answering open-ended questions. XXX has trouble remembering more than three tasks at a time. Although his reading continues to improve, his comprehension skills are poor.

The assessment was scheduled for July 25, 2006.

Testing

This battery of tests was selected to assess various auditory processing skills as noted in *California Speech-Language-Hearing Association's Guidelines for the Diagnosis and Treatment for Auditory Processing Disorders* document. This document was approved and accepted by the California Speech-Language-Hearing Association in October 2004. This test battery is intended to assess auditory-based language weaknesses in the following areas: auditory perception and discrimination, immediate auditory memory, auditory sequential memory, phonemic awareness, auditory closure, auditory analysis, auditory synthesis, auditory comprehension, and auditory cohesion.

Testing consisted of administration of the following standardized instruments:

1. The Lindamood Auditory Conceptualization Test (LAC-3)
2. The Token Test for Children
3. The Test of Auditory Processing Skills—Third Edition (TAPS-3)
4. The Auditory Processing Abilities Test (APAT)
5. The Wide Range Achievement Test (WRAT-3)
6. The Listening Inventory

Findings

The results of this battery indicate that XXX experiences moderate to significant difficulty with skills of auditory processing. Auditory processing is a hierarchy of skills that are basic to the listening and communication process that affect the acquisition and mastery of both spoken and written language skills. Children with auditory processing disorders are a heterogeneous group of people who have difficulty using auditory information to communicate and learn. Auditory processing disorder is a set of problems that occurs in different listening tasks. It is a deficit in the processing of auditory input, which may be exacerbated in unfavorable acoustic environments and is associated with difficulty listening, speech understanding, language development, and learning.

The results of this battery indicate that XXX experiences difficulty with the following auditory processing skills:

1. auditory discrimination
2. auditory attention
3. immediate auditory memory
4. auditory sequential memory
5. auditory conceptualization
6. auditory cohesion
7. auditory comprehension
8. auditory reasoning
9. interpretation and following directions.

The following behaviors were noted and recorded throughout testing:

1. auditory latency
2. working overtime to listen
3. auditory overload
4. auditory fatigue.

The *Lindamood Auditory Conceptualization Test—Third Edition* (LAC-3. was administered to assess skills of auditory perception, discrimination, and auditory conceptualization. The results are summarized as follows:

Sum of RS	SS	Percentile	Rating	Age Equiv	Grade Equiv
23	76	5	Poor	6.6	1.7

The results of this battery indicate that XXX is experiencing significant difficulty with skills of perception, discrimination, and conceptualization as exhibited by attained standard scores and percentile rankings. There is a greater than 3-year discrepancy between his chronologic age level and his age-level equivalent. There is a greater than 3-year discrepancy between his current grade-level and his grade-level equivalent. Response behaviors included auditory latency and frequent requests for repetitions (which are not allowed). Auditory latency at the perceptual and discrimination level suggests an inefficient auditory processing system. Analysis of XXX's responses indicates that he is unable to effectively perceive the number of sounds in a pattern (e.g., syllable or a word), the number of syllables in a multisyllable word, and has difficulty discriminating the differences between similar sounding sounds or words. Assessment of XXX's auditory conceptualization skills (e.g., the ability to hold and compare two spoken patterns) indicated significant weaknesses. Auditory conceptual function is a part of the language development process during infancy and toddlerhood. This skill ability enables a child to understand, conceptualize, and process spoken information in addition to enabling one to give order and organization to new and ongoing information. Impairment with these aforementioned skills may result in reading and spelling problems as well as the inability to effectively store and retrieve information in a learning situation. The results of testing suggest that XXX is experiencing significant difficulty with skills of auditory perception, auditory discrimination, and auditory conceptualization. Furthermore, these skills are not functional for his learning and communication needs.

The *Token Test for Children* was administered to assess XXX's ability to follow spoken directions of increasing length and complexity. The Token Test is a five subtest battery with each subtest becoming increasingly difficult in terms of stimulus length and complexity. The results are summarized as follows:

Subtest	Raw Score	SS—Age	SS—Grade
Part I	9	455	451
Part II	9	496	491
Part III	8	487	488
Part IV	4	488	485
Part V	14	493	491
Overall Score	44	487	486

The results indicate that XXX experiences significant difficulty with auditory processing skills that enable him to follow spoken directions. These skills are interpreted as being in the third negative standard deviation based on age and the third negative standard deviation based on grade levels. In addition, the presence of auditory latency was documented throughout the evaluation. Specific weaknesses in this area that may be affecting his ability to follow directions include: auditory memory, auditory sequential memory, auditory discrimination, auditory association, and auditory latency. These skills may not be functional for his needs. Response delays were present on 22 of the 44 correct responses (50%). Some delays were as much as 6 seconds in duration. The frequency and duration of processing delays places him at risk for missing information presented through the auditory modality. That is, when a child "stops" to process particular input stimuli, the ongoing information continues and when he picks up at the point of input, he has missed a part of the message. As such, when the information is then assimilated, the child will have only partial information and will not understand the information or request that has been presented. Furthermore, by observation, it may appear that these children are "not listening" when, in fact, they are listening, but receiving pieces of the input stimuli rather than the entire message. It was additionally observed that XXX subvocalized most instructions; that is, he repeated the instruction as a retention strategy.

Analysis of these results indicates that XXX is most successful when following simple one-step commands or directions with up to two specific units of information. When presented with two or more step directions, XXX would omit one step or do something entirely different. Frequently, XXX would request a repetition of directions for successful task completion. As the length and complexity of the stimulus items increased, XXX's error and delays increased proportionately. Furthermore, XXX may be at risk for auditory fatigue and auditory overload. That is, he most likely might benefit from short breaks from listening during the academic day. Short breaks will give his auditory system a rest so that further demands for listening and processing can be productive. Repetition of directions will help ensure success for XXX.

Finally, it should be noted that this battery was administered in a "sterile" environment. That is, one that is free of ambient noise and distractions. The difficulty that XXX experienced under these conditions would, most likely, be exacerbated in a normal classroom environment. These skills may not be functional for his learning needs at this time.

The *Test of Auditory Processing Skills—Third Edition* (TAPS-3) was administered to assess Word Discrimination, Phonological Segmentation, Phonological Blending, Auditory Memory, Auditory Comprehension, and Auditory Reasoning. The results are summarized as follows:

Subtest	Raw Score	Percentile	Standard Score
Word Discrimination	22	<1	2
Phonological Segmentation	31	50	10
Phonological Blending	20	25	8
Number Memory Forward	13	9	6
Number Memory Reversed	6	5	5
Word Memory	12	5	5
Sentence Memory	20	16	7
Auditory Comprehension	15	9	6
Auditory Reasoning	1	<1	2
Overall Standard Score:	78		
Phonologic Standard Score:	83		
Memory Standard Score:	79		
Cohesion Standard Score:	70		

Auditory Word Discrimination is the ability to perceive differences between similar sounding words. XXX is at below the 1st percentile, reflecting a significant weakness. Examples of words that XXX heard, without visual clues, as being the same are: *card* and *cart*; *rot* and *rut*; *run* and *fun*; *saddle* and *settle*; *compute* and *commute*; and so on. When present, weaknesses with auditory discrimination can result in difficulty understanding information being presented, difficulty understanding and following directions, and simply being able to accurately process new and ongoing information presented through the auditory channel. Weaknesses with auditory discrimination skills can have significant implications in a listening/classroom situation and are exacerbated in unfavorable listening environments. This skill is the ability to "hear" differences between similar sounding words. This difficulty can exist when listening to paired words as well as sentence length material. The effects can result in "misunderstanding" of what is being said. Furthermore, these weaknesses may exacerbate processing delays as an individual is trying to "figure out" what is being said in order to understand. These skills are not functional for his learning and communication needs at this time.

Phonological Segmentation assesses a child's ability to manipulate phonemes within words. This is a skill fundamental to the development of written language skills. Auditory processing skills that can affect a child's ability to perform this task would include perception and discrimination, immediate auditory memory, auditory latency, and auditory association. XXX is at the 50th percentile indicating skills within the average range. These skills affect the ability to acquire and master written language skills. The results indicate that these skills meet age and grade-level norms and expectations.

Phonological Blending assesses a child's ability to synthesize a word given the individual phonemes. This is a skill fundamental to the development of written language skills. Auditory processing skills that can affect a child's ability to perform this task would include auditory perception and discrimination, immediate auditory memory, and auditory closure. XXX's is at the 25th percentile. Analysis of XXX's responses indicates that he is able to synthesize up to five sounds. Furthermore, the errors tend to be with vowel and consonant omissions, substitutions, and reversals. The results of this subtest indicate a mild weakness with this skill area and may be affecting XXX's ability to acquire and master written language skills. The results indicate that XXX's skills fall within the borderline low-average range.

Auditory Number Memory Forward, Auditory Number Memory Reversed, Auditory Word Memory, and *Auditory Sentence Memory* are measures of basic memory processes, including sequencing. Memory is another process that underlies most processing abilities; if one cannot retain what has been heard and maintain it in correct sequence, one cannot process that information accurately. Numbers Forward taps immediate memory processing in a straightforward manner, whereas Numbers Reversed taps working memory—the ability to hold information in the mind and manipulate that information. So, even though children are not usually asked to remember the reverse of what is presented in the classroom, they are often required to retain and manipulate information before determining an answer, such as when learning to spell or when learning arithmetic processes; those are tasks that utilize working memory. Word Memory also assesses immediate memory and sequencing using a task that is similar to classroom activities whereas Sentence Memory allows the child to utilize the words within the sentence as cues to aid in recall. Auditory processing skills that can affect immediate auditory memory include auditory discrimination and auditory association. Auditory Number Memory Forward and Reversed are at the 9th and 5th percentiles, respectively. Auditory Word Memory is at the 5th percentile. Auditory Sentence Memory is at the 16th percentile. The results indicate that XXX is experiencing a moderate to significant weakness with immediate memory skills. Weaknesses with immediate auditory memory skills will have a significant impact on a child's ability to process new and ongoing information for listening and learning. The results indicate that XXX's skills do not meet age- or grade-level norms and expectations.

Auditory Comprehension assesses a child's ability to understand spoken information. This subtest reflects a child's ability to process new and ongoing information presented through the auditory modality, attend to, and store details in auditory information and recall for later use. Auditory processing skills that can affect a child's ability to perform this task successfully would include auditory discrimination, auditory association, auditory conceptualization, and immediate auditory memory. XXX is at the 9th percentile. Analysis of XXX's responses indicates that he is able to recall general information but is unable to recall specific information. The accuracy of his responses decline as the information that he is processing becomes more complex. The results of this subtest indicate that XXX is experiencing a significant weakness with this skill area and this may be affecting his overall learning ability relative to listening, understanding, and following directions, listening to and understanding instructional material, as well as being able to formulate and organize written language assignments. The results indicate that XXX's skills do not meet age and grade level norms and expectations.

Auditory Reasoning assesses a child's auditory cohesion skill ability. The skills for this subtest reflect higher order linguistic processing and are related to understanding jokes, riddles, inferences, and abstractions. The items on this subtest are intended to determine if the child can understand implied meanings, make inferences, or come to logical conclusions given the information in the sentences presented. Auditory processing skills that can affect a child's ability to perform this task successfully would include auditory perception and discrimination, auditory conceptualization, auditory association, auditory comprehension, and immediate auditory memory. XXX is at below the 1st percentile indicating that XXX is experiencing a significant weakness with this skill area and this may be affecting learning skills requiring abstraction, social pragmatic skills, as well as establishing social relationships. The results indicate that XXX's skills do not meet age- and grade-level norms and expectations.

XXX's overall performance on the TAPS-3 yielded a standard score of 78. He is experiencing difficulty with auditory phonology, auditory memory, and auditory cohesion evident by his respective composite scores of 83, 79, and 70.

The *Auditory Processing Abilities Test* (APAT) is a 10-subtest battery assessing auditory processing skills of auditory memory, auditory discrimination, and auditory cohesion. The APAT was developed to provide clinicians with assessment information in two areas. The first includes the traditional evaluation of skills such as immediate auditory memory, comprehension and processing of sentences and more extended material, understanding grammatical forms, recognition and processing absurdities, and following directions. In addition, the APAT also provides information concerning phonemic processing and awareness, cued recall of words after repeated trials, delayed recall of information, as well as the child's ability to process relationships among words and sentences. Furthermore, interpretation of the APAT results can be generalized to auditory processing in the classroom.

The APAT provides information relative to Global Index for auditory processing, Auditory Memory Index, Linguistic Processing Index, Linguistic Analysis, and Auditory Memory Analysis. The results are summarized as follows:

Composite Index Scores

Subtest		Raw Score	Scaled Score
1. Phonemic Awareness		11	7
2. Word Sequences		5	8
3. Semantic Relationships		7	7
4. Sentence Memory		6	6
5. Cued Recall		4	6
6i. Content Memory, Immed.		6	6
6d. Content Memory, Delayed		6	7
7. Complex Sentences		2	4
8. Sentence Absurdities		7	9
9. Following Directions		5	9
10. Passage Comprehension		11	9
Composite Index Scores	**Global AP**	**Auditory Memory**	**Linguistic Processes**
Index of Standard Scores	89	88	84
Percentile Rank	23	21	14

The Global composites represent performance across the range of skills assessed by the APAT. Because this index measures and represents many different auditory processing abilities, it is typically the best predictor of overall auditory processing abilities and how a child processes auditory information in various environments. The results yielded a Global composite index standard score of 89 with a percentile ranking of 23. This score is a reflection of XXX's overall auditory processing ability and suggests moderate difficulty with the skills measured by the APAT.

The results indicate that XXX experiences moderate difficulty with auditorily memory skills with a composite index standard score of 88 and percentile ranking of 21. Auditory latency was present with many of his responses, which may be affecting his ability to store and recall immediate information. The results indicate that these skills fall below age-level norms and expectations.

XXX experiences significant difficulty with the ability to process auditorily presented linguistic information as reflected by an index standard score of 84, placing him at the 14th percentile. Processing delays, most likely, affect his performance in addition to auditory discrimination. Processing delays were present on many of the correct responses. In order to accurately determine how his specific weaknesses affect this overall performance, one must examine specific response behaviors in specific subtests and refer to the auditory processing skills hierarchy. In this case, the specific subtest results of the APAT indicate difficulty with auditory discrimination and immediate auditory memory. Discrimination weaknesses can affect what one "hears." These skills are not functional for XXX's processing needs and do not meet age-level normative data.

Overall, these results indicate that XXX experiences moderate to significant difficulty with the skills measured by the APAT. It was also noted that XXX's auditory processing endurance declined as the test continued and its effect on performance must be considered when determining the effects of fatigue on classroom performance.

The *Wide Range Achievement Test* (WRAT-3) was administered to assess XXX's skills for reading and spelling isolated words. The results are summarized below:

Subtest	Raw Score	Standard Score	Percentile	Grade Equivalent
Reading	34	99	47	4
Spelling	32	110	75	6

The results yielded a decoding (reading) standard score of 99 and percentile ranking of 47, and an encoding (spelling) standard score of 110 and a percentile ranking of 75. XXX's grade equivalent is fourth grade for reading and sixth grade for spelling. Both of these scores meet age-level norms and expectations.

The Listening Inventory (TLI) is an initial screener for use by speech-language pathologists, parents, and teachers to identify children who may be at risk for having auditory processing deficits. TLI assesses specific behaviors in six categories that can be associated with auditory processing skill weaknesses. TLI captures and quantifies specific behaviors that are typically reported anecdotally. The categories of behaviors include: linguistic organization, decoding and language mechanics, attention and organization, sensory-motor skills, social and behavioral skills, and auditory processes. Furthermore, auditory processing deficits can occur with other problems such as attention deficit disorder (AD/HD) and language and learning disorders. The high rate of co-morbidity of auditory processing deficits with other disorders can affect the precision of the correct diagnosis. After all, if one cannot listen very well and misunderstands what is being said, then one's ability to stay focused and attend to the spoken message wanes and dissipates and vice versa. Children don't listen to what they don't understand. Problems with listening and attention are reflected by behaviors such as daydreaming, fidgeting, tuning out, not paying attention, and drifting away. Children with auditory processing deficits often experience difficulties with learning, speech, language (including reading and spelling), social behavior, and related functions. TLI assists in differentiating from among the various disorders that mask or coexist with auditory processing deficits. The results of the TLI are summarized as follows:

	LO	DL	AO	SM	SB	AP
Parent Rating:	77	40	108	27	25	83
Teacher Rating:	NA	NA	NA	NA	NA	NA
Cutoff Score*	41	32	78	27	51	44

*Scores higher than this signify a "red flag" within the applicable category.
LO = Linguistic Organization, DL = Decoding/Language Mechanics,
AO = Attention/Organization, SM = Sensory/Motor, SB = Social/Behavioral,
AP = Auditory Processes.

The results of XXX's TLI suggest he is experiencing weaknesses with linguistic organization, decoding and language mechanics, attention and organization, sensory and motor processes, social and behavioral skills, and auditory processes.

Discussion

Auditory processing skill weaknesses result in difficulty in the ability to use auditory information to communicate and learn. Auditory processing disorder is a set of problems that occur in different listening tasks. It is a deficit in the processing of auditory input that may be exacerbated in unfavorable acoustic environments and is associated with difficulty listening, reduced speech understanding, and reduced language development and learning. These exist as a hierarchy of skills that are basic to the listening, communication, and learning processes. Although sequential in development, these skills overlap and are essentially inseparable. The results of this battery indicate that XXX experiences weaknesses with: auditory discrimination, auditory attention, immediate auditory memory, auditory sequential memory, auditory latency, auditory conceptualization, auditory cohesion, interpretation and following directions, working overtime to listen, auditory overload, and auditory fatigue.

Auditory attention is the ability to maintain purposeful auditory focus over an extended period of time. This skill is necessary for a child to stay focused on a task, listen to extended amounts of auditory input (age-level appropriate), and to be able to filter out background information and noise. Auditory attention has significant implications for classroom performance. This is a skill, which appears to be developmental to some degree, and may involve several considerations. Issues of interest and volition arise; that is, even when a child is not interested in the auditory stimuli, is the child able to maintain attention, as needed to complete the task? Conversely, when a child has tuned-out or has become distracted, is it because of choice or because of the inability to maintain focus? XXX appears to demonstrate difficulty with auditory attention that may be further affected by auditory overload, auditory endurance, and the acoustic environment. XXX is at risk for auditory overload and would benefit from frequent brief "breaks" from listening to restore auditory attention in a learning situation.

Auditory memory and auditory sequential memory is the ability to retain auditory information as immediately presented. Auditory sequential memory is the ability to recall the order of a series of details. Weaknesses in this can have significant implications in a learning situation. For example, XXX is able to successfully retain four to five digits or four unrelated words in a sequence. Often, classroom instructions may contain two steps with up to six units of information. As a result, XXX may only be able to do one of the steps, do both but leave out a part of the direction, or do a task out of sequence. This skill ability is affected by auditory discrimination, auditory association, auditory latency, and the acoustic environment of the situation. Further considerations would include; rate of presentation, phonemic complexity of the spoken language, and the appropriateness of the language that is used. At this time, XXX experiences significant difficulty with immediate auditory and immediate auditory sequential memory.

Auditory latency is a lapse or delay in response time when presented with an auditory stimulus. It is evident that XXX's auditory latency tendencies increase as the length and complexity of the stimulus increases. Furthermore, delays will become more significant as XXX's overall listening time increases. That is, as his endurance diminishes, processing delays may increase with frequency and duration. When auditory overload is present, persistent auditory latency may increase and be exacerbated. Problems with auditory latency can have implications in a learning situation. What may appear to be weaknesses with following directions, understanding new and ongoing information, and higher level processing will, most likely, be as a result of receiving partial information due to processing delays.

Auditory cohesion is the ability to interpret, organize, and synthesize auditory information on a high-order level of functioning necessary for listening comprehension, organization, semantic, and linguistic organization, and the understanding of ambiguous information.

Summary

XXX XXX is a 10-year-old boy who was referred for an auditory processing assessment by his physician, Dr. XXX, MD, and his parents, XXX and XXX XXX. The assessment was scheduled for July 25, 2006.

The results of this assessment indicate that XXX experiences moderate to significant difficulty with skills of auditory processing. Auditory processing skills are a hierarchy of skills that are basic to the listening and communication process that affect the acquisition and mastery of both spoken and written language skills. These skills are sequential in development. However, the boundaries of each are not well defined, resulting in overlap, and are, essentially, inseparable (Educational Audiology Association, 1996).

Jerger and Musiek (2000) state that "Children and adults with Auditory Processing Disorder (APD) are a heterogeneous group of people who have difficulty using auditory information to communicate and learn. APD is a set of problems that occurs in different listening tasks. It is a deficit in the processing of auditory input which may be exacerbated in unfavorable acoustic environments and is associated with difficulty listening for speech-language understanding, language development and learning."

The American Speech-Language and Hearing Association (ASHA, 1996) stated that Auditory Processing Disorders are deficits in the information of processing of audible signals not attributed to impaired peripheral hearing or intellectual impairment. This processing involves perceptual, cognitive, and linguistic functions that, with appropriate interaction, result in effective receptive communication of auditorily presented stimuli. Specifically, APD refers to limitations in the ongoing transmission, analysis, organization, transformation, elaboration, storage, retrieval, and use of information contained in audible signals. APD involves both active and passive abilities.

According to the CSHA document "an auditory processing disorder is specific to the auditory modality. That is, it may be associated with difficulties in listening, speech understanding, language development and learning, but in its pure form, it is conceptualized as a deficit as a deficit in the processing of auditory input. Yet, the concept of the brain as a compartmentalized system is perhaps simplified, as there is a complex interactive neural network that makes a 'pure' auditory processing disorder the exception, rather than the rule. The differential diagnosis of APD from related problems, including ADHD, language impairment, reading disability, learning disability, autism spectrum disorder, and reduced intellectual functioning is often challenging, but important since children with these disorders may exhibit similar behaviors. In many cases, the diagnosis of APD co-occurs with dysfunction in other modalities." Furthermore, because there is such a wide range of auditory skills assessed, one child with an auditory processing disorder may present with a very different set of symptoms than another.

Review of the research reveals that as brainstem auditory neurons do not develop fully without adequate sound stimulation, and that these neurons may continue to develop into the second and third years of life, auditory deprivation during this period may have "devastating consequences for the development of auditory processing" and "adversely affect later central auditory functioning" (Spreen, Riser, & Edgell, 1995). Otitis media most often results in a temporary conductive hearing loss, specifically while there is significant fluid in the middle ear. Conductive hearing loss may impede a person's hearing threshold by as much as 50 dB, depending on the degree of impedance. In addition, conductive hearing loss resulting from otitis media usually affects hearing in the higher frequencies, most closely associated with sounds of the English language. As XXX experienced chronic otitis media throughout his first and second years of life, the resultant auditory deprivation is the most likely etiology for his current processing deficits.

The results of the evaluation indicate that XXX experiences moderate to significant difficulty with auditory processing skills. XXX presents with weaknesses in auditory discrimination, auditory attention, immediate auditory memory, auditory sequential memory, auditory latency, auditory conceptualization, auditory cohesion, interpretation and following directions, working overtime to listen, auditory overload, and auditory fatigue. Auditory latency is an underlying factor affecting all auditory processing skills. The results of the LAC-3 indicate weaknesses with auditory memory, auditory discrimination, and auditory conceptualization. The results of the TAPS-3 and APAT reflect weaknesses with auditory memory, auditory sequential memory, auditory discrimination, auditory cohesion, phonological processing, and interpretation of directions.

Auditory processing disorder affects a number of skills. Often children have difficulty distinguishing certain sounds. At times, this difficulty with discrimination of individual sounds can present itself as a speech problem or in learning the code for written language. Both reading and spelling can be affected. In addition, auditory processing disorder can affect the way that they are able to listen. Children are frequently accused of having "selective hearing." However, because of the amount of energy the process of listening and storing auditory information requires, the child can do only so much listening before he tunes out because of the auditory overload. At times, these children are incorrectly diagnosed as having ADD when actually their attention is dependent on the amount of auditory processing that is required for a situation.

XXX appears to be working "overtime" to listen and process for learning purposes. The behaviors that were observed during this evaluation will be exacerbated in a classroom where there is ambient noise, competing noise, questionable acoustics, and changes in the quality of the auditory signal. XXX's auditory fatigue and overload will, most likely, appear as tuning out, being easily distracted, or daydreaming.

Recommendations

Currently, the best practices management of auditory processing disorder targets three specific areas: direct therapeutic intervention, modifications, and/or the development of compensatory strategies. To ensure that XXX obtains the maximal benefit from management strategies, it is recommended that these be done concurrently. Direct intervention for remediation should be conducted within a clinical setting. Environmental modifications and/or compensatory strategies should be incorporated within the classroom and clinical setting, as well as at home.

Sound-Based Therapy

It is recommended that XXX participate in the XXX Method of auditory intervention. This intervention is a clinical application of auditory stimulation that can improve auditory processing. This 90-hour protocol has been effective in improving one's ability to perceive, discriminate, associate, and organize auditory input for purposes of receptive and expressive communication and overall auditory processing of input information. The XXX Method has demonstrated to be clinically effective in improving skills of auditory perception, auditory discrimination, auditory attention, auditory association, immediate auditory memory, auditory conceptual function, receptive language, expressive communication skills, and reducing auditory latency.

The XXX Method is not intended to replace traditional speech and language therapy or occupational therapy. Rather, this method is a supplemental and complimentary therapy that can enhance one's response to the therapy process.

Speech and Language Therapy

In addition to the XXX Method, it is recommended that XXX receive individual speech and language therapy twice weekly for 1-hour length sessions. Based on an auditory processing skills hierarchy, specific goals would include:

1. Improved attending to speech (including auditory awareness/vigilance, recognizing pitch changes and patterns, attending to the direction of sound and gap detection)
2. Improved initiating specific clarification and active listening
3. Improved auditory memory of linguistic information (improving the length of time for retaining a verbal message through the development of subvocalization, chunking, and visualization)
4. Improved auditory cohesion (reasoning, paraphrasing, predicting, cause-effect, idioms, humor, etc.).

For further information on specific auditory processing strategies, it is recommended that the speech-language pathologist providing the therapy refer to *A Metacognitive Program for Treating Auditory Processing Disorders* by Patricia McAleer Hamaguchi, published by Pro-Ed Publishers in Austin, Texas. This publication provides comprehensive intervention strategies that are both practical and effective.

PACE

It is recommended that XXX be evaluated for the PACE (Processing and Cognitive Enhancement) Program. The PACE Program is an intense one-on-one training program that develops the skills vital for fast and efficient learning. The PACE Program improves learning skills such as attention, memory, speed, reasoning, comprehension, and visual and auditory processing required for reading and spelling.

Environmental Modifications

Environmental modifications should be incorporated in the classroom as well as at home. The following are suggested:

1. XXX's attention should be obtained before addressing him or preparing him for a listening activity so that he is available to completely attend to what is being said without missing important information. I suggest using the phrase "It's time to listen" when preparing for a listening activity.

2. The use of visual cues is recommended as a way for XXX to compensate for his auditory difficulties. Sitting across from the speaker rather than next to him or her would enhance his access to visual cues. Having him look directly at the speaker when spoken to will further assist XXX.
3. When addressing XXX, the purpose of the communication should be stated in clear, age-level appropriate and sequential terms to allow him to prepare to focus on the appropriate information.
4. Auditory processing difficulties can contribute to trouble with understanding auditory information. Therefore, when addressing XXX, the speaker should watch for signs of lack of attention, concentration, or understanding, and ask for responses from him to pinpoint areas of confusion or misunderstanding. Yes/no questions are not useful for this purpose.
5. Repeat what is said in order to help with understanding is helpful.
6. Reduce the signal-to-noise ratio by having XXX sit closer to the teacher or speaker.
7. Reduce extraneous background noise.
8. Eliminate both visual and auditory distractions.
9. Determine and implement preferential seating. XXX should be seated near the teacher and at a table or part of the classroom where "quiet" students are seated.
10. All auditory information should be produced at a normal rate of speech with good use of pitch variation and vocal expression.
11. Short breaks will give XXX's auditory system a rest so that further demands for listening and processing can be productive. Repetition of directions will help ensure success for him.

Finally, following the completion of the recommended interventions, a formal re-evaluation of auditory processing skills and speech and language skills should be performed using the same standardized measures used for the basis of the findings of this evaluation. Recommendations for further intervention will be made based on those findings.

Should you have any questions regarding the findings of this evaluation and/or the content of this report, please contact this office at (XXX) XXX-XXXX.

Appendix

Web References and Resources

Donna Geffner

These Web sites represent a variety of resources, information, and links to additional sources. The viewpoints on auditory processing (AP), central auditory processing disorders, and related topic are solely those of the individual sites and their Web masters.

Arkansas Department of Education
http://arked.state.ar.us
Site contains: Understanding the Arkansas Department of Education Guidelines.

Audiology Online
http://www.audiologyonline.com
Search for auditory processing disorder. Site contains interviews and articles by experts in AP assessment, management, and treatment of CAPD. The site also compares CAPD to ADHD.

Auditory Processing Down Under—Deb's Homepage
http://d93.k12.id.us/~sservice/Auditory_Processing.html
Site contains links, chat rooms, and message boards to assist parents in finding information, help, and assessment of CAPD and related disorder overseas. The Web site is maintained by a parent whose child was diagnosed with APD at age 11.

Auditory Processing
http://d93.k12.id.us/~sservice/Auditory_Processing .html
Site includes informational articles such as Dealing with an Auditory Processing Disorder, Management of an Auditory Processing Disorder; and Coping with Central Auditory Processing Disorder.

Auditory Processing Disorder Facts
http://www.homestead.com/agertner/HOMEPAGE.html
Professional Web site organized by Alan B. Gertner; Kean University; Union, NJ. Examples of topics: What Is APD? How Does APD Present? What Causes APD? Attention and Memory and APD.

Bala-Metrics, Inc.
http://www.balametrics.com/school/capd.htm
Site discusses: definition of CAPD and its symptoms and the type of products Bala-metrics offer for Children with CAPD. Central Auditory Processing Disorder in schools.

CAPD Parents Page
http://pages.cthome.net/cbristol/
Site contains resources for Parents of Children with Central Auditory Processing Disorders. Contains information on the most recent technology used with children with CAPD. Web site hosted by a parent of a 13-year-old girl with CAPD.

Center for Central Auditory Disorder & Attention Deficit Disorders Information
http://home.earthlink.net/~mcoleman/cpdadd.html
Site contains links to many resources, some of which are designed for parents of children with CAPD.

Central Auditory Disorder and Auditory Neuropathy
http://www.tsbvi.edu/Outreach/seehear/winter01/capd.htm
Statement by Jim Durked, Audiologist and Statewide Staff Development Coordinator, Texas School for the Blind and Visually Impaired (TSVBI), Outreach with help from Kate Moss, Family Support Specialist, Texas Deafblind Outreach Written for the TSVBI Online Newsletter.

Children Today
http://childrentoday.com/resources/articles/capd.htm
The Web site is intended for parents of children with CAPD. This site includes information on what is CAPD; symptoms of the disorder, hints for parents of children with CAPD, and links to resources and articles. Web site maintained by Mindy Hudon, M.S., CCC-SLP.

Colorado Department of Education
http://www.cde.state.co.us/cdesped/download/pdf/CI-APD-Gu.pdf
Site contains guideline document: "APD: A Team Approach to Screening, Assessment, and Intervention Practices."

Deafness/Hard of Hearing
http://deafness.about.com/cs/featurescauses/a/capd.htm
Web site defines CAPD and lists symptoms of CAPD. The Web site gives links to several articles on CAPD. Central Auditory Processing Disorder—When a hearing person is deaf or vice versa.

Delphi Forums: Current Research in ADHD and CAPD
http://forums.delphiforums.com/
Search: ADHD
Web site offers a forum to promote awareness of current research studies being conducted on Attention Deficit (Hyperactivity) Disorder (ADD/ADHD) and/or Central Auditory Processing Disorder (CAPD).

ERIC Digests
http://www.ericec.ed.gov/portal/home.portal
Search: CAPD
Web site includes definition of Central Auditory Processing Disorder (CAPD), characteristics, diagnosis, various classroom modifications for students with CAPD, and the relationship of CAPD to ADHD.

Family Village Web Site
http://www.familyvillage.wisc.edu/lib_capd.html
Links to articles on CAPD and other reference sites. Web site offers links to discussion groups of professionals involved in the area of CAPD.

Florida Department of Education
http://www.firn.edu/doe/commhome
Web site consists of the Technical Assistance Paper on Auditory Processing Disorder (74 pp.). This paper was intended to assist audiologists in educational settings during audiological auditory processing evaluations.

Frank Musiek's Web page
http://speechlab.coms.uconn.edu/faculty/musiek/
Listing of recent publications, research, groups and programs.

Healthy Hearing
http://www.healthyhearing.com/
Search site for CAPD.
Site contains many links with information on CAPD and questions answered from professionals in the field of audiology. Web site also contains an advisory board.

HERDEWE
http://members.aol.com/HERDEWE/
The Web site is maintained by Dr. Gary Pillow who is Teacher of the Deaf and Hard of Hearing Audiologist Speech-Language Pathologist Reading Specialist. The Web site contains information on APD, reading, spelling, and Dr. Pillow's perspective on the relevance of all three.

Home Page for Classroom Acoustics
http://www.classroomacoustics.com/
This Web site contains information on classroom acoustics. The site is intended for both, parents and professionals.

Internet Guide to Understanding CAPD
http://www.angelfire.com/bc/capd/
Web site contains information links on CAPD and links to support groups.

Kids Health for Parents
http://kidshealth.org/parent/medical/ears/central_auditory.html
Web site contains information on Central Auditory Processing Disorder (CAPD); the signs, symptoms, causes, and diagnosis of CAPD.

Ladle Rat Rotten Hut
http://www.exploratorium.edu/exhibits/ladle/
Simulation Web site. The simulation was not designed to actually simulate CAPD, although it is a good example of how some adults with CAPD say they hear.

LD Online
http://www.ldonline.org/
Search Web site for APD.
Web site offers articles on APD periodically; as well as many links.

Listen Up
http://www.listen-up.org/htm/toc.htm
Web site provides us with links to other CAPD sites; information and tip sheets.

Minnesota Department of Education
http://education.state.mn.us/
Web site search: CAPD
The Web site contains information on CAPD and how it is different from other learning and attention problems. Minnesota's Guidelines for Auditory Processing Disorders.

National Coalition on Auditory Processing Disorders
http://www.ncapd.org/
Web site contains professional and consumer information, some very good simulations of APD, and an online chat. The NCAPD is dedicated to assisting

individuals affected by auditory processing disorders through education, public awareness, support, and advocacy and by promoting auditory access of information.

NCEF
http://edfacilities.org/rl/acoustics.cfm
Classroom Acoustics. This Web site displays many links, articles, papers, and books on classroom acoustics.

NIDCD
http://www.nidcd.nih.gov/health/voice/auditory.asp
Auditory Processing Disorder in Children; What Does It Mean? What Causes Auditory Processing Difficulties? What are the symptoms of possible auditory processing difficulty? How is suspected auditory processing difficulty diagnosed in children? What current research is being conducted?

Professor Hafter's Auditory Perception Lab
http://ear.berkeley.edu/
U.C. Berkeley, Department of Psychology Web site contains information on research currently being conducted in the Auditory Lab concerned primarily with information, especially as it impacts listening in real world situations.

Scientific Learning Research
http://www.scilearn.com/
Search Web site for APD
Web site contains links with information on Fast ForWord program effects on various individuals with APD.

Tartan Products
http://www.capdtest.com/keith.cfm
Dr. Robert Keith's Web site contains information about tests he has developed (e.g., SCAN, Compressed Speech Test, RGDT), case studies, and other useful information about APD.

Teaching Research Institute
http://www.tr.wou.edu/tr/dbp/pdf/sept99.pdf
Search site for CAPD
Blind and Deaf Perspective: Central Auditory Processing Disorder; Assessment and Management Practices by Mignon M. Shrninky and Jane A. Baran.

Texas Auditory Processing Disorder Laboratory
http://www.texasapd.org/
Web site contains links to professional research articles on CAPD; addresses the laboratory's goal to develop a better method for diagnosis of APD; and information about new frontiers in AP assessment.

The Hearing Journal
http://www.findarticles.com/cf_0/m0BPK
Search for useful articles on AP, and CAPD, such as the popular Page 10 articles written by experts in APD.

The Hearing Office
http://hearingoffice.com/badown.htm
This site contains a downloadable brochure and information sheets on AP assessment and management and compares Auditory Processing Disorder to Attention Deficit Hyperactivity Disorder.

Tri-City Herald
http://www.tri-cityherald.com/HEARNET/disorders.html
Site contains fact sheet about CAPD and its associated behaviors, diagnostic procedures as well as rehabilitation options.

Wright's Law
http://www.wrightslaw.com/advoc/articles/tests_measurements.html#anchor744732
Understanding Tests and Measurements for Parents and Advocates is an informative piece that reviews psycho-educational evaluations, basic statistics relevant to reporting test results, etc. This is helpful information for the audiologist when comparing APD test results to other evaluations that are a part of the multidisciplinary assessment.

Yahoo Groups: Auditory Processing
http://groups.yahoo.com/group/AuditoryProcessing/
Web site contains an APD discussion board.

Index

Note: APD, (C)APD, and CAPD are considered synonymous in this book

A

D

E

F

G

H

I

J

K

L

M

N

O

Q

R

S

T